MULTIPLE SCLEROSIS: EXPERIMENTAL AND CLINICAL ASPECTS

ANNALS OF THE NEW YORK ACADEMY OF SCIENCES
Volume 436

MULTIPLE SCLEROSIS: EXPERIMENTAL AND CLINICAL ASPECTS

Edited by Labe Scheinberg and Cedric S. Raine

The New York Academy of Sciences
New York, New York
1984

The cover shows damage done to myelin sheaths in a patient with multiple sclerosis (page 19).

Library of Congress Cataloging in Publication Data

Main entry under title:

Multiple sclerosis.

(Annals of the New York Academy of Sciences, ISSN 0077-8923; v. 436)
Papers presented at a conference held by the New York Academy of Sciences on Nov. 29 to Dec. 1, 1983.
Includes bibliographies and index.
1. Multiple sclerosis—Congresses. I. Scheinberg, Labe C., 1925– II. Raine, Cedric S., 1940– III. New York Academy of Sciences. IV. Series.
[DNLM: 1. Multiple Sclerosis—congresses.
W1 AN626YL v.436 / WL 360 M9564 1983]
Q11.N5 vol. 436 500 s 85-3005
[RC377] [616.8′34]
ISBN 0-89766-266-0
ISBN 0-89766-267-9 (pbk.)

SP
Printed in the United States of America
ISBN 0-89766-266-0 (cloth)
ISBN 0-89766-267-9 (paper)
ISSN 0077-8923

ANNALS OF THE NEW YORK ACADEMY OF SCIENCES

Volume 436

December 28, 1984

MULTIPLE SCLEROSIS: EXPERIMENTAL AND CLINICAL ASPECTS[a]

Editors and Conference Organizers

LABE SCHEINBERG and CEDRIC S. RAINE

CONTENTS

[a]The papers in this volume were presented at a conference entitled Multiple Sclerosis: Theory and Practice, which was held by the New York Academy of Sciences on November 29 to December 1, 1983.

Part II. Immunology of Multiple Sclerosis

Part III. Clinical Manifestations of Multiple Sclerosis

Part V. Psychosocial and Economic Features in MS

Poster Papers

Financial assistance was received from:

- The Schmulka Aronson Charitable Trust
- CIBA-GEIGY Corporation
- Davis, Brody and Associates
- Mr. and Mrs. Andrew Golden
- Mr. Clifford Goldsmith
- Hoffmann-La Roche, Inc.
- Mr. and Mrs. Irving Moskovitz
- National Institute of Handicapped Research
  Research and Demonstration Project (no. G008006808)
  Comprehensive Continuing Care and Rehabilitation Program for MS Patients and Medical Rehabilitation Research and Training Center for MS (no. G008300040)
- National Multiple Sclerosis Society
- National Multiple Sclerosis Society—New York City Chapter
- Paralyzed Veterans of America
- Mr. and Mrs. William Rybnick
- Mr. and Mrs. Gerald Stern
- The Upjohn Company

Preface

LABE SCHEINBERG AND CEDRIC S. RAINE

Albert Einstein College of Medicine
Bronx, New York 10461

In 1964, the New York Academy of Sciences held a three-day conference entitled Research in Demyelinating Diseases, the proceedings[a] of which are still a basic reference in the field of multiple sclerosis (MS) research.

Although the cause of MS and other demyelinating diseases remains unknown, in the last 20 years, virologists, immunologists and neuropathologists have collected an impressive body of information on the pathogenesis and physiological manifestations of these conditions. Clinicians have meanwhile gained considerable experience in the areas of diagnosis and management. In most instances, MS can now be diagnosed earlier in its course and without invasive neuroradiological procedures. The average life expectancy of patients has risen. Because the public-at-large is aware of MS to a greater degree than ever before, less of a stigma is attached to its diagnosis. Public and private health agencies and private industries are investing larger sums in basic research and clinical trials. Because interest in MS has grown considerably in recent years, we sensed an important need for another conference on the subject. Entitled Multiple Sclerosis: Theory and Practice, it was held from November 29 to December 1, 1983. Several hundred scientists from around the world participated, and a number of health agencies lent support. The result was a comprehensive forum on MS-related issues.

The ultrastructure, biology and chemical composition of myelin were just being defined in 1964, and the principal experimental model of MS, experimental allergic encephalomyelitis, was undergoing intensive examination. Clinical diagnostic criteria for MS had been established, the basic details of its epidemiology defined, and the problems of clinical trials elucidated.

In the intervening years, virologic and immunologic investigations further clarified MS etiology and pathogenesis. We understand better the function of viruses as possible causes of MS lesions and as triggers of their exacerbations. The cellular elements that play a major role in the pathogenesis of MS and its experimental model have been studied extensively. There is now a general consensus that myelin damage is the primary event in MS and that it results from a viral infection early in life expressed later on as an immune process.

In clinical areas, we have used our knowledge of the neurophysiology of central myelin conduction as an important diagnostic tool for the development of evoked potential techniques that make possible the detection of additional silent lesions. The field of neuroimaging has been advanced by the development of computerized tomography and magnetic resonance and nuclear magnetic resonance imaging. The visualization of silent plaques not only facilitates diagnosis but provides a major tool for evaluation of the course of the disease and the effect of therapeutic interventions.

Clinicians have investigated, and continue to evaluate, many new therapies that range from improved symptomatic treatments to potent immunosuppression. They have also developed new approaches to patient assessment that take into account not

[a]Ann. N.Y. Acad. Sci. 1965. **122**(1).

only neurologic impairment but also activities of daily living and psychosocial and economic effects. This conference brought together some of the principal workers in the field, and the conference organizers wish to thank the supporters and participants. We feel these proceedings present a timely overview of the current status of MS research. The increased emphasis on inquiries concerning the disease itself vis-à-vis therapy, management and possible immunologic anomalies as compared to 20 years ago reflects the latest scientific and medical thinking on MS.

We believe the findings collected herein will influence the many avenues of research on this crucial problem in neurology for years to come.

Opening Remarks

SYLVIA LAWRY

National Multiple Sclerosis Society
and
International Federation of Multiple Sclerosis Societies
New York, New York 10017

I'm happy to welcome you all to this long overdue general medical and scientific conference on multiple sclerosis (MS). The last comprehensive meeting on the disease was held 20 years ago here at the Academy.[a] Since that time there has been a great deal of important new research going on; you will be hearing about it at this meeting.

The high standards of research on MS today are a tribute to the neurological profession. Right from the start, the leading neurologists of this country have stood four-square behind our development, helping us in every way possible. I remember the first medical advisory board meeting of the National Multiple Sclerosis Society at the Academy of Medicine in New York in 1947, a year after the Society was born. Only a handful of neurologists was then interested in MS research. We managed an excellent attendance despite the fact that the neurologists had to weather the worst snowstorm in New York's history. You may recall that blizzard; planes were grounded and airports closed. But somehow the neurologists managed to make it, from as far away as Montreal, San Francisco, Baltimore, and Rochester, Minnesota. They had agreed to serve on the board, and they served well, under the chairmanship of Dr. Tracy J. Putnam, then director of the Columbia Presbyterian Neurological Institute and one of the few people doing research on MS at the time. Dr. Thomas Rivers, director of the Rockefeller Institute, was vice-chairman.

At the end of that first meeting it was evident that we were dealing with a very confusing disease. There was no consensus on anything. We didn't even know how prevalent the problem was. It was not till later that Dr. Leonard Kurland, now of the Mayo Clinic, launched the epidemiological studies pointing to high prevalence areas in temperate zones—work for which he recently earned the Charcot Award of the International Federation of Multiple Sclerosis Societies.

There was one thing we knew: The Society would invest as much as it could in research. The first grant was awarded in 1947 to Dr. Elvin Kabat of Columbia University in the amount of $10,725 to study "The Immunological and Allergic Etiology of Multiple Sclerosis and Disseminated Encephalomyelitis." Even then we were on the trail of immunology! At the outset we established the policy of budgeting at least 50% of the national society's income on research and over the years more than that has been spent. As of August 1983, a total of $73,683,000 in research and fellowship grants has been approved.

At the start of our grants program, our medical board recognized we were on something of a fishing expedition. We had no basis on which we could focus MS research. Very little was known about the nervous system of healthy people, let alone those with MS. So what we did, in effect, was support good basic research in neurology and wait for clues to surface that would lead us into the areas that seemed most promising for the disease. Our research advisers were recommending we expand our programs in virology, immunology, genetics and epidemiology.

[a] Published as Ann. N.Y. Acad. Sci. 1965. **122**(1).

From the beginning we always needed more money for research. In casting about for possible sources of support, I tried to find out what the government had been giving to MS. I found that by 1949 NIH had made only one grant for MS research, in the sum of $14,000. At just about that time we learned that the daughter of Senator Charles Tobey of New Hampshire was diagnosed as having MS. We turned to him to find out what help he could give us in persuading the government to support our research. We decided to move in the direction of establishing what was initially the National Institute of Neurological Diseases and Blindness as part of NIH. At that time the major funding was going into the heart and cancer institutes—I don't think this has changed—whereas all of neurology was buried in what was called the National Institute for Mental Health. Its governing council and review committees were composed largely of psychiatrists. Members of our board testified, chapters wrote their congressmen, and when Mrs. Lou Gehrig testified before Congress on behalf of amyotrophic lateral sclerosis she made front-page headlines. We also had no small amount of help from New York philanthropist Mary Lasker. Thus was the institute born in 1951, signed into law by President Harry Truman.

Today, after several changes in nomenclature, the body is called the National Institute of Neurological and Communicative Disorders and Strokes (NINCDS). With the establishment of the new institute, government appropriations for neurological diseases went up accordingly. The first government appropriation in 1953 was $1.5 million. For fiscal 1984 it is about $335 million. Total appropriations during the 32-year span have amounted to almost four billion dollars.

Dr. H. Houston Merritt, former director of the Columbia Presbyterian Neurological Institute and past vice-chairman of our medical advisory board, stated publicly that this institute was the greatest single factor in raising the level of neurology in our country.

The National Committee for Research in Neurological and Communicative Disorders (NCR), which has been evolving since the institute was established, provides an orderly and effective projection of needs to Congress and the administration to justify increased appropriations. It now numbers over 60 members, equally divided among national voluntary health agencies and professional associations. Its recent formalization increased its effectiveness, which was dramatically evidenced by a 13.3% increase in funds to NINCDS for fiscal 1984. The cooperation of its members was excellent. No larger percentage increase was granted to any of the major disease-related institutes.

By 1970 I was feeling more and more that we needed a commission on MS; other health agencies had been successful in establishing commissions that focused scientific attention on a problem and engendered public interest. So, with the encouragement of our neurological advisors, we brought about the establishment of the National Advisory Commission on Multiple Sclerosis, created by an Act of Congress in 1972 in a bill introduced by Margaret Heckler of Massachusetts. (She is now, as you may know, Secretary of Health and Human Services.)

A director was needed for the commission. In 1967 Dr. Harry M. Weaver, who had been master architect of the polio research program of the national foundation that led to the development of the Salk vaccine, was enjoying his retirement. We liked everything we had heard about him, so we pulled him out of retirement to come and reorganize the society research programs. In 1972 he went to Washington for a year as executive director of the MS Commission. He brought together leading scientists from all over the world to participate. At the end of the commission he issued a report that was applauded by Caspar Weinberger, then Secretary of HEW. The report emphasized the various areas of research that needed further investigation. On the heels of the report, a ground swell of grant applications poured in. The meetings that were held generated many new ideas, and scientists went back to their institutions to carry out the ideas.

Early on we began to see that about one-third of our grants were going to overseas investigators—all outstanding scientists doing high-caliber work. Some were Nobel laureates. Because they could not get funds in their countries, they were turning to us. In the early fifties, on a visit to Britain's Medical Research Council, I asked how much money was being spent on MS research; the answer was none. I wondered why not, since MS was known to be a serious problem in Britain. The director said there were no applications for grants. I replied, "That's strange, because we're supporting research at Oxford."

The fact was that British scientists were coming to us because the favorable climate in the U.S. towards MS research did not exist in Great Britain. So the Medical Research Council was supportive of the establishment of a national MS society in Great Britain. Today the Council awards about $1.5 million annually for MS research in addition to the significant support of its own national society. Similar developments were encouraged in other countries.

By the 1960s it became evident that overseas research and exchange of medical and patient service information would be of direct benefit to us, so in 1965 I recommended to our board that a seed money grant of $100,000 be made to establish an international federation of MS societies that would act as a stimulating force on research abroad and an information clearinghouse on patient management. Today the Federation's committees meet twice a year and a satellite research symposium is held in conjunction with each annual meeting. Scientists from a broad range of surrounding countries—and farther afield—gather to interpret their research activities. MS societies in 29 countries are members. The known level of annual research funding abroad by national societies, their governments and private sources is now over $12,800,000, a minimal figure, but encouraging for a comparatively young program. In the lead are Canada, Germany, Great Britain and Northern Ireland, with annual expenditures well over $1,000,000. Dr. Reginald Kelly of Great Britain is chairman of the international medical adivisory board.

As Dr. Scheinberg likes to say, our society has become a flagship among voluntary health organizations, a model for others to emulate. I think our research program under Dr. Byron H. Waksman and medical and community services program under Dr. Robert J. Slater are among the best to be found in any voluntary health agency. As for Dr. Scheinberg, he himself is something of a flagship! As chairman of the medical advisory board he brought this conference into being, and he has committed his entire professional life to the problems of MS.

The nationwide income of the society has grown annually. It has almost tripled in the past ten years, from the level of $12 million to a peak of about $35 million in 1982 (a percentage increase of 215%). The annual income to national headquarters out of which research is funded increased by 153% during the same ten years. The support of grants for research and research fellowships also tripled during this time to reach a peak of $5.5 million in 1982. This represents a percentage increase of 225% (indeed, a more rapid rate of growth for grants than for income). The stimulating force of the society has succeeded to such a substantial degree that there is a burgeoning interest in the problems of MS in the scientific community. Despite the steady growth of income and grants, the society is currently receiving more meritorious applications for research than available funds can support.

In 1973 the Society established the Ralph I. Straus Award, in an amount equivalent to the most recent Nobel prize in physiology and medicine. It is to be given "to that scientist or those scientists of any nationality whatsoever whose published research shall be judged to have resulted in the development of effective and specific methods for preventing or arresting multiple sclerosis."

In turning over the helm of our society to the distinguished Vice Admiral Thor Hanson a year ago, as founder-director, I am now able to concentrate my efforts on our international program through the International Federation of Multiple Sclerosis Societies. As its secretary, I hope it, too, becomes the flagship among international health agencies. Additionally, representing our society on the board of directors of NCR, I hope that all the funds required for productive research and training in the neurosciences will become available through government, and that the National Multiple Sclerosis Society will resume its long-standing record of funding all approved grants.

I'd like to close with a quote from Dr. A. B. Baker of Minneapolis. He trained most neurologists in the central states and was a distinguished member of the medical advisory board. He said, in substance, "multiple sclerosis is the nub of neurology. If we crack the MS problem, it's going to clarify the whole field of neurology." We fervently hope so—and that this conference moves us well along toward that goal.

When multiple sclerosis joins the ranks of solved medical problems, the role of the neurological profession in bringing this about will have been a prime factor. Until then its continued magnificent support is earnestly sought and appreciated by those suffering from MS — patients and family members — so that they can continue to live in hope, worldwide.

PART I. PATHOGENETIC MECHANISMS

Recent Advances in Myelin Biochemistry[a]

WILLIAM T. NORTON

The Saul R. Korey Department of Neurology
and
Department of Neuroscience
Albert Einstein College of Medicine
Bronx, New York 10461

Twenty years ago at the previous New York Academy of Sciences meeting on demyelination I reported our first detailed lipid analyses of purified bovine myelin.[1] Other reports at that meeting described the composition of rat[2] and guinea pig[3] myelin, some metabolic properties of rat myelin,[2] the protein constituents of myelin,[4,5] and some chemical studies of the basic, encephalitogenic protein.[6] Biochemical studies of isolated myelin had only begun to appear two years previously. Although we then knew with more certainty what myelin was from the chemical point of view it was comforting to realize that at least three decades of careful analytical studies of the nervous system had anticipated most of the findings.

For those wishing detailed information on all aspects of myelin the forthcoming book edited by Morell[7] is recommended. I will only outline selected advances in myelin biochemistry of the past twenty years and discuss briefly the contributions of neurochemistry to demyelination and multiple sclerosis.

MYELIN COMPOSITION[b]

Lipids

Myelin is one of the most lipid-rich membranes, containing 70–80% lipid by weight. The general features of the lipid composition were established by 1964. The distinguishing feature of myelin lipids is the high content of the galactosphingolipids, cerebroside (galactosyl ceramide) and sulfatide. All analytical work points to cerebroside as a universal marker for myelin and oligodendroglia in all vertebrates. Glycosphingolipids are lipid haptens and specific antibodies can be raised to cerebroside and sulfatide. Immunohistochemical studies using these antibodies show that cerebroside is a specific marker for oligodendroglia in central nervous system (CNS) cultures[9] and is restricted to these cells and myelin in sections.[10,11] Sulfatide, however, may also be present in Bergmann glia and ependymal cells.[11]

The gangliosides, complex glycosphingolipids containing sialic acid, also deserve special attention. Mammalian myelin contains these lipids in concentrations ranging from 0.3 to 0.7% of the total lipid.[12] Myelin is the only brain fraction that has a characteristic ganglioside pattern. In mature animals ganglioside GM_1 is always the major species and can account for 70 mole percent of the total gangliosides.[12,13,14] Myelin gangliosides from some species have in addition sialosylgalactosylceramide

[a]Work from the author's laboratory was supported by U.S. Public Health Service grant nos. NS–02476 and NS–03356, and by grant no. 1089 from the National Multiple Sclerosis Society.

[b]See ref. 8 for review.

(GM_4) as a major component. This ganglioside, which is derived from cerebroside, is specific in the CNS for myelin and oligodendroglia.[8,12]

Proteins[c]

Studies of myelin proteins, which have been extensive in the past fifteen years, have been aided by the application of polyacrylamide gel electrophoresis of myelin dissolved in sodium dodecylsulfate solutions. Proteolipid protein (PLP) and basic protein (BP) and its relatives are the major myelin proteins in the CNS. Basic protein has been studied most extensively. Most mammals have two basic proteins, a major one of 18,500 daltons and a minor one of 21,500 daltons. Rats and mice have two additional basic proteins of 17,000 daltons and 14,000 daltons. The small basic protein of 14,000 daltons is the predominant basic protein in these species. The sequences of the 18,500 dalton protein of many species have been determined and minor differences have been reported. All four of these basic proteins are related by deletions or insertions of sequences in the 18,500 dalton protein. Recently the gene for basic protein has been cloned, using recombinant DNA technology, and the cDNA probe has been used to show that the shiverer mutant mouse lacks mRNA for all basic protein species, possibly as a result of a complete gene deletion.[16]

Other less prominent proteins of CNS myelin are MAG, the major myelin glycoprotein of 110,000 daltons, and the Wolfgram group. The lower molecular weight doublet of the Wolfgram proteins, W1 (about 42,000–50,000 daltons) has been shown to be identical to the myelin enzyme 2′,3′-cyclic nucleotide 3′phosphodiesterase (CNP).[17,18]

Proteins of peripheral nervous system (PNS) myelin are quite different from those of CNS myelin. PNS myelin does not have PLP, but has Po protein, a glycoprotein of 28,000 daltons. The 18,500 dalton BP is present as is a basic protein called P_2 of 15,000 daltons, which is not present in the CNS. Rats have a protein called Pr, which may be the same as small basic protein of the CNS.

Enzymes[d]

One of the most exciting new developments in myelin chemistry is the discovery that highly purified myelin contains a number of enzymes. Two of these enzymes, CNP and a cholesterol ester hydrolase, are found at much higher specific activities in myelin than in brain homogenates and it appears that these enzymes are specific to myelin and oligodendroglia. Many other enzymes are found that are not specific to myelin. Some of these, however, such as 5′-nucleotidase and carbonic anhydrase may have specific activities equal to or somewhat greater than those found in brain homogenates. Altogether more than 20 enzyme activities have now been reported in myelin.[8] Besides the four already mentioned, they include nine enzymes involved with lipid metabolism, several protein kinases, a basic protein phosphatase, peptidases, esterases and a neutral proteinase.

The exact function of any of these enzymes is not yet known. Ledeen and co-workers[22–24] have speculated that the enzymes of phospholipid synthesis are involved in the labeling of certain myelin lipids in the optic tract when radiolabeled serine is injected in the eye.[25] They proposed that transported macromolecules are degraded in

[c]See refs. 8 and 15 for reviews.
[d]See refs. 8, 19, 20, and 21 for reviews.

the axon and labeled precursors migrate into the surrounding myelin where they are incorporated.

The presence of the three transport enzymes, carbonic anhydrase, 5′-nucleotidase and Na^+,K^+-ATPase, has significant implications for neuron-glial interactions. It is possible that carbonic anhydrase in myelin facilitates the removal of axonal carbonic acid resulting from intraaxonal metabolism, and that 5′-nucleotidase facilitates the transport of the putative transmitter, adenosine, from axons since AMP is less permeant than adenosine.

The endogenous neutral proteinase degrades MAG and BP, but not other myelin proteins.[26] It is more active in human myelin than in rat myelin. This enzyme may be involved in normal catabolism and could have a role in some forms of demyelination.

MOLECULAR ARCHITECTURE[e]

Some of the lipids, and all of the proteins of myelin are antigens. Specific antibodies raised to these components and reactive chemical probes have been used to determine the localization of some selected components within the sheath. These data show that PLP is localized to the intraperiod line (the fusion of exterior sides of the membrane) and BP is localized to the major dense line or the cytoplasmic side of the membrane. Immunochemical staining shows that these proteins are evenly distributed throughout the sheath.

Studies of Wolfgram proteins and MAG have not been so precise, but they show that these proteins are not uniformly distributed. Immunochemical staining with anti-Wolfgram sera is restricted to inner and outer layers of myelin, and anti-MAG staining is confined to periaxonal regions of myelinated fibers. This is a matter of some controversy, however, and recent ultrastructural studies show that MAG may be uniformly distributed.

METABOLISM[f]

Turnover

The concept that myelin, once formed, is metabolically stable was largely developed by Davison and colleagues. Smith and co-workers confirmed that myelin was relatively stable, but found that individual components turned over at quite different rates. More recent studies have clarified this long-standing problem. The confusion in the literature can be traced to several experimental variables: the precursor used, the time period after injection during which metabolism is studied, and the age of the animal on injection. Davison's earlier postulate of long-term metabolic stability of most myelin components has been verified. Some components, however, do turn over much faster than others and all components show both a fast and a slow turning-over pool.

These data indicate that myelin formed early in life is the most stable, and that newly formed myelin is catabolized faster than "old" myelin. These data may be explained by the geometry of the sheath. Newly formed myelin, which is presumably

[e]See ref. 27 for review.
[f]See refs. 28–31 for reviews.

added to regions of myelin adjacent to cytoplasm, is also more available to degradative enzymes than components sequestered in compacted layers.

Synthesis and Assembly

Studies primarily by Benjamins and colleagues[28,31] show that BP enters the sheath with almost no lag after synthesis, whereas PLP enters myelin after a lag of 30–40 min after synthesis. Moreover, after protein synthesis is stopped with cycloheximide, entry of BP halts immediately, but PLP continues to be incorporated into myelin for 30 min. It is also interesting that lipids continue to be incorporated into myelin for hours after protein synthesis has stopped. These data indicate that myelin is not assembled synchronously as a unit and that BP and PLP are assembled by different mechanisms with PLP possibly taking a longer and more circuitous route through the cytoplasm. Recent studies by Colman and colleagues indicate that polysomes bearing mRNA for BP are concentrated very near the myelin sheath, implying that BP is inserted into the membrane soon after synthesis.

Myelin Components in Culture[g]

Many problems of differentiation of oligodendrocytes, the expression of specific myelin constituents, the temporal sequence of that expression and the biosynthesis of these constituents may be studied in various culture systems in which oligodendroglia thrive. Viable cells can be obtained either from newborn rats or from adult animals such as cows and sheep. Cells from newborn rats do differentiate and express cerebroside, sulfatide, BP, CNP, carbonic anhydrase, and glycerol phosphate dehydrogenase. These properties do not develop simultaneously. Cerebroside and CNP are detectable much earlier than BP. It does appear, however, that the expression of myelinogenic properties is programmed into the cell and will develop in culture in the absence of axons and their presumptive signals.

MULTIPLE SCLEROSIS AND DEMYELINATION[h]

Myelin, rather than the oligodendrocyte, appears to be the primary vulnerable target in multiple sclerosis (MS). These studies of normal myelin furnish an organizing framework for our studies of chemical pathology, but by themselves offer few clues to the disease.

The early neurochemical studies of MS brain were largely confined to defining compositional changes. These were, in all cases, consistent with myelin loss and subsequent gliosis. More refined studies show considerable widespread pathology apart from plaques in the normal-appearing white matter. Myelin is isolated in consistently lower yields from these areas, the myelin enzyme CNP is decreased, MAG appears to be lost in areas where BP is present, and hydrolytic enzymes, including acid proteinases, are increased. All of these changes indicate a diffuse disease process and the possible presence of microscopic lesions in apparently normal white matter. It is interesting that the increased lysosomal enzymes appear to arise more from astrocytes

[g] See refs. 32 and 33 for reviews.
[h] See ref. 34 for review.

than from infiltrating inflammatory cells. Although myelin is obtained in lower yield from the normal-appearing white matter, its composition, with few exceptions, has been found to be normal. The exceptions have exhibited a nonspecific abnormal composition found in several other diseases where myelin is being degraded. One can assume that MS white matter contains normal myelin together with myelin in various stages of degradation. In most isolation methods the abnormal myelin would be discarded, unless the amount is large.

Neurochemists have defined the gross chemical alterations but have found little that could be considered specific to MS. They should be able to contribute to defining details of the early events in demyelination that are unique to MS and that would serve to differentiate it biochemically from other conditions involving myelin degradation by phagocytic cells. Initial events in demyelination must involve hydrolytic enzymes, presumably proteinases and lipases acting extracellularly. There is good evidence that in model systems the macrophage is the source of these enzymes. Recent findings that myelin fixes complement in the absence of antibody and incorporates the membrane attack complex are very promising leads. Proteinases, lipases and complement acting in concert may be what is needed to initiate degradation. Definition of these events could lead to rational methods of interference in the destructive process.

REFERENCES

1. NORTON, W. T. & L. A. AUTILIO. 1965. The chemical composition of bovine CNS myelin. Ann. N.Y. Acad. Sci. **122:** 77–85.
2. CUZNER, M. L., A. N. DAVISON & N. A. GREGSON. 1965. Chemical and metabolic studies of rat myelin of the central nervous system. Ann. N.Y. Acad. Sci. **122**: 86–94.
3. THOMPSON, E. B. & M. W. KIES. 1965. Current studies on the lipids and proteins of myelin. Ann. N.Y. Acad. Sci. **122**: 129–147.
4. WOLFGRAM, F. 1965. Macromolecular constituents of myelin. Ann. N.Y. Acad. Sci. **122**: 104–115.
5. LEES, M. B. 1965. The solubility properties of proteolipids. Ann. N.Y. Acad. Sci. **122**: 116–128.
6. KIES, M. W. 1965. Chemical studies on an encephalitogenic protein from guinea pig brain. Ann. N.Y. Acad. Sci. **122**: 161–170.
7. MORELL, P., Ed. 1984. Myelin. 2d ed. Plenum Press. New York.
8. NORTON, W. T. & W. CAMMER. 1984. Isolation and characterization of myelin. *In* Myelin. 2d ed. P. Morell, Ed. Plenum Press. New York. In press.
9. RAFF, M. C., R. MIRSKY, K. L. FIELDS, R. P. LISAK, S. H. DORFMAN, D. H. SILVERBERG, N. A. GREGSON, S. LIEBOWITZ & M. KENNEDY. 1978. Galactocerebroside is a specific cell-surface antigenic marker for oligodendrocytes in culture. Nature **274**: 813–816.
10. DUPOUEY, P., B. ZALC, M. LEFROIT-JOLY & D. GOMES. 1979. Localization of galactosylceramide and sulfatide at the surface of the myelin sheath: An immunofluorescence study in liquid medium. Cell. Mol. Biol. **25**: 269–272.
11. ZALC, B., M. MONGE & N. BAUMANN. 1980. Immunohistochemical localization of galactosylceramide and sulfogalactosylceramide in the cerebellum of the quaking, shiverer and jimpy mice. *In* Neurological Mutations Affecting Myelination. N. Baumann, Ed: 263–268. Elsevier/North Holland. Amsterdam.
12. LEDEEN, R. W., F. B. COCHRAN, R. K. YU, F. G. SAMUELS & J. E. HALEY. 1980. Gangliosides of the CNS myelin membrane. Adv. Exp. Med. Biol. **125**: 167–176.
13. SUZUKI, K., S. E. PODUSLO & W. T. NORTON. 1967. Gangliosides in the myelin fraction of developing rats. Biochim. Biophys. Acta **144**: 375–381.
14. COCHRAN, F. B., R. K. YU & R. W. LEDEEN. 1982. Myelin gangliosides in vertebrates. J. Neurochem. **39**: 773–779.
15. LEES, M. B. & S. W. BROSTOFF. 1984. Proteins of myelin. *In* Myelin. 2d ed. P. Morell, Ed. Plenum Press. New York. In press.

16. ROACH, A., K. BOYLAN, S. HORVATH, S. B. PRUSINER & L. E. HOOD. 1983. Characterization of cloned cDNA representing rat myelin basic protein: Absence of expression in brain of shiverer mutant mice. Cell **34**: 799–806.
17. DRUMMOND, R. J. & G. DEAN. 1980. Comparison of 2′,3′-cyclic nucleotide 3′-phosphodiesterase and the major component of Wolfgram protein W1. J. Neurochem. **35**: 1155–1165.
18. SPRINKLE, T. J., M. R. WELLS, F. A. GARVER & D. B. SMITH. 1980. Studies on the Wolfgram high molecular weight CNS myelin proteins: relationship to 2′,3′-cyclic nucleotide 3′-phosphodiesterase. J. Neurochem. **35**: 1200–1208.
19. NORTON, W. T. 1980. Myelin enzymes: Indicators of noninsulating functions. *In* Search for the Cause of Multiple Sclerosis and Other Chronic Diseases of the Central Nervous System. A. Boese, Ed.: 64–75. Verlag Chemie. Weinheim.
20. SUZUKI, K. 1980. Myelin-associated enzymes. *In* Neurological Mutations Affecting Myelination. N. Baumann, Ed.: 333–347. Elsevier/North Holland. Amsterdam.
21. LEES, M. B. & V. S. SAPIRSTEIN. 1983. Myelin-associated enzymes. *In* Handbook of Neurochemistry, vol. 4. 2d ed. A. Lajtha, Ed.: 435–460. Plenum Press. New York.
22. LEDEEN, R. 1984. Phospholipid synthesis in myelin: Putative role of the axon. *In* Phospholipids in the Nervous System. II. Physiological Roles. G. Porcellati, L. A. Horrocks & J. N. Kanfer, Eds. Raven Press. New York. In press.
23. WU, P.-S. & R. W. LEDEEN. 1980. Evidence for the presence of CDP-ethanolamine: 1,2-diacyl-sn-glycerol ethanolamine phosphotransferase in rat central nervous system myelin. J. Neurochem. **35**: 659–660.
24. KUNISHITA, T. & R. W. LEDEEN. 1984. Phospholipid biosynthesis in myelin: Presence of CTP:ethanolamine phosphate cytidyltransferase in purified myelin of rat brain. J. Neurochem. In press.
25. HALEY, J. E. & R. W. LEDEEN. 1979. Incorporation of axonally transported substances into myelin lipids. J. Neurochem. **32**: 735–742.
26. SATO, S., R. H. QUARLES & R. O. BRADY. 1982. Susceptibility of the myelin-associated glycoprotein and basic protein to the neutral proteinase in highly purified myelin from human and rat brain. J. Neurochem. **39**: 97–105.
27. BRAUN, P. E. 1984. Molecular architecture of myelin. *In* Myelin. 2d ed. P. Morell, Ed. Plenum Press. New York. In press.
28. BENJAMINS, J. A. & M. E. SMITH. 1984. Metabolism of myelin. *In* Myelin. 2d ed. P. Morell, Ed. Plenum Press. New York. In press.
29. NORTON, W. T. 1981. Biochemistry of myelin. *In* Demyelinating Disease: Basic and Clinical Electrophysiology. S. G. Waxman & J. M. Ritchie, Eds.: 93–121. Raven Press. New York.
30. MORELL, P. & A. D. TOEWS. 1984. *In vivo* metabolism of oligodendroglial lipids. *In* Oligodendroglia. W. T. Norton, Ed. Plenum Press. New York.
31. BENJAMINS, J. A. 1984. Protein metabolism of oligodendroglial cells *in vivo*. *In* Oligodendroglia. W. T. Norton, Ed.: 87–124. Plenum Press. New York.
32. NORTON, W. T. 1983. Recent advances in the neurobiology of oligodendroglia. *In* Advances in Cellular Neurobiology, vol. 4. S. Fedoroff & L. Hertz, Eds.: 3–55. Academic Press. New York.
33. PFEIFFER, S. E. 1984. Oligodendrocyte development in culture systems. *In* Oligodendroglia. W. T. Norton, Ed.: 233–298. Plenum Press. New York.
34. NORTON, W. T. & W. CAMMER. 1984. Chemical pathology of diseases involving myelin. *In* Myelin. 2d ed. P. Morell, Ed. Plenum Press. New York.

Continual Breakdown and Regeneration of Myelin in Progressive Multiple Sclerosis Plaques[a]

J. W. PRINEAS,[b,c] E. E. KWON,[b] EUN-SOOK CHO,[d] AND L. R. SHARER[d]

[b]*Neurology Service*
Veterans Administration Medical Center
East Orange, New Jersey 07901

[c]*Department of Neurosciences*
[d]*Department of Pathology*
University of Medicine and Dentistry of New Jersey
New Jersey Medical School
Newark, New Jersey 07103

Depending on the amount and type of myelin breakdown products present, multiple sclerosis lesions may be classified as old, inactive lesions with little or no evidence of recent myelin breakdown, subacute lesions with numerous lipid macrophages present at the edges of the demyelinated tissue, and acute, hypercellular lesions in which numerous lipid macrophages and macrophages containing undigested myelin debris are present throughout the demyelinated tissue. Acute plaques are seen only rarely in patients who die more than a few years after the onset of the disease. Subacute lesions, however, are much more common and are not rare even in cases of 20 years duration.

In the present study, we describe changes seen in myelin sheaths at the edges of subacute plaques in patients in whom the duration of the disease ranged from ten months to 20 years. The findings indicate that remyelination and active demyelination frequently coexist in such lesions. The study also adds to existing evidence implicating infiltrating macrophages as the agent primarily responsible for myelin destruction at the edge of progressive lesions.

MATERIALS AND METHODS

The tissue examined in the present study was obtained at autopsy from the following five cases of multiple sclerosis, one of which (Case 2) has been reported previously.[26] Case 1 was a male, aged 61 years, who had impaired vision in one eye for several weeks when aged 20 years. At age 54 the left arm was weak and clumsy for several weeks. At age 59 he lost vision in each eye over the course of several days, and a few weeks later became quadriparetic with signs of an acute cervical cord lesion. Vision improved moderately but there was no improvement in motor or sensory signs until his death twenty months after the onset of quadriparesis. Case 2 was a 34-year-old man in whom the neurological illness progressed, without remission, to death three years and

[a]This investigation was supported by the Medical Research Service of the Veterans Administration and by the National Multiple Sclerosis Society.

eleven months after onset. Case 3 was a woman aged 29 years who developed impaired memory, weakness of the left arm and urinary incontinence over a period of several weeks in January 1979. With steroids there was a substantial clinical improvement which lasted three months. Over the next few months her balance deteriorated, there was bilateral visual impairment with bilateral optic atrophy, and following the onset of coma vigil, she died in November 1979, ten months after the onset of the neurological illness. Case 4 was a 60-year-old man in whom signs and symptoms of the disease had been present for twenty years. After an initial relapsing and remitting course, he developed a static paraplegia and showed little evidence of disease activity during the five years prior to death. Case 5 was a woman aged 30 years in whom the neurological illness ran a relapsing and remitting course until it became progressive four years before her death eleven years after the onset of the disease.

At autopsy, typical old and/or subacute plaques were found throughout the central nervous system in each case except Case 1, where they were restricted to the spinal cord (all segments), lower medulla, and optic nerves and chiasm.

The interval between death and autopsy was 30 minutes in Case 5, three hours in Case 2, and between 12 and 22 hours in Cases 1, 3 and 4. Tissue for epoxy embedding was fixed by immersion (Cases 1–4) or by *in situ* perfusion through the abdominal aorta (Case 5) with 3 or 3.5 percent glutaraldehyde in 0.1 M cacodylate buffer. Blocks of tissue 0.5 × 4 × 4 mm were subsequently fixed in 2 percent osmium tetroxide and embedded in Spurr's epoxy resin. Toluidine blue-stained 1 μm sections were prepared from 20 to 60 blocks from each case for light microscopy and to select areas for electron microscopy. Frozen sections stained for lipids (hematoxylin and oil red O), and paraffin sections stained for myelin (Luxol fast blue and PAS; Heidenhain), axons (Bodian) and with hematoxylin and eosin, were prepared from formalin-fixed tissue.

Longitudinally disposed myelin internodes were studied in appropriately orientated epoxy blocks using 1 μm toluidine blue-stained sections and differential interference contrast microscopy of 6 μm thick unstained sections of osmium-fixed tissue.

The plaques selected for the present study were lesions containing moderate to large numbers of lipid-containing macrophages within the demyelinated zone. All exhibited relatively good myelin fixation, and, although not a criterion for selection, all were found to be active lesions in the sense that some macrophages contained, in addition to lipid or lipid vacuoles, particles with the morphology and staining characteristics of myelin as seen in toluidine blue-stained sections. Confirmation that this material was undigested myelin was obtained by electron microscopy and by immunocytochemical staining for myelin basic protein using deplasticized 1 μm sections from representative lesions. In all lesions studied, perivasular mononuclear cell cuffing was inconspicuous. The lesions studied were obtained from the spinal cord (Case 1-5, Case 2-4, Case 3-3, Case 4-2), cerebellar white matter (Case 5-1) and centrum ovale (Case 2-3, Case 5-1).

RESULTS

Remyelination

All 14 spinal cord plaques and two of the other five lesions examined revealed thinly myelinated fibers of central nervous system type (*i.e.,* unassociated with Schwann cell nuclei) in demyelinated tissue amongst lipid-containing macrophages. The number varied from a few fibers scattered around plaque margins to large numbers present throughout demyelinated zones up to a millimeter or more in diameter which appeared as shadow plaques on naked eye examination (FIGURE 1).

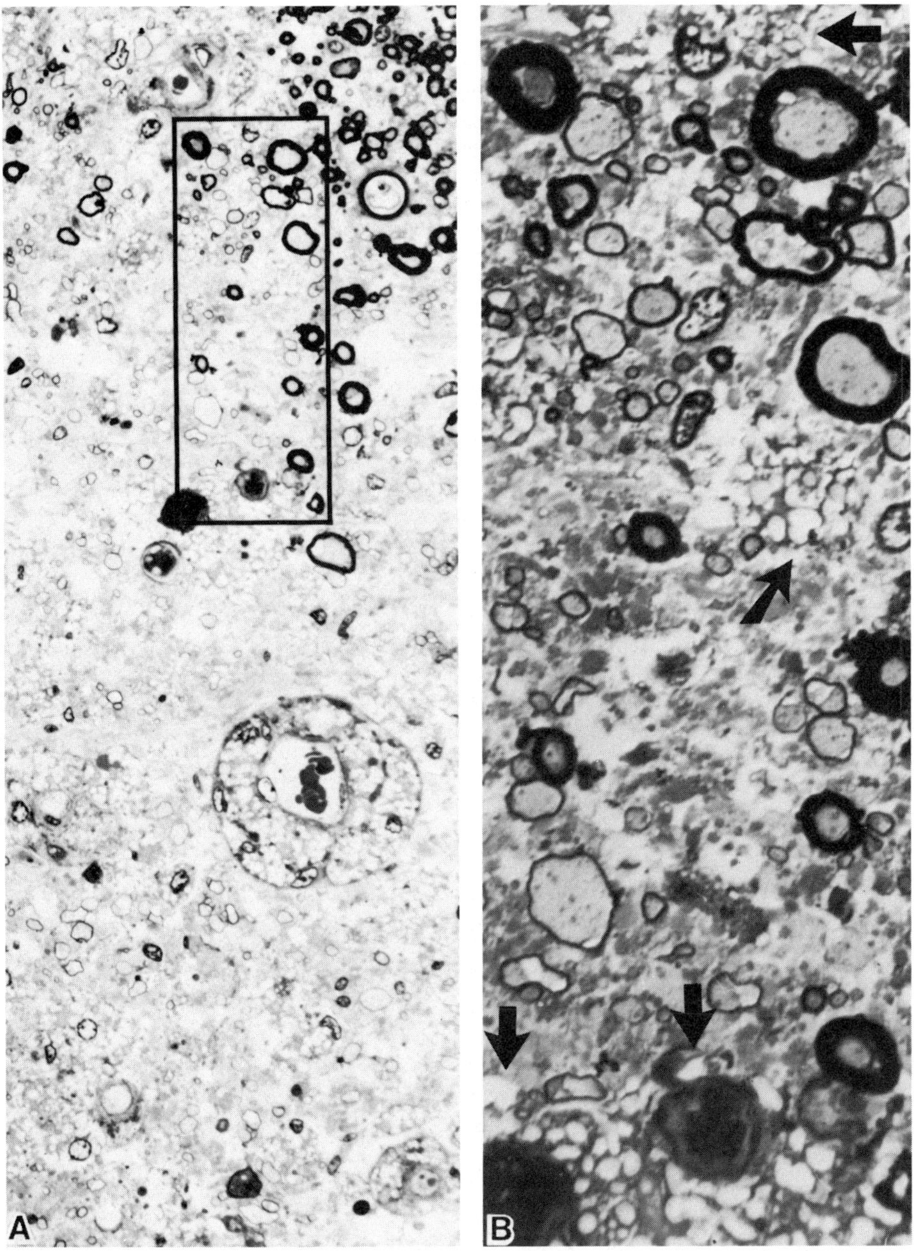

FIGURE 1. Edge of a plaque in dorsal columns of spinal cord. (**A**) Thinly myelinated fibers are present throughout the plaque. (**B**) Enlargement of boxed area in (**A**) shows thinly myelinated fibers in the presence of macrophages containing lipid vacuoles and myelin debris (*arrows*). Case 1, toluidine blue, (**A**) ×360, (**B**) ×1160.

When fibers ensheathed in peripheral nervous system myelin (*i.e.*, associated with Schwann cell nuclei) were also present in the same lesion (about one-third of the spinal cord lesions examined), they were located usually in bundles under the pia and they had thicker sheaths than the other thinly myelinated fibers present.

Examination of the same plaques orientated to allow the thinly myelinated fibers of central type located in demyelinated tissue to be observed in longitudinal sections revealed that the great majority had uniformly thin, short internodes, frequently less than 30 μm in length. They occurred (a) as isolated segments on long stretches of bare axon, (b) adjacent to normal paranodes from which they were separated by a normal nodal gap, (c) in rows in which they were separated from each other by normal nodal gaps (FIGURE 2), or (d) contiguous with degenerate internodes of the type illustrated in FIGURE 8B. The thin internodes were not infrequently in contact with macrophages (FIGURE 2A, FIGURE 7D). Oligodendrocytes were present, usually in reduced numbers. In the patient with acute multiple sclerosis with a duration of ten months, central type remyelination was as prominent as in the other cases including the formation of chains of short internodes separated by normal nodal gaps.

Short, uniformly thin, central-type myelin internodes were observed with some frequency in two other locations, namely around small veins in the myelinated margin of plaques, and amongst normally myelinated fibers at plaque margins. In both of these locations, however, other types of thinly myelinated fibers were also present as described below.

In the few plaques examined in which no remyelinating fibers of central type could be identified, it is uncertain that these were in fact absent. These particular lesions were located in white matter in which small, normal nerve fibers with relatively thin sheaths and running in all directions were common, which made it difficult to recognize an abnormally thin sheath or to examine large numbers of longitudinally sectioned fibers. Thus while it would have been of interest to identify histological features associated with noninitiation of central remyelination, if this exists in multiple sclerosis, the present study provides no reliable information on this point.

Demyelination

The selection of lesions for examination in the present study was based on the presence in the plaque of moderate to large numbers of macrophages containing lipid vacuoles (foamy macrophages). In all of the lesions so selected, it was observed by light microscopy of epoxy sections that some foamy macrophages also contained undigested myelin fragments, most often in the form of myelin balls. These macrophages were located chiefly in myelinated tissue bordering the plaque, and especially around small veins in myelinated tissue. Their number ranged from very few (*e.g.*, six in a single plaque) to many hundreds present in a single section. Lesions of the latter type were found in Cases 1 (FIGURES 3 and 4), 3 and 5 (FIGURE 5).

Virtually all discrete myelin fragments that were seen lying between nerve fibers, when examined by bright field microsocpy in 1 μm toluidine blue-stained sections or in thick, osmium-stained sections examined by differential interference contrast microscopy, appeared to be located within macrophages and not extracellularly. The often numerous normal myelinoid bodies present[9] could be distinguished by their relationship to thick myelin sheaths (FIGURES 6A, B).

Many myelin sheaths in areas infiltrated by macrophages containing undigested myelin fragments appeared normal (FIGURES 3, 4, 5A, B). Others were abnormally thin (FIGURE 4), and a few were irregularly swollen. Sectioned longitudinally, the thinly myelinated fibers were found to be of several types: (a) fibers with normally

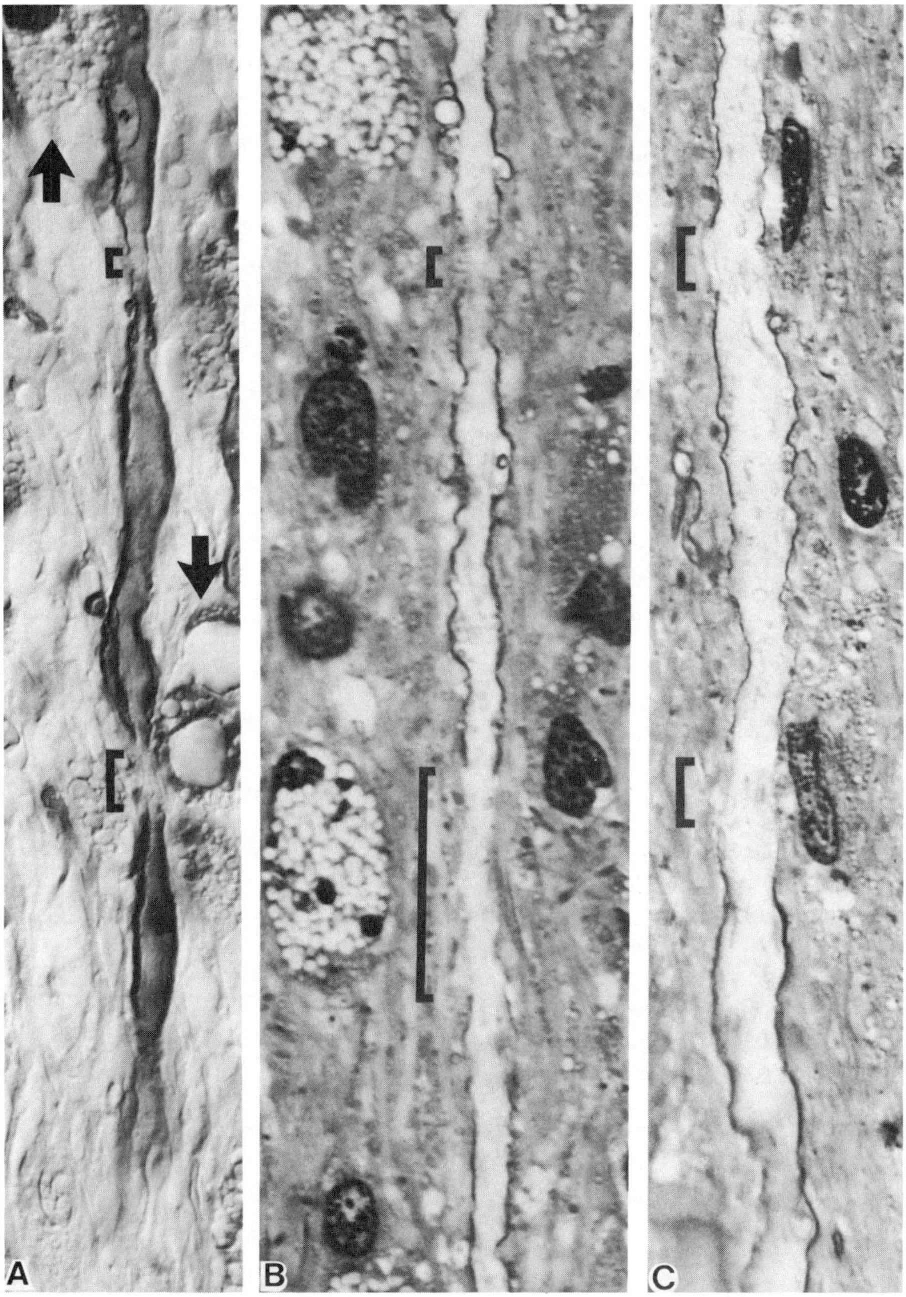

FIGURE 2. Remyelinating internodes separated by stretches of bare axon that may represent regenerating nodes of Ranvier (*bars*). (**A**) Case 1, osmium tetroxide, ×860. *Arrows* indicate macrophages in contact with new sheath. (**B**) and (**C**), Case 2, toluidine blue, ×1460.

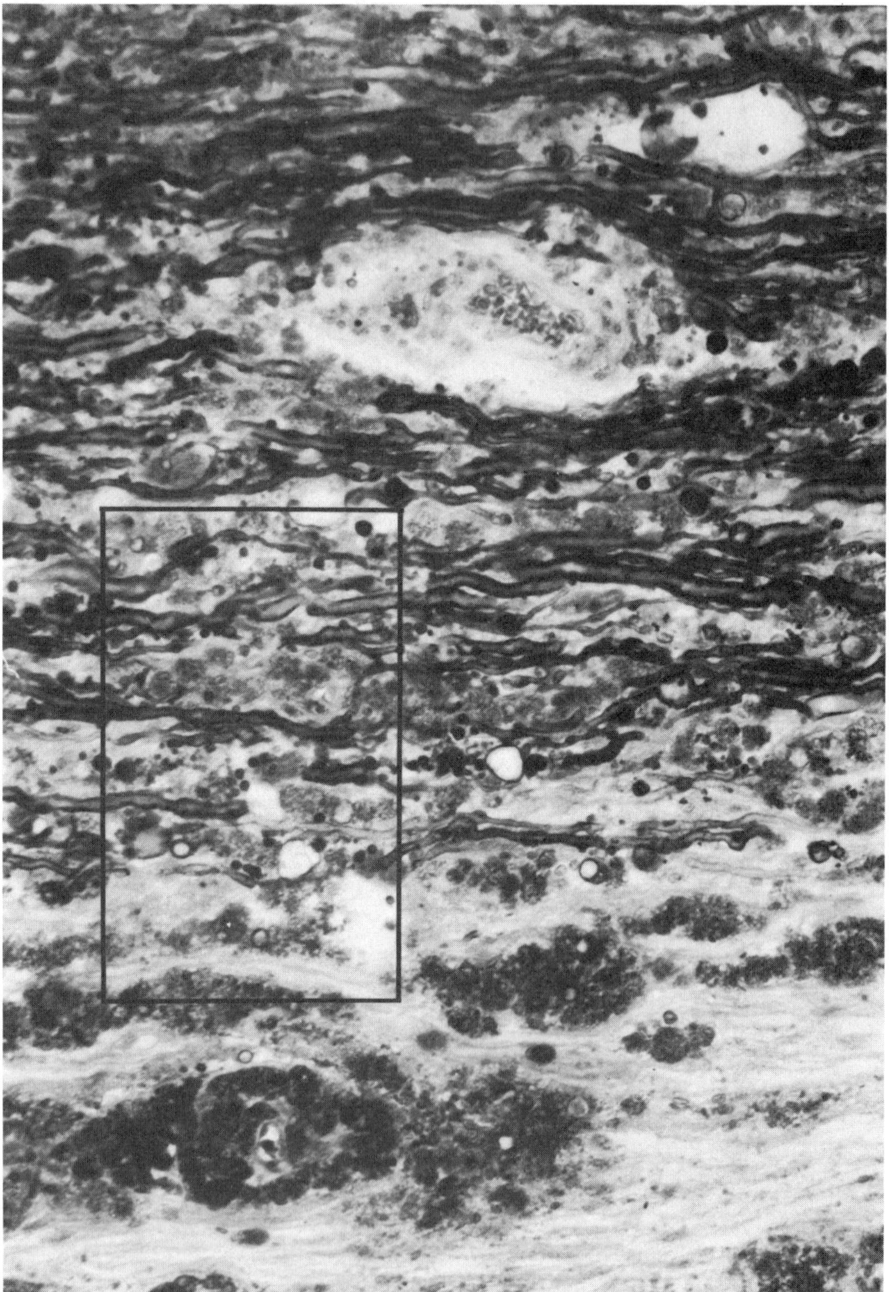

FIGURE 3. Longitudinal section of spinal cord plaque showing osmiophilic debris in demyelinated zone. Case 1, osmium tetroxide, ×340.

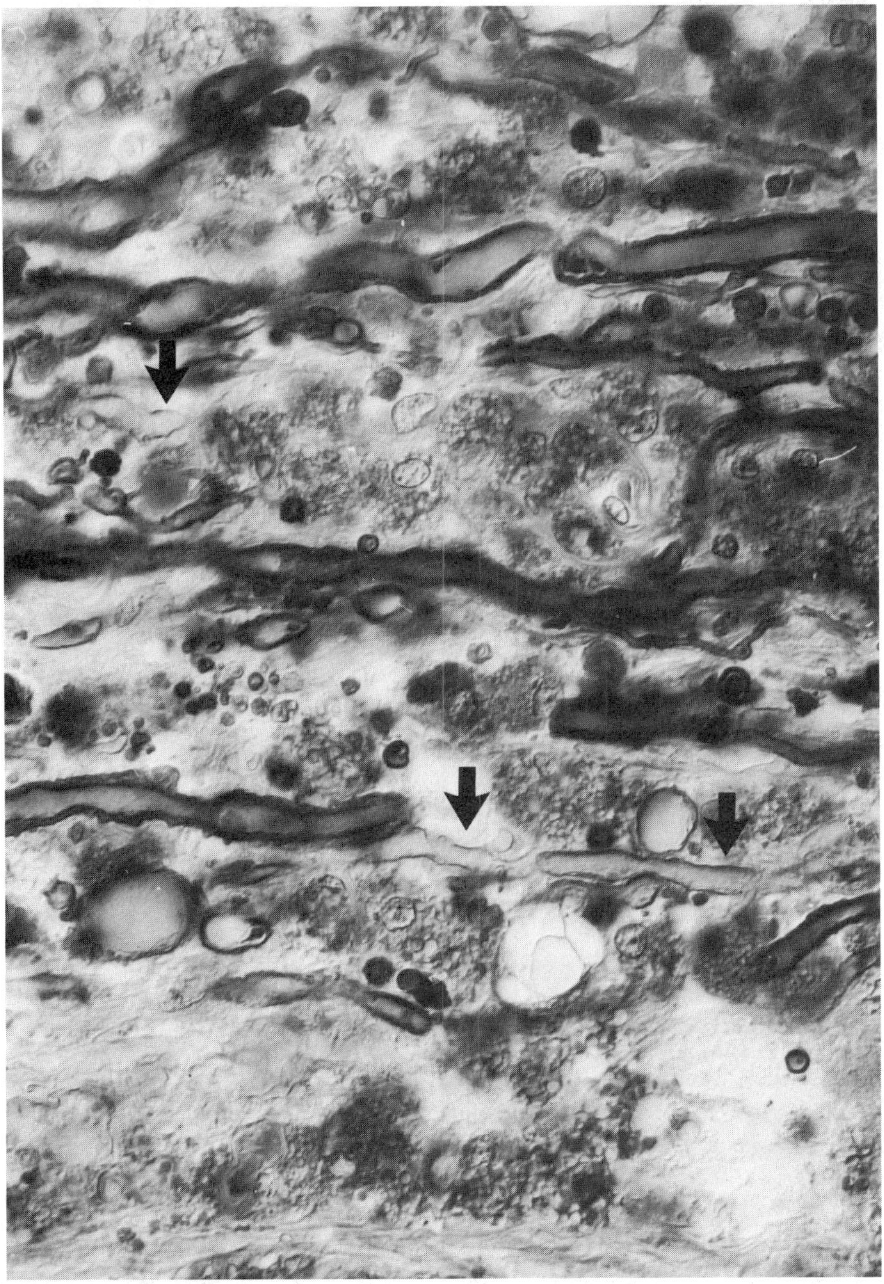

FIGURE 4. Enlarged view of boxed area in FIGURE 3. Rows of macrophages together with numerous particles of myelin (myelin balls and myelinoid bodies) can be seen among myelinated nerve fibers, most of which appear normal. *Arrows* indicate thinly myelinated fibers. ×540.

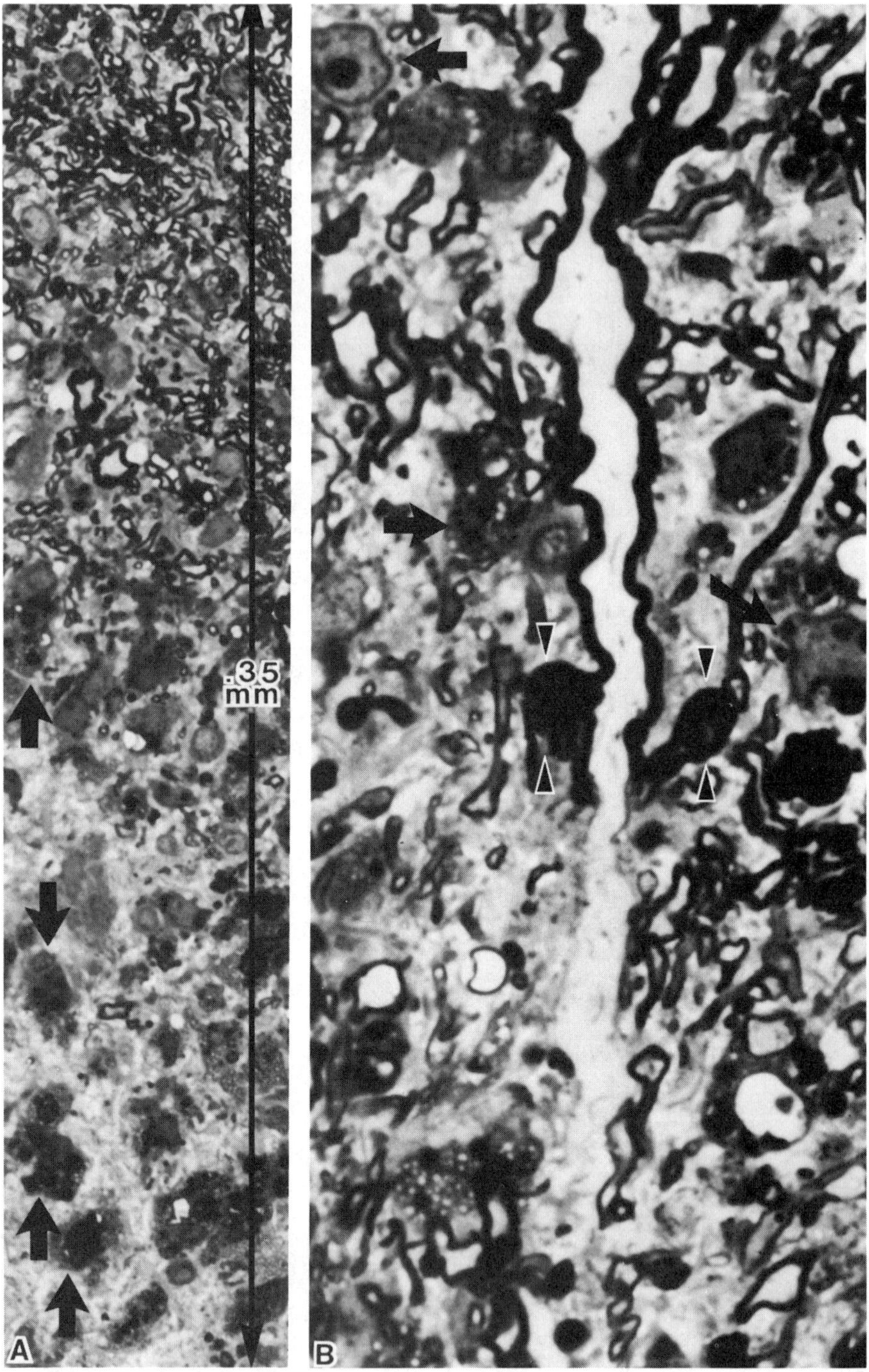

FIGURE 5. (**A**), (**B**) Macrophages (*arrows*) containing undigested myelin fragments at plaque margin. Myelin sheaths are normally compact. The large myelin internode in (**B**) ends in what appear to be redundant folds of myelin (*arrow points*) where the axon enters demyelinated zone. Cell counts determined electron microscopically across the edge of the plaque illustrated in (**A**) are shown in TABLE 1. Case 5, toluidine blue, (**A**) ×540, (**B**) ×1690.

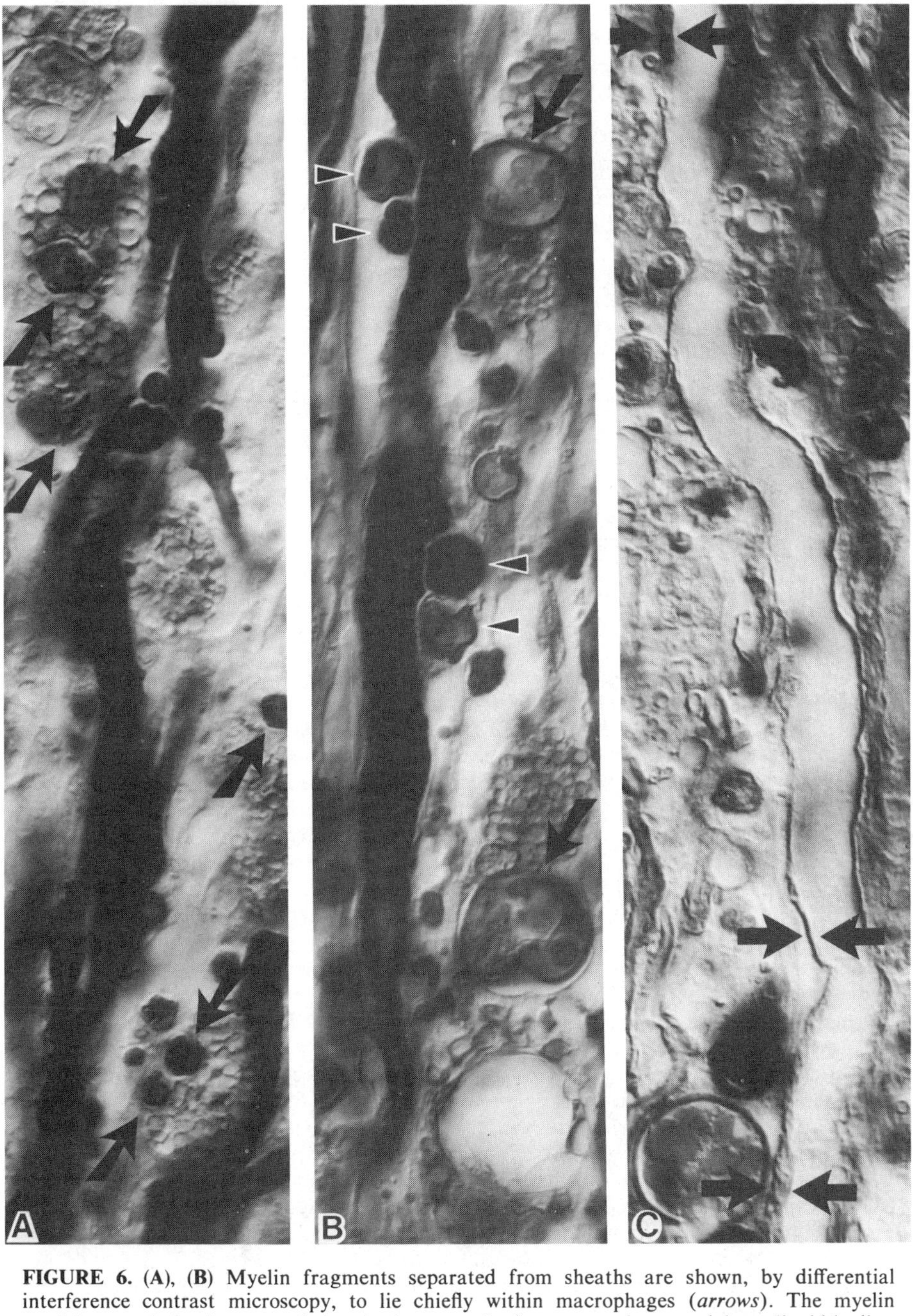

FIGURE 6. (**A**), (**B**) Myelin fragments separated from sheaths are shown, by differential interference contrast microscopy, to lie chiefly within macrophages (*arrows*). The myelin particles seen indenting normal sheaths (*arrow points*) are normal paranodal myelinoid bodies. (**C**) Nonuniform thinning (*arrows*) of a fiber in an area of active demyelination. Foamy cytoplasm of macrophages contact the sheath at several points. Case 1, osmium tetroxide, (**A**) ×870, (**B**) ×870, (**C**) ×860.

thick myelin sheaths which became progressively thinner along the course of the fiber (FIGURE 6C), (b) fibers in which the sheath was swollen at one point as described below and which showed nonuniform thinning of the sheath on one side of the swelling, and (c) remyelinating fibers (fibers with uniformly thin, short internodes). The relative number of each variety was different in different plaques. In the plaque illustrated in FIGURES 3 and 4 there were numerous thinly myelinated fibers in the zone infiltrated by macrophages. Some of these were remyelinating fibers but the great majority were of type (a) or (b). In contrast, in other plaques in the same case, with macrophages containing undigested myelin debris present amongst myelinated fibers at the plaque margin, most of the thinly myelinated fibers present were of the remyelinating type with only a few fibers of type (a) or (b) present. Macrophages containing myelin fragments and lipid vacuoles were frequently observed contacting thin myelin segments of all three types (FIGURE 6C, FIGURE 7).

The focally swollen sheaths exhibited a widened periaxonal space around an intact axon together with splitting and distortion of the sheath (FIGURE 8A). Macrophages were commonly present inside the swellings (FIGURE 8B). Macrophages were also observed inside compact sheaths (FIGURE 8C). As described above, the swollen segments were sometimes observed to continue along the fiber as an abnormally thin sheath (FIGURE 8C). Some swollen segments were seen to be separated by a normal nodal gap from a remyelinating internode.

In several cases, phagocytosis of corpora amylacea was observed (FIGURE 8D).

Electron Microscopy

Of the 19 lesions examined light microscopically, fine structure was best preserved in two lesions located in the cerebellum and cerebrum in Case 5 where tissue was fixed by perfusion 30 minutes after death. The following observations were made on sections from blocks trimmed from the edges of these two plaques, both of which exhibited, light microscopically, macrophages containing undigested myelin fragments in bordering myelinated tissue (FIGURE 5). Unlike most of the other plaques examined in the present study, no thinly myelinated fibers were discernible by light microscopy. However they were detected electron microscopically.

Scanning systematically towards the plaque from normal white matter, apart from mild fibrous astrogliosis, the first abnormality encountered was the appearance of occasional small macrophages containing lipid vacuoles, laminated inclusions and myelin debris in tissue in which the number and morphology of myelin sheaths, including their inner and outer tongues, and oligodendrocyte perikarya appeared normal.

Approaching closer to the plaque the next abnormality seen was the appearance of occasional naked axons together with fibers with abnormally thin myelin sheaths embraced by macrophages containing myelin debris (FIGURES 9 and 10). It was frequently observed that these thin internodes were not uniformly thin but revealed superficial lamellae that terminated prematurely along the internode. Particular attention was paid to inner and outer tongues of oligodendrocyte cytoplasm in these sheaths but nothing abnormal was discovered. Normal oligodendrocyte perikarya were present but in reduced numbers (FIGURES 10 and 11). Rare, necrotic cells were present.

Passing into the demyelinated zone, numerous oligodendrocyte perikarya could still be identified in the absence of myelin sheaths.

Rare plasma cells were observed, chiefly in perivascular spaces. Also observed were rare, medium-sized lymphocytes with few polysomes and with very little granular

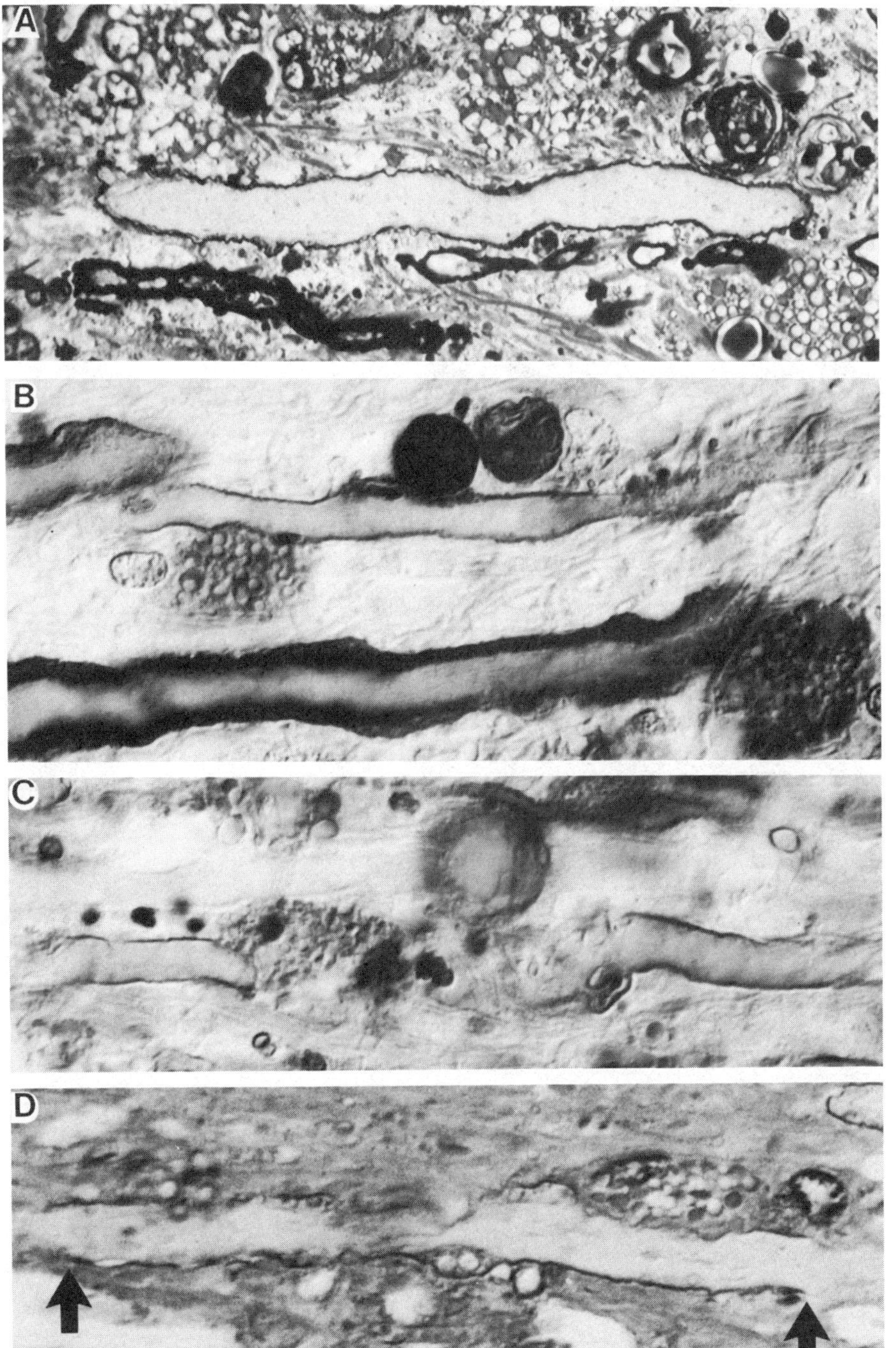

FIGURE 7. Nerve fibers with abnormally thin sheaths in plaque margins are shown contacting macrophages, some of which contain myelin balls. The internode (*arrows*) seen in (**D**) is probably a remyelinating internode. (**A**) Case 1, toluidine blue, ×870. (**B**), (**C**) Case 1, osmium tetroxide, ×860. (**D**) Case 2, toluidine blue, ×1450.

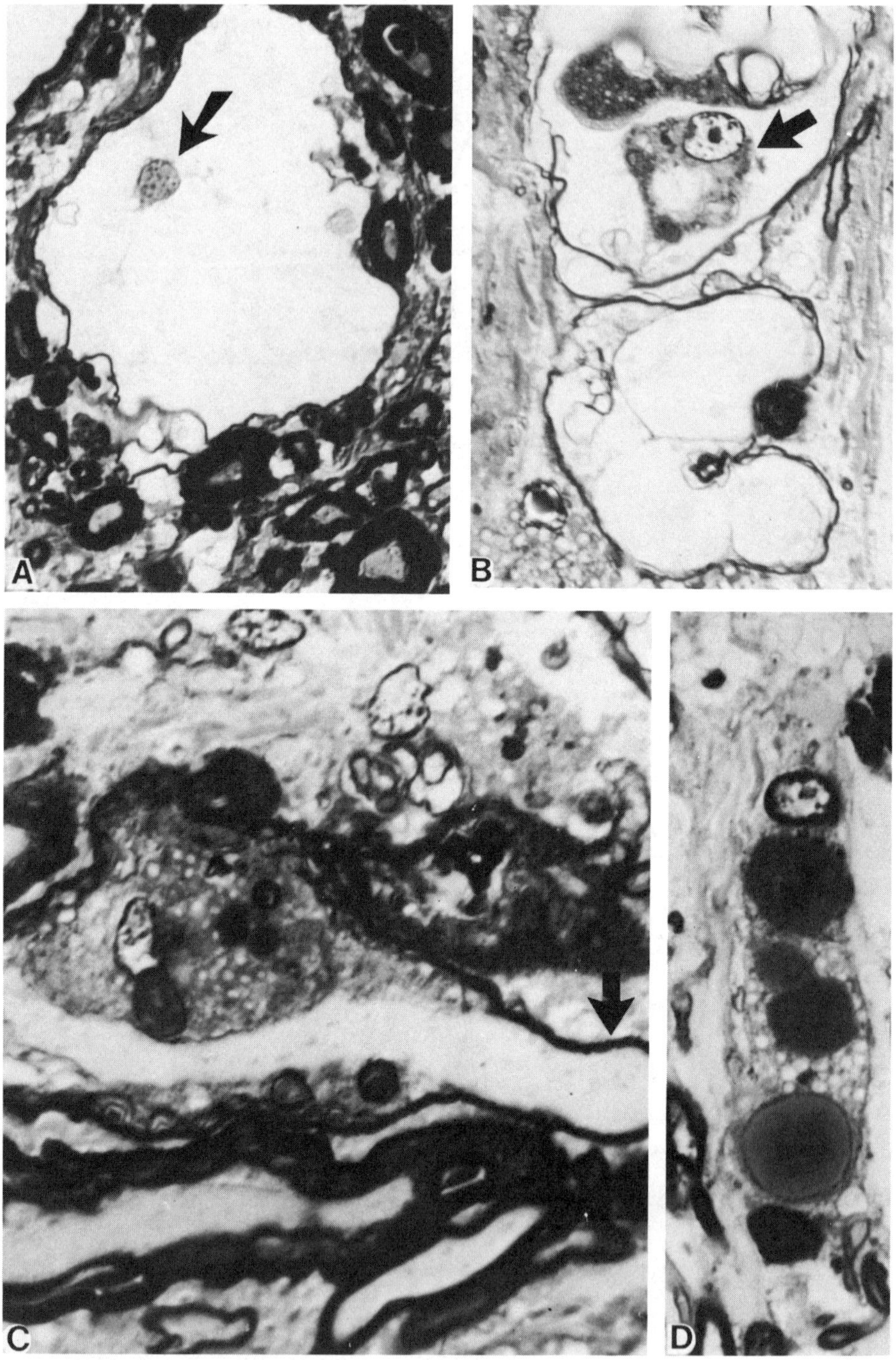

FIGURE 8. (**A**), (**B**) Swollen myelin sheaths. Affected fiber is seen in cross section. The axon is indicated by the *arrow*. (**B**) Affected fiber sectioned longitudinally. *Arrow* points to a macrophage within the distended sheath. (**C**) A macrophage containing myelin debris lies inside part of a myelin sheath which is continuous with an abnormally thin myelin segment (*arrow*). (**D**) Phagocytosed corpora amylacea. Case 1, toluidine blue, (**A**) ×1010, (**B**) ×900, (**C**) ×1310, (**D**) ×1400.

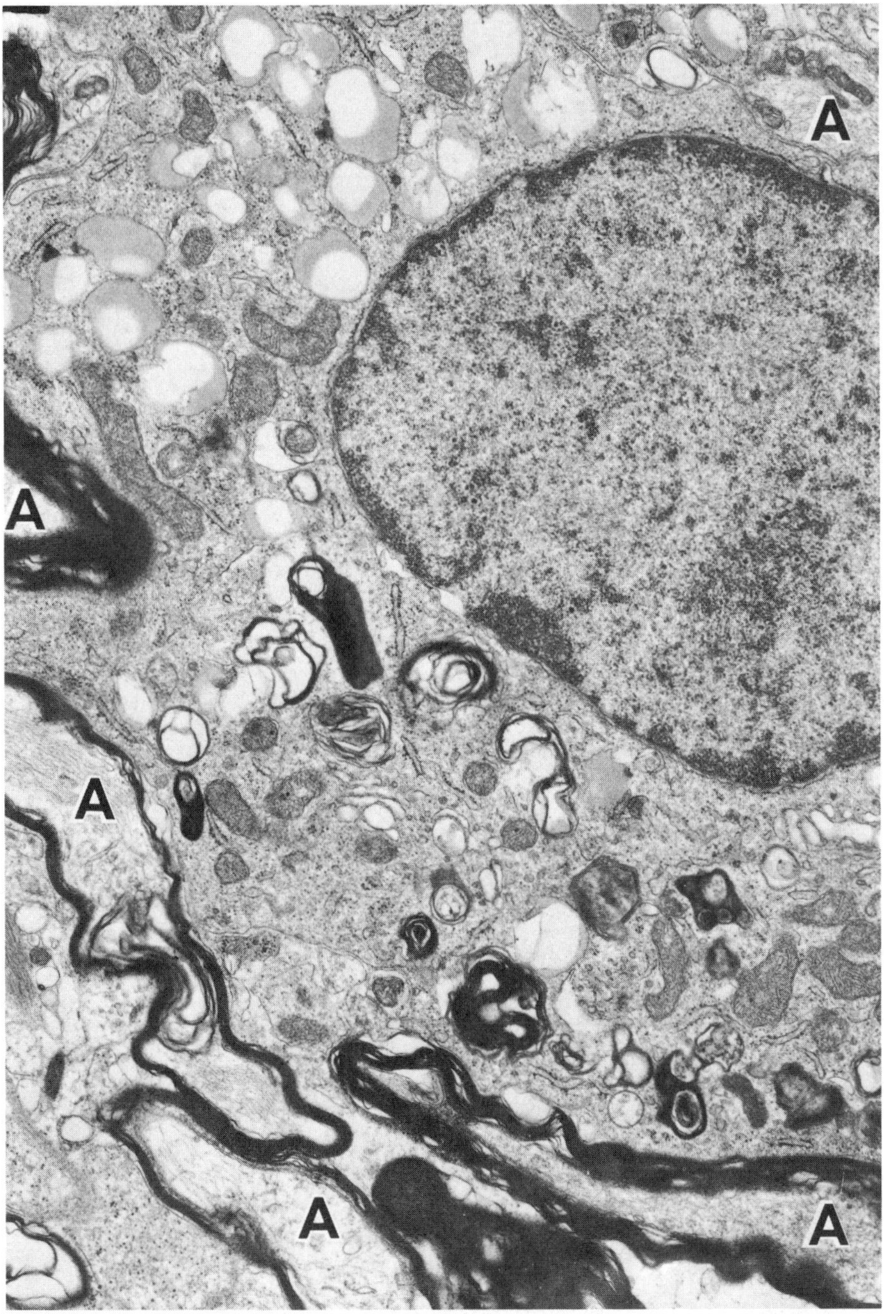

FIGURE 9. A macrophage containing myelin fragments invests normally myelinated, thinly myelinated, and demyelinated axons. *A* = axon. Case 5, ×14,000.

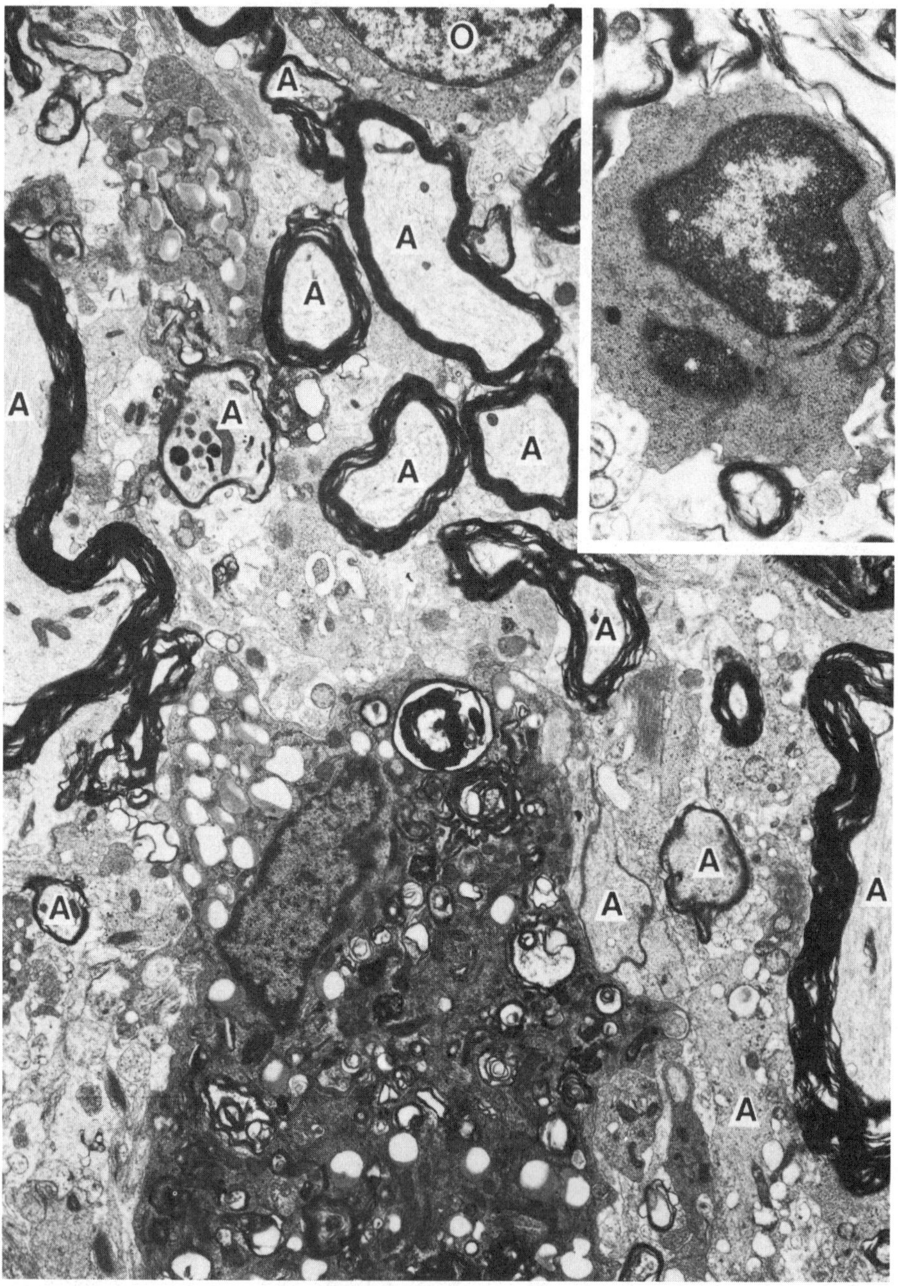

FIGURE 10. Normally myelinated, thinly myelinated, and demyelinated axons (*A*) are seen near a macrophage filled with myelin debris. A normal oligodendrocyte (*O*) is present. Inset shows a lymphocyte with sparse granular endoplasmic reticulum closely contacting normal myelinated nerve fibers. Case 5, ×7000. Inset ×12,000.

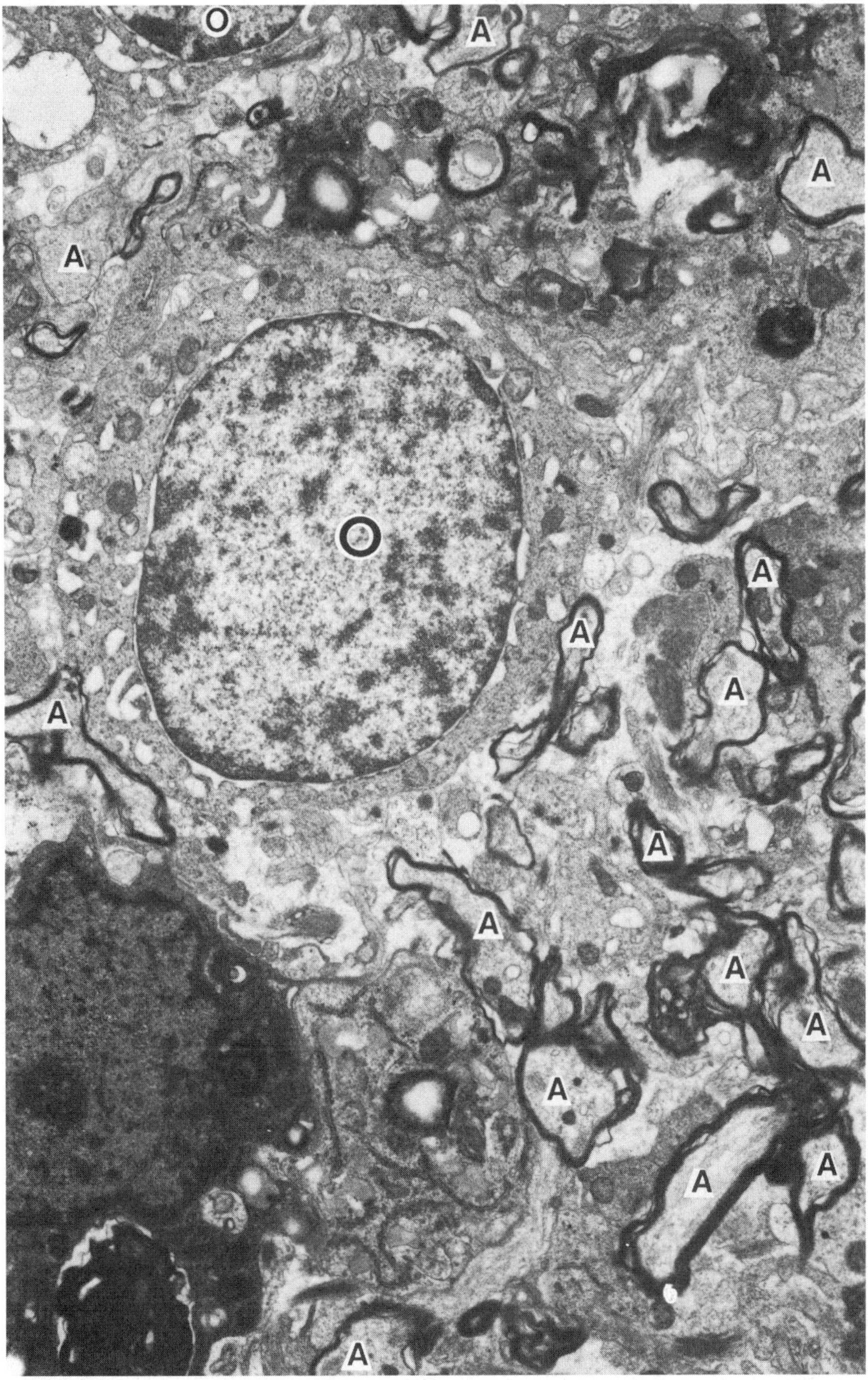

FIGURE 11. Two normal oligodendrocytes (*O*) can be seen in tissue infiltrated by macrophages containing myelin debris. Some myelin sheaths may be abnormally thin. *A* = axon. Case 5, ×10,000

endoplasmic reticulum in both the parenchyma and perivascular spaces in demyelinated tissue and in bordering white matter (FIGURE 10). In the latter situation they were observed intimately contacting both myelin sheaths and oligodendrocyte perikarya but no morphological changes were observed that correlated with their presence.

Because of the small size and random orientation of nerve fibers in the margins of these plaques, it was not possible to study a sufficient number of longitudinally sectioned thinly myelinated fibers to determine whether or not any were remyelinating fibers. Most appeared to be undergoing active demyelination.

An attempt was made to determine the relative numbers of the different types of cells in each of the zones just described. A 1 mm × 1 mm electron microscope section from a block trimmed from the edge of the plaque illustrated in FIGURE 5A was collected on a 200 mesh/inch grid and all nucleated cells present in 40 grid spaces extending on either side of the plaque margin were examined and photographed. The total area examined was 0.34 sq.mm (the grid spaces measured 0.093 mm × 0.093 mm and each was separated from its neighbor by a bar 0.035 mm wide). The results are shown in TABLE 1.

DISCUSSION

Demyelination

Earlier descriptions of degenerating myelin in multiple sclerosis refer to changes which, according to Greenfield,[7] are not too dissimilar to those seen in Wallerian degeneration, namely initial, irregular swelling of sheaths followed by fragmentation into particles and balls of myelin which are later phagocytosed by scavenging microglia. In the first electron microscope study of recent lesions obtained at autopsy from a multiple sclerosis patient, Lumsden[15] observed pronounced myelin changes (transformation of the sheath into extracellular vesicular and lamellar debris) in the absence of microglia and he concluded that this supported "... the current view that microglia play no role whatsoever in the pathogenesis of the disease, chiefly because there is no hint of preliminary activation in the tissue prior to myelin breakdown. ..." However more recent ultrastructural studies have failed to confirm this and the present evidence strongly favors an initiating role for macrophages in myelin destruction in multiple sclerosis. In an electron microscope study of 34 plaques from five multiple sclerosis patients, in two of whom improved fixation for electron microscopy was obtained by *in situ* perfusion with glutaraldehyde within 20 minutes of death, 12 lesions were examined which appeared to be active or recently active (plaques in which hypercellular white matter bordered demyelinated areas containing moderate to large numbers of lipid macrophages).[23] The myelin alterations observed electron microscopically in the margins of these lesions bore little resemblance to previous light microscope descriptions of myelin breakdown in multiple sclerosis. The most common change was the presence of abnormally thin myelin internodes in which superficial lamellae terminated prematurely along the length of the internode. This change, described previously in chronic lesions,[30] was restricted to areas infiltrated by cells of uncertain origin containing laminated inclusions and, on occasion, lipid droplets and myelin fragments. As these cells were commonly seen contacting the abnormal internodes, it was concluded that the myelin change was related in some way to the presence of these cells. The ultrastructure of these cells corresponded to later descriptions of normal microglia.[20]

The same picture—of focally attenuated myelin sheaths in contact with infiltrating

TABLE 1. Edge of an Active Mature Plaque. Numbers of Cells[a] and Myelin Morphology Determined Electron Microscopically in a Single 1 mm × 1 mm Section

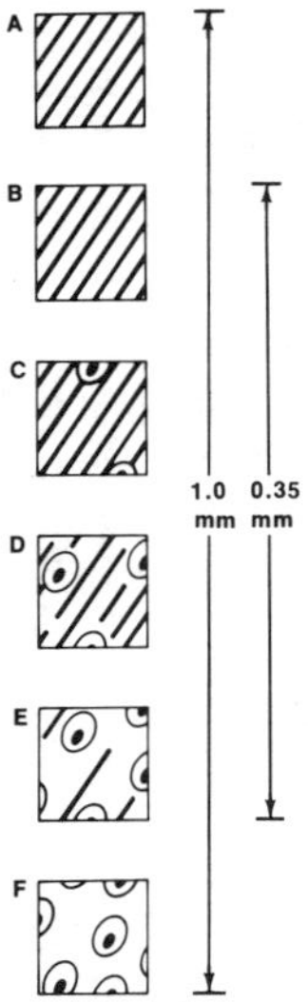

	Myelin Sheaths	Oligodendrocytes		Macrophages Containing Myelin Debris	Lymphocytes[b] PV Space	Lymphocytes[b] Parenchyma	Plasma Cells[c] PV Space	Plasma Cells[c] Parenchyma
Grid spaces[e] further than B from plaque (number examined = 5) (A)	normal	+++[f]	(2.4)[d]	0	0	±	0	0
Grid spaces immediately adjacent to C or D in which myelin debris was absent (number examined = 6) (B)	normal	+++	(2.8)	0	0	±	0	0
Grid spaces in which myelin debris was detected in presence of close to normal number of myelin sheaths (number examined = 11) (C)	normal	+++	(2.5)	+++	±	±	±	0
Grid spaces which had mild to moderate loss of myelin (number examined = 10) (D)	normal and abnormal	++	(1.5)	++++	0	±	0	0
Grid spaces immediately adjacent to C or D in which myelin was largely gone (number examined = 3) (E)	normal and abnormal	++	(1.5)	++++	0	±	±	0
Grid spaces in which there was no myelin (number examined = 5) (F)	absent	++	(1.2)	++++	0	0	0	0

[a]Only those cells in which a nucleus was seen were counted. Not all cells observed are shown in the table. Other cells present included astrocytes, some neurons, unidentified cells, and rare necrotic cells.

[b,c]In the total number of 40 grid spaces examined, 6 lymphocytes and 4 plasma cells were observed.

[d]Average number of oligodendrocytes/grid space.

[e]Each grid space measured 0.093 × 0.093 mm in area and was separated from its neighbor by a bar 0.035 mm wide.

[f]0 = 0; ± = <0.5; + = 0.5–1; ++ = 1–2; +++ = 2–3; ++++ = 3 < nucleated cells per grid space.

debris-containing microglia—was observed in a subsequent study of active lesions in a case of acute multiple sclerosis in which the total duration of the clinical illness was three months and where autopsy was carried out within three hours of death.[27] In this case, some infiltrating cells were also observed within myelin sheaths. Immunocytochemical studies of tissue from this case confirmed that extensive infiltration of white matter bordering active plaques by microglia (macrophages) preceded any detectable reduction in staining for myelin basic protein.[26]

In tissue fixed within a few minutes of death, it has been possible to show that myelin lamellae are removed directly from the surface of intact sheaths by an unusual type of phagoctyosis involving attachment of superficial lamellae to coated pits on the macrophage surface and their entry into the cell in the form of vermiform vesicles[24] (FIGURE 12). The entry of materials into cells which do not require initial binding to specific surface receptors occurs mainly via smooth-walled vesicles and larger vacuoles. In contrast, entry via coated pits, which are now recognized to be the major pathway for receptor-mediated endocytosis,[17] implies that macrophages engaged in myelin breakdown in multiple sclerosis have surface receptors that bind to a ligand present on the myelin surface (extracellular face of minor dense line). A similar mechanism of myelin destruction has now been observed in acute lesions in experimental allergic encephalomyelitis.[4,28] Whether the ligand is the same in the two conditions remains to be determined.

Another type of phagocytosis, namely that mediated by Fc receptors, has been implicated as a mechanism of myelin destruction in multiple sclerosis by the observation that macrophages engaged in myelin breakdown exhibit Fc receptors[16] and capping of surface IgG.[26] How this fits in with phagocytosis via coated pits is at present unknown.

The present findings and those reported in a recent study of tissue obtained at biopsy from the edge of an active lesion[29] further suggest that removal of myelin lamellae from the surface of compact myelin sheaths, resulting in local reduction in the thickness of the sheath, is the common pattern of myelin destruction in multiple sclerosis.

Two other major patterns of myelin breakdown have been described in multiple sclerosis, namely extracellular vesicular dissolution and splitting of myelin,[12–15, 22] and intramyelin edema with invasion of the swollen sheath by macrophages.[14] The former change is rare in tissue obtained at biopsy or soon after death and is probably caused by autolysis. It is most pronounced, however, in white matter close to plaques.[12]

Whereas plasma cells have often been seen in the parenchyma in multiple sclerosis plaques, the present study represents one of the few instances in which lymphocytes have been observed by light or electron microscopy outside perivascular spaces in multiple sclerosis tissue. In the one other morphological study in which lymphocytes have been identified in the parenchyma in an active multiple sclerosis lesion, Raine *et al.*[29] identified fewer than ten lymphocytes along a three millimeter length of active plaque margin. Though these authors found no relation between the area of myelin breakdown and infiltrating lymphocytes, in the present study rare lymphocytes were found amongst myelinated nerve fibers ahead of the zone of active myelin breakdown, which is in keeping with recent immunocytochemical data reported by Traugott *et al.*[31] No blast forms were seen, and, on the basis of their ultrastructure, the infiltrating lymphocytes observed in the present study could have been either B or T cells.

In the present study, no change in the fine structure or number of oligodendrocytes was detected in white matter beyond the zone infiltrated by macrophages. This, together with the fact that oligodendrocytes, although reduced in number, remained numerous in the zone of active myelin breakdown and in the demyelinated zone, support previous morphological evidence that myelin destruction in multiple sclerosis

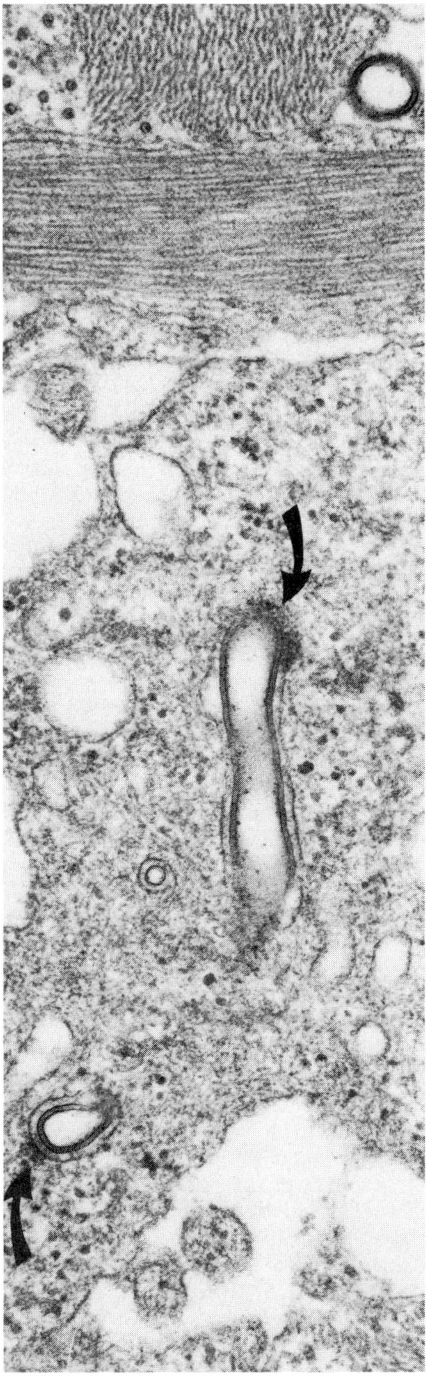

FIGURE 12. Myelin entering a macrophage in the form of "micropinocytosis vermiformis." The myelin lamellae are attached to coated pits, one cut tangentially (*arrows*) at the blind end of each tubular invagination of the macrophage plasma membrane. Multiple sclerosis, ×104,000.

is not secondary to oligodendrocyte loss.[24,29] The present electron microscope observations, however, contrast with previous light microscope studies that have suggested that oligodendrocytes are present in increased numbers at the edges of expanding lesions.[5,10,29]

Remyelination in Actively Demyelinating Lesions

Thinly myelinated nerve fibers may be observed in paraffin sections[3,11] and by electron microscopy[19,25,30] at the edges of old multiple sclerosis plaques that show little evidence of recent demyelinative activity. When such fibers are examined in longitudinal sections it is apparent that some are remyelinating fibers (fibers with uniformly thin, short internodes) whereas others exhibit focal thinning limited to the paranode or affecting longer stretches of the internode.[25,30] It is likely that the latter are partially demyelinated fibers ("partial thickness demyelination"[6,8]).

As noted in the present study and in a number of previous studies, thinly myelinated nerve fibers may also be seen at the edges of plaques considered to be active or recently active because of a short clinical illness,[12,27] or the presence of lipid macrophages or macrophages containing undigested myelin debris.[2,13,14,23,27,29] While some authors have regarded these as remyelinating fibers,[13,29] others have noted that many of these fibers exhibit nonuniform thinning and have suggested that they are degenerating or damaged fibers.[1,2,23,30] It is now known that some of these thinly myelinated fibers are fibers in the process of losing their myelin sheaths.[24,27,29] In others, this process appears to have been arrested, resulting in partially demyelinated fibers. Here we document the fact that when such lesions are sectioned to show whole myelin internodes, it is apparent that many of the thinly myelinated fibers present at the edges and in the demyelinated zone of actively demyelinating and recently active lesions are remyelinating internodes.

The occurrence of regenerating sheaths and myelin destruction in the same plaque raises new questions about plaque growth and also about the relationship of these two processes. It cannot be concluded, from the present results, that both processes necessarily proceed simultaneously in the sense that new myelin internodes are forming and increasing in thickness in regions of continuing breakdown; it may be that these processes recur at different intervals, or that they have an inverse relationship. Some conclusions, however, are possible on the basis of the present findings. Firstly, whether remyelination and demyelination occur together or at different times in the same plaque, the balance between these two processes will determine whether the plaque increases in size, remains the same size, or becomes smaller; secondly, it may be assumed that in some expanding lesions, possibly even in the majority, enlargement of the plaque involves destruction of both new and original myelin internodes at the plaque margin; thirdly, those shadow plaques that are composed of remyelinating nerve fibers represent lesions in which, for some unknown reason, extensive areas of damaged tissue retain remyelinative capacity. Perhaps the most likely possibility is preservation of some oligodendrocyte perikarya in acutely demyelinated areas.

Of the various sorts of shadow plaques that occur in multiple sclerosis, one group is distinguished by the presence of nerve fibers with myelin sheaths that stain less intensely than normal[7,15,21] and that appear thinner than normal.[7,13,18] Such lesions have been described with and without gliosis and with and without the presence of lipid macrophages.[7] Although it has been considered that these possibly represent remyelinating lesions,[13,15] usually they have been regarded as areas of incomplete myelin destruction.[7,15] The present findings indicate that some shadow plaques composed of thinly myelinated fibers are in fact regions of extensive remyelination, and that they may appear within ten months of the onset of clinical signs.

SUMMARY

Plaques with lipid macrophages and macrophages containing undigested myelin fragments from five multiple sclerosis patients were studied by light microscopy of epoxy-embedded tissue (five cases) and electron microscopy (one case). Cell counts determined electron microscopically revealed that oligodendrocytes were reduced in number in areas of commencing myelin breakdown. The major mechanism of myelin destruction was phagocytosis by macrophages of intact myelin sheaths in the presence of very small numbers of lymphocytes and plasma cells.

When plaques were orientated to allow examination of whole myelin internodes, it was found that most lesions, including lesions known to have been present for less than ten months, contained remyelinating internodes, sometimes in numbers large enough to form shadow plaques. It is concluded that the two processes of sometimes massive remyelination and active demyelination frequently coexist in "fatty" subacute plaques filled with lipid-containing macrophages, and that myelin breakdown at the edges of progressive lesions includes destruction of remyelinating internodes.

REFERENCES

1. ANDREWS, J. M. 1972. The ultrastructural neuropathology of multiple sclerosis. *In* Multiple Sclerosis. Immunology, Virology and Ultrastructure. F. Wolgram, G. W. Ellison, J. G. Stevens & J. M. Andrews, Eds.: 23–52. Academic Press. New York and London.
2. ANDREWS, J. M. & P. A. CANCILLA. 1973. Subacute demyelinating disease in an adult (diffuse-disseminated sclerosis). Electron microscopic findings. Bull. Los Angeles Neurol. Soc. **38:** 49–59.
3. DAWSON, J. W. 1916. The histology of multiple sclerosis. Trans. R. Soc. Edin. **L:** 517–740 (with plates). Reproduced by the Montreal Neurological Institute. Montreal, 1973.
4. EPSTEIN, L. G., J. W. PRINEAS & C. S. RAINE. 1983. Attachment of myelin to coated pits on macrophages in experimental allergic encephalomyelitis. J. Neurol. Sci. **61:** 341–348.
5. FRIEDE, R. L. 1961. Enzyme histochemical studies in multiple sclerosis. Arch. Neurol. (Chicago) **5:** 433–443.
6. GLEDHILL, R. F. & W. I. MCDONALD. 1977. Morphological characteristics of central demyelination and remyelination: A single-fiber study. Ann. Neurol. **1:** 552–560.
7. GREENFIELD, J. G. 1958. *In* Neuropathology. J. G. Greenfield, W. Blackwood, W. H. McMenemey, A. Meyer & R. M. Norman, Eds.: 441–474. Edward Arnold. London.
8. HARRISON, B. M., W. I. MCDONALD, J. OCHOA & G. D. OHLRICH. 1972. Paranodal demyelination in the central nervous system. J. Neurol. Sci. **16:** 489–494.
9. HILDEBRAND, C. & S. SKOGLUND. 1971. Histochemical studies of adult and developing feline spinal cord white matter. Acta Physiol. Scand. Suppl. **364:** 145–166.
10. IBRAHIM, M. Z. M. & C. W. M. ADAMS. 1963. The relationship between enzyme activity and neuroglia in plaques of multiple sclerosis. J. Neurol. Neurosurg. Psychiatry **26:** 101–110.
11. ITOYAMA, Y., H. DEF. WEBSTER, E. P. RICHARDSON, JR. & B. D. TRAPP. 1983. Schwann cell remyelination of demyelinated axons in spinal cord multiple sclerosis lesions. Ann. Neurol. **14:** 339–346.
12. KIRK, J. 1979. The fine structure of the CNS in multiple sclerosis. II. Vesicular demyelination in an acute case. Neuropath. Appl. Neurobiol. **5:** 289–294.
13. LASSMANN, H. 1983. Comparative Neuropathology of Chronic Experimental Allergic Encephalomyelitis and Multiple Sclerosis. Springer. Berlin, Heidelberg, New York, and Tokyo.

14. LASSMANN, H., H. BUDKA & G. SCHNABERTH. 1981. Inflammatory demyelinating polyradiculitis in a patient with multiple sclerosis. Arch. Neurol. **38**(2): 99–102.
15. LUMSDEN, C. E. 1970. The neuropathology of multiple sclerosis. *In* Handbook of Clinical Neurology. Multiple Sclerosis and Other Demyelinating Diseases, vol. 9. P. J. Vinken & G. W. Bruyn, Eds.: 217–309. North Holland. Amsterdam.
16. NYLAND, H., R. MATRE & S. MØRK. 1980. Fc receptors on microglial lipophages in multiple sclerosis. N. Engl. J. Med. **302:** 120–121.
17. PASTAN, I. H. & M. C. WILLINGHAM. 1981. Journey to the center of the cell: Role of the receptosome. Science **214:** 504–509.
18. PERIER, O. 1969. Electron microscopic observations on human demyelinating diseases. Int. Arch. Allergy **36:** 452–462.
19. PÉRIER, O. & A. GRÉGOIRE. 1965. Electron microscopic features of multiple sclerosis lesions. Brain **88:** 937–952.
20. PETERS, A., S. L. PALAY & H. DEF. WEBSTER. 1976. The Fine Structure of the Nervous System. The Neurons and Supporting Cells. W. B. Saunders. Philadelphia, London, and Toronto.
21. PETERS, G. 1968. Multiple sclerosis. *In* Pathology of the Nervous System, vol. 1. J. Minckler, Ed.: 821–843. McGraw-Hill Book Co. New York.
22. PRINEAS, J. 1972. Paramyxovirus-like particles associated with acute demyelination in chronic relapsing multiple sclerosis. Science **178:** 760–763.
23. PRINEAS, J. 1975. Pathology of the early lesion in multiple sclerosis. Hum. Pathol. **6:** 531–554.
24. PRINEAS, J. W. & F. CONNELL. 1978. The fine structure of chronically active multiple sclerosis plaques. Neurology **28**(9, Part 2): 68–75.
25. PRINEAS, J. W. & F. CONNELL. 1979. Remyelination in multiple sclerosis. Ann. Neurol. **5:** 22–31.
26. PRINEAS, J. W. & J. S. GRAHAM. 1981. Multiple sclerosis: Capping of surface immunoglobulin G on macrophages engaged in myelin breakdown. Ann. Neurol. **10:** 149–158.
27. PRINEAS, J. W. & C. S. RAINE. 1976. Electron microscopy and immunoperoxidase studies of early multiple sclerosis lesions. Neurology **26**(2): 29–32.
28. RAINE, C. S., L. B. BARNETT, A. BROWN, T. BEHAR & D. E. MCFARLIN. 1980. Neuropathology of experimental allergic encephalomyelitis in inbred strains of mice. Lab. Invest. **43:** 150–157.
29. RAINE, C. S, L. SCHEINBERG & J. M. WALTZ. 1981. Multiple sclerosis. Oligodendrocyte survival and proliferation in an active established lesion. Lab. Invest. **45**(6): 534–546.
30. SUZUKI, K.,J. M. ANDREWS, J. M. WALTZ & R. D. TERRY. 1969. Ultrastructural studies of multiple sclerosis. Lab. Invest. **20:** 444–454.
31. TRAUGOTT, U., E. L. REINHERZ & C. S. RAINE. 1983. Multiple sclerosis: Distribution of T cell subsets within active chronic lesions. Science **219:** 308–310.

Experimental Autoimmune Demyelination

Chronic Relapsing Models and Their Therapeutic Implications for Multiple Sclerosis[a]

CEDRIC S. RAINE AND UTE TRAUGOTT

Departments of Neuropathology, Neuroscience and Neurology
and
The Rose F. Kennedy Center for Research
in Mental Retardation and Human Development
Albert Einstein College of Medicine
Bronx, New York 10461

INTRODUCTION

Interpreted either against a backdrop of studies on the localization of immunologic components within the central nervous system (CNS) or against similarities to its major laboratory analogue, experimental allergic (autoimmune) encephalomyelitis (EAE), investigations on demyelinated multiple sclerosis (MS) plaques invariably invoke immune-mediated demyelination.[1-4] In some circles, the concept of a cell-mediated response within the CNS might seem antediluvian, having been implied for many years, but it has only been in the past two or three years that direct evidence for such a process has been documented. Indeed the major efforts of investigators have been targeted towards the elucidation of destructive events, and commonplace in the MS literature are references to studies purporting to contribute to the understanding of lesion pathogenesis. A notable omission from most treatises on the subject is consideration of CNS remyelination and its potential significance to MS. This is particularly significant in view of the fact that CNS remyelination[5-13] and oligodendroglial cell sparing[13,14] are now widely accepted phenomena occurring after a variety of primary demyelinating insults including EAE and MS. Therefore, since myelin regeneration and oligodendrocyte sparing are known to exist in MS, it is possible that CNS remyelination might be enhanced if lesion progression and/or the reported defects in immunoregulation could be abrogated. Although the latter have been major goals in MS research in the past, the concept of induced remyelination has rarely been discussed and some pioneer workers in the field even considered CNS demyelination to be an inexorable lesion.[1]

To approach the problem of CNS myelin regeneration with conventional acute EAE serves little purpose as most forms are monophasic and fatal.[15,16] However, in some species, like the rat, clinical recovery and remyelination do occur spontaneously.[8] The growing trend in the past decade towards the establishment of models of chronic relapsing EAE has yielded several that lend themselves to a wider spectrum of MS-related problems including the analysis of lesion development, myelin regeneration, and therapy.[17-24] Preeminent among the chronic relapsing autoimmune demyelinating disease models is a form first described as "chronic" by Stone and Lerner[25] and later revealed to have relapsing activity.[17,21,26] This model, induced in Strain 13 guinea

[a]This work was supported in part by NMSS grant no. RG 1001-D-4; and USPHS grant nos. NS 08952, NS 11920 and NS 07098.

pigs, possesses more features in common with MS than any other currently available.[4,27] However, although affording a broad platform for the analysis of demyelination and the testing of therapeutic protocols, it is sometimes hampered by the relative paucity of specific T cell subset markers in the guinea pig. This deficiency renders hazardous the precise monitoring of T cell events within the circulation and the target organ, the CNS, and represents a handicap with considerable import since EAE is a known T cell-mediated disease.[28] This is further substantiated from work on both chronic relapsing EAE and MS in which T cells have been shown *in situ* to be involved early in lesion formation.[29,30] However, the application of recently described forms of chronic relapsing EAE in the mouse,[22–24,31,32] a species for which there is available a large battery of phenotypically well-characterized T cell markers, might overcome some of the deficiencies of the Strain 13 guinea pig model.

The present report will outline briefly the contributions of the various models of chronic relapsing EAE in the guinea pig, rat and mouse to the understanding of the genesis of demyelinated CNS plaques, will document the frequency of CNS remyelination and will demonstrate, where appropriate, similarities to MS lesions. Furthermore, with the Strain 13 model we shall highlight its clinical applications to MS and show that with this model, clinical improvement can be achieved after treatment with a mixture of myelin components. Furthermore, this clinical amelioration correlates structurally in the CNS with an enhancement of remyelination.[33,34] These latter studies support the hypothesis that demyelination in MS might be the result of an autoimmune response to a combination of myelin components[35] and that the appropriate application of such components might have therapeutic value in the chronic progressive inflammatory demyelinating conditions.

MATERIALS AND METHODS

Strain 13 Model

For the induction of chronic relapsing EAE in Strain 13 guinea pigs (Strain 13N from NIH), juvenile males with body weights less than 250 g are given a single inoculation in the nuchal area with an emulsion of syngeneic spinal cord in complete Freund's adjuvant (CFA), according to previously published techniques.[17] Animals thus sensitized develop signs 1–3 months postinoculation (PI) that invariably remit and after which clinical relapses occur at irregular intervals up to more than 36 months PI.

Hartley Strain Model

For the induction of chronic relapsing EAE in Hartley Strain guinea pigs, a similar protocol is used except that animals are inoculated into the dorsum of each hind foot.[20] About 30% of animals thus injected go on to develop a chronic relapsing course, the remaining 70% succumbing to a hyperacute EAE in the first month PI.

Strain 2 Model

Chronic relapsing EAE in Strain 2 guinea pigs is induced by the injection of syngeneic spinal cord in CFA in the nuchal area,[36] a protocol similar to that employed in the Strain 13 model. It has previously been reported that 25% of injected Strain 2 females develop clinically apparent chronic relapsing EAE, whereas 75% of females and all males fail to display signs.

Lewis and Sprague-Dawley Rat Models

Chronic relapsing EAE can be induced in the Lewis or Sprague-Dawley rat[18,19] by a single inoculation in the hind footpads with guinea pig myelin basic protein or spinal cord in CFA, respectively. Some inoculated animals develop a sometimes fatal acute EAE 10–20 days PI. In survivors, a single second episode of clinical worsening follows thereafter between 20 and 70 days PI but this bout is mild and does not compare well with relapses in guinea pigs. More than one bout is not described.

SJL/J Mouse Models

Chronic relapsing EAE is induced in the mouse either by active sensitization or by adoptive transfer in eight-week-old female SJL/J mice. For chronic relapsing EAE induced by active sensitization, mice for the present review were given subcutaneous injections of syngeneic spinal cord homogenate in CFA on two occasions one week apart, according to previously published procedures.[23,24] Pertussis vaccine, a prerequisite in a similar model,[22] was not involved. Mice thus sensitized invariably develop clinical signs of EAE 14–21 days PI, recover from the initial episode, and go on to display several relapses over 6–12 months. For adoptively transferred chronic relapsing EAE,[31,32] donor animals are sensitized with rat or mouse myelin basic protein (MBP) in CFA[37] and, after signs are manifest, lymph node cells are removed and cultured for 4 days in RPMI 1640 medium (GIBCO) containing 100 μg/ml rat MBP. Recipient animals are given either 3×10^7 or 6×10^7 cells into a tail vein. Clinical disease is usually evident 7–10 days PI and long-term maintained animals display remissions and relapses.

Therapeutic Studies

To date, only the form of chronic relapsing EAE in the Strain 13 guinea pig has been applied to any great extent to therapeutic studies. These investigations have either involved the suppression of the disease before signs developed using a course of intramuscular injections containing myelin basic protein in incomplete Freund's adjuvant (IFA),[38,39] or the treatment of the condition after several relapses had been documented.[33,34] For treatment, injections contained either MBP alone in IFA or MBP plus galactocerebroside (GC). Fuller details are given elsewhere.[33,34]

RESULTS

Guinea Pig Models

During the latent period preceding the onset of overt clinical signs in Strain 13 juvenile guinea pigs inoculated for chronic relapsing EAE, a period of transient weakness is often observed, a manifestation accompanied morphologically by the presence of inflammatory changes and small foci of subpial demyelination in the lumbar spinal cord.[17] Inflammatory infiltrates consist initially of small mononuclear cells that are gradually replaced by large mononuclear cells as lesions enlarge. By the time overt neurological signs are manifest (8–12 weeks PI), large CNS plaques of varying disease activity can be seen, sometimes on gross examination, randomly scattered throughout the spinal cord and cerebral white matter.[17,19,26,27,40] The majority of these lesions can be classed as chronic progressive and are composed of a demyelinated, gliotic center with margins displaying inflammation and active phagocytosis (FIGURE 1). Other lesions can be identified that are chronic silent, being either chronically demyelinated (but noninflammatory) or largely remyelinated. Not infrequently, some are seen that are acutely demyelinating with dense, recent infiltrates and scattered demyelinated axons but little gliosis. When animals are sampled soon after a relapse, areas of chronic demyelination can be seen that contain superimposed episodes of recent inflammatory activity around vessels that previously displayed fibrotic changes within the Virchow-Robin space (FIGURE 2). In all cases where disease activity subsides and where the extent of the lesion is not widespread, CNS remyelination is common (FIGURE 3). This remyelination is most apparent along the perimeter of large lesions and not infrequently is accompanied by a moderate increase in the number of oligodendrocytes. On some occasions, demyelinated CNS axons become myelinated by Schwann cells that invade the CNS from root entry zones.

Myelin breakdown in the Strain 13 model is similar to that observed in acute EAE[17,41] and involves dissolution of myelin lamellae in the vicinity of mononuclear cells (FIGURE 4), the uptake of myelin debris either as lamellar aggregates or by a stripping process, and the degradation of phagocytosed material into lamellar stacks and, eventually, neutral lipid droplets. Commonly seen, but only recently appreciated since its observation in active MS lesions,[42] is a process of myelin uptake by macrophages in

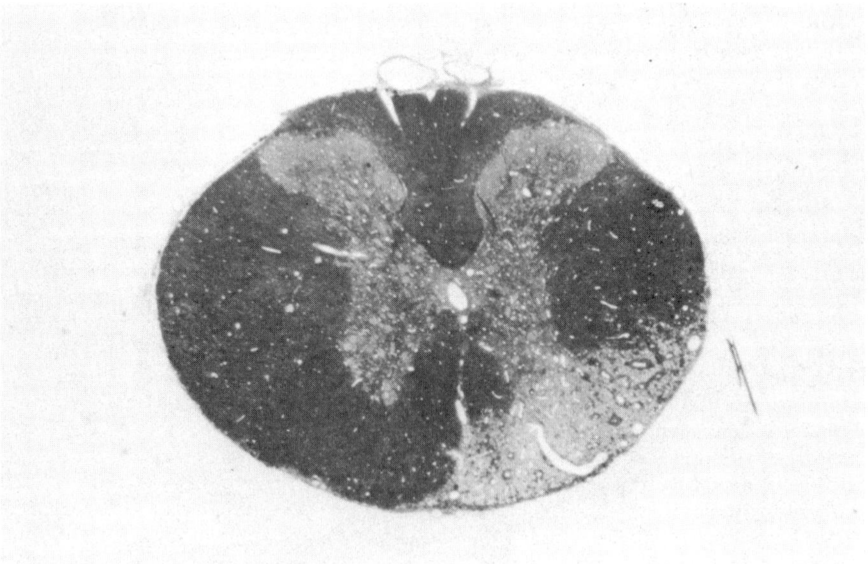

FIGURE 1. Strain 13 chronic relapsing EAE, 20 weeks PI. An anterior column of the spinal cord at L6 contains a large demyelinated lesion of the chronic progressive type, extending inwards from the meningeal surface (*below*). Around the margins of the plaque, perivascular cuffing is apparent. One micron, toluidine blue-stained, epoxy section. Magnification: ×22.

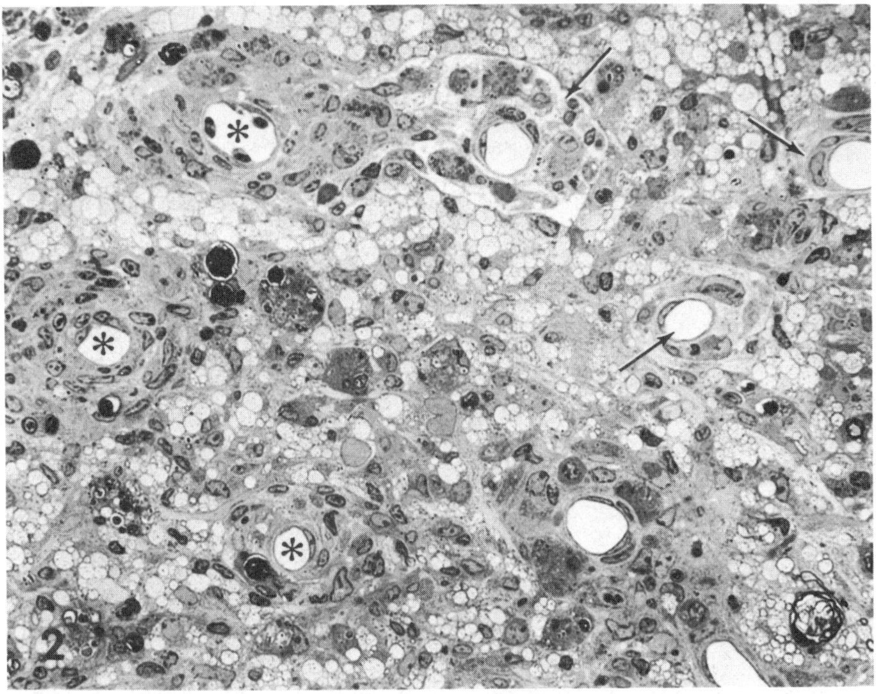

FIGURE 2. Strain 13 chronic relapsing EAE, 24 weeks PI. Detail from a spinal cord plaque, taken from an animal shortly after a clinically documented relapse, shows a gliotic CNS background matrix containing many chronically demyelinated axons among which blood vessels are seen. Some vessels (*) display active inflammatory activity while others (*arrows*) display vascular fibrosis. Magnification: ×400.

EAE that involves the attachment of small lamellar droplets to coated pits on the surface of the macrophage and the uptake of these droplets into the cell body (FIGURE 5). This process results in membranous channels at the bases of which myelin debris can be detected. Described recently in rabbit acute EAE,[43] this mechanism has also been seen previously in EAE in the guinea pig and mouse.[36,44] Though very common in autoimmune demyelinating states, it is not specific for them and is also seen during virus-induced demyelination.[45]

The pathology of lesions in Hartley Strain guinea pigs with chronic relapsing EAE contrasts markedly with that of Strain 13 animals in that hemorrhage and polymorphonuclear leukocyte (PMN) infiltration are not unusual.[20,46] These features are consistent with more severe damage to the blood-brain barrier than the Strain 13 model and a picture reminiscent of hyperacute EAE. It also may explain why the lesions are often more readily detectable macroscopically than they are in the Strain 13 model (FIGURE 6). Myelin degradation is similar to that described in other animal models of EAE and variable amounts of axonal damage are encountered. Other parameters are similar to the Strain 13 model[17] except that by 12 months PI, the disease process in Hartley guinea pigs is invariably burnt out, after which lesion progression is not seen.

Chronic relapsing EAE in Strain 2 guinea pigs compares favorably with the Strain

13 model in the small percentage (25%) of females who are clinically susceptible. However, chronic lesions are demonstrable at the microscopic level in all inoculated animals (male and female), irrespective of clinical picture.[36] The majority of these lesions were of the chronic, silent type and displayed remyelinative changes (see FIGURE 3). Thus, the concept of resistance to EAE by Strain 2 remains only a clinical phenomenon in that, at the level of the target organ, disease is always demonstrable.

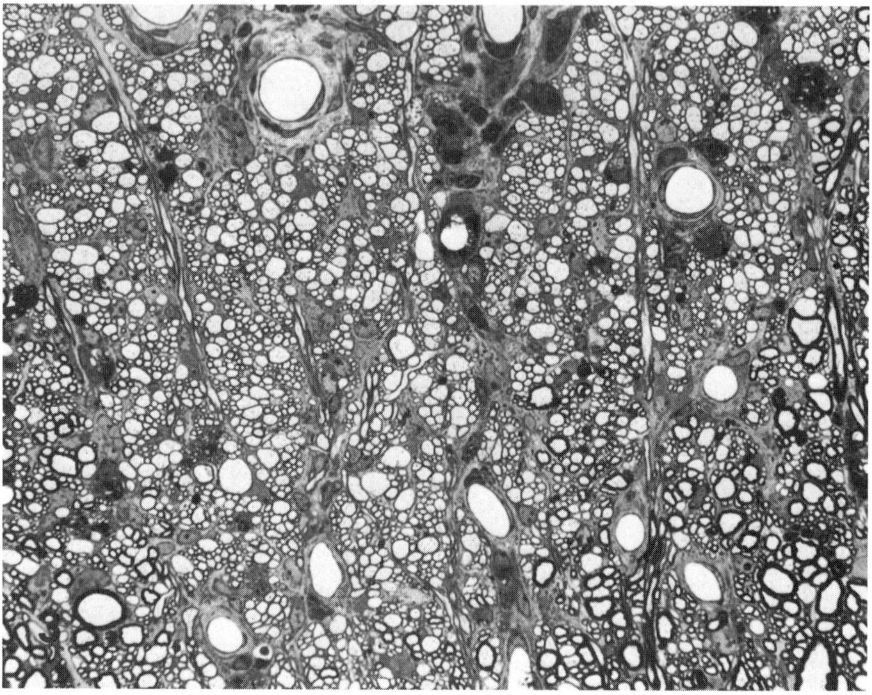

FIGURE 3. A subpial lesion from a Strain 13 guinea pig displays nerve fibers most of which have been uniformly, thinly remyelinated. A few macrophages and some background gliosis are apparent. Magnification: ×400.

Immunologic Studies

Detailed immunocytochemical examination of inflammatory events during autoimmune demyelination[29,47,48] has only been performed on the Strain 13 model and has revealed that prior to the period of clinical signs and frank demyelination, T cells enter the CNS (after about five days PI) and migrate to the white matter parenchyma. A little later, just before signs are manifest in the acute disease (in adults, 10–11 days PI), B cells and IgG-bearing macrophages enter the CNS. Unlike T cells, B cells and macrophages remain mainly in perivascular locations except where more extensive damage to the vasculature is noted. These events *in situ* are mirrored somewhat by results from studies on circulating T cell subpopulations in EAE that display increases prior to signs and decreases as signs develop.[40,49] Studies on infiltrating cells isolated from the CNS of affected animals have confirmed that T cell migration to the CNS correlates with clinical worsening.[50]

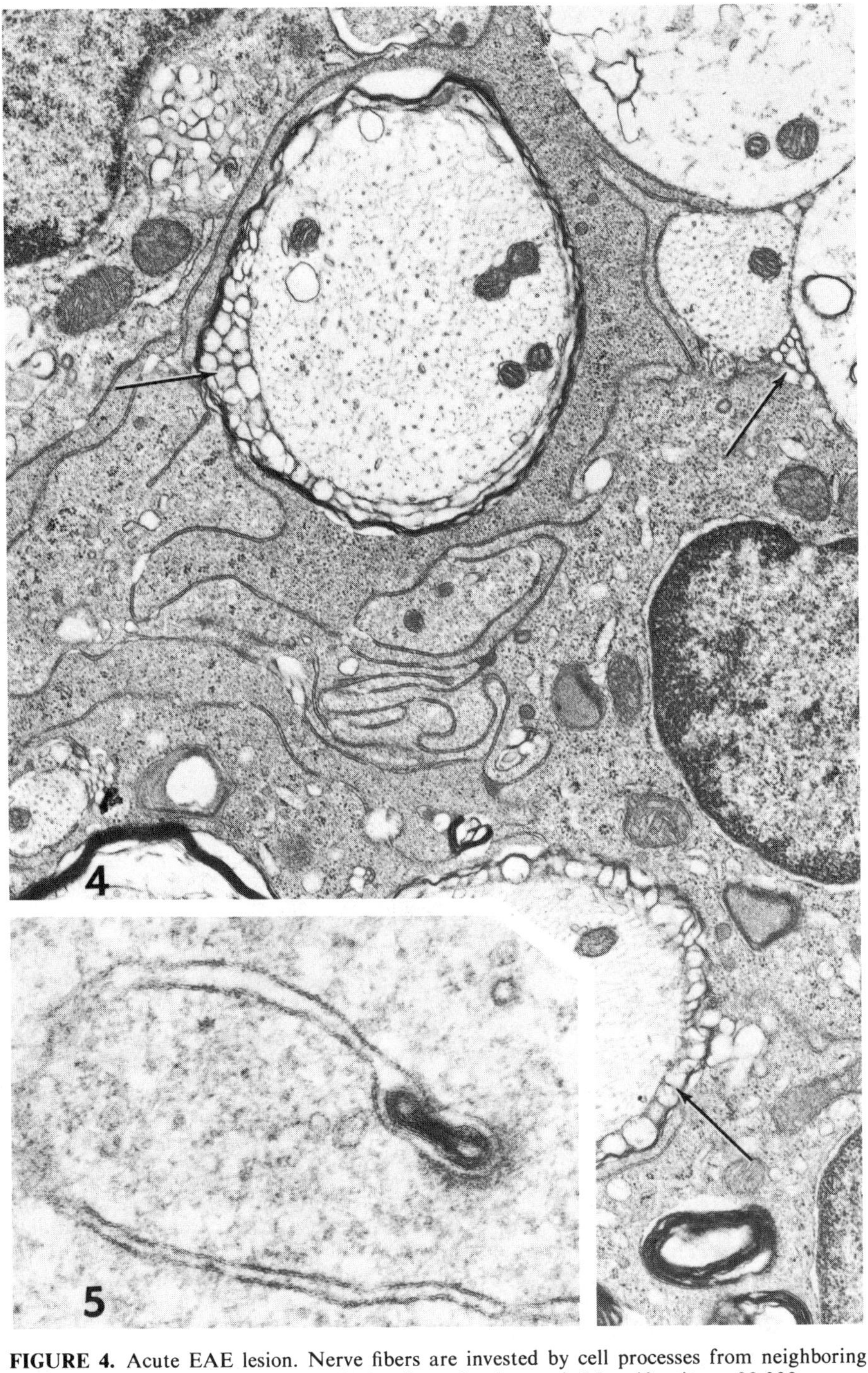

FIGURE 4. Acute EAE lesion. Nerve fibers are invested by cell processes from neighboring macrophages and myelin displays vesicular disruption (*arrows*). Magnification: ×20,000.

FIGURE 5. A droplet of myelin debris lies at the base of a crypt formed from the surface of a macrophage and is closely associated with a coated pit, an appearance interpreted as being representative of receptor-mediated phagocytosis. Magnification: ×80,000.

In the circulation of chronic relapsing EAE animals, decreases are seen in the level of active T cells[38,39] that increase during remissions. As chronic CNS lesions develop in Strain 13 guinea pigs, there is initially an abundance of T cells and B cells and these decrease with time as lesions become established. Macrophages become concentrated towards the lesion edge, and within the CNS of animals in remission, only occasional T cells can be located. Corresponding to the onset of clinical relapses are fresh waves of T cells and a few B cells in lesion areas.[51]

While a primary causative role for the major encephalitogen of CNS myelin, MBP, is well-known in EAE, its precise role in the establishment of demyelinated lesions in the guinea pig has recently been investigated.[52] This facet of autoimmune demyelination was reexamined in studies *in vivo* in the guinea pig[52] *in vitro* using myelinated CNS cultures,[53] and in the myelinated retina of the rabbit eye.[54] Myelinated cultures have been applied to the examination of immune-mediated demyelination for many years (see refs. 6 and 55) and to the rabbit retina since the work of Wray *et al.*[56] The

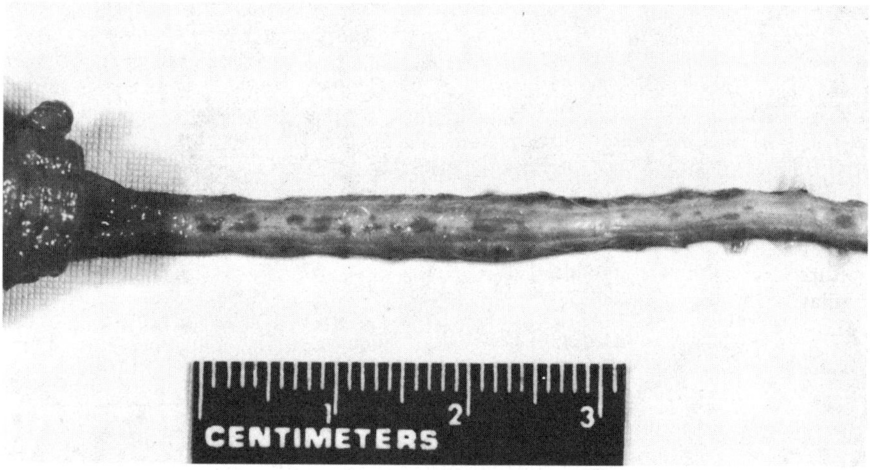

FIGURE 6. Hartley Strain chronic relapsing EAE. A macroscopic picture of the spinal cord of an animal sensitized 12 weeks earlier. Note the numerous punctate areas of demyelination. Figure taken from ongoing work in collaboration with Dr. William Lyman.

net conclusions of our three approaches[52–54] were that MBP was necessary in EAE for T cell recruitment to the CNS whereas a myelin lipid hapten, *e.g.*, galactocerebroside (GC), caused an accompanying B cell response only in the presence of which was extensive demyelination produced. Antibody to MBP had no apparent effect on CNS myelin whereas anti-GC has been shown by several studies in addition to our own to have strong demyelinative properties. More recent studies[57] have documented a similar augmenting role of other myelin lipids on the encephalitogenic effect of MBP in guinea pigs. In summary, the combined effect of MBP plus a myelin lipid is necessary for demyelination in the guinea pig with MBP eliciting a T cell and the lipid, a demyelinating B cell response.

The enhancement of autoimmune CNS demyelination by antibody to a lipid hapten has thus far only been demonstrated in the guinea pig. In some species (*e.g.*, mouse and monkey), it has been demonstrated that both inflammation and demyelination occur after sensitization with MBP alone,[31,32,52] a consequence possibly of a more extensive damage to the blood-brain barrier during EAE in these species. For example, mouse and monkey EAE lesions are typified by extravasation of circulating elements, hemorrhage and PMNs,[44,59] rare features in guinea pig EAE.

Mouse Models

Chronic relapsing EAE in the SJL mouse is somewhat less spectacular than in the Strain 13 guinea pig since lesions are usually less extensive, limited in extent, and display a significantly greater amount of axonal pathology and depletion. Actively induced chronic relapsing EAE in the mouse, induced by two sets of injections of spinal cord in CFA in the absence of pertussis,[23,24] begins as an acute disease some 14–21 days PI, during which the CNS (subpial spinal cord, paraventricular white matter, cerebellar white matter) is heavily infiltrated by waves of hematogenous elements. This infiltration begins with small lymphocytes, hemorrhage, and PMNs and is followed by successive waves of large mononuclear cells that become involved in nerve fiber phagocytosis. Later, plasma cells are seen in increasing numbers. As the initial acute episode subsides, CNS lesions undergo fibrillary astrogliosis and although naked (demyelinated) axons persist, it is apparent that many have been lost during the initial immunologic assault upon the tissue (FIGURES 7–9). Subsequent episodes of disease can usually be matched by recurrent inflammation. Remyelination is a common component of chronic lesions. Particularly noticeable in the mouse model is a predilection for involvement of spinal nerve root entry zones.[24]

Adoptively transferred chronic relapsing EAE in the mouse,[31,32] induced after a single transfer of lymph node cells from MBP-sensitized SJL/J mice (subsequently cultured for four days *in vitro* and given a boost of guinea pig or mouse MBP) has more similarities to the guinea pig model than has actively induced chronic relapsing EAE in the mouse in that axonal pathology is less marked. Nevertheless, lesions are small and still display PMN invasion, features typical of neither the Strain 13 model nor of MS.

Suppression Experiments

Manipulation of the course of chronic relapsing EAE has involved experiments on the Strain 13 model where the disease was suppressed before clinical onset with a course of intramuscular injections containing MBP in IFA.[27,38–40] In our own studies on animals in which the disease was suppressed with MBP, clinical signs failed to develop and although some changes were noted in the CNS of long-term suppressed animals, they were relatively minor, noninflammatory and largely reparatory. The latter suggested that the suppressive regimen had not completely prevented cellular invasion of the CNS but that further development of lesions had been prevented and therefore, lesion repair was possible.

Treatment Experiments

A situation more analogous to that in MS has been the protocol followed in recent experiments on the treatment of chronic relapsing EAE[33,34] where manipulation was commenced after animals had shown evidence of several clinical relapses. These treatment experiments involved the comparison of the effect of intramuscular injections of MBP alone in IFA with that of injections containing MBP plus GC in IFA

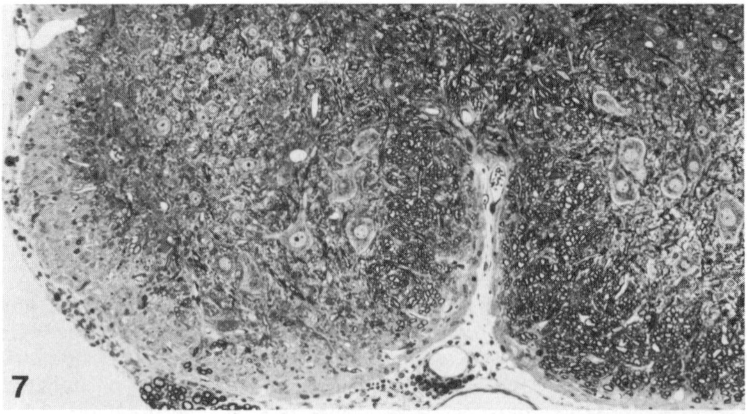

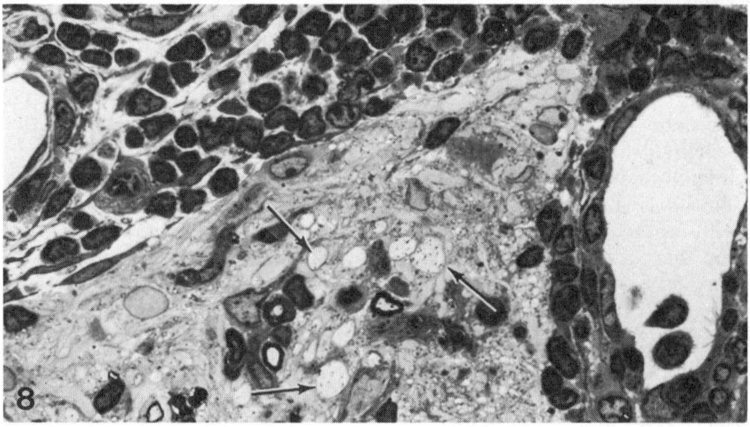

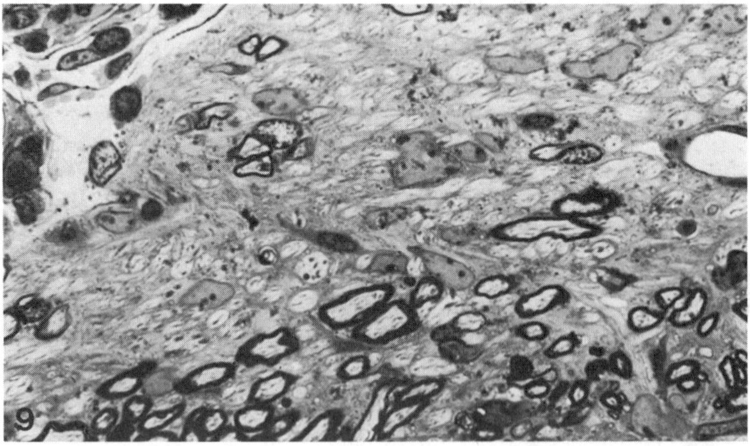

FIGURE 7. SJL mouse chronic relapsing EAE by active sensitization, 7 months PI. Note the broad rim of subpial demyelination (*left*) and the residual inflammatory activity within the meningeal space over the spinal cord. FIGURES 7–9 are taken from collaborative work with Dr. Dale E. McFarlin. Magnification: ×120.

FIGURE 8. SJL mouse chronic relapsing EAE. A portion of spinal cord from an animal sampled shortly after a relapse. Note the active inflammatory response and the scattered, somewhat depleted, demyelinated axons (*arrows*). Magnification: ×750.

FIGURE 9. In this area of mouse spinal cord demyelination is apparent and most axons are preserved (*above*). Magnification: ×750.

upon the course of the disease.[33,34,51] MBP/IFA treatment was found to cause some clinical improvement (usually for 4–12 months) that was visualized morphologically by lesions lacking extensive inflammation and displaying perhaps a greater degree of remyelination than that seen in untreated animals. The clinical improvement after MBP/IFA treatment was usually short-lived, and by 6–12 months after treatment commenced, clinical relapses were once more apparent.[33] These relapses could be

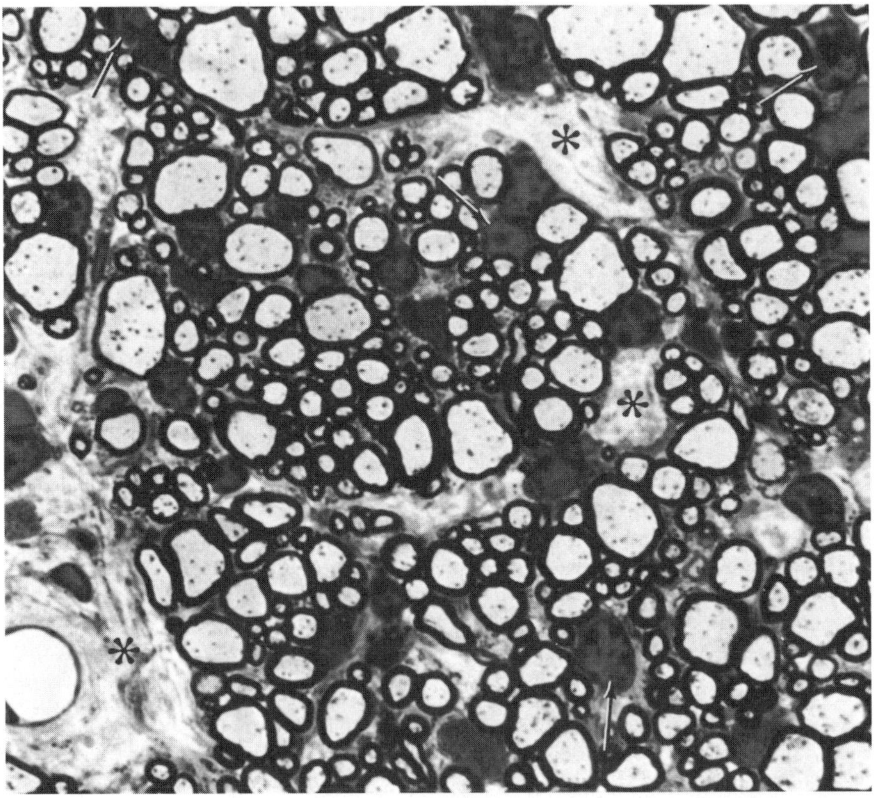

FIGURE 10. Strain 13 chronic relapsing EAE, 27 months PI after 3 months of treatment with MBP/GC in IFA during which time marked clinical improvement was noted. Note widespread remyelination and unusually large numbers of densely staining interfascicular oligodendroglia (*arrows*). Some parenchymal collagen deposition and vascular fibrosis is present (∗). Magnification: ×1,000.

matched morphologically by the presence of fresh perivascular infiltrates within the CNS.

In contrast to the MBP/IFA group, animals treated with MBP/GC/IFA demonstrated a more dramatic clinical improvement that has proven long-lasting. The CNS of MBP/GC-treated animals has demonstrated widespread proliferation of oligodendrocytes and extensive remyelination in previously affected areas (FIGURE 10). Inflammatory cells were absent from perivascular spaces and by immunofluorescence, only an occasional T cell could be seen.[51,60] Tg cell (suppressor) levels were elevated for longer periods in MBP/GC-treated animals than after treatment with MBP alone and there was an increase in the level of anti-GC antibody. Ultrastructural examination revealed that many oligodendrocytes contained centrioles, evidence for recent or impending mitosis, and were connected to the myelin sheaths of remyelinated fibers (FIGURE 11). Mitotic figures in oligodendrocytes and connections with myelin sheaths are never seen in the normal adult CNS. The observed remyelination after MBP/GC treatment had occurred against a background of fibrous astrogliosis and parenchymal deposition of collagen, features not usually conducive to CNS repair.

DISCUSSION

With the proliferation in recent years of different models of chronic relapsing EAE, it has become necessary for investigators to recognize within each model those features which are reminiscent of MS, those which bear promise for future MS research, and those which distinguish one model from another. Although all models are in some way applicable to MS, no two are identical and none is ideal, *i.e.,* satisfies all the criteria. Thus, the repertoire of chronic relapsing EAE models available to the experimentalist can be summarized as follows: (a) one inbred guinea pig model, Strain 13,[17,21,25,26] with striking clinical and pathologic similarities to MS, disease activity throughout life, well tested immunologically and therapeutically, but with a limited battery of immunologic probes; (b) one inbred guinea pig model, Strain 2,[36] which has most potential for investigations on clinically silent demyelination and possible disparities between clinical manifestations and CNS damage; (c) one outbred guinea pig model, Hartley Strain,[20] that has a more severe acute course, high mortality, large CNS lesions, and frequent relapses but a duration of about 12 months only; (d) two rat models (one inbred) which display small lesions and a single relapse[18,19] but which may have some applications since a large battery of immunologic probes exists for the rat; (e) two inbred mouse models (SJL Strain), induced by active sensitization, one of which requires boosting with pertussis vaccine,[22] one that requires double sensitization but no pertussis[23,24] and both displaying more severe, acute pathology than MS, smaller lesions, good relapses, and an available, veritable fusillade of well-tested immunologic probes; and finally, still in its infancy, (f) one adoptively transferred model in the SJL mouse[31,32] that lays to rest discussions on relapses being attributable to antigenic depôts and that promises much for finer dissection of cellular events in this disease. The respective properties of the various models are summarized in TABLE 1 and show that although none can approach the longevity of MS, the Strain 13 model has most points of similarity. The low mortality, clinical course, immunologic patterns, genetic predisposition, large lesions and profound sparing of axons are key points of similarity and have been the basis for this model being the most heavily applied to therapeutic investigations relevant to MS.[4,51]

A major question in MS and its various autoimmune laboratory analogues is that, assuming that initial sensitization (a putative virus in MS, CNS myelin in EAE) occurs peripherally, what causes cells to cross the CNS barrier and trigger the cascade of events leading the plaque formation? To satisfy current immunologic dogma one would have to invoke class II MHC antigens, helper T cells and the concomitant network. However, to demonstrate this *in situ* represents a task of mammoth proportions. One might speculate perhaps that the lesion begins at the CNS endothelium where, because of some antecedent sensitizing event against myelin or an agent, antigen is presented. This is then recognized by the appropriately sensitized T helper

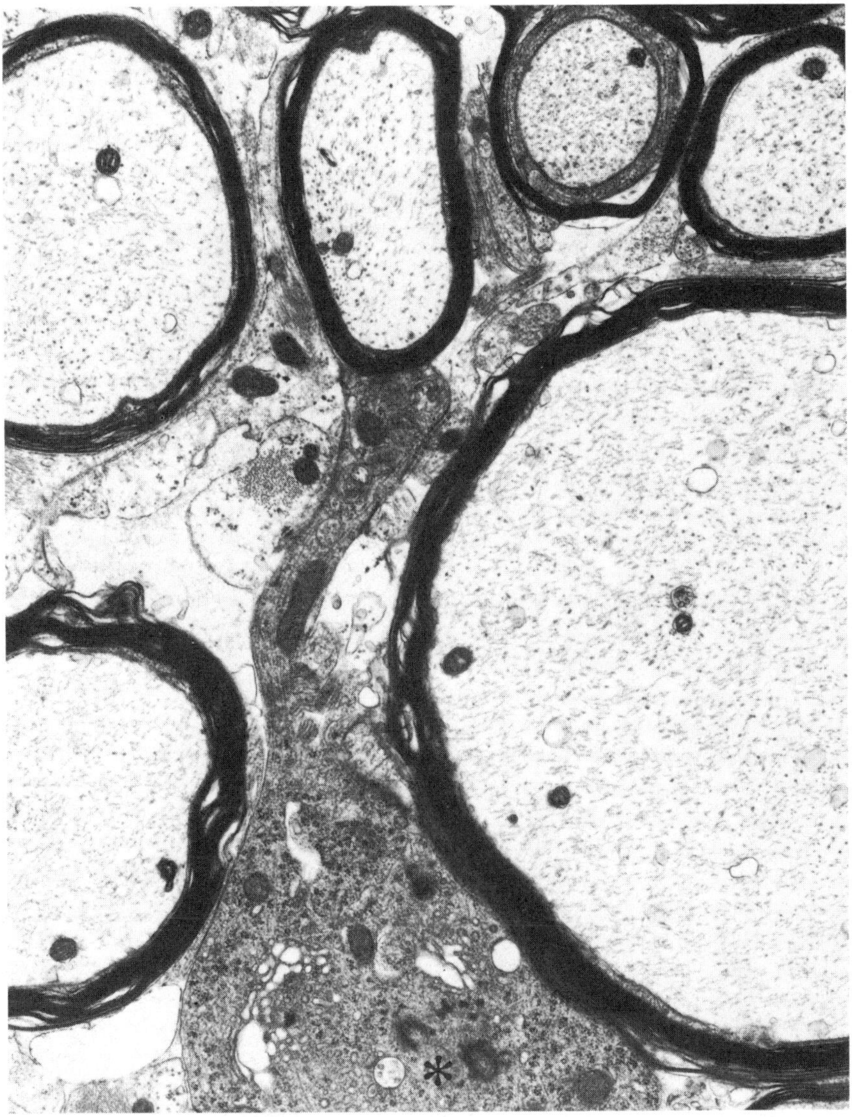

FIGURE 11. Same animal as FIGURE 10. Ultrastructural appearance of an oligodendrocyte close to mitosis (centrioles at *) which is connected to a remyelinated fiber by a cell process. Other CNS remyelinated fibers are also seen. Magnification: ×20,000.

TABLE 1. Comparative Pathology of MS and Chronic Relapsing EAE in the Guinea Pig and Mouse

	Multiple Sclerosis	Strain 13 Guinea Pig	Strain 2 Guinea Pig	Hartley Strain Guinea Pig	SJL/J Mouse (active)	SJL/J Mouse (passive)
Duration (years)	20–40	2–4	2–3	0.5–1	0.5–1	0.5–1
Genetic predisposition	+	+	+	+	+	+
Subclinical disease	+	+	+	–	–	–
Age and sex dependency	+	+	+	+	+	+
Mortality (%)	<10	<25	<10	70	<25	<10
Macroscopic lesions	+	+	–	+	–	–
Axonal sparing	±	+	+	+	±	±
Oligodendrocyte sparing	±	±	+	±	±	±
Remyelination	+	+	+	+	+	+
Circulating T cell changes	+	+	ND	ND	ND	ND
T cells in CNS	+	+	ND	ND	+	ND
Autoimmunity to myelin antigens	+	+	ND	+	ND	ND
Oligoclonal bands in CSF	+	+	ND	+	ND	ND
IgG synthesis in CNS	+	+	ND	+	+	ND

cell and the chain of events leading up to B cell stimulation is initiated. No direct evidence for such a mechanism exists in MS or any of its analogues but the observations of Ia-bearing endothelial cells around the perimeter of active chronic MS lesions[61] and Ia-positive macrophages closely associated in adjacent normal white matter with T cells smack strongly of antigen presentation *in situ*. Obviously, in the absence of the simultaneous demonstration of antigen, these observations should remain speculative but might perhaps channel attention to the endothelial cell surface which has been known for some time from *in vitro* studies to be capable of expressing Ia antigen.[62]

From the standpoint of lesion pathogenesis, there is unequivocal evidence that T cells play a cardinal role in both acute and chronic relapsing EAE lesions and are the first elements to enter the tissue as an attack becomes imminent.[47,48] With the Strain 13 guinea pig model and the presently available markers, it is impossible to define precisely which subset of T cells is involved in the CNS damage but indirect evidence from the mouse models based on adoptive transfer techniques[37,63] and preliminary results on CNS lesions *in situ*[64,65] imply a role for Lyt-1^+2^- cells. However, since the Lyt-1^+2^- subset is mixed and consists both of helper and DTH populations (among others), further dissection will be needed before conclusive, functional claims can be made.

Although T cell involvement has rarely been disputed in EAE, a central role for antibody has traditionally been a bone of contention. The latter has its roots in the phenomenon of serum-induced demyelination *in vitro*[55] and anti-GC antibody-induced demyelination *in vivo*.[66,67] It has now become apparent from our own investigations[52–54] that in addition to MBP sensitization, an antibody response to a myelin lipid is necessary for CNS demyelination in the guinea pig. Antibody involvement in EAE has also received support from experiments in rats on μ-suppression which led to the prevention of EAE.[68,69] Thus, the work on the causative roles of MBP and GC in EAE in the guinea pig, in CNS cultures and in the rabbit eye model[52–54] appears to indicate that autoimmune demyelination is the result of an antibody dependent cell-mediated cytotoxic type of reaction to two different myelin components—one (MBP) sensitizing the T cell arm of the immune response to recruit cells to the CNS, the other (GC), the B cell arm to induce demyelination. This concept fits in well with MBP suppression of EAE in which the T cell response is suppressed prior to signs, cells fail to migrate to the CNS and lesions do not develop. The unsuccessful outcome of MBP treatment of Strain 13 chronic relapsing EAE (which commences after signs and lesions are established) might reflect an inability of MBP alone to abrogate the ongoing complex immunologic cascade. On the other hand, it appears that our double-barreled treatment with MBP in combination with GC leads to a successful modulation of both arms of the immune response (changes in suppressor T cells and anti-GC levels have been noted[51,60]) and to the clearance of inflammatory cells from the CNS.[33,34] The net results of this treatment were cessation of lesion progression, massive proliferation of oligodendrocytes and widespread CNS remyelination.

The observation that CNS remyelination usually occurs in chronic relapsing EAE and that it is enhanced following treatment should encourage investigators to research ways in which lesion progression might be prevented in MS since, in this condition also, CNS remyelination and oligodendrocyte survival have been noted.[12,13] Whether or not the observed remyelination after treatment of chronic relapsing EAE in Strain 13 is antigen-specific, related to alterations in T cell subsets, antibody type, or the consequence of conformational changes in the MBP molecule, must remain issues in need of further exploration. The availability of chronic relapsing EAE models in the SJL mouse for the testing of our treatment regimen and the large retinue of haplotype and mouse markers promise to be an interesting avenue for future investigations.

ACKNOWLEDGMENTS

We thank Sanford H. Stone, Dale E. McFarlin and Ethan Shevach of NIH for their collaboration, Everett Swanson, Miriam Pakingan, Howard Finch and Patricia Kennedy for technical expertise, and Nanci E. Legg for secretarial assistance.

REFERENCES

1. LUMSDEN, C. E. 1970. The neuropathology of multiple sclerosis. *In* Handbook of Clinical Neurology, vol. 9. P. J. Vinken & G. W. Bruyn, Eds.: 217–309. North-Holland Publishing Co. Amsterdam.
2. PRINEAS, J. W. 1975. Pathology of the early lesion in multiple sclerosis. Human Pathol. **6:** 531–554.
3. PATERSON, P. Y. 1977. Autoimmune neurological diseases: Experimental animal systems and implications for multiple sclerosis. *In* Autoimmunity. Genetic, Immunologic, Virologic and Clinical Aspects. N. Talal, Ed.: 643–692. Academic Press. New York.
4. RAINE, C. S. 1983. Multiple sclerosis and chronic EAE: Comparative ultrastructural neuropathology. *In* Multiple Sclerosis. J. F. Hallpike, C. W. M. Adams & W. W. Tourtellotte, Eds.: 413–460. Chapman & Hall. London.
5. BUNGE, M. B., R. P. BUNGE & H. RIS. 1961. Ultrastructural study of remyelination in an experimental lesion in adult cat spinal cord. J. Biophys. Biochem. Cytol. **10:** 67–94.
6. BORNSTEIN, M. B. & S. H. APPEL. 1961. The application of tissue culture to the study of experimental "allergic" encephalomyelitis. I. Patterns of demyelination. J. Neuropath. Exp. Neurol. **20:** 141–157.
7. RAINE, C. S. 1978. Pathology of demyelination. *In* Physiology and Pathobiology of Axons. S. G. Waxman, Ed.: 283–310. Raven Press. New York.
8. LAMPERT, P. W. 1965. Demyelination and remyelination in experimental allergic encephalomyelitis: Further electron microscopic observations. J. Neuropath. Exp. Neurol. **24:** 371–385.
9. PRINEAS, J., C. S. RAINE & H. WISNIEWSKI. 1969. An ultrastructural study of experimental demyelination and remyelination. III. Chronic experimental allergic encephalomyelitis in the central nervous system. Lab. Invest. **21:** 472–483.
10. RAINE, C. S. 1976. Experimental allergic encephalomyelitis and related conditions. *In* Progress in Neuropathology, vol. 3. H. M. Zimmerman, Ed.: 225–251. Grune & Stratton. New York.
11. SUZUKI, K., J. M. ANDREWS, J. M. WALTZ & R. D. TERRY. 1969. Ultrastructural studies of multiple sclerosis. Lab. Invest. **20:** 444–454.
12. PRINEAS, J. W. & F. CONNELL. 1979. Remyelination in multiple sclerosis. Ann. Neurol. **5:** 22–31.
13. RAINE, C. S., L. C. SCHEINBERG & J. M. WALTZ. 1981. Multiple sclerosis: Oligodendrocyte survival and proliferation in an active, established lesion. Lab. Invest. **45:** 534–546.
14. MOORE, G. R. W., U. TRAUGOTT & C. S. RAINE. 1984. Survival of oligodendrocytes in chronic relapsing experimental encephalomyelitis. J. Neurol. Sci. In press.
15. WAKSMAN, B. H. & R. D. ADAMS. 1962. An histologic study of the early lesion in experimental allergic encephalomyelitis in the guinea pig and rabbit. Am. J. Pathol. **41:** 135–150.
16. LEVINE, S. 1974. Hyperacute, neutrophilic and localized forms of experimental allergic encephalomyelitis: A review. Acta. Neuropathol. (Berlin) **28:** 179–189.
17. RAINE, C. S., D. H. SNYDER, M. P. VALSAMIS & S. H. STONE. 1974. Chronic experimental allergic encephalomyelitis in inbred guinea pigs: An ultrastructural study. Lab. Invest. **31:** 369–380.
18. MCFARLIN, D. E., S. E. BLANK & R. F. KIBLER. 1974. Recurrent experimental allergic encephalomyelitis in the Lewis rat. J. Immunol. **113:** 712–715.
19. LASSMANN, H., K. KITZ & H. M. WISNIEWSKI. 1980. Chronic relapsing experimental allergic encephalomyelitis in rats and guinea pigs: A comparison. *In* Search for the Cause

of Multiple Sclerosis and Other Chronic Diseases of the Central Nervous System. A. Boese, Ed.: 96–104. Verlag Chemie. Weinheim.
20. Wisniewski, H. M. & A. B. Keith. 1977. Chronic relapsing experimental allergic encephalomyelitis: An experimental model of multiple sclerosis. Ann. Neurol. **1:** 144–147.
21. Raine, C. S. & S. H. Stone. 1977. Animal model for multiple sclerosis. Chronic experimental allergic encephalomyelitis in inbred guinea pigs. N.Y. State J. Med. **77:** 1693–1696.
22. Lublin, D., H. Maurer, R. G. Berry & D. Tippett. 1981. Delayed, relapsing experimental allergic encephalomyelitis in mice. J. Immunol. **126:** 819–822.
23. Brown, A. & D. E. McFarlin. 1981. Relapsing experimental allergic encephalomyelitis in SJL mouse. Lab. Invest. **45:** 278–285.
24. Brown, A., D. E. McFarlin & C. S. Raine. 1982. The chronologic neuropathology of relapsing experimental allergic encephalomyelitis in the mouse. Lab. Invest. **46:** 171–185.
25. Stone, S. H. & E. M. Lerner. 1965. Chronic disseminated allergic encephalomyelitis in guinea pigs. Ann. N.Y. Acad. Sci. **122:** 227–241.
26. Snyder, D. H., M. P. Valsamis, S. H. Stone & C. S. Raine. 1975. Progressive and reparatory events in chronic experimental allergic encephalomyelitis. J. Neuropath. Exp. Neurol. **34:** 209–221.
27. Raine, C. S., U. Traugott & S. H. Stone. 1980. Applications of chronic relapsing experimental allergic encephalomyelitis to multiple sclerosis. *In* Progress in MS Research. H. Bauer, S. Poser & G. Ritter, Eds.: 3–10. Springer Verlag. Berlin.
28. Weigle, O. 1980. Analysis of autoimmunity through experimental models of thyroiditis and allergic encephalomyelitis. *In* Advances in Immunology, vol. 30. Frank J. Dixon & Henry G. Kunkel, Eds.: 159–273. Academic Press. New York.
29. Traugott, U., E. Shevach, J. Chiba, S. H. Stone & C. S. Raine. 1981. Autoimmune encephalomyelitis: Simultaneous identification of T and B cells in the target organ. Science **214:** 1251–1253.
30. Traugott, U., E. L. Reinherz & C. S. Raine. 1983. Multiple sclerosis: Distribution of T cell subsets within active chronic lesions. Science **219:** 308–310.
31. Mokhtarian, F., D. E. McFarlin & C. S. Raine. 1983. Induction of chronic relapsing experimental allergic encephalomyelitis (EAE) by adoptive transfer of lymph node cells. J. Neuropath. Exp. Neurol. **42:** 359 (Abstract).
32. Mokhtarian, F., D. E. McFarlin & C. S. Raine. 1984. Adoptive transfer of myelin basic protein sensitized cells produces chronic relapsing demyelinating disease in mice. Nature **309:** 5966–5969.
33. Traugott, U., S. H. Stone & C. S. Raine. 1982. Chronic relapsing experimental autoimmune encephalomyelitis: Treatment with combinations of myelin components promotes clinical and structural recovery. J. Neurol. Sci. **56:** 65–73.
34. Raine, C. S. & U. Traugott. 1983. Chronic relapsing autoimmune encephalomyelitis: Ultrastructure of the CNS of animals treated with combinations of myelin components. Lab. Invest. **48:** 275–284.
35. Raine, C. S. & U. Traugott. 1982. The pathogenesis and therapy of multiple sclerosis is based upon the requirement of a combination of myelin antigens for autoimmune demyelination. J. Neuroimmunol. **2:** 83–91.
36. Stone, S. H., U. Traugott & C. S. Raine. 1983. Chronic experimental allergic encephalomyelitis in Strain 2 guinea pigs: Sex dependence of clinical disease and absence of resistance to nervous system changes. J. Neuroimmunol. **4:** 187–199.
37. Pettinelli, C. B. & D. E. McFarlin. 1981. Adoptive transfer of experimental allergic encephalomyelitis in SJL/J mice after *in vitro* activation of lymph node cells by myelin basic protein: Requirement for Lyt $1^{+}2^{-}$ T lymphocytes. J. Immunol. **127:** 1420–1423.
38. Raine, C. S., U. Traugott & S. H. Stone. 1978. Suppression of chronic allergic encephalomyelitis: Relevance to multiple sclerosis. Science **201:** 445–448.
39. Traugott, U., S. H. Stone & C. S. Raine. 1979. Chronic relapsing experimental allergic encephalomyelitis: Correlation of circulating lymphocyte fluctuations with disease activity in suppressed and unsuppressed animals. J. Neurol. Sci. **41:** 17–29.

40. RAINE, C. S., U. TRAUGOTT & S. H. STONE. 1980. Lymphocyte studies in acute and chronic relapsing EAE during suppression. *In* The Suppression of Experimental Allergic Encephalomyelitis and Multiple Sclerosis. A. N. Davison & M. L. Cuzner, Eds.: 119–140. Academic Press. New York.
41. LAMPERT, P. W. & S. CARPENTER. 1965. Electron microscopic studies on the vascular permeability and the mechanisms of demyelination in experimental allergic encephalomyelitis. J. Neuropath. Exp. Neurol. **24:** 11–24.
42. PRINEAS, J. W. & F. CONNELL. 1978. The fine structure of chronically active multiple sclerosis plaques. Neurology **28:** 68–75.
43. EPSTEIN, L. G., J. W. PRINEAS & C. S. RAINE. 1983. Attachment of myelin to coated pits on macrophages in experimental allergic encephalomyelitis. J. Neurol. Sci. **61:** 341–348.
44. RAINE, C. S., L. B. BARNETT, A. BROWN, T. BEHAR & D. E. MCFARLIN. 1980. Neuropathology of experimental allergic encephalomyelitis in inbred strains of mice. Lab. Invest. **43:** 150–157.
45. FLEURY, H. J., R. D. SHEPPARD, M. B. BORNSTEIN & C. S. RAINE. 1980. Further ultrastructural observations of virus morphogenesis and myelin pathology in JHM virus encephalomyelitis. Neuropath. Appl. Neurobiol. **6:** 165–179.
46. WISNIEWSKI, H. M., H. LASSMAN, C. F. BROSNAN, P. D. MEHTA, A. A. LIDSKY & R. E. MADRID. 1982. Multiple sclerosis: Immunological and experimental aspects. *In* Recent Advances in Clinical Neurology, vol. 3. W. B. Matthews & G. H. Glaser, Eds.: 95–124. Churchill, Livingstone. Edinburgh.
47. TRAUGOTT, U., E. SHEVACH, J. CHIBA, S. H. STONE & C. S. RAINE. 1982. Chronic relapsing experimental allergic encephalomyelitis: Identification and dynamics of T and B cells within the central nervous system. Cell. Immunol. **68:** 261–265.
48. TRAUGOTT, U., E. SHEVACH, J. CHIBA, S. H. STONE & C. S. RAINE. 1982. Acute experimental allergic encephalomyelitis: T and B cell distribution in the target organ. Cell. Immunol. **70:** 345–356.
49. TRAUGOTT, U. & C. S. RAINE. 1977. Experimental allergic encephalomyelitis in inbred guinea pigs. Correlation of decrease in early T cells with clinical signs in suppressed and unsuppressed animals. Cell. Immunol. **34:** 146–155.
50. TRAUGOTT, U., S. H. STONE & C. S. RAINE. 1978. Experimental allergic encephalomyelitis: Migration of early T cells from the circulation to the central nervous system. J. Neurol. Sci. **36:** 55–61.
51. RAINE, C. S. & U. TRAUGOTT. 1984. The application of chronic relapsing experimental allergic encephalomyelitis to the study of remyelination. *In* Pathology of the Myelinated Axon. Current Trends in Neuroscience, vol. 3. M. Adachi, Ed. Igaku-Skoin. New York.
52. RAINE, C. S., U. TRAUGOTT, M. FAROOQ, M. B. BORNSTEIN & W. T. NORTON. 1981. Augmentation of immune-mediated demyelination by lipid haptens. Lab. Invest. **45:** 174–182.
53. RAINE, C. S., A. B. JOHNSON, D. MARCUS, A. SUZUKI & M. B. BORNSTEIN. 1981. Demyelination *in vitro:* Absorption studies demonstrate that galactocerebroside is a major target. J. Neurol. Sci. **52:** 117–131.
54. BROSNAN, C. F., U. TRAUGOTT & C. S. RAINE. 1983. Analysis of humoral and cellular events and the role of lipid haptens during CNS demyelination. Acta Neuropathol. Suppl. (Berlin) **9:** 59–70.
55. RAINE, C. S. & M. B. BORNSTEIN. 1970. Experimental allergic encephalomyelitis: An ultrastructural study of experimental demyelination *in vitro*. J. Neuropath. Exp. Neurol. **29:** 177–191.
56. WRAY, S. H., D. G. COGAN & B. G. W. ARNASON. An *in vivo* model of demyelination of intraocular myelin in the rabbit. Proc. Assoc. Res. Vis. Ophthalmol. April 1974. p. 260 (Abstract).
57. MOORE, G. R. W., U. TRAUGOTT, M. FAROOQ, W. T. NORTON & C. S. RAINE. 1983. Comparison of the augmenting effects of different myelin lipids upon autoimmune demyelination in the CNS. J. Neuropath. Exp. Neurol. **42:** 357 (Abstract).
58. ALVORD, E. C., G. M. SHAW, S. HRUBY & L. R. SIRES. 1980. The ambiguity of our clinico-pathological, enzymological and immunochemical evidences concerning the agent(s) responsible for multiple sclerosis. *In* Search for the Cause of Multiple Sclerosis

and Other Chronic Diseases of the Central Nervous System. A. Boese, Ed.: 454–465. Verlag Chemie. Weinheim.

59. FLIED, E. J. & C. S. RAINE. 1969. Experimental allergic encephalomyelitis in the Rhesus monkey: An EM study. J. Neurol. Sci. **8:** 397–411.
60. RAINE, C. S. & U. TRAUGOTT. 1984. Therapeutic trials in relapsing autoimmune demyelination. *In* Neuroimmunology. F. Spreafico & P. O. Behan, Eds.: 325–346. Raven Press. New York.
61. TRAUGOTT, U., E. L. REINHERZ & C. S. RAINE. Multiple sclerosis: Distribution of T cells, T cell subsets and Ia-positive macrophages in lesions of different ages. J. Neuroimmunol. **4:** 201–221.
62. BURGER, D. R., D. FORD, R. M. VETTO, A. HAMBLIN, A. GOLDSTEIN, M. HUBBARD & D. C. DUMONDE. 1981. Endothelial cell presentation of antigen to human T cells. Human Immunol. **3:** 209–230.
63. BERNARD, C. C. A. & I. R. MCKAY. 1983. Transfer of murine experimental autoimmune encephalomyelitis and cell-mediated immunity to myelin protein is effected by Lyt-1 cells. J. Neuroimmunol. **4:** 61–65.
64. SRIRAM, S., D. SOLOMON, R. V. ROUSE & L. STEINMAN. 1982. Identification of T cell subsets and B lymphocytes in mouse brain experimental allergic encephalitis lesions. J. Immunol. **129:** 1649–1651.
65. TRAUGOTT, U., D. E. MCFARLIN, F. MOKHTARIAN & C. S. RAINE. 1984. Experimental allergic encephalomyelitis in the mouse: Immunocytochemical analysis of lesion development. J. Neuropath. Exp. Neurol. **43:** 325 (Abstract).
66. SAIDA, T., K. SAIDA, S. DORFMAN, D. H. SILBERBERG, A. J. SUMNER, M. C. MANNING, R. P. LISAK & M. J. BROWN. 1979. Experimental allergic neuritis induced by sensitization with galactocerebroside. Science **204:** 1103–1196.
67. SAIDA, T., K. SAIDA & D. H. SILBERBERG. 1979. Demyelination produced by experimental allergic neuritis serum and anti-galactocerebroside antiserum in CNS cultures. Acta Neuropathol. (Berlin) **48:** 19–25.
68. GAUSAS, J., P. Y. PATERSON, E. D. DAY & M. C. DAL CANTO. 1982. Intact B-cell activity is essential for complete expression of experimental allergic encephalomyelitis in Lewis rats. Cell. Immunol. **72:** 360–366.
69. WILLENBORG, D. O. & S. J. PROWSE. 1983. Immunoglobulin deficient rats fail to develop experimental allergic encephalomyelitis. J. Neuroimmunol. **5:** 99–109.

The Current Status of Multiple Sclerosis Intra-Blood-Brain-Barrier IgG Synthesis

WALLACE W. TOURTELLOTTE, MICHAEL J. WALSH, ROBERT W. BAUMHEFNER, SUSAN M. STAUGAITIS, AND PAUL SHAPSHAK

Neurology and Research Services
VAMC West Los Angeles
Wadsworth Division
Los Angeles, California 90073
and
Department of Neurology
Reed Neurological Research Center
University of California at Los Angeles School of Medicine
Los Angeles, California 90024

In the last year we have published three extensive reviews on multiple sclerosis (MS) intra-blood-brain-barrier (intra-BBB) IgG synthesis.[1,2,3] The reader is referred to these reports for reconsideration of historical aspects, cytological base and restricted heterogeneity, as well as information concerning immunoglobulins other than IgG, immune complexes and complement synthesis. The present report will focus on new data and unanswered questions about intra-BBB IgG synthesis, dealing briefly with its cytologic base, measurement, specificity, and modulation. Finally an immunokinetic model is proposed that unifies some observations on cellular and humoral immunologic disturbances in MS.

The Fountainhead of Intra-BBB IgG Synthesis (Cytological Base)

One of the hallmarks of MS central nervous system (CNS) lesions is multifocal areas of primary demyelination (plaques). Extensive lymphoid infiltration is often found associated with plaques but inflammatory cells are also found in normal-appearing white matter, around venules, and in the leptomeninges. Sometimes, there is extensive cellular infiltration in one region of a plaque with only a few cells in the remaining part, and plaques may be seen without associated inflammatory cells. There is myelin phagocytosis, various degrees of axonal and oligodendroglia cell loss, and gliosis. These changes are a reflection of a dynamic multiphasic process. These pathologic findings place MS in the category of primary inflammatory demyelinating diseases.[4]

Utilizing the electron microscope, Prineas and Wright[5] were the first to quantitate plasma cells, the cell population responsible for *in situ* and *de novo* CNS production of IgG in brains of MS patients. They found no plasma cells in MS normal gray matter, but in the plaque they found about five times more cells than in the adjacent normal-appearing white matter.

Esiri[6] performed a detailed study of plasma cells in the brains of patients with MS. Nonplaque tissue contained very small numbers of plasma cells, whereas plaques categorized as recent by histological criteria contained almost 30 times more. Intermediate numbers of cells were present in the plaques of intermediate age, and chronic plaques had the lowest number, but substantially more than were present in nonplaque tissue. In all plaques and nonplaque areas examined, an excess of light to heavy chains was found. The light chain excess was greatest in recent plaques. A major portion of the heavy chains present belonged to IgG, which accounted for 83% of the intracellular heavy chains in plaques and 93% in nonplaque tissue. IgA heavy chains accounted for almost all the remaining heavy chains (15–17% in plaque and 7% in nonplaque areas). Cells containing IgM were rare except for one patient in whom IgM accounted for 27% of the total heavy chains identified. In chronic plaques and normal tissue, plasma cells were confined almost exclusively to the perivascular spaces, but in recent lesions, plasma cells were found in the surrounding parenchyma as well.

In view of critical new insights in the past decade into T cell regulation of B cell maturation and immunoglobulin synthesis, attempts have been made to identify T cells in brains of MS patients. One qualitative report[7] has described both helper-inducer (OKT4+) and cytotoxic-suppressor (OKT8+) T cells at the margin of active chronic plaques and mainly helper-inducer cells in adjacent normal-appearing white matter. A supplemental report,[8] using quantitative methods, showed the distribution of T cell subsets and macrophages to vary with lesion activity. In acute plaques (TH+) T cells, helper-inducer (T4+) cells, suppressor-cytotoxic (T8+) cells, and macrophages (Ia+) were more numerous at the lesion center with no T cells or Ia+ cells seen in the normal white matter. Active chronic lesions were as described above with close contact between small lymphocytes and Ia+ macrophages commonly seen. Another brief report noted cytotoxic-suppressor cells in plaques.[9] Booss *et al.*[10,10a] studied quantitative aspects of T lymphocytes in CNS parenchyma in a series of patients with MS and related them to histopathological criteria for disease activity. Cytotoxic-suppressor T cells outnumbered helper-inducer T cells by about 3:1 in MS CNS parenchyma. Numbers of cytotoxic-suppressor and helper-inducer cells in plaques did not correlate with plaque activity, but in nonplaque areas there were fewer cytotoxic-suppressor cells in areas near active than near inactive plaques. At the plaque edge[10b] both the cytotoxic-suppressor and the helper-induced subsets peaked. Although the cytotoxic-suppressor subset usually predominated the ratio varied greatly.

Of relevance is a possible correlation of intra-BBB IgG synthesis in MS manifested by oligoclonal IgG banding in the CSF (another independent manifestations of intra-BBB IgG synthesis—see below) and the number of plasma cells in plaques and meninges.[11] Patients without bands had very few or no identifiable plasma cells on routine sections. Every patient with oligoclonal bands had numerous plasma cells in their meninges and plaques.

The question arises whether there are enough plasma cells located intra-BBB to account for average daily intra-BBB IgG synthesis in MS. The average intra-BBB IgG synthesis daily rate in clinical definite MS patient is 30 mg of IgG/day.[12] It has been determined that 10^6 plasma cells produce 22.4 μg IgG/day.[13] Accordingly, 1.3×10^9 plasma cells should be in the CNS, or in the CSF per day to synthesize 30 mg (about 1.5 ml of packed plasma cells distributed throughout the brain and leptomeninges). Since the average MS patient has 24 plasma cells per ml of CSF[14] and 500 ml of CSF turn over per day, these 12,000 cells would contribute about 0.27 μg/day, a miniscule amount.

Prineas and Wright[5] assumed a homogenous distribution of perivascular plasma cells throughout the brain; based on this assumption they calculated 0.13×10^9 plasma cells in the white matter. Even though they were aware of lepto-meningeal plasma cells they made no additional adjustments. Adams,[15] who performed cell counts in the brain parenchyma and cerebral meninges, only recorded lymphocytes. Adams found approximately five times more lymphocytes in the cerebral meninges when compared to brain parenchyma. Assuming that the same ratio of plasma cells to lymphocytes as reported by Prineas and Wright prevails in the cerebral meninges as it does in the brain parenchyma, the plasma count found in the leptomeninges would be $5 \times 0.13 \times 10^9 = 0.65 \times 10^9$. Adding this figure to the plasma count of the brain parenchyma based on electronmicrographs, a figure of 0.78×10^9 plasma cells per average MS brain is calculated. Because of the large number of variables relating to brain cell counts and regulation of IgG synthesis in any regional compartment of the immune system, we believe the close correlation, 0.78×10^9, for Prineas and Wright plus Adams *versus* our estimate of 1.3×10^9 speaks for their validity.

In summary, the hallmark of the MS CNS lesion is multifocal primary demyelination (loss of oligodendroglia with sparing of axon) associated with a dynamic multiphasic chronic inflammation. Plasma cells have been enumerated in relation to active plaques. The presence of helper-inducer and cytotoxic-suppressor T cells intermingled and in the vicinity of plaques suggests that immunoregulation of plasma cell IgG synthesis is plausible in the MS CNS. In those cases of MS where no plasma cells are found in the brain, no intra-BBB IgG synthesis as manifested by IgG oligoclonal bands in the CSF is found. On the other hand, in all cases with plasma cells present, bands are found. On a quantitative basis, the number of plasma cells found in the average MS brain is probably sufficient to account for the average daily intra-BBB IgG synthesis calculated by our formula. Accordingly, these findings are not inconsistent with the view that intra-BBB IgG synthesis, measured quantitatively by our formula or qualitatively by oligoclonal bands, is a marker for persistent MS activity.

Measurement of Intra-BBB IgG Synthesis

Data indicate that the fountainhead of IgG inside the BBB in health is exclusively the blood.[1,2] Blood is also the fountainhead when there is a break in the BBB, but this is accompanied by a proportional elevation in albumin, a natural marker of BBB integrity. Intra-BBB synthesis of IgG in MS occurs in multifocal regions, by plasma cells, mainly at the edges of active plaques of demyelination and perivenous infiltrates. Cellular infiltrates in the leptomeninges are likely to be an additional source of CSF IgG in MS. As previously discussed, the circulating CSF cells, by calculation, contribute essentially nothing to the average daily intra-BBB IgG synthesis rate. Furthermore, after secretion of IgG by plasma cells into the extravascular space of the CNS the IgG sinks by diffusion into the CSF space—a fast-moving 500 ml per day lacuna of the CNS extracellular space—and is returned to blood via the arachnoid villi.

There are three types of methods to detect and measure intra-BBB IgG synthesis: dimensionless quotients, rate of synthesis by formulas, and demonstration of CSF oligoclonal IgG bands. Comparisons among the various measurement systems made for MS showed that of the three different methods of IgG measurement, quotients provide the least satisfactory data.[16–18,18a] Demonstration of IgG oligoclonal bands in the CSF and not in serum is considered a *sine qua non* of intra-BBB synthesis. However, formulas alone provide estimates in mg of IgG synthesized per dl (or mg per day) after correcting for diffusion of blood IgG across the normal and/or abnormal BBB. In a recent study of 78 patients with clinical definite MS, over 99% of the patients had evidence of intra-BBB IgG synthesis by our rate formula and the presence of CSF oligoclonal IgG utilizing isoelectric focusing followed by immunofixation and silver staining.[19]

The dimensionless quotients are CSF IgG/CSF total protein, CSF IgG/CSF albumin and CSF IgG/serum IgG divided by CSF albumin/serum albumin (IgG index). The least sensitive of these quotients is CSF IgG divided by CSF total protein.

In 1983 Caroscio *et al.*[20] compared four ways of measuring intra-BBB IgG synthesis [our intra-BBB IgG synthesis rate formula, IgG index, and IgG concentration (mg/dl), and IgG/albumin] on 106 patients with MS and 127 patients with other neurological diseases. The IgG synthetic rate (our formula) and IgG index were the most sensitive tests. The IgG concentration (mg/dl) and IgG-albumin ratio were less valuable. The IgG synthetic rate was more specific than the IgG index, making it the quantitative measure that best correlated with a diagnosis of clinical definite MS.

In the same year (1983) Mandler *et al.*[21] determined intra-BBB IgG synthesis rate and they detected CSF oligoclonal bands by polyacrylamide gel isoelectric focusing. In 15 normal controls intra-BBB IgG daily synthesis was 0 ± 1.75 mg/day (mean ± 1 SD), and no oligoclonal bands were detected. Eighty-eight percent of the clinical definite patients had increased (>3.59 mg/day) intra-BBB IgG synthesis (mean = 25.4 mg/day), and 92% had oligoclonal bands in the CSF. Sixty-seven percent of probable MS patients had increased intra-BBB IgG synthesis (mean = 20.2 mg/day) and/or oligoclonal bands. Eight percent of other neurological diseases had abnormal synthesis and bands. The correlation between IgG daily synthesis and oligoclonal bands was 92%. The predictive value of a positive test was 92% for both IgG synthesis and oligoclonal bands; the predictive value of a negative test was 93% for IgG synthesis and 95% for oligoclonal bands. These results indicate that both tests are useful diagnostic tools in MS.

Wurster, also in 1983,[22] addressed the issue of mathematical interrelations of five formulas proposed to calculate intra-BBB IgG synthesis and the IgG index. From these analyses our formula fared very well. In addition, the major advantage of our formula over the IgG index was judged to be the expression of results in actual mg IgG (per ml or day) rather than as a dimensionless ratio. It was pointed out that this becomes especially important in serial determinations with fluctuating CSF albumin against which the IgG index shows a nonlinear response (graphically shown in his Figure 1).

A controversial aspect of our formula has been examined by Felgenhauer.[23] He discovered that the filtration line of the BBB for albumin and IgG was stable irrespective of the actual permeability conditions. He selected the albumin concentration as the best permeability parameter, as we had done in our simultaneous double labeled (^{125}I-albumin and ^{131}I-IgG) isotope study.[24] In Table 1 of his publication[23] the limiting ratios of IgG with those of albumin were 0.69, irrespective of the actual barrier state. This is the most convincing experimental proof that our assumption is correct, *i.e.,* the IgG and albumin is transferred in equimolar portions across the BBB. On the other hand, this is not the case for IgA and IgM (also shown in Felgenhauer in his Table 1[23]) where the transfer is strongly dependent on permeability conditions.

Another controversial aspect of our formula relates to the report by Tibbling and Link that CSF albumin concentration increased significantly with advancing age.[25] On the other hand our studies[14] and those of Vatassen *et al.*[26] found no correlation between CSF albumin concentration and age (27–71 years of age).

IgG and albumin can be measured concomitantly in CSF and serum by electroimmunodiffusion[27] or separately by single radial diffusion or by nephrolometry.[28] The formula to quantitate the rate of intra-BBB IgG synthesis is as follows:[29]

$$\left[\left(\mathrm{IgG_{CSF}} - \frac{\mathrm{IgG_{serum}}}{369}\right) - \left(\mathrm{Alb_{CSF}} - \frac{\mathrm{Alb_{serum}}}{230}\right) \times \left(\frac{\mathrm{IgG_{serum}}}{\mathrm{Alb_{serum}}}\right)(0.43)\right] \times 5,$$

where intra-BBB IgG CSF represents the IgG in mg per day in the CSF derived from extravascular sources, *i.e.*, synthesized primarily within the BBB by plasma cells. IgG_{CSF} is the IgG concentration (mg per dl) found in the patient's CSF, and the IgG_{serum} is the patient's serum IgG concentration (mg per dl). The number 369 is a ratio constant that quantitatively determines the proportion of CSF IgG that normally passes by filtration from the serum into the CSF across an intact BBB. It is the quotient of the serum IgG/CSF IgG ratio of a normal healthy population. Thus, $IgG_{serum}/369$ is the IgG that is expected to cross from the serum to the CSF, based on the patient's serum IgG concentration and the normal CSF:serum ratio.

Alb_{CSF} is the albumin concentration (mg per dl) found in the patient's CSF and Alb_{serum} is the patient's serum albumin concentration (mg per dl). The number 230 represents a constant that determines the proportion of CSF albumin that normally passes by filtration from the serum into the CSF across an intact BBB. It is the average of the serum albumin/CSF albumin ratio in a normal healthy population. Thus, $(Alb_{CSF}) - (Alb_{serum}/230)$ is a term that represents the excess CSF albumin that has crossed a damaged BBB. This term is then multiplied by (serum IgG/serum Alb) × (0.43) to convert the excess CSF albumin to excess CSF IgG (on a molar basis) that has crossed a damaged BBB with the albumin, assuming a one-to-one molar equivalence. To calculate the daily IgG synthesis, this entire equation is then multiplied by 5 to convert from concentration in mg per dl to the amount present in 5 dl of CSF which, on the average, is formed each day. This formula has been validated by a radioisotope two compartment study.[24]

SAMPLE CALCULATION

CSF IgG	= 10.5 mg/100 ml	Serum IgG	= 1310 mg/100 ml
CSF Albumin	= 27.3 mg/100 ml	Serum Albumin	= 5070 mg/ml

Daily Intra-BBB

$$IgG_{SYN} = \left[\left(10.5 - \frac{1310}{369}\right) - \left(27.3 - \frac{5070}{230}\right)\left(\frac{1310}{5070}\right)(0.43)\right] \times 5$$

$$= (6.95 - 0.58) \times 5$$

Intra-BBB $IgG_{SYN} = 31.8$ mg/day

The normal range of intra-BBB IgG synthesis is −9 to 3.3 mg/day and the average synthesis in MS patients is 30 mg/day. Elevated rates of synthesis have been reported in over 90% of clinical definite MS patients.[12,29]

The formation of intra-BBB IgG synthesis of 30 mg per day by the average MS patient[12] is really quite significant when compared to the rate of IgG synthesis by the core immune system of a normal individual. According to Janeway *et al.*,[30] the normal 70 kg individual synthesizes 2380 mg of IgG/day. Therefore, the average MS patient is synthesizing within the BBB 1.3% of the total body IgG. The IgG synthesized within the BBB sinks into the CSF that is pumped into the blood via arachnoid villi. Accordingly, in one month a gram of IgG is injected into the body, a dose which is equivalent to that used to maintain agamma globulinemic patients. In about 20% of MS patients there exists a modest significant evaluation of serum IgG of about 20%.[14] Since catabolism of IgG (all subclasses represented in normal proportion) in the core immune system is 7% per day, it is possible that the elevated serum IgG in some MS patients is due to intra-BBB IgG synthesis.

In summary, measurement of intra-BBB IgG synthesis has been achieved in MS and evidence exists that it reflects the degree of chronic inflammatory reaction in the MS CNS. The formula we proposed in 1975 has been shown to be a reliable and valid estimation of intra-BBB IgG production. The average MS patient synthesizes 30 mg of IgG per day within the BBB which is about 1.3% of the total body synthesis. This amount of IgG is probably the result of about 1.3 billion plasma cells located at mulifocal sites in the CNS, such as, in or near active plaques of demyelination as well as in perivenous infiltrates and in the leptomeninges. Recent comparisons of synthesis formulas indicate that our formula best correlates with a diagnosis of clinical definite MS.

Unique CSF Oligoclonal IgG Bands As an Indicator of Intra-BBB IgG Synthesis

The first systematic study and probably the discovery of oligoclonal bands in CSF was made by Drs. Lowenthal, van Sande, and Karcher in 1960.[31] Nobody took it very seriously until 10 years later when Laterre *et al.* in 1970[32] wrote a classic report in which they compared a large number of MS and non-MS patients and found that oligoclonal gamma globulin bands in the CSF discriminated for MS, with some exceptions. Since that time the technique for detection has been refined and numerous studies have confirmed their results (reviewed in refs. 1 and 2). Our studies have shown that over 99% of all clinical definite MS patients have on the average 13 unique IgG (usually cathodic) oligoclonal bands in the CSF when compared to the serum.[19] Accordingly, IgG oligoclonal band analysis has become a standard clinical laboratory test to corroborate the diagnosis of MS.[3,33]

What is the fountainhead of IgG oligoclonal bands in the brain? IgG oligoclonal bands extracted from the MS brain are equivalent to those found in the CSF.[34] Accordingly, unique CSF IgG oligoclonal bands have been interpreted as an indicator of intra-BBB IgG synthesis. We believe that one or a few clones of plasma cells derived from B lymphocytes recruited inside the BBB from the core immune system are the fountainhead. The evidence to support this has recently been reviewed.[1,2,35] Based upon our studies, and those of others, of CSF and serum in clinical definite MS patients and normal individuals, a standardized reproducible method for demonstrating oligoclonal IgG is available. The most sensitive, reliable and valid method is isoelectric focusing electrophoresis combined with immunofixation and silver staining. In order to detect properly CSF oligoclonal IgG bands it is necessary to establish the location and intensity of serum IgG bands for comparison. Details for the determination and interpretation of the results have been reported.[3,36,37]

In a recent study, we examined the stability of CSF oligoclonal bands in MS in 20 chronic progressive patients from whom serial samples were available over periods of 5 to 12 years.[38] The overall IgG spectrotype was essentially unaltered even in patients who had received treatment that drastically reduced total CSF IgG levels. The pattern of IgG light and heavy chains analyzed by two dimensional electrophoresis also showed remarkable stability. These studies demonstrate that the intra-BBB IgG humoral immune response in MS at the clonal level is remarkably stable over time in contrast to the situation in acute inflammatory conditions of the CNS. On the other hand, Thompson[39] found changes in banding pattern of relapsing-remitting, but not in progressive MS patients studied longitudinally.

In summary, the technique for detection of unique CSF oligoclonal IgG bands has been refined in the last three decades, whereas 99% of all clinical definite MS patients have on the average 13 unique IgG (usually cathodic) bands in the CSF when compared to serum. The source of CSF oligoclonal IgG is presumably a few clones of plasma cells which is very stable in chronic progressive MS patients, in contrast to acute inflammatory diseases of the CNS.

Differential Diagnosis of Intra-BBB IgG Synthesis

There is no question that elevated rate of intra-BBB IgG synthesis and oligoclonal IgG have been shown to be of great diagnostic value in recent years. By using these two independent tests of intra-BBB IgG synthesis, we found that 99.8% of 78 clinically definite MS patients showed significant abnormalities ($p < 0.05$); only one patient did not have increased rate of synthesis by our formula or our IgG oligoclonal technique (isoelectric focusing followed by immunofixation and silver nitrate staining).[19] Although these indicators increase the confidence in the diagnosis of MS, they have little relation to various clinical parameters such as gender, age of onset, and duration and activity of the disease.[20]

On the other hand, it can occur in a few normal individuals, and for a while in acute neurological infections and noninflammatory diseases usually of known etiology.[1,2,3,16,20,40] In MS and in chronic infections, such as SSPE neuro-syphilis, fungal and parasitic, unless adequately treated, it persists probably for life,[14] (although this proposal has recently been challenged).[11] Accordingly, it is recommended that serial CSF/blood exams be carried out to assess the degree of persistency of intra-BBB IgG synthesis for each patient, because if the intra-BBB IgG synthesis should disappear, experience indicates the diagnosis of clinical definite MS should be questioned, though there are exceptions.[11]

Numerous reports have indicated that increased intra-BBB IgG synthesis can be caused by diseases other than MS. It is convenient to classify non-MS cases into those caused by inflammatory diseases and other neurologic diseases. The non-MS CNS inflammatory conditions include: SSPE; chronic phases of CNS infection caused by bacteria, spirochetes, parasites (toxoplasmosis, cystericercosis, trypanosomiasis), mycoses, and viruses; Guillain-Barré syndrome; postinfectious and postvaccine vasculomyelinopathies; and CNS vasculitides. The non-MS neurologic conditions include cerebrovascular disease, brain tumor, and many others. The consensus is that 30–50% of patients with non-MS inflammatory disease and 5–10% of patients with non-MS noninflammatory neurologic diseases will have increased intra-BBB IgG synthesis. However, in our experience it is relatively uncommon in clinical practice for these other conditions to cause major confusion with MS.

The rate of intra-BBB IgG synthesis can be depressed by ACTH and corticosteroids for a while, but the unique CSF IgG oligoclonal bands are still present. In our experience this is the only situation in which intra-BBB IgG synthesis has been changed in longitudinal studies.[41,42]

In our experience[1,3,14,16,29] the specificity of elevated intra-BBB IgG synthesis due to the MS process can be enhanced if we exclude patients with distinct pleocytosis (more than 50 leukocytes per cm), a few CSF polymorphonuclear cells, marked albumin elevation (>65 mg/dl), abnormal serum electrophoresis, microorganisms isolated from the CSF, and positive CSF serologic reactions for various infectious diseases, such as for syphilis and SSPE (measles or rubella). In addition, intra-BBB IgG synthesis (rate of formation and/or unique CSF IgG bands) should persist on subsequent examinations.

The predictive value of intra-BBB IgG synthesis was studied by Moulin and co-workers.[40] They reviewed 185 patients with "possible" MS in whom CSF electrophoresis had been performed at the initial diagnostic evaluation. All patients had objective evidence of neurologic disease, and the majority had chronic myelopathy, or metencephalopathy. Of the 102 patients without oligoclonal bands who were followed for an average of 28 months, 8% developed clinically definite MS. Of 83 patients with oligoclonal bands followed for a mean of 29 months, 16% developed definite MS. This indicates that patients with monosymptomatic demyelination who have oligoclonal bands are about twice as likely as those without banding to develop clinically definite MS (over a two-year follow-up). This rate of occurrence is still only one in six, however.

In summary, the presence of intra-BBB IgG synthesis (rate and oligoclonal bands), is the cardinal aspect of CSF profile indicative of clinically definite MS, but it is not specific for MS. From an immunologic as well as a neuropathologic standpoint, it is a consequence of inflammation of the CNS, a feature shared with other neurological diseases. However, it should be found in almost all cases of clinically definite MS and persist. On the other hand, it has been found for a while in 30–50% of acute infections and in 3–5% of noninflammatory non-MS cases. It is more persistent in chronic untreated infections, such as neurosyphilis and SSPE. In addition, it is necessary to determine in a standardized way unique IgG oligoclonal bands in the CSF, one of the most sensitive and stable indicators of intra-BBB IgG synthesis in clinical definite MS. With the most sensitive techniques in our hands (isoelectric focusing followed by immunofixation and silver nitrate staining), oligoclonal bands appear in nearly 100% of cases and persist in spite of ACTH and/or corticosteroid therapy. It is recommended that serial CSF and blood exams be carried out to assess the degree of persistence of intra-BBB IgG synthesis for a given patient. Experience indicates that if the intra-BBB IgG synthesis should disappear the diagnosis of MS should be re-examined.

Antibody Specificity of Intra-BBB IgG Synthesis

Despite more than a generation of systematic study of CSF IgG in MS, the specificity of about 90% of the CSF IgG synthesis is unknown.[1,2] A small portion has antiviral activity, especially measles[43]; a portion is directed against brain tissue,[44] possibly myelin basic protein, oligodendrocytes and glycolipids; and a portion is directed against other autoantigens, including nucleic acids, erythrocytes, and smooth muscle antigens.[2] A portion may have rheumatoid factor-like activity.[2]

At present, it appears that a portion of the elevated CSF IgG in MS is nonspecific. It may be the result of polyclonal activation of B cells that are recruited to the CNS by the event that caused MS or due to bystander demyelination. The specificities of this portion of IgG produced as a result of polyclonal B cell activation reflect those of the systemic core immune system, and is identified by the presence of IgG bands in CSF or diffusely dispersed zones of IgG that correspond with the bands and zones found in serum as demonstrated by electrophoresis, isoelectric focusing, or capillary isotachophoresis.[42] Possibly, bands accentuated in CSF compared with serum represent a focal polyclonal B cell activation within the CNS. The presence of IgG bands unique to the CSF, *i.e.*, oligoclonal IgG, is postulated to represent the intra-BBB synthesis of IgG with specificity for a putative MS antigen directly related to the cause of MS,[1,2] and not an epiphenomenon. Determining the specificity of oligoclonal IgG remains a major objective of research in MS. For example, in SSPE, a disease that has marked evidence of intra-BBB IgG synthesis, we have shown that 59–82% of the intra-BBB IgG synthesis is directed at measles virus. Furthermore, a precise diagnostic test for MS may depend on the identification of the specificity of IgG synthesized within the BBB.

Monitoring Intra-BBB IgG Synthesis As an Outcome Measure in the Evaluation of a Putative Therapy for MS

We have proposed the measurement of intra-BBB IgG synthesis as one monitor for the effects of putative therapies in MS[46] for several reasons. Firstly, intra-BBB IgG synthesis can be determined simply, quickly, reliably and validly, and it occurs in over 99% of clinically definite MS patients.[19] The IgG synthesis rate tends to remain stable in clinically stable patients. Confidence limits can be established for individuals,[41] and changes in intra-BBB IgG synthesis rate can then be assessed statistically in a single patient. Since measurement of IgG synthesis rate can be conducted reliably, it represents a common basis for comparisons of drug efficacy between laboratories.[27,28] The sensitivity of detection and quantification of IgG oligoclonal band pattern is improving, and this technique may eventually provide even more specific and sensitive diagnostic, prognostic, and evaluative indicators of the MS disease process.[38]

Secondly, there is considerable evidence to support the hypothesis that intra-BBB IgG synthesis reflects one of the cardinal pathologic manifestations of active MS, namely multi-focal areas of white matter inflammation (see the first section of this review).

Thirdly, it is now generally accepted that the clinical signs and symptoms of MS represent only the tip of the iceberg of the active MS disease process. Signs and symptoms are a combination of residual effects of old lesions, as well as direct expressions of currently active lesions. Autopsy studies of MS brains often reveal extensive areas of active lesions that were without obvious clinical expression.[47] There is also increasing laboratory evidence for the presence of "subclinical" lesions, and these may also be considered either old and inactive or new and active. As new objective laboratory procedures are developed, such as an ever-increasing array of evoked potential techniques, nuclear magnetic resonance imaging and double-dose delayed contrast CT scans, the frequency and severity of subclinical pathology will become more evident.

Hence as experience is gained in the uses and limitations of measures of subclinical pathology in MS, we may find that they will be the outcome measures of choice in evaluating therapies in patients with mild neurological disabilities or early MS.[48]

The main point is that we must not place undue reliance on clinical signs and symptoms as the only or even major outcome measure in MS, especially in preliminary evaluations of putative therapies. To do so may lead us to reject potentially efficacious treatments because of overly insensitive outcome measures. Since it may require years of serial evaluations in patient, or shorter periods in large groups of patients, to document substantive changes in clinical course it behooves us to utilize the most sensitive measures we can find. At the current stage of investigation of treatments in MS, we argue strongly for inclusion of objective measures of subclinical pathology, as well as more direct measures of MS disease state or process including intra-BBB IgG synthesis.

If intra-BBB IgG synthesis is an indicator of CNS inflammation, an important goal of putative treatment in MS could be the eradication of intra-BBB IgG synthesis. With this purpose in mind we have recently presented our experience with immunosuppressive agents over the last years.[48] The treatments involved were ACTH, oral corticosteroids, pulse corticosteroids, intrathecal corticosteroids, cytosine arabinoside, cyclophosphamide, 5-fluorouracil, CCNU, and CNS irradiation. The most effective treatments were intramuscular ACTH gel and ACTH gel followed by prednisone[41]; all patients had a significant reduction in intra-BBB IgG synthesis rate, which became normal in 70% of patients. The order of effectiveness of the corticosteroids used was: oral dexamethasone, intrathecal methylprednisolone acetate, prednisone, pulse intra-

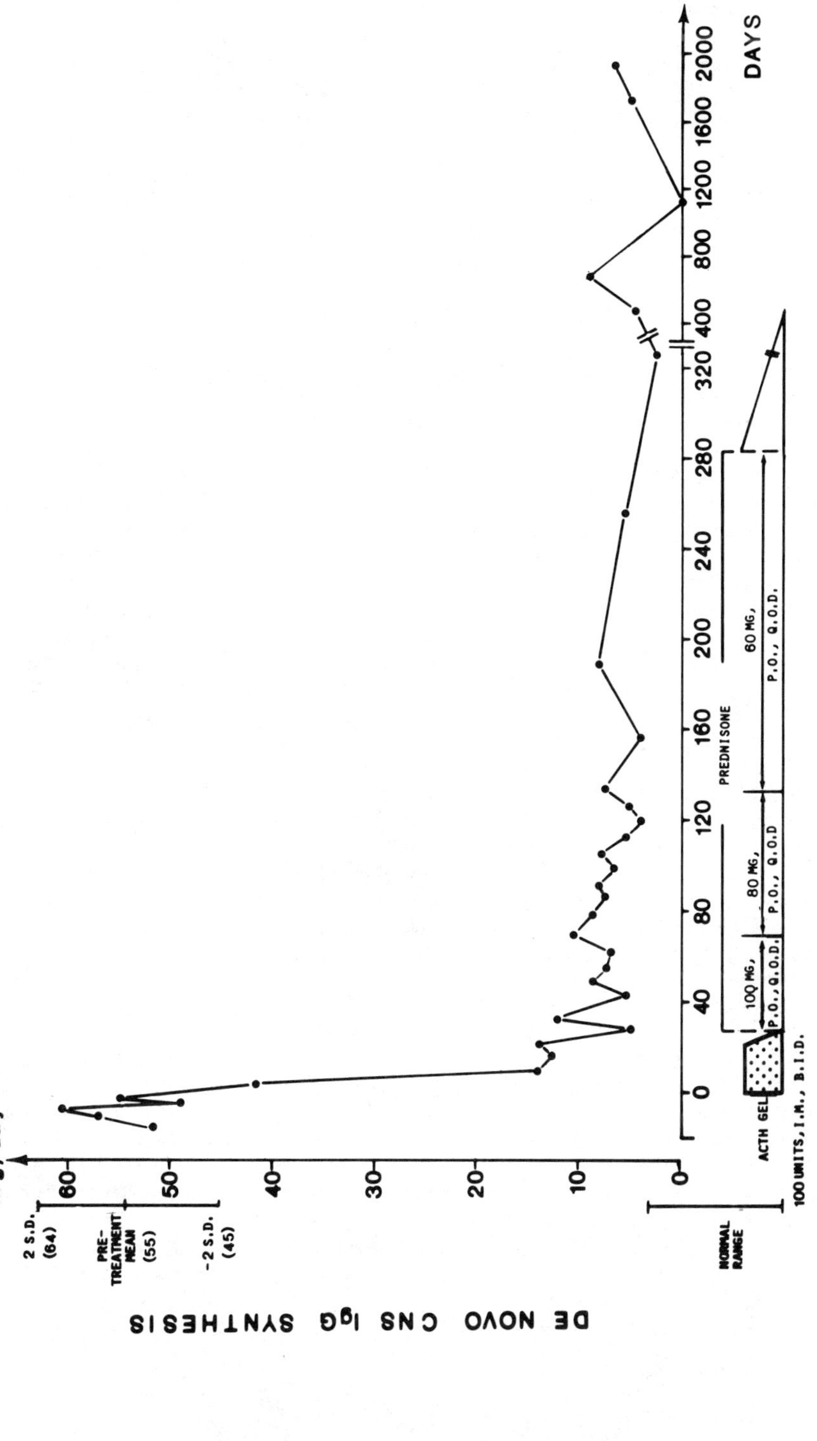

FIGURE 1. Effect of ACTH gel followed by alternate-day prednisone on intra-blood-brain-barrier (*de novo* central nervous system) IgG synthesis rate in a multiple sclerosis patient (ID 3536). Reprinted with permission from Tourtellotte *et al.*[41]

venous methylprednisolone sodium succinate, and hydrocortisone administered intrathecally. For most treatments, reduction of the rate of intra-BBB IgG synthesis occurred within days and persisted for months after cessation of treatment (FIG. 1). The MS CNS immune reactions was not eradicated when IgG synthesis rate became normal, because CSF IgG oligoclonal bands persisted. None of the chronic progressive, severely disabled patients demonstrated significant change in neurologic function or persistent adverse effects. All other treatments had no effect on intra-BBB IgG synthesis except CNS irradiation, which produced enhancement at 1,800 rads[49] and intrathecal cytosine arabinoside,[50] and oral CCNU which produced a modest transient depression,[51] as did 1,200 rads.[49]

Immunokinetic Model for MS

Based in part on the results for our immunopharmacologic trials and information presented in this report, we have proposed a model of the MS immune reaction.[48] The essential elements of this model are: (1) an initial lesion produced by a virus and/or autoimmune reaction, (2) continuous recruitment of B cells, T cells and monocytes from the peripheral circulation into the CNS, probably by nonspecific chemotaxic mechanisms generated by the preexisting inflammatory response, (3) lymphoid cell (B and T cell) interaction, (4) B cell to plasma cell conversions generating viral and/or autoimmune antibody as well as nonspecific preprogrammed antibodies, (5) monocyte-macrophage activation, (6) lysosomal enzyme liberation causing destruction of myelin (bystander demyelination), (7) antibody-antigen complexes possibly blocking destruction of myelin or virus eradication by sensitized T cells.

Our studies so far have led us to postulate that ACTH and corticosteroids decrease intra-BBB IgG synthesis by reducing recruitment of mononuclear cells in the CNS, possibly by decreasing the production of chemotaxic factors or lymphokins, such as interleukin 1. In addition, because intra-BBB IgG synthesis was markedly reduced though not eradicated, and IgG oligoclonal bands persisted, albeit reduced in intensity, two sources of intra-BBB IgG may exist. One of these is from recently recruited B cells that may be more steroid sensitive and the other from resident plasma cells, relatively steroid resistant and/or longer lived.[12]

Since cytosine arabinoside inhibits cell reproduction by preventing DNA synthesis and it had no effect on intra-BBB IgG synthesis, it is possible that cellular proliferation at least over the short term is not necessary for intra-BBB IgG synthesis. In addition, cell recruitment may not be affected by cytosine arabinoside since peripheral lymphocytic counts were virtually unchanged. On the other hand, peripheral blood monocytes were significantly lowered so it is possible that the turnover of monocyte-phagocyte is slow (<3 weeks) and/or has little to do with intra-BBB IgG synthesis.

Our study with CCNU, a modest modulator of intra-BBB IgG synthesis, indicates that another feature that may be important in selecting an immunosuppressive agent for MS is BBB penetration.[51] Part of the reason for the failure of cyclophosphamide and 5-FU, both protein synthesis inhibitors which interfere with transcription, to affect intra-BBB synthesis is perhaps the lack of adequate penetration into the CNS.[51]

One important aspect of our studies to date is that remarkable decreases in peripheral blood monocytes and lymphocytes for up to three weeks do not have any significant effect on intra-BBB IgG synthesis.[48–51] Accordingly, the MS CNS inflammatory reaction is independent for a time of the core immune system. It is still possible that suppression of the core immune system for a longer period would prove effective in the eradication of intra-BBB IgG synthesis.

Questions Raised by This Review and Suggested Experimentation

The following are some questions raised by this report with suggested experiments to advance further our understanding of intra-BBB IgG synthesis as it relates to the etiopathogenesis of MS.

1. Is the site of immunoregulation of intra-BBB IgG synthesis within the BBB?

   Suggested experiments: (1) Determine cell mediators such as interleukin 1 and 2 and correlate with T subsets, macrophages, B cells, and NK cells in fresh autopsy material. (2) Determine IL1 and IL2 in blood/CSF and relate to intra-BBB IgG synthesis.

2. Can active plaques of MS synthesize intra-BBB IgG *in vitro?* Does this IgG have the same oligoclonal pattern when compared with CSF IgG from the same patient?

   Suggested experiments: Culture fresh plaques and extract IgG synthesized; correlate *in vitro* synthesized IgG with histological activity and pre- and postmortem unique CSF oligoclonal bands.

3. Will further studies of intra-BBB IgG synthesis be correlated with intra-BBB plasma cells intra-BBB, as proposed by Ebers *et al.*?[11]
4. Will intra-BBB IgG synthesis be correlated with the size and activity of NMR lesions?
5. Will further systematic immunopharmacologic studies as proposed in this report disclose a treatment that will eradicate intra-BBB IgG synthesis?

   Suggested experiments: (1) Try repetitive cyclic treatment with ACTH and prednisone (burst of ACTH every four months followed by prednisone q.o.d.). (2) Try cyclosporine A with or without corticosteroids. (3) Try different types of interferon by different routes and different doses.

6. If prolonged or persistent eradication of intra-BBB IgG synthesis occurs, will a blood-CSF IgG isotope two compartment study, the benchmark for intra-BBB IgG synthesis, also demonstrate no synthesis?

   Suggested experiments: Use same design as we did to validate our formula.[24]

7. What is the specificity of intra-BBB IgG synthesis in MS?

   Suggested experiments: Apply ELISA technology[44] to calculate mg of antibody per ml and utilize our intra-BBB IgG synthesis formula as we have done for SSPE.[45]

8. Can the detection of unique CSF oligoclonal IgG be improved by performing isoelectrofocusing on agarose, followed by electrophoretic transfer to nitrocellulose paper, and immunoenzyme detection?

9. Can an improved technique mentioned in question 8 be used to screen for putative MS antigens?

10. Can virus be detected in MS brain using the technology of *in situ* hybridization?

    Suggested experiments: Do *in situ* hybridization with as many viral complementary probes as are available.[52]

SUMMARY

The status of the central nervous system as an immunologic organ synthesizing IgG in several neurological diseases has been established convincingly in the past two decades. The measurement of intra-BBB IgG synthesis has been accomplished. It has been demonstrated that this synthesis is a potential marker for an abnormal immunologic process within the CNS which if manipulated may be a quantifiable aspect of disease modulation. Modulation of intra-BBB IgG synthesis is feasible, but there is no evidence yet that modulation of this synthesis is an index of effective disease control in MS. Only ACTH and corticosteroids lead to a significant and lasting depression of intra-BBB IgG synthesis, even though clonal eradication is not achieved. Based on our immunopharmacologic studies in MS we have proposed an immunokinetic model. The qualitative analysis of the specificity of IgG synthesized intra-BBB in MS has not led to the etiology of MS, but utilization of quantitative methods may. Questions raised by this review with suggested experiments to advance further our understanding of intra-BBB IgG synthesis as it relates to the etiopathogenesis of MS are included.

REFERENCES

1. Walsh, M. J., W. W. Tourtellotte, A. R. Potvin & J. H. Potvin. 1983. The cerebrospinal fluid in multiple sclerosis. *In* Multiple Sclerosis. Pathology, Diagnosis and Management. J. F. Hallpike, C. W. M. Adams & W. W. Tourtellotte, Eds. Chapman and Hall. London.
2. Walsh, M. J., W. W. Tourtellotte & A. R. Potvin. 1983. Central nervous system immunoglobulin synthesis in neurological disease. Quantitation, specificity, and regulation. *In* Neurobiology of Cerebrospinal Fluid, vol. 2. J. H. Wood, Ed.: 331–368. Plenum Press. New York.
3. Tourtellotte, W. W. & M. J. Walsh. 1984. Cerebrospinal fluid profile indicative of clinical definite multiple sclerosis. *In* Diagnosis of Multiple Sclerosis. C. Poser, Ed. Thieme-Stratton, Inc. New York. In press.
4. Adams, C. M. W. 1983. The general pathology of multiple sclerosis: Morphological and chemical aspects of the lesions. *In* Multiple Sclerosis. Pathology, Diagnosis and Management. J. F. Hallpike, C. W. M. Adams & W. W. Tourtellotte, Eds. Chapman and Hall. London.
5. Prineas, J. W. & R. G. Wright. 1978. Macrophages, lymphocytes, and plasma cells in the perivascular compartment in chronic multiple sclerosis. Lab. Invest. **38:** 409–421.
6. Esiri, M. M. 1980. Multiple sclerosis. A quantitative and qualitative study of immunoglobulin-containing cells in the central nervous system. Neuropathol. Appl. Neurobiol. **6:** 9–21.
7. Traugott, U., E. G. Reinherz & C. S. Raine. 1983. Multiple sclerosis: Distribution of T-cell subsets within active chronic lesions. Science **219:** 308–310.
8. Traugott, U., E. L. Reinherz & C. S. Raine. 1983. Multiple sclerosis. Distribution of T cells, T cell subsets, and Ia-positive macrophages in lesions of different ages. J. Neuroimmunol. **4:** 201–221.
9. Nyland, H., R. Matre, S. Mork, J.-R. Bjerke & A. Naess. 1982. T-lymphocyte subpopulations in multiple sclerosis lesions. (Letter). N. Engl. J. Med. **307:** 1643–1644.
10. Booss, J., M. M. Esiri, W. W. Tourtellotte & D. Y. Mason. 1983. Immunohistological analysis of T lymphocyte subsets in the central nervous system in chronic progressive multiple sclerosis. J. Neurol. Sci. **62:** 219–232.

10a. Weiner, H. L., A. K. Bhan, J. Burks, F. Gilles, C. Kerr, E. Reinherz & S. L. Hauser, 1984. Immunohistochemical analysis of the cellular infiltrate in multiple sclerosis lesions. Neurology **34**(Suppl. 1):112.

10b. McCallum, K., M. M. Esiri, W. W. Tourtellotte & J. Booss. 1984. T cell subsets in the border of multiple sclerosis plaques peak exactly on the edge. Ann. Neurol. **16:** 139.
11. Ebers, G. C., M. Farrell & J. C. Kaufmann. 1983. Oligoclonal bands in MS: Clinical pathological correlation. Neurology **33** (Suppl. 2): 141.
12. Tourtellotte, W. W. & B. I. Ma. 1978. Multiple sclerosis: The blood-brain-barrier and the measurement of *de novo* central nervous system IgG synthesis. Neurology **28**(9, Part 2): 76–83.
13. Schubert, D., A. Munro & S. Ohno. 1968. Immunoglobulin biosynthesis. I. A myeloma variant secreting light chain only. J. Mol. Biol. **38:** 253–262.
14. Tourtellotte, W. W. 1970. Cerebrospinal fluid in multiple sclerosis. *In* Handbook of Clinical Neurology, vol. 9. P. Vinken & G. W. Bruyn, Eds: 324–382. North-Holland Publishing Co. Amsterdam.
15. Adams, C. W. M. 1977. Pathology of multiple sclerosis: Progression of the lesion. Br. Med. Bull. **33:** 15–20.
16. Tourtellotte, W. W., P. Shapshak, R. W. Baumhefner *et al.* 1984. Laboratory aids in the diagnosis of multiple sclerosis. *In* Experimental Allergic Encephalomyelitis: A Useful Model for Multiple Sclerosis. E. C. Alvord, Jr., M. W. Kies & A. J. Suckling, Eds.: 313–321. Alan R. Liss, Inc. New York.
17. Tourtellotte, W. W., A. R. Potvin & M. J. Walsh. 1982. Measurement of intra-blood-brain-barrier IgG synthesis in multiple sclerosis. A review. *In* Multiple Sclerosis East and West. Y. Kuroiwa & L. T. Kurland, Eds: 235–248. Kyushu University Press. Fukuoka, Japan.
18. Tourtellotte, W. W., M. J. Walsh, S. M. Staugaitis *et al.* 1984. Scientific basis of intra-blood-brain-barrier IgG synthesis. Ann. Neurol. In press.
18a. Bocci, L., H. Goren & R. Valenzuela. 1984. Quantitation of intrathecal IgG synthesis in multiple sclerosis: Comparison between Tourtellotte's and Schuller's formulas, link index, and cerebrospinal fluid IgG/albumin ratio. Ann. Neurol. **16:** 143.
19. Tourtellotte, W. W., P. Shapshak, S. M. Staugaitis *et al.* 1983. Do all clinical definite multiple sclerosis patients have evidence of intra-blood-brain-barrier IgG synthesis. Neurology **33** (Suppl 2): 197.
20. Caroscio, J. T., S. Kochwa, H. Sacks *et al.* 1983. Quantitative CSF IgG measurements in multiple sclerosis and other neurological diseases. An update. Arch. Neurol. **40:** 409–413.
21. Mandler, R., R. Valenzuela, H. Goren & S. Slaughter. 1983. Diagnosis of multiple sclerosis using laser immunophelometry and isoelectric focusing. Neurology **30** (Suppl. 2): 123.
22. Wurster, U. 1983. Comparison of formulas for the calculation of intrathecal IgG. *In* Actual Problems in Multiple Sclerosis Research. E. Pedersen, J. Clausen & L. Oades, Eds.: 298–301. Fadl's Forlag. Copenhagen.
23. Felgenhauer, K. 1982. Differentiation of the humoral immune response in inflammatory diseases of the central nervous system. J. Neurol. **228:** 223–237.
24. Tourtellotte, W. W., A. R. Potvin, J. O. Fleming *et al.* 1980. Multiple sclerosis: Measurement and validation of central nervous system IgG synthesis rate. Neurology **30:** 240–244.
25. Tibbling, G., H. Link & S. Ohman. 1977. Principles of albumin and IgG analyses in neurological disorders. I. Establishment of reference values. Scan. J. Clin. Lab. Invest. **37:** 385–90.
26. Vatassery, G. T., T.-Y. Chiang & E. J. Tourje. 1982. Relationship of total lipids, proteins, and albumin in human cerebrospinal fluid with age. Biochem. Med. **27:** 161–167.
27. Tourtellotte, W. W., B. Tavolato, J. A. Parker & P. Comiso. 1971. Cerebrospinal fluid electroimmunodiffusion. An easy, rapid, sensitive, reliable, and valid method for the simultaneous determination of immunoglobulin-G and albumin. Arch. Neurol. **25:** 345–350.
28. Mandler, R., H. Goren & R. Valenzuela. 1982. Value of central nervous system IgG daily synthesis determination in the diagnosis of multiple sclerosis. Neurology **32:** 296.

29. TOURTELLOTTE, W. W. 1975. What is multiple sclerosis? Laboratory criteria for diagnosis. *In* Multiple Sclerosis Research. A. N. Davison, J. H. Humphrey, A. L. Liversedge, W. I. McDonald & J. S. Porterfield, Eds: 9–26. Elsevier. New York.
30. JANEWAY, C. A., F. S. ROSEN, E. MERLER & C. A. ALPER. 1966. The Gamma Globulins. Little, Brown & Co. Boston.
31. LOWENTHAL, A., M. VAN SANDE & D. KARCHER. 1960. The differential diagnosis of neurological diseases by fractionating electrophoretically the CSF G-globulins. J. Neurochem. **6:** 51–56.
32. LATERRE, E. C., A. COLLEWAERT, J. F. HEREMANS & Z. SFAELLO. Electrophoretic morphology of gamma globulins in cerebrospinal fluid of multiple sclerosis and other diseases of the nervous system. Neurology **20:** 982–990.
33. EBERS, G. C. & D. W. PATY. 1980. CSF electrophoresis in one thousand patients. Can. J. Neurol. Sci. **7:** 275–280.
34. MEHTA, P. D., J. A. MILLER & W. W. TOURTELLOTTE. 1982. Oligoclonal IgG bands in plaques from multiple sclerosis brains. Neurology **32:** 372–376.
35. TOURTELLOTTE, W. W., P. SHAPSHAK, S. M. STAUGAITIS & R. E. SAXTON. 1984. Hypothesis: Multiple sclerosis cerebrospinal fluid IgG multiple bands are derived from one or a few IgG secretor cell clones. *In* Experimental Allergic Encephalomyelitis. A Useful Model for Multiple Sclerosis. E. C. Alvord, Jr., M. W. Kies & A. J. Suckling, Eds. Alan R. Liss, Inc. New York.
36. WALSH, M. J., S. M. STAUGAITIS, P. SHAPSHAK & W. W. TOURTELLOTTE. 1982. Ultrasensitive detection of IgG in unconcentrated cerebrospinal fluid utilizing silver nitrate staining after isoelectric focusing and immunofixation. Ann. Neurol. **12:** 114.
37. TOURTELLOTTE, W. W. 1984. CSF studies in EAE and MS. Introductory remarks. *In* Experimental Allergic Encephalomyelitis. A Useful Model for Multiple Sclerosis. E. C. Alvord, Jr., M. W. Kies & A. J. Suckling, Eds.: 329–333. Alan R. Liss, Inc. New York.
38. WALSH, M. J. & W. W. TOURTELLOTTE. 1983. IgG, IgM, and IgA temporal clonal stability in multiple sclerosis. Neurology **33** (Suppl. 2): 123.
39. THOMPSON, E. J., P. KAUFMANN & P. RUDGE. 1983. Sequential changes in oligoclonal patterns during the course of multiple sclerosis. J. Neurol. Neurosurg. Psychiatry **46:** 546–550.
40. MOULIN, D. W., D. W. PATY & G. C. EBERS. 1982. The predictive value of cerebrospinal fluid in "possible" multiple sclerosis. Ann. Neurol. **12:** 104.
41. TOURTELLOTTE, W. W., R. W. BAUMHEFNER, A. R. POTVIN *et al.* 1980. Multiple sclerosis *de novo* CNS IgG synthesis: Effect of ACTH and corticosteroids. Neurology **30:** 1155.
42. TOURTELLOTTE, W. W., A. R. POTVIN, B. I. MA *et al.* 1982. Isotachophoresis quantitation of subfractions of MS intra-BBB IgG synthesis modulated by ACTH and/or steroids. Neurology **32:** 261–266.
43. ALBRECHT, P., W. W. TOURTELLOTTE, J. T. HICKS *et al.* 1983. Intra-blood-brain-barrier measles virus antibody synthesis in multiple sclerosis patients. Neurology **33:** 45–50.
44. VANDENBARK, A. A., F. VAN ROMPAEY, D. NIJST, H. HEYLIGEN & J. RAUS. 1984. Cerebrospinal fluid antibodies detect brain antigens. *In* Immunological and Clinical Aspects of Multiple Sclerosis. R. E. Gonsette & P. Delmotte, Eds. MTP Press. Lancaster.
45. TOURTELLOTTE, W. W., B. I. MA, D. W. BRANDES *et al.* 1981. Quantification of *de novo* central nervous system IgG measles antibody synthesis in SSPE. Ann. Neurol. **9:** 551–556.
46. TOURTELLOTTE, W. W., K. SYNDULKO, R. W. BAUMHEFNER & A. R. POTVIN. 1984. Neuroimmunologic pharmacology of multiple sclerosis. I. A comprehensive protocol for preliminary clinical trials in MS. *In* Immunosuppressive Therapy in Multiple Sclerosis. O. R. Hommes, J. Mertin & W. W. Tourtellotte, Eds. Clinical Trials Journal (Suppl.). In press.
47. GILBERT, J. J. & M. Sadler. 1983. Unsuspected multiple sclerosis. Arch. Neurol. **40:** 533–536.
48. BAUMHEFNER, R. W., W. W. TOURTELLOTTE, K. SYNDULKO *et al.* 1984. Neuroimmunologic pharmacology of multiple sclerosis. II. The evaluation of immunosuppressive

agents. *In* Immunosuppressive Therapy in Multiple Sclerosis. O. R. Hommes, J. Mertin & W. W. Tourtellotte, Eds. Clinical Trials Journal (Suppl.). In press.

49. TOURTELLOTTE, W. W., A. R. POTVIN, R. W. BAUMHEFNER *et al.* 1980. Multiple sclerosis *de novo* CNS IgG synthesis. Effect of CNS irradiation. Arch. Neurol. **37:** 620–624.
50. TOURTELLOTTE, W. W., A. R. POTVIN & M. MENDEZ *et al.* Failure of intravenous and intrathecal cytarabine to modify central nervous system IgG synthesis in multiple sclerosis. Ann. Neurol. **8:** 402–408.
51. SHIH W. W. H., R. W. BAUHEFNER, W. W. TOURTELLOTTE *et al.* 1983. Difference in effect of single immunosuppressive agents (cyclophosphamide, CCNU, 5-FU) on peripheral blood immune cell parameters and central nervous system immunoglobulin synthesis rate in patients with multiple sclerosis. Clin. Exp. Immunol. **53:** 122–132.
52. HAASE, A. T., P. VENTURA, C. J. GIBBS, JR. & W. W. TOURTELLOTTE. 1981. Measles virus nucleotide sequences: Detection by hybridization *in situ*. Science **212:** 672–675.

Pathophysiology of Demyelination[a]

MICHAEL RASMINSKY

Neurosciences Unit
Montreal General Hospital
and
Department of Neurology and Neurosurgery
McGill University
Montreal, Quebec, Canada

Much of the symptomatology of both peripheral and central demyelinating disease can now be satisfactorily explained on the basis of the known physiologic properties of demyelinated nerve fibers.[1–9] These properties reflect not only abnormal morphology, but also changes in the distribution of voltage-sensitive ion channels within demyelinated axon membranes.

ORGANIZATION OF THE AXON MEMBRANE OF MAMMALIAN MYELINATED NERVE FIBERS

Early voltage clamp studies of the voltage and time-dependent permeability properties of squid axon membrane and nodal axon membrane of amphibian myelinated fibers, together with subsequent pharmacological studies of these axons, indicated the coexistence of sodium and potassium channels in these membranes, repolarization during the action potential being enhanced by an increase in potassium permeability which lags the initial explosive increase in sodium permeability.[10] Recent voltage clamp studies have shown the absence of potassium channels from mammalian nodal axon membranes[11,12] and from the nodal axon membranes of small diameter amphibian fibers.[13] Potassium channels are, however, present in internodal axon membrane.[14–16] This exclusion of potassium channels from the nodal axon appears to occur in the course of normal development in both the peripheral nervous system (PNS) and central nervous system (CNS).[17,18]

Our current picture of the axon membrane of myelinated nerve fibers is thus one of highly specialized regionalization, the nodal axon membrane containing sodium channels but excluding potassium channels, and the internodal and paranodal axon membrane containing potassium channels but excluding sodium channels. This concept of regional specialization of the axon membrane is strongly supported by: (1) binding studies with saxitoxin, a drug with high affinity for sodium channels, which indicate a high concentration of sodium channels ($\sim 10^5/\mu m^2$) at nodes and very few, if any, channels ($\leq 25/\mu m^2$) in internodal axon[19]; (2) freeze fracture electron microscopy that reveals high local concentrations of E-face particles at nodes of Ranvier and low concentrations in internodes[20]; and (3) cytochemical staining techniques that are highly specific both for nodal axon membrane and for other membranes assumed to have high sodium channel densities such as the initial segment of CNS neurons and the excitable but not the inexcitable nodes of Ranvier of *Stenarchus* axons.[21]

This orderly division of the axon membrane of myelinated fibers into specific

[a]This work was supported by the Medical Research Council of Canada.

domains presumably reflects one facet of the complex interaction between myelin-producing glial cells—Schwann cells and oligodendroglia—and axons. During demyelination, or in axons in which myelination is congenitally abnormal, absence of this normal interaction is reflected in changes in the normal periodicity of organization of ion channel distribution in the axon membrane.

CONDUCTION IN DEMYELINATED FIBERS

Nerve impulses are conducted in demyelinated axons with reduced conduction velocity, and conduction block is the extreme physiologic consequence of demyelination in both the PNS and CNS.[22,23] It is becoming increasingly apparent that there is no simple correlation between the severity of demyelination as assessed morphologically and the degree of impairment of conduction of nerve impulses. In acute lesions, minimal pathology may be associated with blockage of conduction,[24,25] whereas in more chronic lesions, persistent segmental demyelination is compatible with preserved conduction.[26] It is instructive to consider individually abnormalities of conduction that have been found in a number of different states in which myelination is disrupted, either by acquired pathology, or genetically.

Acute Conduction Block

Serum-mediated Conduction Block

When rabbit antiserum to galactocerebroside (GC), a component of myelin, is injected into rat sciatic nerve, a complete conduction block ensues within a few hours.[24] Pathological changes in the sciatic nerve at the time of onset of the conduction block are limited to minimal paranodal demyelination, widening of Schmidt-Lanterman clefts and some vacuolation and swelling of myelin in the paranodal region and in the region of the Schmidt-Lanterman clefts.[24] In order to elucidate the mechanism of conduction block in the anti-GC lesion, conduction was studied in single rat spinal root fibers subjected to focal application of anti-GC serum over lengths of only a few mm.[25] In the region of serum exposure, conduction time from node to node rose from the normal 20 μec to more than 200 μsec before conduction block eventually ensued (FIGS. 1 and 2). The antiserum acts more quickly on smaller diameter fibers, conduction block occurring within as little as 60 minutes in the more slowly conducting fibers but requiring at least three or four hours in the larger diameter, more rapidly conducting fibers in the roots. That conduction block was due to change in cable properties of serum-exposed fibers in this lesion was inferred from simultaneous recordings of membrane current and extracellular potential (FIG. 3), which showed that conduction block occurred at nodes where relatively large outward currents were associated with relatively small displacements of membrane potential. This finding is consistent with an increased nodal capacitance due to an increase in nodal surface area, but could also reflect an alternate pathway of current to the exterior through the capacitance of the internodal axon, then along the submyelinic periaxonal space and finally through the periaxonal space at the paranode. Hirano and Dembitzer[27] have suggested that an early change in demyelination may be disruption of the transverse bands sealing the terminal loops of the myelinating cell to the axonal membrane. Our previous calculations[25] of an order of magnitude increase in the capacitance (and thus nodal area) of nodes at which conduction block ensued were based on the implicit assumption that the second pathway was not of significance.

Whatever the pathways of current flow, it is clear that acute paranodal demyelination is a sufficient morphologic substrate for conduction block. That this pathology may be insufficient to give rise to conduction block in a more chronic lesion will become apparent in the subsequent discussion.

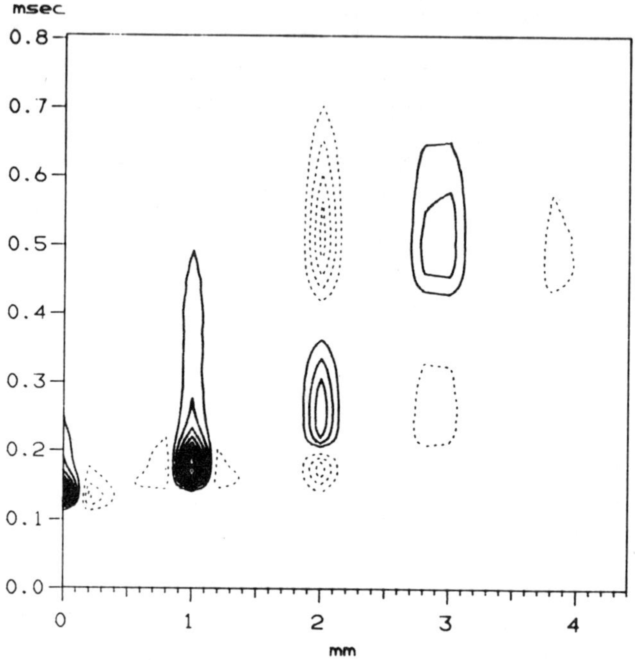

FIGURE 1. Contour plots of membrane current from a rat spinal root fiber after three hours exposure to antiserum to galactocerebroside. The direction of transmission of the nerve impulse is from left to right and time is shown on the ordinate. Inward membrane current is denoted by filled contours, outward membrane current by dotted contours each representing 1.5 nA/200 μm (see ref. 26 for details of the contour-plotting display technique). The sites of inward membrane current indicate the sites of nodes of Ranvier at 0, 1, 2 and 3 mm. Internodal conduction times are successively 40, 85, and 235 μsec in contrast to the normal 20 μsec. Conduction is blocked at the node at 4 mm as indicated by the absence of a phase of inward current following the early outward (depolarizing) current. Note the late outward current following activation of the node at 2 mm. This is presumably potassium current associated with early paranodal demyelination. (From an unpublished experiment by M. Rasminsky, A.J. Sumner and S. Lafontaine.)

Cell-mediated Conduction Block

Yarom *et al.*[28] have recently found that exposure of rat optic nerve to syngeneic T lymphocytes specifically reactive to myelin basic protein causes conduction block in the optic nerve. The effect is highly specific, the sensitized lymphocytes having no effect on conduction in allogeneic optic nerve or syngeneic peripheral nerve. The block is reversible if the sensitized lymphoctes are withdrawn from the optic nerve within two hours. These preliminary experiments did not address the mechanism of the conduc-

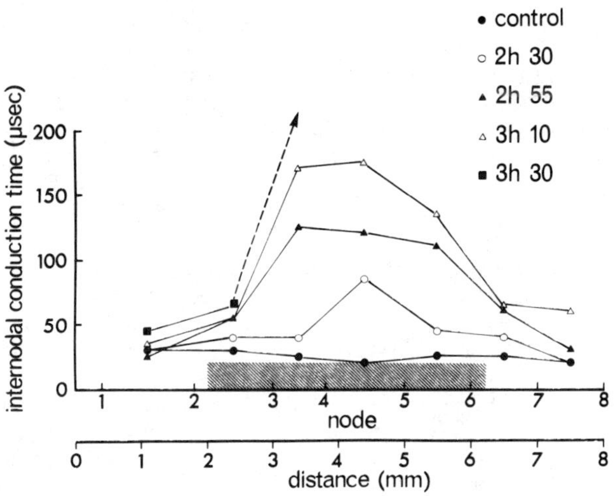

FIGURE 2. Internodal conduction time between eight successive nodes of Ranvier of a rat spinal root fiber exposed to antiserum to galactocerebroside in the region indicated by cross-hatching. There is a monotonous increase in internodal conduction time with increasing duration of exposure to the antiserum until conduction block ensues after 3 hours and 30 minutes. (Reproduced with permission from ref. 25.)

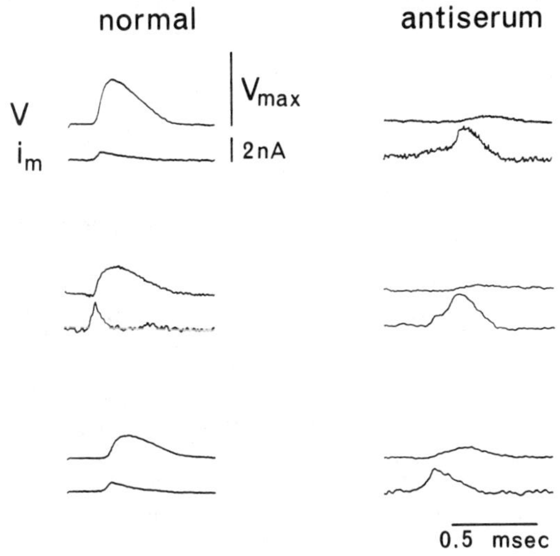

FIGURE 3. Extracellular potential (*upper traces*) and membrane current (*lower traces*) recorded from normal nodes at which conduction was blocked with local anesthetic or tetrodotoxin (*left*) or following exposure to antiserum to galactocerebroside (*right*). Voltage scale shows amplitude of the action potential in a normally conducting portion of the same fiber. Upward deflection in current records is outward membrane current. (Reproduced with permission from ref. 25.)

tion block. Because of the marked specificity of the lymphocytes for a myelin antigen, it is likely that the physiologic effect of these lymphocytes is due to conduction abnormalities similar to those resulting from exposure to anti-GC serum. It is tempting to speculate that the effect and its reversibility are related to loss and reestablishment of the normal close apposition of glial terminal loops to paranodal axonal membrane. Plasticity of structure of the paranodal region may be a feature of normal nerve fibers.[29]

Conduction of Nerve Impulses in Demyelinated Fibers

More than twenty years ago, McDonald[22] demonstrated conduction slowing and conduction block in peripheral nerve fibers of cats subjected to systemic intoxication with diphtheria toxin. McDonald and Sears[23] subsequently showed similar conduction abnormalities in central nerve fibers exposed to focal injection of diphtheria toxin and also demonstrated the increased refractory period of these fibers and their inability to transmit trains of impulses at high frequency. In our initial studies of the mode conduction in diphtheria demyelinated spinal root fibers, we[30] observed preservation of saltatory conduction in slowly conducting demyelinated nerve fibers, the variably increased delay in depolarization of successive nodes to threshold for excitation being attributed to the variably increased capacitance of successive demyelinated internodes.

Bostock and Sears[26] subsequently found that conduction was not invariably saltatory in axons demyelinated by diphtheria toxin. They observed continuous conduction at greatly reduced conduction velocity over lengths of $\geqslant 1$ mm in some axons a few days after exposure to diphtheria toxin. This implies a density of sodium channels in the demyelinated axon adequate to sustain continuous conduction. In light of our current understanding of the partitioning of myelinated axon membrane into sodium channel-rich nodal axon and sodium channel-poor internodal axon, this demonstration of continuous conduction in diphtheria demyelinated axons constitutes very strong evidence for reorganization of the distribution of sodium channels in demyelinated axon membrane. It is likely that resumption of continuous conduction is favored in smaller diameter axons with smaller membrane capacitance.

Bostock and Sears[26] observed relatively normal action potentials at some nodes with increased capacitance in diphtheria toxin demyelinated fibers and inferred that the widening of the node in chronic paranodal demyelination was compensated by increased numbers of sodium channels. This prediction was explicitly confirmed by voltage clamp studies of isolated fibers with paranodal demyelination.[31] Unlike the case of the *acute* anti-GC lesion, *chronic* paranodal demyelination probably is not a sufficient morphological substrate for conduction block.

Resumption of conduction in axons demyelinated by lysolecithin differs somewhat from that in diphtheria toxin demyelinated axons.[32] For the first few days following segmental demyelination by lysolecithin, conduction is blocked in rat spinal root fibers. After about four days the demyelinated axon membrane appears to be electrically excitable but impulses die out within a few hundred μm after entering the region of demyelination, presumably because of an insufficient density of sodium channels to sustain propagation in the highly capacitive bare axon membrane. By six days, before remyelination has begun, propagation becomes more secure, probably because of recruitment of further sodium channels into the axon membrane.[32] However, rather than being continuous, as is the case for diphtheria demyelinated axons, excitation jumps in a saltatory fashion between sites of excitability 100–200 μm apart which Smith *et al.*[32] have called physiologic nodes or ϕ-nodes. As remyelination ensues, the separation between sites of electrical excitability increases, corresponding to the lengthening of internodes.

Potassium Currents in Demyelinated Fibers

During excitation of demyelinated axons, the inward membrane current carried by sodium ions is succeeded by a late outward membrane current that can be eliminated by application of the potassium channel blockers 4-aminopyridine (4AP) or tetraethylammonium (TEA).[33] This implies the presence of potassium channels in chronically demyelinated paranodal or internodal axon membrane. An example of such late outward current at an acutely demyelinated node is shown in FIGURE 1. Postassium channels are present in normal paranodal and internodal axon[14–16]; it is not known if they undergo redistribution as a consequence of demyelination as do sodium channels.

Dystrophic Mouse Axons

In the lumbosacral spinal roots of dystrophic mice, many large diameter axons congenitally lack ensheathment over lengths of up to several mm.[34,35] Those axons that are ensheathed have widened nodes, internodes inappropriately short for the axon diameter and inappropriately thin myelin.[35,36] Both continuous and saltatory conduction have been observed in these unusual axons,[36,37] but the distribution of ion channels is somewhat different from that observed in demyelinated nerves. Although a uniform distribution of sodium channels is seen in the bare axons of dystrophic mice, appreciable late outward current is seen only at widely separated foci. Potassium channels in these congenitally unmyelinated axons thus appear to be less ubiquitous than in demyelinated axons, although they are found at many nodes of Ranvier, occasionally even in the absence of sodium channels.[37]

Organization of Axon Membrane in Demyelinated Fibers

As noted above, there are impressive differences in the patterns of (re)organization of axon membranes in various pathological states of myelination. Sodium channels appear to become uniformly distributed in diphtheria demyelinated axons[26] in contrast to their segregation into ϕ-nodes in the early stages of lysolecithin demyelination.[32] There also appear to be differences in the distribution of potassium channels when comparisons are made between the bare axons of dystrophic mice and demyelinated axons. The existence of these differences in the patterns of axon membrane organization suggests the possibility that the nature of the interaction (or lack of it) with potential myelin-forming glial cells is an important determinant of the channel organization of axon membranes.

In addition to the evidence from physiological studies, there is some inferential morphologic evidence suggestive of axonal reorganization in the wake of demyelination. Foster *et al.*[38] have observed changes in patterns of axonal staining with the Fe^{+++}/ferrocyanide stain following demyelination and Rosenbluth[39] has observed freeze fracture specializations in axon membranes of mutant mice that can be related to the proximity of glial cells. More precise information concerning the distribution of ion channels in pathological axons will undoubtedly soon be forthcoming from the application of staining techniques using monoclonal antibodies to ion channels.

ENHANCEMENT OF CONDUCTION IN DEMYELINATED FIBERS

Conduction is blocked in demyelinated axons at sites where depolarizing current is insufficient to depolarize axon membrane to threshold for excitation or at sites where the denuded axon membrane contains an insufficient complement of sodium channels to regenerate a propagated action potential despite depolarization to threshold. Conduction can be restored in demyelinated fibers by remyelination, by manipulation of the currents generated by demyelinated axons and, as noted above, by changes in the ion channel distribution in demyelinated axons.

Remyelination

Schwann cells readily remyelinate demyelinated peripheral axons, and conduction velocity in such axons increases dramatically as myelin thickness and internodal length increases.[40] Remyelination is also associated with increased security of conduction as assessed by decreased refractory period of transmission.[40] Remyelination of peripheral nerves is accompanied by formation of new nodes of Ranvier with an apparently normal complement of sodium channels.[41] Remyelination by oligodendroglial cells occurs in some CNS demyelinating lesions,[42] and secure conduction is restored in the CNS lysolecithin lesion coincident with remyelination.[43] Theoretical considerations[44] suggest that relatively little remyelination is necessary for dramatic increases in conduction velocity and security of conduction in demyelinated axons. Except for the rather impractical expedient of transplanting Schwann cells into the CNS,[45] no way has yet been found to promote remyelination in the CNS.

Manipulation of Currents Generated by Demyelinated Fibers

Conduction block in some demyelinated fibers can be overcome by small reductions in temperature.[46] Decreasing temperature increases the duration of the nerve action potential and increases the time integral of inward membrane current generated by excited membrane. The adjacent membrane can thus be more depolarized by the additional inward membrane current and this slight additional depolarization may represent the difference between secure conduction and conduction block.

Two other procedures have been used experimentally to delay the repolarization phase of the action potential and thus to enhance the security of conduction in regions of demyelination. The action potential of mammalian nerve fibers can be markedly prolonged by application of *Leiurus* toxin which blocks sodium inactivation and thus prolongs the inward sodium current. Application of this drug consistently increases the blocking temperature of demyelinated nerve fibers.[47] A more physiologic approach to prolongation of the action potential of demyelinated fibers is the application of 4AP or TEA.[33] The drugs increase the net inward current generated by demyelinated axons by blocking the delayed late outward current flowing through potassium channels. Unlike *Leiurus* toxin, the potassium channel blockers have no effect on normal nodal axon membrane which has no functional potassium channels.

ECTOPIC GENERATION OF IMPULSES IN PATHOLOGICALLY MYELINATED AXONS

Nerve impulses are ordinarily generated only at cell bodies or at nerve terminals specialized for this purpose. However, in several types of pathological axons impulses arise in mid-axon either spontaneously, or in response to mechanical stimuli that would be ineffective in normal axons.

Peripheral axons demyelinated by the experimental granuloma technique,[48] or central axons demyelinated by focal microinjection of lysolecithin,[49] become exquisitely mechanosensitive, generating showers of impulses in response to minimal mechanical stimuli. Single impulses propagating into the site of hyperexcitability in such axons may give rise to a burst of impulses in response, this manifestation of hyperexcitability being enhanced by decreased Ca^{++} or pCO_2.[50] In spinal root axons of dystrophic mice, hyperexcitability is manifested by spontaneous generation of impulses, ephaptic transmission between adjacent single fibers and by repetitive responses to single stimuli.[51–53] In contrast, axons demyelinated by exposure to diphtheria toxin manifest little or no spontaneous ectopic activity and do not have local sites of decreased threshold to electrical stimulation.[54]

The differences in pathological excitability among various types of abnormally myelinated axons may be related to the above noted differences in ion channel distributions. Chiu and Ritchie[15,16] have suggested that retention of potassium channels in normal paranodal and internodal axon membrane serves as a protection against repetitive firing at nodes in the eventuality of demyelination. This suggestion is reinforced by the finding that blockage of potassium channels in developing,[55] regenerating,[56,57] or lysolecithin demyelinated central[49] or peripheral[58] nerve fibers leads to increased excitability manifested by increased spontaneous activity or multiple responses to single stimuli.

Although the precise mechanism of spontaneous impulse generation or repetitive firing in the various axons described above remains to be elucidated, it appears likely that it is somehow related to a relative paucity of functioning potassium channels (either congenitally as in some portions of some dystrophic mouse spinal root axons, or because of pharmacologic blockade) near areas of membrane where spontaneous excitation or repetitive firing occur, areas where there must be substantial local densities of sodium channels. Differences in ectopic excitability of various pathological axons may reflect differences in the patterns of distribution of sodium and potassium channels.

CLINICAL IMPLICATIONS

Conduction Block

The importance of conduction block in giving rise to negative symptoms of demyelination such as blindness, sensory loss, motor weakness and ataxia need not be belabored. Fatiguability of muscle may reflect the inability of demyelinated fibers to transmit trains of impulses at high frequency.[7] Transient negative symptomatology such as that frequently seen with increased body temperature is satisfactorily accounted for on the basis of reversible conduction block in the appropriate population of demyelinated central nerve fibers.[46]

Slowing of Conduction

The importance of decreased conduction velocity of demyelinated fibers in symptom production is much less clear-cut. Several lines of evidence suggest that this may be of limited importance. Conduction velocity in regions of demyelination may be locally slowed up to 40-fold without conduction block.[26,30] Conduction block with increased temperature occurs only in demyelinated fibers with substantial preexisting slowing of conduction at the site of block.[46] In pathways containing relatively short axons such as some of those subserving eye movements or vision, involvement of only a few internodes with demyelination sufficient to give rise to a temperature-sensitive conduction block will thus result in substantial decreases in end-to-end average conduction velocity. The abrupt onset of signs or symptoms such as nystagmus or visual blurring with small increases in body temperature in some individuals suggests that such reductions in conduction velocity are clinically well tolerated until conduction block ensues.

Further evidence of the ability of the nervous system to tolerate slowed central conduction velocity comes from evoked potential studies of individuals with MS in whom increased latencies are often found in the absence of corresponding clinical deficits. This poor correlation between conduction slowing and symptomatology suggests caution in the use of evoked potential techniques as a tool for assessing the efficacy of putative therapeutic regimes in MS. The use of evoked potentials in confirming clinically apparent deficits is usually unnecessary[59]— and abnormalities in evoked potentials are unlikely to disappear completely even in the face of clinical resolution of a deficit.[60] Changes in latency of evoked potential waves recorded from clinically normal portions of the CNS may reflect differences in myelination and/or ion channel distributions but give no necessary indication of clinical improvement. This predictable lack of correlation between clinical status and findings in evoked potential studies is now being confirmed with empirical longitudinal studies.[61]

Some functions of the nervous system do depend on very precise timing and here abnormalities of conduction velocity may be of crucial importance. The best documented of these in the clinical context of MS is the loss of stereoscopic vision experienced by some patients on recovery from optic neuritis despite excellent visual acuity in the recovered eye. This presumably reflects failure of input from the two eyes to impinge upon relevant cortical neurons with the required degree of simultaneity.[7] Fine sensory discrimination may also be dependent upon temporal coherence of sensory input.[7]

Recovery Processes in Multiple Sclerosis

One of the most striking clinical features of multiple sclerosis is the frequent dramatic improvement in symptomatology within short periods of time. This presumably reflects resumption of conduction in populations of fibers in which there had previously been conduction block. The most likely explanation of resumed conduction is reorganization of axon membrane with the insertion of new sodium channels at widened notes or in bared internodal axon membrane. That continuous conduction does indeed occur in demyelinated central axons is strongly suggested by pathologically documented cases of preserved vision in individuals with totally demyelinated optic nerves.[7] There are now many reports of individuals with so-called "silent MS" who are found at autopsy to have extensive demyelinating lesions with no historical evidence of neurologic deficit. It is likely that demyelination in such individuals is, at least to some extent, compensated by axon membrane reorganization.

Remyelination in experimental CNS demyelination is associated with return of function.[43] However, since remyelination in multiple sclerosis is not impressive, it is unlikely that this is usually a major factor in recovery.

The importance of the role of CNS edema in causing acute conduction block remains unclear. It is theoretically arguable that axonal compression would increase axial resistance to forward current flow and thus further compromise conduction in demyelinated axons with low safety factor. This would be particularly likely to occur in a confined space such as the optic nerve where swelling of the nerve is limited by the optic nerve sheath. In this situation, relief of compression might theoretically predispose towards resumption of conduction and resolution of symptoms.

The role of "circulating factors" in MS sera temporarily affecting conduction in demyelinated fibers is even more problematic. Although such factors were originally suggested almost twenty years ago on the basis of tissue culture studies,[62] there is still no evidence that factors in MS sera have any specific deleterious effect on conduction in demyelinated nerve fibers.[63] It has, however, been suggested that such factors might have some effect on synaptic function.[63]

Positive Symptoms

Positive symptoms of MS can be understood in relation to the ectopic excitability and sensitivity to mechanical stimulation of demyelinated nerve fibers.[4] Paresthesias experienced on neck flexion (Lhermitte's phenomenon) probably reflect excitation due to mechanical deformation of demyelinated fibers in the dorsal columns in the cervical spinal cord.[49] Some patients with optic neuritis "see" flashes of light in the affected eye on eye movement. These visual phosphenes can also be accounted for by mechanical stimulation of demyelinated fibers in the affected nerve.[64]

Other positive symptoms such as tic douleureux, facial myokymia, muscle spasms, and dysesthesias of various types, may arise spontaneously and paroxysmally, particularly in relation to anxiety or hyperventilation.[65–68] The reduction in ionized serum calcium caused by hyperventilation may be an important factor in increasing the excitability of already hyperexcitable foci in fibers coursing through plaques of demyelination. The occurrence of ephaptic transmission has not been experimentally proven in demyelinated nerve fibers; the suggestion that this has a role in production of positive symptoms is supported only by the inferential clinical evidence.[4]

Positive symptoms frequently respond well to treatment with diphenylhydantoin or carbamazepine. It is likely that these drugs act by suppressing ectopic generation in demyelinated fibers.[4] As noted above, the excitability of some demyelinated fibers is enhanced by exposure to potassium channel blockers such as 4AP. Administration of such drugs could theoretically be of value as a means of alleviating negative symptoms of MS.[3,5,33] However, production of positive symptoms may prove to be a major limiting factor in their use.

CONCLUSION

Much of the symptomatology of MS can now, at least in broad outline, be understood in relation to the known properties of demyelinated nerve fibers. In the last few years it has become clear that the physiologic properties of demyelinated fibers are not predictable solely on the basis of their morphology. Demyelination must be regarded simply as the first of a sequence of events affecting not only glial cells but also the axons ensheathed by them. The distribution of ion channels within axon membranes is a major determinant of the physiologic properties of nerve fibers. As yet we have little insight into the reasons for the apparent differences in the distribution of these channels in different types of pathologically myelinated or demyelinated axons.

REFERENCES

1. HALLIDAY, A. M. & W. I. MCDONALD. 1977. Pathophysiology of demyelinating disease. Br. Med. Bull. **33:** 21–27.

2. RASMINSKY, M. 1978. Physiology of conduction in demyelinated axons. *In* Physiology and Pathobiology of Axons. S. G. Waxman, Ed.: 361–376, Raven Press. New York.
3. SEARS, T. A., H. BOSTOCK & M. SHERRATT. 1978. The pathophysiology of demyelination and its implications for the symptomatic treatment of multiple sclerosis. Neurology (Minneap.) **28**(2): 21–26.
4. RASMINSKY, M. 1981. Hyperexcitability of pathologically myelinated axons and positive symptoms in multiple sclerosis. Adv. Neurol. **31:** 289–297.
5. SEARS, T. A. & H. BOSTOCK. 1981. Conduction failure in demyelination: Is it inevitable? Adv. Neurol. **31:** 357–75.
6. WAXMAN, S. G. 1981. Clinicopathological correlations in multiple sclerosis and related diseases. Adv. Neurol. **31:** 169–182.
7. MCDONALD, W. I. 1982. Clinical consequence of conduction defects produced by demyelination. *In* Abnormal Nerves and Muscles as Impulse Generators. W. J. Culp & J. Ochoa, Eds.: 253–270. Oxford University Press. New York.
8. RASMINSKY, M. 1982. Physiologic properties of demyelinated nerve fibers. *In* Disorders of the Motor Unit, D. L. Schotland, Ed.: 61–74, John Wiley & Sons. New York.
9. WAXMAN, S. 1982. Membranes, myelin, and the pathophysiology of multiple sclerosis. N. Eng. J. Med. **306:** 1529–1533.
10. HILLE, B. 1977. Ionic basis of resting and action potentials. *In* Handbook of Physiology: Section I. The Nervous System. E. R. Kandel, Ed.: **1:** 99–136, Williams & Wilkins Co. Baltimore.
11. CHIU, S. Y., J. M. RITCHIE, R. B. ROGART & D. STAGG. 1979. A quantitative description of membrane currents in rabbit myelinated nerve fibres. J. Physiol. (London) **292:** 149–166.
12. BRISMAR, T. 1980. Potential clamp analysis of membrane currents in rat myelinated nerve fibres. J. Physiol. (London) **298:** 171–184
13. SMITH, K. J. & C. L. SCHAUF. 1981. Size-dependent variation of nodal properties in myelinated nerve. Nature (London) **293:** 297–299.
14. CHIU, S. Y. & J. M. RITCHIE. 1980. Potassium channels in nodal and internodal axonal membrane of mammalian myelinated fibres. Nature (London) **284:** 170–171.
15. CHIU, S. Y. & J. M. RITCHIE. 1981. Evidence for the presence of potassium channels in the paranodal region of acutely demyelinated mammalian single nerve fibres. J. Physiol. (London) **313:** 415–437.
16. RITCHIE, J. M. & S. Y. CHIU. 1981. Distribution of sodium and potassium channels in mammalian myelinated nerve. Adv. Neurol. **31:** 329–342.
17. RITCHIE, J. M. 1982. Sodium and potassium channels in regenerating and developing mammalian myelinated nerves. Proc. R. Soc. Lond. **B 215:** 273–287.
18. FOSTER, R. E., B. W. CONNORS & S. G. WAXMAN. 1982. Rat optic nerve: Electrophysiological, pharmacolgical and anatomical studies during development. Dev. Brain Res. **3:** 371–386.
19. RITCHIE, J. M. & R. B. ROGART. 1977. Density of sodium channels in mammalian myelinated nerve fibers and nature of the axonal membrane under the myelin sheath. Proc. Nat. Acad. Sci. U.S.A. **74:** 211–215.
20. ROSENBLUTH, J. 1976. Intramembranous particle distribution at the node of Ranvier and adjacent axolemma in myelinated axons of the frog brain. J. Neurocytol. **5:** 731–745.
21. WAXMAN, S. G. 1981. Plasticity in the ontogeny and pathophysiology of myelinated fibers. Adv. Neurol. **31:** 69–92.
22. MCDONALD, W. I. 1963. The effects of experimental demyelination on conduction in peripheral nerve: A histological and electrophysiological study. II. Electrophysiological observations. Brain **86:** 501–524.
23. MCDONALD, W. I. & T. A. SEARS. 1970. The effects of experimental demyelination on conduction in the central nervous system. Brain **93:** 583–598.
24. SUMNER, A. J., K. SAIDA, T. SAIDA, D. H. SILBERBERG & A. K. ASBURY. 1981. Acute conduction block associated with experimental antiserum-mediated demyelination of peripheral nerve. Ann. Neurol. **11:** 469–477.
25. LAFONTAINE, S., M. RASMINSKY, T. SAIDA & A. J. SUMNER. 1982. Conduction block in rat myelinated fibres following acute exposure to anti-galactocerebroside serum. J. Physiol. (London) **323:** 287–306.

26. Bostock, H. & T. A. Sears. 1978. The internodal axon membrane: Electrical excitability and continuous conduction in segmental demyelination. J. Physiol. (London) **280:** 273–301.
27. Hirano, A. & H. M. Dembitzer. 1978. Morphology of normal central myelinated axons. *In* Physiology and Pathobiology of Axons. S. G. Waxman, Ed.: 65–82. Raven Press. New York.
28. Yarom.Y., Y. Naparstek, V. Lev-ram, J. Holoshitz, A. Ben-nun & I. R. Cohen. 1983. Immunospecific inhibition of nerve conduction by T lymphocytes reactive to basic protein of myelin. Nature (London) **303:** 246–247.
29. Moran, O. & L. Mateu. 1983. Loosening of paranodal myelin by repetitive propagation of action potentials. Nature (London) **304:** 344–345.
30. Rasminsky, M. & T. A. Sears. 1972. Internodal conduction in undissected demyelinated nerve fibres. J. Physiol. (London) **227:** 323–350.
31. Brismar, T. 1981. Specific permeability properties of demyelinated rat nerve fibres. Acta Physiol. Scand. **113:** 167–76.
32. Smith, K. J., H. Bostock & S. M. Hall. 1982. Saltatory conduction precedes remyelination in axons demyelinated with lysophosphatidyl choline. J. Neurol. Sci. **54:** 13–31.
33. Bostock, H., T. A. Sears & R. M. Sherratt. 1981. The effects of 4-aminopyridine and tetraethyl-ammonium ions on normal and demyelinated mammalian nerve fibres. J. Physiol. (London) **313:** 301–315.
34. Bradley, W. G. & M. Jenkison. 1973. Abnormalities of peripheral nerve in murine muscular dystrophy. J. Neurol. Sci. **18:** 227–247.
35. Bray, G. M. & A. J. Aguayo. 1975. Quantitative ultrastructural studies of axon-Schwann cell abnormality in spinal nerve roots from dystrophic mice. J. Neuropathol. Exp. Neurol. **34:** 517–530.
36. Rasminsky, M., R. E. Kearney, A. J. Aguayo & G. M. Bray. 1978. Conduction of nervous impulses in spinal roots and peripheral nerves of dystrophic mice. Brain Res. **143:** 71–85.
37. Bostock, H. & M. Rasminsky. 1983. Potassium channel distribution in spinal root axons of dystrophic mice. J. Physiol. (London) **340:** 145–156.
38. Foster, R. E., C. C. Whalen & S. G. Waxman. 1980. Reorganization of the axon membrane in demyelinated peripheral nerve fibers: Morphological evidence. Science **210:** 661–663.
39. Rosenbluth, J. 1981. Freeze-fracture approaches to ionophore localization in normal and myelin-deficient nerves. Adv. Neurol. **31:** 391–418.
40. Smith, K. J. & S. M. Hall. 1980. Nerve conduction during peripheral demyelination and remyelination. J. Neurol. Sci. **48:** 201–19.
41. Ritchie, J. M., H. P. Rang & R. Pellegrino. 1981. Sodium and postassium channels in demyelinated and remyelinated mammalian nerve. Nature (London) **294:** 257–259.
42. Ludwin, S. K. 1981. Pathology of demyelination and remyelination. Adv. Neurol. **31:** 123–168.
43. Smith, K. J., W. F. Blakemore & W. I. McDonald. 1981. The restoration of conduction by central remyelination. Brain **104:** 383–404.
44. Koles, J. Z. & M. Rasminsky. A computer simulation of conduction in demyelinated nerve fibres. J. Physiol. (London) **227:** 351–364.
45. Harrison, B. H. 1980. Remyelination by cells introduced into a stable demyelinating lesion in the central nervous system. J. Neurol. Sci. **46:** 63–81.
46. Rasminsky, M. 1973. The effects of temperature on conduction in demyelinated single nerve fibers. Arch. Neurol. **28:** 287–292.
47. Bostock, H., R. M. Sherratt & T. A. Sears. 1978. Overcoming conduction failure in demyelinated nerve fibers by prolonging action potentials. Nature (London) **274:** 385–387.
48. Howe, J. F., J. D. Loeser & W. H. Calvin. 1977. Mechanosensitivity of dorsal root ganglia and chronically injured axons: A physiological basis for the radicular pain of nerve root compression. Pain **3:** 25–41.
49. Smith, K. J. & W. I. McDonald. 1982. Spontaneous and evoked electrical discharges from a central demyelinating lesion. J. Neurol. Sci. **55:** 39–47.

50. BURCHIEL, K. J. 1981. Ectopic impulse generation in demyelinated axons: Effects of P_aCO_2, pH and disodium edetate. Ann. Neurol. **9:** 378–383.
51. HUIZAR, P., M. KUNO & Y. MIYATA. 1975. Electrophysiological properties of spinal motoneurons of normal and dystrophic mice. J. Physiol. (London) **248:** 231–246.
52. RASMINSKY, M. 1978. Ectopic generation of impulses and cross-talk in spinal nerve roots of "dystrophic" mice. Ann Neurol. **3:** 351–357.
53. RASMINSKY, M. 1980. Ephaptic transmission between single nerve fibres in the spinal nerve roots of dystrophic mice. J. Physiol. (London) **305:** 151–169.
54. BOSTOCK, H., T. A. SEARS & R. M. SHERRATT. 1983. The spatial distribution of excitability and membrane current in normal and demyelinated mammalian nerve fibres. J. Physiol. (London) **341:** 41–58.
55. KOCSIS, J. D., J. A. RUIZ & S. G. WAXMAN. 1983. Maturation of mammalian myelinated fibers: Changes in action potential characteristics following 4-aminopyridine application. J. Neurophysiol. **50:** 449–463.
56. KOCSIS, J. D., S. G. WAXMAN, C. HILDEBRAND & J. A. RUIZ. 1982. Regenerating mammalian nerve fibres: Changes in action potential waveform and firing characteristics following blockage of potassium conductance. Proc. R. Soc. London **B 217:** 277–287.
57. KOCSIS, J. D. & S. G. WAXMAN. 1983. Long-term regenerated nerve fibres retain sensitivity to potassium channel blocking agents. Nature **304:** 640–642.
58. WAXMAN, S. G., J. D. KOCSIS, D. L. ENG & R. J. PRESTON. 1983. Demyelinated nerve fibers: Burst activity following blockage of G_K. Soc. Neurosci. Abstr. **9:** 1103.
59. EISEN, A. & R. Q. CRACCO. 1983. Overuse of evoked potentials: Caution. Neurology **33:** 618–621.
60. HALLIDAY, A. M. 1981. Visual evoked potentials in demyelinating disease. Adv. Neurol. **31:** 201–215.
61. DAVIS, S. L., M. J. AMINOFF & H. S. PANITCH. 1983. Serial somatosensory evoked potentials in multiple sclerosis: Limited correlation with clinical disease activity. Ann. Neurol. **14:** 147.
62. BORNSTEIN, M. D. & S. M. CRAIN. 1965. Functional studies of cultured brain tissues as related to demyelinative disorders. Science **148:** 1242–1244.
63. SCHAUF, C. L. & F. A. DAVIS. 1981. Circulating toxic factors in multiple sclerosis: A perspective. Adv. Neurol. **31:** 267–280.
64. DAVIS, F. A., D. BERGEN, C. SCHAUF, I. MCDONALD & W. DEUTSCH. 1976. Movement phosphenes in optic neuritis: A new clinical sign. Neurology (Minneap.) **26:** 1100–1104.
65. EKBOM, K. A., C-E. WESTERBERG & P. O. OSTERMAN. 1968. Sensory-motor seizures of spinal origin. Lancet **1:** 67.
66. MATTHEWS, W. B. 1975. Paroxysmal symptoms in multiple sclerosis. J. Neurol. Neurosurg. Psychiatry **38:** 617–623.
67. OSTERMAN, P. O. & C-E. WESTERBERG. 1975. Paroxysmal attacks in multiple sclerosis. Brain **98:** 189–202.
68. TOYOKURA, Y., M. SAKUTA & T. NAKANISHI. 1978. Painful tonic seizures in multiple sclerosis. Neurology (Minneap.) **26** (6, Part 2): 18–19.

GENERAL DISCUSSION

M. APPEL (*Cornell University*): First I want to caution against the treatment of multiple sclerosis with desensitization by myelin basic protein. We have tried this in dogs and using Dr. Raine's regimen, have produced classical EAE. So one species may respond differently from another. Then I have a question to Dr. Prineas. There seems to be a basic difference between early lesions in EAE and in MS. The EAE situation was invasion of T cells, and if they find the target, the consequence is logical. In MS, we have seen that antibody is present and macrophages invade first. My question is, can one of the components alone, macrophages or antibody, in the presence of complement initiate demyelination? If macrophages invade alone, the vascular leakage may be explainable. If not, what causes vascular damage and what is the target of antibody?

J. W. PRINEAS (*University of Medicine and Dentistry of New Jersey, Newark*): The material that I examined doesn't allow me to make any comment as to what numbers and types of lymphocytes are there concurrently with a macrophage or indeed whether or not they precede in appearance the macrophage. Everything I've shown is entirely consistent with there being quite a large population of mononuclear cells there. The only evidence that I offered as to the number and types of cells was morphological and there's no doubt that there are lymphocytes there which have a morphology consistent with that of T cells. With regard to time, I don't think that you can discuss that with regard to the chronic progressive lesion. With regard to the early lesion, it's a useful question to ask, does the lymphocyte precede the macrophage? And I have no data on that. I understand Drs. Traugott and Raine have some data on that in terms of what cells appear first based on a few cases and on plaques that have been there for several weeks. We have no data at present as to when the lymphocyte appears in the acute MS lesion, in particular whether it precedes the appearance of macrophages and changes in the blood-brain barrier.

R. M. HERNDON (*University of Rochester Medical Center, Rochester, NY*): Dr. Raine, if I remember correctly, you showed some time ago in a tissue culture system that antibody to myelin basic protein would split the intra-period line. . . .

C. S. RAINE (*Albert Einstein College of Medicine, Bronx, NY*): Antibody to whole myelin would split the intra-period line.

HERNDON: I mis-remembered then, that is consistent then with the localization of BP in the major dense line. The second question is also directed to you. You indicated that if you induced EAE with myelin basic protein you did not get demyelination. Does that apply only to the minimal dosage level or does that apply to even higher doses with MBP?

RAINE: It goes up to about 150 μg of MBP per animal. I haven't tried higher doses and it only works reliably in the guinea pig and the rat. Other species have different responses. The mouse in particular shows both demyelination and inflammation after MBP. Most mouse models are given about 400 μg of MBP, so it is a larger dose. Although there is no direct comparison, I have the feeling that the dose has got to be relatively small in order to dissect inflammation from demyelination.

HERNDON: Then that's also consistent with the idea that the basic protein is not exposed on the surface of the myelin.

RAINE: It's consistent with that.

HERNDON: This is directed to both Drs. Raine and Rasminsky. The statement was made that remyelination was not clinically significant in MS and I think the physiologic evidence would contradict that if what I understand is correct. That is, that if you get demyelination and you get no small segments of remyelination at the plaque edge, that you will have an impedance mismatch and will have in effect a conduction block. We know that you can conduct in demyelinated segments from the work on optic nerve. I wonder if you'd care to comment on this very small, probably significant, amount of remyelination near the plaque margin and on the physiologic effect.

RAINE: I think Dr. Prineas would agree with me that remyelination is always there and one can always find it. Its amount is small; it's a very thin rim around most lesions. Perhaps Dr. Rasminsky could address the physiology of that and the clinical significance.

M. RASMINSKY (*Montreal General Hospital and McGill University, Montreal*): It's certainly the case, one shouldn't denigrate the importance of remyelination. In fact Zolly, Pose and I years ago did computer simulations and the figures, which shouldn't be taken seriously (though the idea should), showed that a very small amount of remyelination may make a difference between conduction block and secure conduction. That every little bit helps, I think, is the answer to the question about remyelination. As far as impedance mismatch is concerned, I find that a difficult question. This is an idea that was introduced by Dr. Waxman, who showed from computer simulations that even if one had axon membrane with a reasonable amount of sodium channels there was no guarantee that conduction was going to proceed. It depends very much how you do the simulation and you can get out of a computer simulation whatever you like. It is the case that conduction does appear to resume more quickly, or more easily in smaller diameter demyelinated fibers than in larger diameter myelinated fibers and that speaks in favor of Drs. Bostock and Sears who have pointed out the impedance mismatch idea. I think only when we have techniques for staining axon membranes with monoclonal antibodies to sodium channels shall we see what is actually happening in axon membranes, not inferentially from physiology, but actually see it by morphology. One should probably reserve discussion about the importance of impedance mismatch in concentrations of sodium channels.

J. N. WHITAKER (*Memphis Veterans Administration Medical Center*): Dr. Tourtellotte, in your study and those of the morphology or the changes of perivascular infiltration after ACTH, one might infer that the oligoclonal band-secreting plasma cells are out in the parenchyma, whereas those producing the bulk amount of IgG that you detect through your synthetic rate determination are produced in the perivascular compartment. Is that inference right? Did you mean to imply that or is that just speculation at this point?

W. W. TOURTELLOTTE (*Veterans Administration Wadsworth Medical Center, Los Angeles, CA*): Well, that's a question that I think we can only extract from our data and the way we come up with our two compartment system is based on our immunopharmacological studies and our proposal is that perhaps the B lymphocytes or the cell that's going to mature into the plasma cell is the one that is blocked by the steroid. Then you end up with a plasmacyte type of inflammation in the brain and perhaps this plasmacyte has a longer half-life than what we usually assign to the plasmacyte because the IgG oligoclonal bands are very difficult to eradicate. But then, take somebody who's synthesizing 150 mg down to 20 mg. We can bring most of these people down to about 5 mg of IgG per day. Sometimes we'll peak down to normal in the rate formulation and then come back up again but the bands are just exactly like they were before. There's no question that the bands go down because we put the same amount of IgG on the plates. So each one of the bands has gone down and the pattern in a band is exactly like that of your fingerprints.

D. W. PATY (*University of British Columbia, Vancouver*): I have two questions, the first is to Dr. Raine. Did you have myelin basic protein controls for your treatment regimen in chronic relapsing EAE?

RAINE: Yes. That was the essential control and animals treated identically to the group I showed but with myelin basic protein alone in IFA showed short-term improvement and then subsequent return of the relapsing clinical disease. So MBP had a temporary improving effect upon the disease but not long lasting, as was the case of MBP/GC.

PATY: Drs. Raine or Prineas, do you feel that the oligodendrocytes, which seem to be proliferating in your recovery phase, are coming from migration of oligodendrocytes from other portions of the nervous system or are there purely potential cells present within the lesion that might be stimulated?

RAINE: In the interest of fairness, I'll let Dr. Prineas answer that one.

PRINEAS: There's no reported evidence that oligodendrocytes proliferate in multiple sclerosis. All the data that Dr. Raine referred to is from the EAE model. The evidence that he presented this morning suggested that those cells remyelinating were the cells that were dividing. It looked to me as if they were a progeny of mature oligodendrocytes in the vicinity of the lesion.

R. J. SLATER (*National Multiple Sclerosis Society, New York*): Was I correct in hearing Dr. Prineas describe lesions in the cortex?

PRINEAS: It's really astonishing to a neuropathologist that that question is frequently asked by clinicians, but I don't know where the ideas come from that you don't get plaque formation in the cortex in multiple sclerosis. It's one of the most common areas to be affected. The lesions are exquisitely specific to multiple sclerosis and there are cases of MS in which all of the plaques are restricted to the cerebral cortex. One perhaps has to qualify that and explain this lack of knowledge or misapprehension on the part of non-neuropathologists. That is, the cortex has a lot of myelin in it and by "cortical plaque" we refer to a punched out area of myelin loss located within the cortex.

SLATER: Is there any relationship between those cortical lesions and the presence of cognitive problems?

PRINEAS: The cognitive problems in multiple sclerosis have been best correlated with changes in total brain weight and atrophy of the cerebral white matter. As far as I'm aware, there are no clinical correlates to the cortical location of cortical lesions. With regard to remyelination, we have recently examined material that suggests that one may get very extensive remyelination in subacute plaques, not the oldest plaques, and we have definite evidence of destruction of remyelinating fibers.

RAINE: We recently studied a case of acute MS which came to us in June 1983. One of the striking features in this case of acute MS, which also had features of Balo's concentric sclerosis, were significant waves of remyelination within relatively acute lesions.

A. VANDENBARK (*Portland VA Hospital, Portland, ORE*): Dr. Norton mentioned molecules which seem to be specifically related to myelin. My question is, what are the differences between myelin membrane components and the actual membranes of the oligodendroglial cells and where do you make the distinction in terms of the processes of the cell that are producing the myelin and the actual membrane of that cell?

W. T. NORTON (*Albert Einstein College of Medicine, Bronx, NY*): I should have been more general and talked about molecules that are in both the cell membrane and the myelin sheath. Obviously, there's nothing in myelin that's not in the oligodendrocyte, and we know much more about myelin than we do about the membrane of the oligodendrocyte.

VANDENBARK: So in fact then, both may in terms of composition serve as identical targets?

NORTON: Yes except the oligodendrocyte membrane is probably a good bit more complicated. It has more things in it than myelin.

VANDENBARK: My second question is related to the immunoglobulin content in plaques and relationships to macrophages. What is the role of complement and is there any distinction between alternative or classical complement pathways and activation?

PRINEAS: There's no information as to the presence or absence of complement in the MS lesion. It would certainly fulfill the same role that IgG-mediated phagocytosis would—that it's a very potent ligand for phagocytosis.

VANDENBARK: Is Dr. Raine's system with anti-lipid antibodies complement dependent?

RAINE: Yes, it is complement dependent, particularly in tissue culture.

F. DAVIS (*Rush Medical School, Chicago, IL*): Question for Dr. Prineas, I wonder if you would comment on the possibilities that rather than a primary attack of macrophage on myelin there could be some dystrophic effect of oligodendroglial cell or myelin leading to injured myelin and then what you really are seeing is the secondary event.

RAINE: Dr. Prineas, the old question—metabolic defect in the oligodendrocyte?

PRINEAS: Well it's one of the major possibilities that we keep in mind but what's impressive here is that there's no myelin debris or deformation of the myelin sheath prior to the arrival of this inflammatory contingent. We are very familiar with myelin diseases secondary to oligodendrocyte disease such as progressive multifocal leukoencephalopathy and all of the leukodystrophies and one of the characteristics of those diseases is that one sees myelin debris lingering in the lesion and being quietly phagocytosed over a long period. In MS, one is looking at a disease process in which the myelin vanishes before we actually see any significant changes in it. So the evidence that we have I believe is against this simply being dead myelin being phagocytosed subsequent to oligodendrocyte injury.

R. MADRID (*Institute for Basic Research, Staten Island, NY*): Dr. Raine, you appear to have succeeded in transferring a demyelinating condition in the mouse by passive transfer of lymph node cells from MBP-sensitized animals. Now that was one of the five models you showed during your presentation, then at the end of your presentation you stated "autoimmune demyelination requires a combination of myelin components." My question is, to answer this contradiction, was the myelin basic protein contaminated?

RAINE: There was no contradiction. The point was made throughout the talk that the rule applied to guinea pig and the mouse was an exception. The passively transferred model is in the mouse. EAE in the mouse is totally different from EAE in other species, so there is a proviso there. I would address the contamination comment to Dr. McFarlin, I assume he knows how clean his preparations are. Was your myelin basic protein clean, Dale, or did it have a tiny drop of GC or something in it?

D. E. MCFARLIN (*NINCDS, Bethesda, MD*): Well, it's the same as we've used the last 15 years and its interesting how this question always comes up. There was no indication of any lipid contamination.

RAINE: I must also emphasize that Dr. McFarlin's dose of MBP in this model is higher than the dose given in the Strain 13 model, so there could be something in that too.

J. R. RICHERT (*Georgetown University Medical Center, Washington, D.C.*): Dr. Raine, when you treat your chronic relapsing EAE with a combination of BP and galactocerebroside, do they have to be present in the same emulsion?

RAINE: They are present in the same emulsion. We have not tried separating them. We have inoculated healthy animals with the various mixtures without effect.

F. D. LUBIN (*Thomas Jefferson University, Philadelphia, PA*): Dr. Raine, I was wondering if you wanted to speculate on the mechanism of demyelination in the mice where myelin basic protein alone was used and raise the possibility whether there couldn't be a secondary sensitization to other myelin lipids following initial inflammatory response against myelin basic protein?

RAINE: A good question. I think the mouse is a tricky species in that there is so much damage experienced at the level of the endothelium and so much extravasation of all kinds of components that it makes interpretation of events very difficult. The mouse is an exceptionally hard model in which to interpret those very early events and before one could speculate on secondary sensitization to other components, one would have to reduce the amount of damage which theoretically should cause sensitization to any number of things.

G. HASHIM (*St. Lukes Hospital, New York*): Dr. Raine, in regard to your concept of an antigenic depôt and its relationship to relapsing EAE including the mouse, I think your experiments with Dr. McFarlin do not rule out the involvement of an antigenic depot. Might I suggest that the brain itself is a depôt.

RAINE: Previous discussion on antigenic depôt generally related to the subcutaneous site of injection, and here in the mouse is a model of intravenous injection of cells which dispenses with that aspect of the argument.

HASHIM: Alright, I agree with that if you restrict it to the footpad, but the depôt concept remains more general than a local injection.

A. ECKER (*Syracuse University, Syracuse, NY*): Dr. Rasminsky, it is delightful to see that your work deals with the mechanism of tic douloureux trigeminal neuralgia. Your work with the demyelinated mouse or unmyelinated mouse is supplemented by this mechanical business. Do you know the common causes of either multiple sclerosis plaque at a root or caused by nearby pressure from an artery? My question is, do you go along with these as good mechanisms for trigeminal neuralgia and has anything been done about the mechanism of glycerol in relieving pain promptly and persistently like a spontaneous remission without producing anesthesia?

RASMINSKY: We've talked about this before. My answer before was, I don't know; my answer still is I don't know. I have no specific comment about glycerol.

R. P. LISAK (*University of Pennsylvania School of Medicine, Philadelphia*) Cedric, what happens when you give just Gal-C, you told us about Gal-C and MBP and MBP by itself in your chronic model? Does Gal-C by itself cause any changes?

RAINE: At this moment we have seen no effect caused by Gal-C alone.

Mechanisms and Consequences of Virus Persistence in the Human Nervous System[a]

V. TER MEULEN, M. J. CARTER, H. WEGE, AND R. WATANABE

Institute for Virology and Immunobiology
University of Würzburg
Würzburg, Federal Republic of Germany

INTRODUCTION

The central nervous system (CNS) consists of highly complex tissues. Although intracellular communication is observed throughout the body, nowhere else does this property take on such significance and reach such a level of refinement. Cells of nervous tissue possess an unusual morphology and are highly elongated or branched to maximize cell/cell contacts, and cell membranes reveal a spectacular degree of specialization. The metabolism of these neuro-functional cells is rendered subservient to cell function, and cell division does not occur. It is therefore to be expected that persistent infection by viruses could have a profound effect on cell function. The production of viral proteins and their insertion into cell membranes could disrupt vital processes, and render the cells susceptible to immunological attack. Since neuronal tissue does not divide, cells destroyed either by immune responses or directly by the virus cannot be replaced. Similarly, damage induced in supportive tissue could also affect the neurons and so the function of the CNS as a whole could be impaired. It is the purpose of this review to consider briefly the mechanisms by which viruses may persist in the CNS and to assess the effects of this process. To this end we shall consider events in the human CNS, although results obtained from animal experiments will be discussed where relevant.

In the context of this discussion, a persistent infection is any infection that is not eliminated by the host immune response. This definition therefore encompasses persistent infections that may be termed latent or slow virus infections.

MECHANISMS OF PERSISTENCE

The CNS is well protected anatomically and consequently does not normally constitute the site of primary infection. Most viruses reach the CNS by the hematogenous route, and the duration and extent of viremia are significant in the success of CNS invasion. Some viruses, such as canine distemper virus, invade the CNS through infected lymphocytes[3] and the related human pathogen, measles virus, probably achieves invasion in the same way.[4] Other viruses (rabies) enter the CNS through the peripheral nerves following initial replication at the site of infection.[1,2]

[a]The authors acknowledge the financial support of the Deutsche Forschungsgemeinschaft.

DNA Viruses

Two virus groups, herpes and papovaviruses, will be considered in this section.

Herpes viruses that most commonly establish persistent infections of the human CNS are herpes simplex (HSV) and varicella zoster. Most data have been gathered concerning HSV persistence in the sensory ganglia, but this virus may also persist in the CNS of rodents[5,6,7] and man.[8,9] Both HSV and varicella establish a persistent infection that exhibits occasional reactivation. Virus particles then migrate along peripheral nerve fibers to cause a recurrent infection of tissue served by those nerves. This results in cold sores and mouth ulcers in the case of HSV and shingles in the case of varicella. Animal experiments have shown that virus enters the nervous system through peripheral nerves[1] and establishes a latent infection in the sensory ganglia. There is no evidence that cells in the ganglion infected with virus actually display any surface antigens recognizable by the immune system, and virus-specific intracellular inclusions cannot be found. However, virus-specific DNA and RNA can be detected by *in situ* hybridization,[10,11] suggesting that limited virus expression may occur. Persistent virus at this site can be rescued by cultivation of explants *in vitro* or co-cultivation of this tissue with cells susceptible to herpes virus. Human ganglia cells subjected to this technique did not always respond by induction of infectious virus. However, ganglia that failed to respond were obtained from individuals expressing a strong anti-HSV immune response which suggested that these persons were in fact infected.[12] This was confirmed by superinfection experiments in which temperature-sensitive (ts) mutants of HSV were used. Virus growth was then observed at the nonpermissive temperature, which was interpreted as the complementation of the ts lesion by viral genetic information residing in the cell of the ganglion, but which was itself defective in some other function.[9] The "defectiveness" of the persistent virus may contribute to the carriage of the virus in the absence of any detectable cytopathic effect. Nondefective virus information is presumably carried in an inactive state or one in which virus replication is so slow as to be undetectable by present techniques. The manner in which this is achieved is at present unknown and it is also not certain whether the DNA is carried in an integrated or episomal form. However, unlike persistent infections, CNS cells maintained *in vitro* are nondividing, and therefore virus can be efficiently maintained as an episome in the absence of replication.[13]

Papovaviruses that persist in the CNS are associated with the slow virus disease progressive multifocal leukoencephalopathy (PML). The two viruses so far associated with this condition are JC virus and SV40 PML, which are closely related both serologically and by DNA sequence. JC virus grows very poorly in tissue cultures and this has hampered research. Both viruses can be isolated from PML brain and large numbers of particles can be demonstrated in infected tissue by biochemical or electron microscopic studies.[14,15] Therefore, unlike herpes virus persistence, virus antigens are expressed in the CNS. The majority of PML cases occur following some underlying immunodeficiency. This is also true of virus isolation from extraneural tissue, where successful isolation has only been possible in subjects exhibiting a reduced immune response during pregnancy or immunosuppressive regimes following organ transplantation.[16,17]

RNA Viruses

RNA viruses establishing persistent infections in the human CNS include arena, echo, rubella and measles virus.

Rubella CNS infection is normally only important in congenital infections.[18] However, in rare instances the virus can give rise to a slowly progressive rubella panencephalitis (PRP) that emerges some ten years after childhood or congenital rubella.[19,20] Infectious virus could be recovered from the brain both with and without co-cultivation procedures[21] and also from infected lymphocytes.[22] However, virus antigens could not be detected in the CNS. *In vitro,* rubella virus gives rise to a limited cytopathic effect and readily establishes persistently infected cultures in which defective interfering (DI) particles may be involved.[23] The relevance of this to the CNS infection is not known.

Arena and echovirus persistence in the CNS is uncommon. Lymphocytic choriomeningitis (LCM) virus is associated with acute aseptic meningitis, meningoencephalitis or an influenza-like syndrome. The disease is normally controlled, but very occassionally it may take a chronic course.[24] There are no data available concerning the production of this condition, nor concerning the mechanism of virus persistence. It is, however, well established that LCMV is able to produce a life-long persistent infection in congenitally or neonatally infected rodents. In this case virus persists despite a humoral anti-virus immune response.[25] The cell-mediated immune system, however, is tolerized towards the virus and this is thought to provide the basis for virus persistence and the failure to eliminate the infection. The virus replication process may be held in check by the production of DI particles that can be detected in many organs, and whose appearance correlates with the cessation of the acute phase of the disease.[26] However, in the rodent, this infection is generalized and there is as yet no evidence for immunological tolerance, or DI particles in the chronic human CNS infection.

Immunodeficiency is better characterized by the case of chronic echovirus CNS infections. Echovirus infections are ordinarily easily controlled by the body's own defense mechanisms, but in patients with severe immunodeficiency and a lack of B cells a chronic echovirus infection may be produced.[27–31] This infection results in a chronic meningoencephalitis and infectious virus has been recovered from the CSF. Occasionally virus can also be isolated from extraneural tissue.

Measles virus is a member of the morbilliviruses, and before the advent of vaccination procedures, was ubiquitous amongst human populations large enough to sustain it. Acute measles is a self-limiting condition controlled by a strong immune response, but involvement of neural tissue is well known. The virus exhibits a marked lymphotropism resulting in a transient hyporesponsiveness during the disease, and it is thought the virus gains access to the CNS either by viremia or inside infected lymphocytes. Virus penetration may result in acute encephalitis, but occasionally a persistent infection is established that leads to a fatal slowly progressing disease, subacute sclerosing panencephalitis (SSPE). During this condition inclusion bodies are present in the CNS cells that consist of measles virus nucleocapsids.[32–35] However, cell fusion that is characteristic of measles virus-induced CPE is not observed, and mature virus particles are absent. However, virus expression may sometimes be rescued from this infected tissue by co-cultivation procedures.[36] These experiments have therefore confirmed that measles virus is the etiological agent of SSPE and also indicated that virus persistence may be based on some defect in the virus maturation process that could involve some form of host effect. Viruses rescued from SSPE tissue revealed some structural differences from wild-type measles strains. Some of these concern electrophoretic migration differences between measles and SSPE virus polypeptides but the advent of monoclonal antibodies has permitted the detection of more subtle differences in structure.[37,38] Many of these concern the matrix (M) protein[39] and may arise as a consequence of the acquisition of mutations during persistence.[40] Indeed this process has been detected in persistent infections *in vitro*.[41,42] Most SSPE viruses grow more poorly than wild-type measles and more readily produce persistent infections in tissue culture. This may be a consequence of the acquisition of mutations, discussed above, and therefore there may be some selection towards a more easily carried virus than during the persistent infection itself. However, none of these mutations seems to be a common characteristic of the persistent measles virus and this suggests that this is a general process. No specific marker has yet been found that differentiates persistent measles viruses from isolates derived from acute measles. Interestingly, many of these mutations involve the M protein[39] and this protein has been strongly implicated in the original establishment of the persistent infection of the CNS.

The SSPE patient displays a strong humoral immune response towards measles virus, and antibodies directed to virus polypeptides are present in both serum and CSF.[43] However, whereas most virus proteins are well recognized, there are no antibodies in the CSF directed towards the matrix protein.[44–46] Current evidence suggests that this situation arises through a lesion in the synthesis of this protein in the CNS,[47] and consequently, M protein is not available to serve as an immunogen. The failure to produce large amounts of this major structural protein is thought to explain the maturation defect observed in the CNS, conferring a cell-associated phenotype of the virus. This in turn is thought to account for the slowly progressing nature of the disease. Attempts to rescue SSPE viruses from infected tissue are not always successful[36] and occasionally a persistently infected cell line is obtained in which capacity to produce M protein is not restored.[48–50] Investigation of these cell lines, known as SSPE cell lines, has shown that in one case failure to produce this protein was accomplished by a defect in translation,[51] but in other cases, mRNA was apparently not produced or rapidly degraded.[52] Some evidence suggests the latter mechanism also occurs in human brain (Baczko *et al.*, in preparation). Since M protein and possibly M protein mRNA are not produced in infected brain, these molecules are presumably subject to no selection pressure. Mutations could be rapidly acquired that might explain the variation observed in matrix proteins whose expression was restored during the rescue of SSPE viruses.[39] Other mutations could have a more profound effect, either on the ability of a rescued mRNA to function in translation reactions or on the ability of genome RNA to act as template for the production of mRNA itself. In these cases rescue of infectious virus by co-cultivation techniques would be impossible and the cell-associated SSPE virus persistent infections could then result. Viewed in this way, study of SSPE cell lines may not necessarily reveal the nature of the original events driving the virus toward persistence.

Recent work with measles virus-infected tissue cultures has suggested that measles antibody may play a crucial role in the establishment of persistence. It was found that antibody could strip virus antigens from the surface of infected cells and thus protect such cells from immunological injury.[53,54] Furthermore, polyvalent antiserum can alter the synthesis of intracellular virus polypeptides, a phenomenon termed antibody-induced antigenic modulation.[55,56] This event is also operative in persistently infected tissue cultures,[57] and could give rise to a virus association in which virus antigen production is apparent.[52] This state, once established, is apparently stable in the absence of antiserum. Since it has been suggested that measles virus may enter the CNS inside invading lymphocytes, it is possible that antibody is synthesized within the CNS at the time of invasion. This antibody may then be more active in inducing a modulation process and persistence than in complement-mediated cytolysis because complement is relatively lacking in the CSF. A modulation process such as that described above is operative on all virus polypeptides, reducing the total expression of virus genetic information. Therefore, this event cannot alone account for the situation observed in SSPE where the effect predominantly concerns just one polypeptide. Other factors, perhaps host-specific, may therefore play a role in establishment and maintenance of measles virus persistence. In this connection the finding of measles virus genetic information in the brains of apparently normal individuals by *in situ* hybridization[58] is of interest. Measles virus may be part of the normal human CNS virological fauna, as suggested by Johnson and Carrigan.[59] Consequently, SSPE or measles encephalitis might result from those rare instances when the modulation process was incomplete or ineffective. Further study of the involvement of the CNS during normal acute measles, and of virus expression in normal or diseased brain will be necessary to clarify this process.

It is apparent from the foregoing discussion that the methods of instigation and maintenance of a persistent infection in CNS tissue may vary, and in no case are these processes fully understood. Infections range from those truly latent infections, such as HSV, where the virus genome is only poorly, if at all, expressed to those in which virus replication is complete, and infectious virus is directly reisolable such as in PML, PRP or echovirus infections. Other infections, such as SSPE, reveal an intermediate state of expression, and although virus antigen is present, infectious virus is not produced. In all of these cases the role of the immune system has been stressed. A neuron latently infected with HSV cannot be attacked by the immune system, and the immune system itself may protect SSPE virus-infected cells from cytotoxic events by stripping off virus-specific cell surface markers. It is not known by what mechanism the herpes virus infection is converted to latency. However, suppression of cell-mediated immunity has been successful in precipitating reactivation in animals,[60] and patients undergoing HSV recurrence often show an impairment of some aspects of cell-mediated immunity.[61–63] Thus the immune system may be to some extent instrumental in controlling this process also.

Immunological dysfunction is involved in the cases of PML or echovirus infection and permits productive virus replication to occur, but in the case of PML it is not known whether the immune system deficiency has prompted the activation of a previously existing but inapparent persistent infection, or if virus invasion occurred as a consequence of a failure in immunological protection. The case of PRP is an exception; infectious virus may be isolated directly despite a strong antibody response in both serum and CSF.[64] Similarly, the cell-mediated immune system does not show any specific deficiency.[20,65] However, the site of rubella virus antigen expression has not yet been identified during this disease process. Consequently, the mechanisms underlying virus persistence in this case are as yet unknown.

THE CONSEQUENCES OF VIRAL PERSISTENCE FOR NEURAL TISSUE

The consequences of a persistent viral infection may be considered under two main headings. Firstly, direct effects result from the action of the persistent virus, either by promoting cell destruction or by interfering with the efficiency with which the host cell may function. Direct destruction of extraneural tissue may also be included in this heading. Secondly, indirect effects arise largely through the response of the immune system to the infection. This may involve an autoimmune reaction that could lead to tissue destruction and consequent inhibition of CNS function.

Direct Effects

In the case of HSV latency, virus persistence does not seem to have any direct consequences on the host cell although subtle effects have been discussed by Sequiera *et al.*[8] Reactivation of the latent virus, however, results in the expression of virus antigens. This has been detected in explanted cervical ganglia from the mouse.[66]

Mature virus particles are formed that migrate along cell processes to reinfect that area of the skin served by the nerve. The original host cell is presumably killed by the virus but latency may be reestablished by spread to a different neurone. Consequently, damage by these events is cumulative.

PML is associated with two papovaviruses, JC and SV40 PML. In common with other papovaviruses infection can take two courses depending upon the permissiveness of the host cell. PML lesions consist of demyelinating plaques in the white matter. Oligodendroglial cells are lost from these areas but those in the periphery are enlarged and contain large numbers of papovavirus particles. Astrocytes, which display various morphological aberrations but rarely contain virus, are observed in the foci of these lesions.[67] This has led to the suggestion that the oligodendroglial cells and astrocytes could constitute permissive and nonpermissive cell populations, respectively. The virus is able to destroy selectively oligodendroglia cells, their cytoplasmic extensions are lost and demyelination follows with resultant damage to the CNS.[68] The astrocytes could then undergo nonpermissive virus replication leading to transformation. Some evidence to support this has been obtained from *in vitro* experiments.[69] No inflammatory lesions have been observed in PML, and since this disease is associated with immune deficiency, it seems that most tissue destruction is accomplished by a direct effect of the virus. Similarly, chronic echovirus infection is associated with immune deficiency, and although inflammatory processes are observed in extraneural tissue, it seems unlikely that CNS damage is largely caused by virus-mediated cell destruction.

However, persistent viruses are able to interfere with cell function in ways other than tissue destruction. Insertion of virus antigens into the membrane or the occurrence of virus maturation processes could well be expected to disturb the activity of structurally refined, highly specialized membrane systems. Studies in tissue culture have shown that neural cells persistently infected with LCM, measles, or even rabies virus, often display altered characteristics related to neural function. The activities of acetyltransferase and acetylcholinesterase were found to be greatly altered.[70,71,72] Recently, it has been shown that glioma cells persistently infected with measles virus have a greatly reduced capacity to respond to catecholamine hormones and produce cyclic AMP (cAMP).[73] Barrett and Koschel[57] used antibody to remove virus antigens from the surface of these infected cells and found that stimulation by these hormones was restored. Furthermore, intracellular virus proteins were not apparently involved in this inhibition, since full function was restored despite the continued presence of intracellular virus antigen. In this case, the actual activity of the cAMP synthetase enzyme was not altered, but virus antigen in the membrane affected the ability of the hormone receptor on the external surface of the plasma membrane to activate the cAMP synthesizing complex on the internal surface.

In none of the above cases was cell growth rate appreciably altered, suggesting that the luxury functions of neural cells may indeed be highly susceptible to this type of interference. Such changes could have a profound effect on brain function and eventually lead to a disease with a clinically defined symptomatology.

Indirect Effects

With the exception of PML, all slow virus diseases associated with conventional viruses reveal some form of inflammatory lesion. The destruction of infected cells by immune mechanisms is therefore to be expected in every case. Although this is a normal function of the immune system, it takes on a further significance in the context of CNS infections because of the lack of regenerative capacity of this tissue. However, a further component to be considered in this context is the production of an autoimmune response that can probably be elicited by a wide variety of viruses resulting in the destruction of uninfected CNS tissues. The most characterized model for such an immune response is experimental allergic encephalomyelitis (EAE), a disease induced by immunization with myelin basic protein or CNS-tissue extracts in combination with adjuvants. The human condition of postinfectious encephalomyelitis reveals many similarities to EAE and may arise weeks or months after virus infection (measles or mumps) or after vaccination (smallpox or rabies). The mechanism by which virus infection brings about this type of reaction has been extensively studied in the mouse and rat.

Theiler's virus (TV) infection in the mouse leads to a demyelination which is very similar to that observed in EAE.[74] Cells surrounding lesions are free of virus antigen, indicating that direct virus-mediated tissue destruction is not important in damage production. Furthermore, immunosuppression with cyclophosphamide results in a decrease in white matter lesions, suggesting that host immune responses are involved.[75]

Recently, the murine coronavirus JHM has been used for infection of rats to produce a condition termed subacute demyelinating encephalomyelitis (SDE) that is characterized by lesions of primary demyelination and can run a relapsing course[78,79] (Wege *et al.*, in press). An EAE-like condition could be induced in normal animals by adoptive transfer of lymphocytes from rats with SDE. Such lymphocytes were found to have been sensitized to myelin basic protein itself, during coronavirus JHM infection of the brain.[76]

The most obvious mechanisms by which a virus could trigger an autoimmune reaction against CNS tissue would be some form of cross-reaction between distinct virus and cellular antigens. Indeed Panitch *et al.*,[77] have reported such a cross-reaction between measles virus and myelin basic protein (MBP). Secondly, it is possible that virus infection causes the release of CNS tissue antigens that might normally be shielded from the immune system. Alternatively, this release of tissue might mimic the action of adjuvant necessary for the induction of EAE by immunization of experimental animals against CNS tissue. Thirdly, it is possible that virus antigen physically associates with the host membrane antigen, resulting in a complex that is recognizably foreign but must also contain a "self" component.

CONCLUSIONS

In the foregoing discussion the immune response has been implicated in both the mechanism of virus persistence in the CNS and in the pathogenic consequences of that infection. Although the virus may be directly pathogenic, it seems likely that immunopathological mechanisms are often involved. These reactions are often similar regardless of the virus concerned, for instance PRP and SSPE show clinical and immunological similarities although the mechanisms of persistence seem to be very different. Observations such as these may explain why it has so far been impossible to identify a single viral etiology for multiple sclerosis. It is possible that a variety of agents are capable of stimulating a host-dependent autoimmune process leading to the onset and perpetuation of disease, even in the absence of viral antigens.

ACKNOWLEDGMENT

The authors thank Helga Kriesinger for typing the manuscript.

REFERENCES

1. STEVENS, J. G. & M. L. COOK. 1971. Latent herpes simplex virus in spinal ganglia of mice. Science **173:** 843–845.
2. COOK, M. L. & J. G. STEVENS. 1973. Pathogenesis of herpetic neuritis and ganglionitis in mice: Evidence for intra-axonal transport of infection. Infect. Immunol. **7:** 272–288.
3. SUMMERS, B. A., H. A. GREISEN & M. J. G. APPEL. 1978. Possible initiation of viral encephalomyelitis in dogs by migrating lymphocytes infected with distemper virus. Lancet **2:** 187–189.
4. FRASER, K. B. & S. J. MARTIN. 1978. Measles Virus and Its Biology. Academic Press. London, New York and San Francisco.
5. COOK, M. L. & J. G. STEVENS. 1976. Latent herpetic infections following experimental viraemia. J. Gen. Virol **31:** 75–80.
6. KNOTT, F. B., M. L. COOK & J. G. STEVENS. 1973. Latent herpes simplex virus in central nervous system of rabbits and mice. J. Exp. Med. **138:** 740–744.
7. CABRERA, C. V., C. WOHLENBERG, H. OPENSHAW, M. REY-MENDEZ, A. PUGA & A. L. NOTKINS. 1980. Herpes simplex DNA sequences in the CNS of latently infected mice. Nature **288:** 288–290.
8. SEQUIERA, L. W., L. C. JENNINGS, L. H. CARRASSO, M. A. LORD, A. CURRY & R. N. P. SUTTON. 1979. Detection of herpes virus genome in brain tissue. Lancet **2:** 609–612.
9. BROWN, S. M., J. H. SUBAK-SHARPE, K. G. WARREN, Z. WROBLEWSKA & H. KOPROWSKI. 1979. Detection by complementation of defective or uninducible (herpes simplex Type I) virus genomes latent in human ganglia. Proc. Natl. Acad. Sci. **76:** 2364–2368.
10. STEVENS, J. G. 1977. Latent characteristics of selected herpes viruses. Adv. Cancer Res. **26:** 227–256.
11. GALLOWAY, D. A., C. PEOGLIO, M. J. SHEVCHUK & K. MCDOUGALL. 1979. Detection of herpes simplex RNA in human sensory ganglia. Virology **95:** 265–268.
12. BARINGER, J. R. 1975. Herpes simplex infection of nervous tissue in animals and man. Prog. Med. Virol. **20:** 1–26.
13. FENNER, F., B. R. MCAUSLAN, C. A. MIMS, J. SAMBROOK & D. O. WHITE. 1974. Biology of Animal Viruses. Academic Press. New York.
14. JOHNSON, R. T., O. NARAYAN, C. P. WEINER & J. E. GREENLEE. 1977. Progressive multifocal leukoencephalopathy. *In* Slow Virus Infections of the CNS. V. ter Meulen & M. Katz, Eds.: 91–100. Springer Verlag. New York, Heidelberg and Berlin.
15. DÖRRIES, K., R. T. JOHNSON & V. TER MEULEN. 1978. Detection of polyomavirus DNA in PML brain tissue by *in situ* hybridization. J. Gen. Virol. **41:** 49–57.
16. COLEMAN, D. V., R. A. DANIEL, S. D. GARDENER, A. M. FIELD & P. E. GIBSON. 1977. Polyomavirus in urine during pregnancy. Lancet **2:** 709–710.
17. GRIFFIN, B. W. 1982. How do papovaviruses persist in their host. *In* Virus Persistence. B. W. J. Mahy, A. C. Minson & G. K. Darby, Eds. **33:** 227–248. Cambridge University Press. London and New York.
18. HORSTMAN, D. M. 1982. Rubella. *In* Viral Infections of Humans: Epidemiology and Control. A. S. Evans, Ed.: 519–539. John Wiley and Sons. New York.
19. TOWNSEND, J. J., J. R. BARINGER, J. S. WOLINSKY, N. MALAMUD, J. P. MEDNICK, H. S. PANITCH, R. A. T. SCOTT, L. S. OSHIRO & N. E. CREMER. 1975. Progressive rubella panencephalitis. Late onset after congenital rubella. N. Engl. J. Med. **292:** 990–993.
20. WEIL, M. L., H. H. ITABASHI, N. E. CREMER, L. S. OSHIRO, E. H. LENNETTE & L. CARRAY. 1975. Chronic progressive panencephalitis due to rubella virus stimulating subacute sclerosing panencephalitis. N. Engl. J. Med. **292:** 994–998.
21. CREMER, N. E., L. S. OSHIRO, M. L. WEIL, E. H. LENNETTE, H. H. ITABASHI & L. CARNAY. 1975. Isolation of rubella virus from brain in chronic progressive panencephalitis. J. Gen. Virol. **8:** 143–153.
22. WOLINSKY, J. S., B. O. BERG & C. J. MAITLAND. 1976. Progressive rubella panencephalitis. Arch. Neurol. **33:** 722–723.
23. STANWICK, T. L. & J. V. HALLUM. 1974. Role of interferon in six cell lines persistently infected with rubella virus. Infect. Immun. **10:** 810–815.
24. LEHMANN-GRUBE, F. 1982. Lymphocytic choriomeningitis. *In* International Textbook of

Medicine, vol. 2. A. H. Samly, L. H. Smith & J. B. Wyngaarden, Eds. W. B. Saunders. Philadelphia, London and Toronto.
25. BUCHMEIER, M. J. & M. B. A. OLDSTONE. 1978. Virus-induced immune complex disease: Identification of specific viral antigens and antibodies deposited in complexes during chronic lymphocytic choriomeningitis virus infection. J. Immunol **120:** 1297–1304.
26. POPESCU, M. & F. LEHMANN-GRUBE. 1977. Defective interfering particles in mice infected with lymphocytic choriomeningitis virus. Virology **77:** 78–83.
27. ZIEGLER, J. B. & R. PENNY. 1975. Fatal echo 30 virus infection and amyloidosis in X-linked hypogammaglobulinemia. Clin. Immunol. Immunopathol. **3:** 347–352.
28. BARDELAS, J. A., J. A. WINKELSTEIN, D. S. Y. SETO, T. TSAI & A. D. ROGOL. 1977. Fatal ECHO 24 infection in a patient with hypogammaglobulinemia: Relationship to dermatomyositis-like syndrome. J. Pediatr. **90:** 396–399.
29. WILFERT, C. M., R. H. BUCKLEY, T. MOHANAKUMAR, J. F. GRIFFITH, S. L. KATZ, J. K. WHISNANT, P. A. EGGLESTON, M. MOORE, E. TREADWELL, M. N. OXMAN & F. S. ROSEN. 1977. Persistent and fatal central-nervous-system echovirus infections in patients with agammaglobulinemia. N. Engl. J. Med. **296:** 1485–1489.
30. WEBSTER, A. D. B., J. H. TRIPP, A. R. HAYWARD, A. D. DAYAN, R. DOSHI, E. H. MACINTYRE & D. A. J. TYRRELL. 1978. Echovirus encephalitis and myositis in primary immunoglobulin deficiency. Arch. Dis. Childhood **53:** 33–37.
31. WEINER, L. S., J. T. HOWELL, M. P. LANGFORD, G. J. STANTON, S. BARON, R. M. GOLDBLUM, R. A. LORD & A. S. GOLDMAN. 1979. Effect of specific antibodies on chronic echovirus type 5 encephalitis in a patient with hypogammaglobulinemia. J. Infect. Dis. **140:** 858–863.
32. CONNOLLY, J. H., I. V. ALLEN, L. J. HURWITZ & J. H. D. MILLER. 1967. Measles-virus antibody and antigen in subacute sclerosing panencephalitis. Lancet **1:** 542–544.
33. FREEMAN, J. M., R. L. MAGOFFIN, E. H. LENNETTE & R. M. HERNDON. 1967. Additional evidence of the relations between subacute inclusion-body encephalitis and measles virus. Lancet **2:** 129–131.
34. TER MEULEN, V., D. MÜLLER & C. JOPPICH. 1967. Fluorescence microscopy studies of brain tissue from a case of subacute progressive panencephalitis. Ger. Med. Meth. **12:** 438–441.
35. TER MEULEN, V., G. ENDERS-RUCKLE, D. MÜLLER & G. JOPPICH. 1969. Immunhistological, microscopical and neurochemical studies on encephalitides. III. Subacute progressive panencephalitis: virological and immunohistological studies. Acta Neurophathol. (Berlin) **12:** 244–259.
36. KATZ, M. & H. KOPROWSKI. 1973. The significance of failure to isolate infectious viruses in cases of subacute sclerosing panencephalitis. Arch. Ges. Virusforsch. **41:** 390–393.
37. TER MEULEN, V., S. LÖFFLER, M. J. CARTER & J. R. STEPHENSON. 1981. Antigenic characterization of measles and SSPE virus haemagglutinin by monoclonal antibodies. J. Gen. Virol. **57:** 357–364.
38. TRUDGETT, A., E. A. GOULD, M. ARMSTRONG, E. S. MINGIOLI & D. E. MCFARLIN. 1981. Antigenic differences in the hemagglutinin of measles and related viruses. Virology **109:** 180–182.
39. SHESHBERADARAN, H., S. N. CHEN & E. NORRBY. 1983. Monoclonal antibodies against five structural components of measles virus. I. Characterization of antigenic determinants on nine strains of measles virus. Virology **128:** 341–353.
40. HOLLAND, J. J., E. A. GRABAU, C. L. JONES & B. L. SEMBER. 1979. Evolution of multiple genome mutations during long-term persistent infection by vesicular stomatitis virus. Cell **16:** 495–504.
41. CARTER, M. J. & V. TER MEULEN. 1983. Subacute sclerosing panencephalitis: Are antigenic changes involved in measles virus persistence? *In* Immunology of Nervous System Infections. Progr. Brain Res. **59:** 163–171.
42. CARTER, M. J., M. M. WILLCOCKS, S. LÖFFLER & V. TER MEULEN. 1983. Comparison of lytic and persistent measles virus matrix proteins by competition radio immunoassay. J. Gen. Virol. **64:** 1801–1805.
43. SEVER, J. L. & W. ZEMAN. 1968. Serological studies of measles and subacute sclerosing panencephalitis. Neurology **18:** 95–97.

44. HALL, W. W., R. A. LAMB & P. W. CHOPPIN. 1979. Measles and subacute sclerosing panencephalitis virus proteins: Lack of antibodies to the M protein in patients with subacute sclerosing panencephalitis. Proc. Natl. Acad. Sci. **76:** 2047–2051.
45. STEPHENSON, J. R. & V. TER MEULEN. 1979. Subacute sclerosing panencephalitis: Characterization of the etiological agent and its relationship to the morbilliviruses. *In* Aspects of Slow and Persistent Virus Infection, vol. 2. New Perspectives in Clinical Microbiology. D. A. J. Tyrrell, Ed.: 61–75. Martinus Nijhoff Publishers. The Hague, Boston and London.
46. WECHSLER, S. L., R. RUSTIGIAN, K. C. STALLCUP, K. B. BYERS, S. H. WINSTON & B. N. FIELDS. 1979. Measles virus-specific polypeptide synthesis in two persistently infected HeLa cell lines. J. Virol. **31:** 677–684.
47. HALL, W. W. & P. W. CHOPPIN. 1981. Measles-virus proteins in the brain tissue of patients with subacute sclerosing panencephalitis. Absence of the M protein. N. Engl. J. Med. **304:** 1152–1155.
48. HALL, W. W. & P. W. CHOPPIN. 1979. Evidence for the lack of synthesis of the M polypeptide of measles virus in brain cells from SSPE. Virology **99:** 443–447.
49. LIN, F. H. & H. THORMAR. 1980. Absence of M protein in a cell-associated subacute sclerosing panencephalitis virus. Nature **285:** 490–492.
50. MACHAMER, C. E., E. C. HAYES & H. J. ZWEERINK. 1981. Cells infected with a cell-associated subacute sclerosing panencephalitis virus do not express M protein. Virology **108:** 515–520.
51. CARTER, M. J., M. M. WILLCOCKS & V. TER MEULEN. 1983. Defective translation of measles virus matrix protein in a subacute sclerosing panencephalitis cell line. Nature **305:** 153–155.
52. CARTER, M. J., P. N. BARRETT, M. M. WILLCOCKS, K. KOSCHEL & V. TER MEULEN. 1984. *In* Mechanisms of Viral Pathogenesis: From Gene to Pathogen. A. Kohn & P. Fuchs, Eds.: 95–114. Martinus Nijhoff. The Hague, Boston and London. Factors involved in measles virus persistence.
53. JOSEPH, B. S. & M. B. A. OLDSTONE. 1975. Immunologic injury in measles virus infection. II. Suppression of immune injury through antigenic modulation. J. Exp. Med. **142:** 864–876.
54. OLDSTONE, M. B. A. & A. TISHON. 1978. Immunologic injury in measles virus infection. IV. Antigenic modulation and abrogation of lymphocyte lysis of virus-infected cells. Clin. Immunol. Immunopath. **9:** 55–62.
55. FUJINAMI, R. S. & M. B. A. OLDSTONE. 1979. Antiviral antibody reacting on the plasma membrane alters measles virus expression inside the cell. Nature **279:** 529–530.
56. FUJINAMI, R. S. & M. B. A. OLDSTONE. 1980. Alterations in expression of measles virus polypeptides by antibody: Molecular events in antibody-induced antigenic modulation. J. Immunol. **125:** 78–85.
57. BARRETT, P. N. & K. KOSCHEL. 1983. Effect of antibody-induced modulation of measles (SSPE) virus membrane proteins on β-adrenergic receptor-mediated adenylate cyclase activity. Virology **127:** 299–308.
58. HAASE, A. T., P. VENTURA, C. J. GIBBS, JR. & W. W. TOURTELOTTE. 1981. Measles virus nucleotide sequences: Detection by hybridization *in situ*. Science **212:** 672–675.
59. JOHNSON, K. P. & D. R. CARRIGAN. 1982. Neurologic diseases caused by measles virus. *In* Proceedings of the 12th World Congress of Neurology. S. Katsuki, T. Tsubaki & Y. Toyokura, Eds.: 404–415. Elsevier. Amsterdam.
60. SEKIZAWA, T., H. OPENSHAW, C. WOHLENBERG & A. L. NOTKINS. 1980. Latency of herpes simplex virus in absence of neutralizing antibody: Model of reactivation. Science **210:** 1026–1028.
61. O'REILLY, R. J., A. CHIBBARO, E. ANGER & C. LOPEZ. 1977. Cell-mediated responses in patients with recurrent herpes simplex infections. II. Infection associated deficiency of lymphokine production in patients with recurrent herpes labialis or genitalis. J. Immunol. **118:** 1095–1102.
62. DONNENBERG, A. D., R. B. BELL & L. AURELIAN. 1980. Immunity to herpes simplex virus type 2. Development of virus-specific lymphproliferative and LIF responses in HSV-2 infected guinea pigs. Cell. Immunol. **56:** 526–539.

63. DONNENBERG, A. D., E. CHAIKOF & L. AURELIAN. 1980. Immunity to herpes simplex virus type 2. Cell mediated immunity in latently infected guinea pigs. Infect. Immun. **30:** 90–109.
64. COYLE. P. K. & J. S. WOLINSKY. 1981. Characterization of immune complexes in progressive rubella panencephalitis. Ann. Neurol. **9:** 557–562.
65. WEIL, M. L., L. PERRIN & E. BUIMOVICI-KLEIN. 1976. Immunologic abnormalities associated with chronic progressive panencephalitis due to congenital infection with rubella virus. Clin. Res. **24:** 185–190.
66. MCLENNAN, J. L. & G. DARBY. 1980. Herpes simplex virus latency: The cellular location of virus in dorsal root ganglia and the fate of the infected cell following virus inactivation. J. Gen. Virol. **51:** 13–243.
67. ASTRÖM, K. E., E. L. MANCALL & E. P. RICHARDSON, JR. 1958. Progressive multifocal leukoencephalopathy: A hitherto unrecognized complication of chronic lymphatic leukaemia and Hodgkin's disease. Brain **81:** 93–111.
68. JOHNSON, R. T., O. NARAYAN & L. P. WEINER. 1974. The relationship of SV40 related viruses to progressive multifocal leukoencephalopathy. *In* Mechanism of Virus Disease. C. W. S. Robinson & C. F. Fox, Eds.: 187–197. W. A. Benjamin. Menlo Park, California.
69. SHEIN, H. M. 1967. Transformation of astrocytes and destruction of spongioblasts induced by simian tumour virus SV40 in cultures of human fetal neuroglia. J. Neuropathol. Exp. Neurol. **26:** 60–76.
70. OLDSTONE, M. B. A., V. A. BOKISCH, F. J. DIXON, L. H. BARBOSA, D. FUCCILLO & J. L. SEVER. 1977. Subacute sclerosing panencephalitis: Destruction of human brain cells by antibody and complement in an autologous system. Clin. Immunol. Immunopath. **4:** 459–472.
71. HALBACH, M. & K. KOSCHEL. 1979. Impairment of hormone dependent signal transfer by chronic SSPE virus infection. J. Gen. Virol. **42:** 615–619.
72. KOSCHEL, K. & M. HALBACH. 1979. Rabies virus infection selectively impairs membrane receptor functions in neuronal model cells. J. Gen. Virol. **42:** 627–632.
73. KOSCHEL, K. & P. MÜNZEL. 1980. Persistent paramyxovirus infection and behaviour of β-adrenergic receptors in C6-rat glioma cells. J. Gen. Virol. **47:** 513–517.
74. DAL CANTO, M. C. & H. L. LIPTON. 1975. Primary demyelination in Theiler's virus infection: An ultrastructural study. Lab. Invest. **33:** 626–637.
75. LIPTON, H. L. & M. C. DAL CANTO. 1976. Theiler's virus-induced demyelination. Prevention by immunosuppression. Science **192:** 62–64.
76. WATANABE, R., H. WEGE & V. TER MEULEN. 1983. Adoptive transfer of EAE-like lesions from rats with coronavirus-induced demyelinating encephalomyelitis. Nature **305:** 150–153.
77. PANITCH, H. S., P. SWOVELAND & K. P. JOHNSON. 1979. Antibodies to measles virus react with myelin basic protein. Neurology **29:** 548–549.
78. NAGASHIMA, K., H. WEGE, R. MEYERMANN & V. TER MEULEN. 1978. Coronavirus induced subacute demyelinating encephalomyelitis in rats: A morphological analysis. Acta Neuropathol. (Berlin) **44:** 63–70.
79. WEGE, H., M. KOGA, R. WATANABE, K. NAGASHIMA & V. TER MEULEN. 1983. Neurovirulence of murine coronavirus JHM temperature-sensitive mutants in rats. Infect. Immun. **39:** 1316–1324.

DISCUSSION OF THE PAPER

W. W. TOURTELLOTTE (*VA Wadsworth Medical Center, Los Angeles*): We too have found it wise to hybridize and we thought that we were the first ones to find that the M genome was present in SSPE brain. I think we're all finding in our material that the M protein is not being formed but now that the genome is there, this means again as you propose, there might be a block somehow in getting it from the gene to the mRNA. Is it possible that we're going to find nucleic acid sequences in some of these acute MS lesions?

R. T. JOHNSON (*The Johns Hopkins University, Baltimore, MD*): Why don't we leave that for the general discussion.

R. S. TINDALL (*Dallas, TX*): With reference to the CSF oligoclonal banding in the JHM-infected mice, I presume that this is an inbred strain?

V. TER MEULEN (*University of Würzburg, Würzburg, FRG*): Lewis rats.

TINDALL: Would you interpret from that data that those immunoglobulins were not directed to similar viral constituents because of the disparity in the response seen but indeed that some of those responses were directed at different, presumably oligo, determinants?

TER MEULEN: The point I want to raise is that in this animal model there are animals that have all viral-specific oligoclonal IgG in the CSF. Later on when they recover, this disappears as in man but then something else occurs, and this has not yet been identified. We can say quite clearly it is not viral. We have to evaluate now whether it's basic myelin protein or another antigen. Certainly, I think it is of interest that the disease process is ongoing and this is reflected by the oligoclonal bands. We can only show this by IgG activity. But it has nothing to do with the virus. I think that's the only point I wanted to make at the present time.

Demyelination and Remyelination in Murine Viral Encephalomyelitis[a]

W. LANG,[b] M. RODRIGUEZ,[c] V. A. LENNON,[c]
AND P. W. LAMPERT[b]

[b]*Department of Pathology*
University of California, San Diego
La Jolla, California 92093

[c]*Departments of Immunology and Neurology*
Mayo Clinic
Rochester, Minnesota 55905

INTRODUCTION

Plaques of demyelination consistently develop in the spinal cord of susceptible mice following intracerebral inoculation at 4–5 weeks of age with either the JHM strain of mouse hepatitis virus (MHV)[1] or the DA strain of Theiler's mouse encephalomyelitis virus (TMEV).[2]

Intracerebral infection with the JHM strain of MHV produces demyelination in Balb/c mice at 6–10 days postinfection (PI),[3,4] following degeneration of MHV-infected oligodendrocytes.[3,5] These early plaques show little relationship to vessels and are extensively remyelinated by 4–5 weeks PI.[4,6] Immunosuppressive measures enhance mortality of infected mice.[1] In contrast, SJL/J mice inoculated with the DA strain of TMEV show perivascular cuffs of inflammatory cells and chronic demyelinated plaques for several months PI.[2,7] Immunosuppressive measures prevent demyelination.[8] Abortive central nervous system (CNS) remyelination is observed at the periphery of plaques,[3,7] which contain persistently infected oligodendrocytes,[7] immunoglobulins and plasma cells.

In this report we will emphasize that remyelination in chronic TMEV-infected mice can be enhanced by treatment with a mixture of myelin components, myelin basic protein (MBP) and galactocerebroside (GC). These observations are similar to findings by Raine and Traugott,[9] who were able to improve remyelination in chronic experimental allergic encephalomyelitis (EAE) after treatment with MBP and GC.

MATERIALS AND METHODS

Four-week-old Balb/c mice were inoculated intracerebrally with 10^4 PFU of the ts8 mutant of JHM strain MHV,[4] and SJL/J mice of the same age were infected in the same manner with 5×10^5 PFU of the DA strain of TMEV.[7]

At three months PI, TMEV-infected animals were divided into four groups consisting each of four mice and treated with the following compounds (10 injections administered subcutaneously every third day, total dosage per animal given in

[a]This work was supported by PHS grant nos. NS 09053, NS 07078, NS 12428 and AG 04342.

parentheses):

1. MBP (0.14 mg, from rat brain) and GC (0.35 mg) in physiological saline (0.5 ml), lecithin (1.4 mg) and bovine serum albumin (BSA, 1.62 mg); emulsified with an equal volume of incomplete Freund's adjuvant (IFA, 0.5 ml).
2. Physiological NaCl (0.5 ml with lecithin and 1.62 mg BSA).
3. No treatment.
4. MBP and GC as above without prior virus inoculation.

Following treatment, the animals survived for four weeks and were subsequently sacrificed by intracardiac perfusion with 3% glutaraldehyde in PBS. Spinal cords were removed, dissected, osmicated, dehydrated in alcohol, and embedded in araldite. One micron sections from 10–15 araldite blocks of each animal were stained with paraphenylenediamine for light and grids with ultrathin sections were stained with uranyl acetate and lead citrate for electron microscopic examination. The MHV-infected animals underwent the same procedure following survival times of 1, 2, 3, 4, and 5 weeks.

For immunohistochemical studies of TMEV-infected mice, immunoelectron microscopic peroxidase-antiperoxidase techniques were used to determine the localization of viral antigen in infected cells, as previously described.[7]

RESULTS

Light microscopic examination of spinal cords from MHV-infected mice revealed areas of demyelination at early stages (6–8 days PI), which showed little relation to vessels and scanty leukocytic infiltrates.[3,4] Later, at 10–20 days PI, larger plaques of demyelination and edema containing numerous macrophages developed (FIG. 1A).

Electron microscopic examination revealed presence of viral particles in the cytoplasm of oligodendrocytes,[3,5] which underwent hypertrophy and subsequent degeneration.[3] Following degeneration of the infected cells, disintegrated myelin sheaths were stripped off axons by invading macrophages.[3] At three weeks PI, some evidence of remyelinating activity was observed at the periphery of lesions, and by 4–5 weeks PI, most demyelinating plaques showed extensive remyelination (FIG. 1B).

By contrast, spinal cords of TMEV-infected mice showed occasional mononuclear infiltrates in the leptomeninges at early states of disease (4–11 days PI),[7] followed by multiple areas of demyelination at 2–3 months PI, which were in close association with perivascular lymphocytes and plasma cells. These plaques contained a large number of macrophages, often filled with myelin debris. Demyelination and inflammation persisted in chronic stages of infection (up to 6–12 months PI).[7] Occasionally, areas of Schwann cell remyelination and scanty oligodendroglial remyelination were observed. Immunohistochemical studies on chronically infected TMEV mice showed viral antigen to be localized mainly in oligodendroglial cells.[7] Spinal cords of untreated and NaCl-treated TMEV-infected mice at five months PI showed multiple plaques of demyelination associated with perivascular mononuclear infiltrates and numerous macrophages with little evidence of CNS remyelination (FIG. 2A).

Spinal cords of all animals treated with MBP and GC showed, along with some demyelinated plaques, multiple areas of extensive CNS remyelination, which were practically devoid of inflammatory cells (FIG. 2B). Some scattered mononuclear infiltrates were observed in adjacent leptomeninges. Noninfected animals treated with MBP and GC showed no evidence of inflammatory activity or demyelination in the CNS.

DISCUSSION

In MHV-induced demyelinating disease in mice, demyelination is caused by lysis of infected oligodendrocytes,[3] and immunosuppressive measures enhance rather than lessen the mortality of infected mice.[1] Rapid extensive CNS remyelination in this disease occurs,[4,6] and has been attributed to oligodendroglial cell proliferation.[6]

By contrast, TMEV-induced demyelination is probably caused by an immune-mediated mechanism,[2,7] in which immunosuppressive measures prevent the development of demyelinating lesions.[8] The morphological appearance of demyelinating plaques shows similarities to chronic EAE, an autoimmune-demyelinating disease.[2] A recent immunohistochemical study[7] suggests that TMEV-induced demyelination occurs as a result of an immune-mediated response to persistently infected oligodendrocytes. Although evidence for Schwann cell remyelination at chronic stages of disease has been reported,[10] spontaneous CNS remyelination is rare. Our untreated and NaCl-treated TMEV-infected mice showed occasionally some abortive remyelination at five months PI at the periphery of lesions. None of them displayed large areas of CNS remyelination as observed in all of the MBP/GC-treated animals (FIG. 2B).

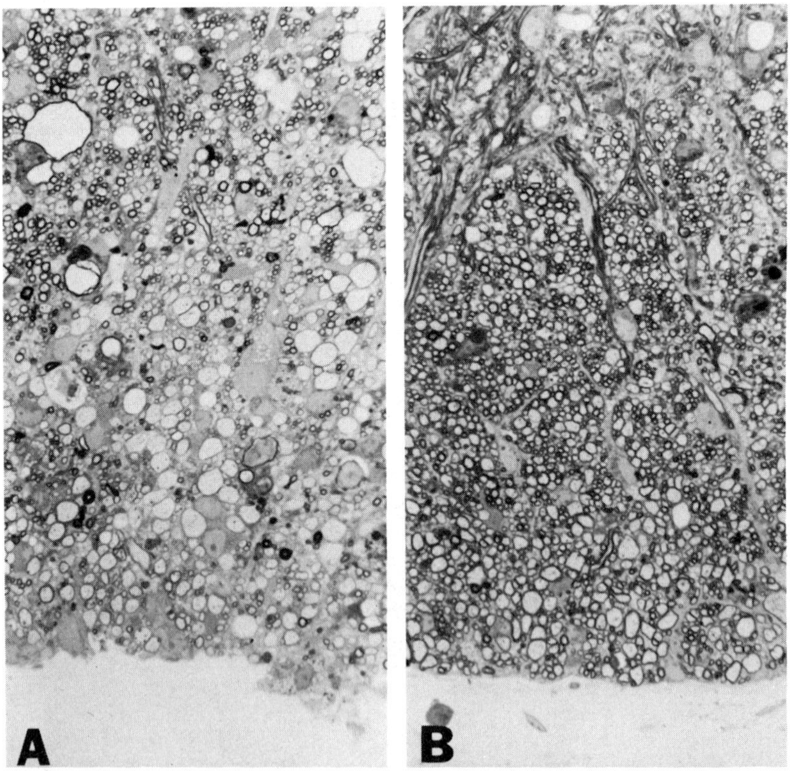

FIGURE 1. Spinal cord white matter lesions of MHV-infected Balb/c mice at two weeks (**A**) and four weeks PI (**B**). Note the extensive remyelination of the lesion in (**B**). (paraphenylenediamine, ×450.)

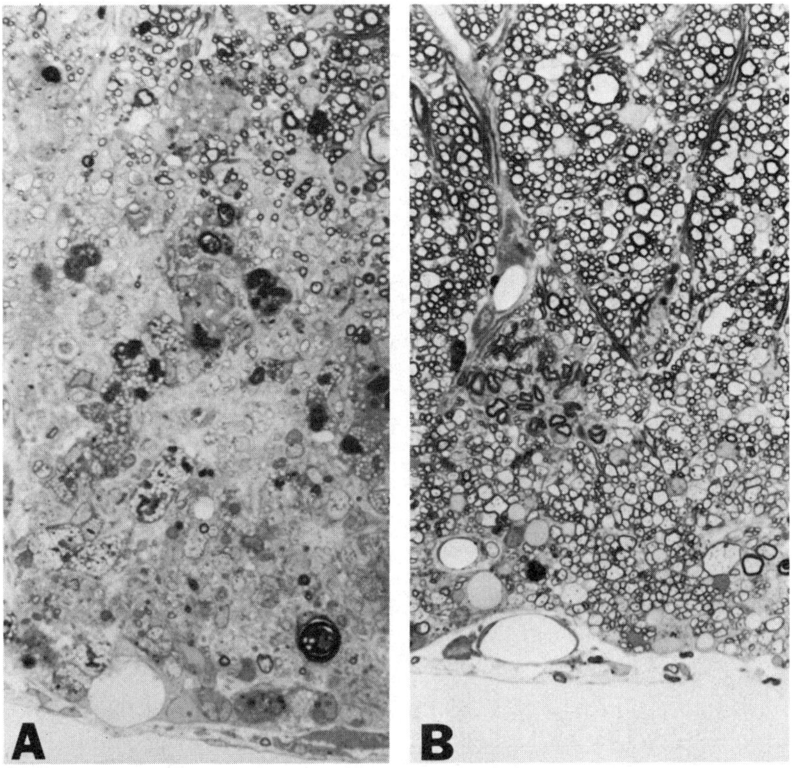

FIGURE 2. Spinal cord white matter lesions of TMEV-infected SJL/J mice at five months PI treated with NaCl (**A**) and with MPB/GC (**B**). Note the area of CNS remyelination with numerous large axons surrounded by thin myelin sheaths in (**B**). (paraphenylenediamine, ×450.)

Similar treatment effects were reported in chronic autoimmune relapsing EAE of guinea pigs.[9] It was suggested that a combined serological and cellular effect was responsible for the extensive CNS remyelination and possible oligodendroglial proliferation observed following MBP/GC administration.[9] Whether similar mechanisms are effective in the marked CNS remyelination observed in our MBP/GC-treated TMEV-infected mice is currently being investigated.

REFERENCES

1. Weiner, L. P. 1973. Pathogenesis of demyelination induced by a mouse hepatitis virus (JHM virus). Arch. Neurol. **28:** 298–303.
2. dal Canto, M. C. & H. L. Lipton. 1975. Primary demyelination in Theiler's virus infection. Lab. Invest. **33:** 626–637.
3. Lampert, P. W., J. K. Sims & A. J. Kniazeff. 1973. Mechanisms of demyelination in JHM virus encephalomyelitis. Acta Neuropathol. **24:** 76–85.
4. Haspel, M. V., P. W. Lampert & M. B. Oldstone. 1978. Temperature-sensitive mutants

of mouse hepatitis virus produce a high incidence of demyelination. Proc. Nat. Acad. Sci. U.S.A. **75:** 4033–4036.

5. Powell, H. P. & P. W. Lampert. 1975. Oligodendrocytes and their myelin-plasma membrane connections in JHM mouse hepatitis virus encephalomyelitis. Lab. Invest. **33:** 440–445.
6. Herndon, R. M., D. L. Price & L. P. Weiner. 1977. Regeneration of oligodendroglia during recovery from demyelinating disease. Science **195:** 693–694.
7. Rodriguez, M., J. L. Leibowitz & P. W. Lampert. 1983. Persistent infection of oligodendrocytes in Theiler's virus-induced encephalomyelitis. Ann. Neurol. **13:** 426–433.
8. Lipton, H. L. & M. C. dal Canto. 1976. Theiler's virus-induced demyelination: Prevention by immunosuppression. Science **192:** 62–64.
9. Raine, C. S. & U. Traugott. 1983. Chronic relapsing experimental autoimmune encephalomyelitis: Ultrastructure of the central nervous system of animals treated with combinations of myelin components. Lab. Invest. **48:** 275–284.
10. dal Canto, M. C. & H. L. Lipton. 1980. Schwann cell remyelination and recurrent demyelination in the central nervous system of mice infected with attenuated Theiler's virus. Am. J. Pathol. **98:** 101–122.

DISCUSSION OF THE PAPER

R. T. Johnson (*The Johns Hopkins University, Baltimore, MD*): Specific questions to clarify a specific point?

B. G. Arnason (*University of Chicago, Chicago, IL*): We tried cyclophosphamide and it didn't work.

P. W. Lampert (*University of California at San Diego, La Jolla, CA*): It's not published yet but I'm afraid the results of our suppression experiments have turned out to be negative. We are treating these animals with MBP before we infect them. This prevents disease in EAE but did not prevent disease in TMEV-infected mice. We did not repeat the cyclophosphamide studies reported by Lipton.[8]

Arnason: Is that your work or the literature?

Lampert: The immunosuppression work is quoted from Lipton.

Arnason: I disagree.

Lampert: Our studies on preventing disease by prior desensitization with myelin basic protein failed to affect TMEV-induced demyelination.

Detection by Hybridization of Viral Infection of the Human Central Nervous System[a]

ASHLEY T. HAASE,[b] LINDA STOWRING,[c]
PETER VENTURA,[d] JACK BURKS,[e] GEORGE EBERS,[f]
WALLACE TOURTELLOTTE,[g] AND KENNETH WARREN[h]

[b]*Department of Microbiology*
University of Minnesota
Minneapolis, Minnesota 55455

[c]*Department of Laboratory Medicine*
University of California
San Francisco, California 94117

[d]*Bio-Response, Inc.*
Hayward, California 94545

[e]*Center for Neurological Diseases*
Rocky Mountain Multiple Sclerosis Center
Denver, Colorado 80262

[f]*University of Western Ontario*
London, Ontario, Canada

[g]*Veterans Administration Wadsworth Medical Center*
Los Angeles, California 90073
and
University of California at Los Angeles School of Medicine
Los Angeles, California 90024

[h]*Faculty of Graduate Studies and Research*
University of Alberta
Edmonton, Alberta, Canada

INTRODUCTION

Studies of animal models of demyelination and investigation of the epidemiology of multiple sclerosis (MS) both point to the possibility of virus infection as one inciting factor in the disease, but until recently there has been little evidence for the central prediction of this hypothesis, persistence of viruses in the human brain. Advances in technology, particularly in methods for detecting virus genes by hybridization, have now provided us with our first glimpse of an indigenous viral flora of the brain, and

[a]This work was supported by grants from the ACS, NMSS, NIH and the Veterans Administration. Dr. Haase was a medical investigator of the Veterans Administration.

thus offer some support for the view that MS might be an immunopathological response to infection in susceptible individuals. In this article we describe the background that led to the discovery of virus genes in the brain; the current status of the ongoing search for virus genetic material in chronic diseases; and some findings on the relationship between infected cells and pathology that place some restraints on theories of virus infection as the cause of MS.

RESTRICTED GENE EXPRESSION AS A GENERAL THEME IN CHRONIC VIRUS INFECTIONS

The rationale and the means for the search for virus genes in the CNS are an outgrowth of studies of slow infections of man and animals. One of the important lessons we have learned in the course of these investigations is that the infected cell is a minority species in the tissue as a whole, and in infected cells virus gene expression is restricted. From the implied limits on the production of virus particles and proteins we can understand how viruses can satisfy the two logical preconditions for persistent infections *in vivo:* (1) survival of virus in the face of host immune surveillance, (2) survival of the host for extended periods in the face of infection by viruses that in other situations, permissive infection of tissue culture cells, kill the cells in hours to a few days. We can also reopen the question of virus infection in disease like MS where viruses have been suspected, but for which there has been no evidence of viral antigens or particles in the tissues.

This concept of restricted gene expression in chronic virus infections is a derivative of analysis of the slow infection in sheep caused by visna virus, and the slow infection in man, subacute sclerosing panencephalitis, caused by measles virus. Visna[1] is a slowly progressive demyelinating condition of sheep that occurs months to years after introduction of the etiological agent, a virus of the retrovirus family.[2] The virus provokes an inflammatory response in the lungs and CNS of infected sheep, and in the CNS the attendant destruction of cells is responsible for secondary demyelination. In some animals there is also evidence of a primary demyelinative process, the causes of which are presently unknown.[3] Infection by visna virus stimulates both a cellular and humoral immune response, but in most instances the virus is not eradicated because the genome is harbored in most cells in a lysogenic state.[4] The synthesis of viral RNA[5] and protein subcomponents is greatly reduced compared to productive infections in tissue culture, and consequently the infected cell escapes detection and destruction by immune surveillance.

The unveiling of this covert relationship between virus and host cell depended on refinements in cytological hybridization methods that are now approaching extraordinary levels of sensitivity in the attogram (10^{-18} g) range. We can detect in a cell, for example, a single copy of the genomes of visna virus,[6] measles virus,[7] or hepatitis B virus [8] and this already has enlarged our view of the host range of common viruses. *In situ* hybridization is also a quantitative technique,[6] so that by counting rains over cells we can enumerate the number of transcripts and assess the level of gene expression. We believe this aspect of the method will have the greatest impact on our understanding of virus infections at the molecular level.

Application of this technology in visna disclosed first of all virus genomes in cells that had too little antigen to be detected by immunofluorescent methods[4]; and, second, about a two order of magnitude decrease in the number of copies of viral RNA compared to permissive infections *in vitro.*[5] We also came to appreciate with this technique the focal nature of virus infection in real life — only about 0.1–1.0% of the cells in a section from an infected animal actually carried viral genetic information.

This observation provided the explanation for our previous inability to detect virus infection by hybridization methods that relied on nucleic acid extracted from the tissues, for in the extraction process nucleic acids from uninfected cells diluted viral genetic material beyond the limits of detection.

The focal nature of infection and the limited synthesis of viral genome and transcripts has turned out to be a general theme of slow virus infections. In TABLE 1 we have summarized a comparison of visna and measles virus infection assessed at the single cell level. In both measles and visna productive infections in tissue culture are characterized by the synthesis of thousands of copies of viral RNA and readily detectable concentrations of antigens in most cells. Similar results obtain in hamsters succumbing to measles virus encephalitis, but the proportion of infected cells is much less than in tissue culture. In chronic infections an even smaller fraction of cells are infected, there are only a few copies of viral nucleic acid in the cell, and antigens can be detected only rarely.[9]

TABLE 1. Restricted Synthesis and Expression of Viral Genes in Two Slow Infections

	Frequency of Cells with Viral RNA		Frequency of Cells with Viral DNA	Average Number of Copies of Viral RNA		Frequency of Cells with Viral Antigen	
Type of Infection	Measles	Visna	Visna	Measles	Visna	Measles	Visna
Permissive infection of tissue culture cells	90%	90%	90%	2500	10,000	90%	90%
Acute infections of animals	0.9%	—	—	1500	—	90%	—
Chronic infection of animals	0.3%	1.9%	1.6%	3	140	0–0.01%	0–0.05%
Subacute sclerosing panencephalitis	0.3%	—	—	7	—	0–0.01%	—

The frequencies of cells with viral nucleic acids and copy numbers were determined by *in situ* hybridization; the frequencies of antigen positive cells were evaluated by immunofluorescence. (Data taken from references 5, 9.)

This global repression is, moreover, not the only kind of restriction in SSPE. The figures in the table were derived from analyses of brain biopsy material taken for diagnostic purposes from four patients at a relatively early phase of disease. In material from patients succumbing to SSPE many cells contain inclusion bodies with viral antigens and hundreds of copies of viral RNA (unpublished), but virus can be recovered only with difficulty by explanation. In this stage of infection the restriction in the virus life cycle is at the level of virus assembly, and involves a defect in the synthesis, structure, or stability of the measles virus matrix polypeptide that is responsible for aligning the viral nucleocapsid with the viral envelope components.[10]

MEASLES VIRUS GENES IN MS

Appreciation of the subtlety of the relationship between virus and host cell in slow infections logically leads to a reevaluation of the role of virus infection in chronic diseases of man like MS where previous attempts to demonstrate viral antigens, particles or infectivity predictably would have been unsuccessful. We therefore undertook a search for virus genes in MS, and initially looked for measles virus genes because of the prominent immunological response to this virus in MS.[11] In the first four cases we examined we found two foci in one brain with fewer than ten copies of viral RNA in several cells.[7] We could not detect viral antigens by immunofluorescence in these foci, in accord with many other negative results in MS, even the most contemporary where extremely sensitive assays for measles virus proteins have been employed.[12,13]

A PROGRESS REPORT

In the past two years we have continued these investigations and have found measles virus genes in the brains of both MS and controls. (See TABLE 2A).

In MS in plaques and in areas that had no obvious pathological changes we found cells that contained the equivalent of five to ten copies of the measles genome. We found similar foci in control material (other neurological and nonneurological diseases and trauma). Initially it appeared that the proportion of positive cases might be higher in MS, but in the past year with control material with shorter autolysis times no significant differences were observed between the two groups.

VIRUSES OTHER THAN MEASLES IN HUMAN BRAIN

As one of the criteria for the specificity of hybridization we routinely anneal visna virus probe to sections since it is likely a virus restricted to ruminants[1] and would not be expected to bind to human tissues (TABLE 2B). In work in progress we also have hybridized, to subjacent sections to those positive for measles, probes specific for cytomegalovirus, poliovirus, or a picornavirus, Theiler's agent, that causes a demyelinating disorder in mice. Thus far these surveys have been negative, but there is one report of detection by liquid hybridization of poliovirus sequences in nervous tissue,[15] and Michel Brahic (personal communication) has detected by *in situ* hybridization polio and Theiler's virus sequences in one brain from a control. The other virus for which there is now good evidence of spread to the CNS is herpes simplex. From analyses of animal models of herpetic infections it appears that the virus establishes

TABLE 2A. Detection of Measles Virus Genes in Human Brain

Diagnosis	Fraction of Cases with Positive Hybridization: All Cases	Fraction of Cases with Positive Hybridization: Cases with Less than Six Hours of Autolysis
MS	13/25	8/18
plaque	8/13	
nonplaque	5/13	
Non-MS	5/18	4/7

Sections of frozen tissues were hybridized *in situ* with a measles virus-specific probe labeled with ^3H to a specific activity of 4×10^8 dpm per μg.[7] A positive result indicates that with a radioautographic exposure of two weeks there were cells in foci that had grain counts severalfold higher than background—equivalent to five to ten copies of the viral RNA genome per cell. The probability that the increased number of grains could have occurred by chance was less than 0.01.[14] Criteria for the specificity of hybridization are summarized in TABLE 2B.

TABLE 2B. Specificity of Hybridization

Probe	Hybridization Result
Measles	
Hybridization on Section One	positive
Two	positive
Three	positive
Second piece of tissue, coded	positive
After digestion with ribonuclease	negative
Visna	negative
Theiler's virus	negative
Polio virus types 1, 2, 3	negative
Cytomegalovirus	negative

Specificity criteria illustrated with one case of MS: (1) Measles virus-specific probe reproducibly bound to cells in two foci in one fragment of tissue, and to cells in one focus in a second fragment sent under code. (2) Digestion of the tissue with ribonucleases A, T_1 reduced binding of probe to background levels. (3) Probes specific for the other viruses listed were labeled with ^{3}H, ^{35}S, or ^{125}I to specific activities comparable to the measles probe sufficient to detect a single copy of the virus genome with an exposure of two weeks. Grain counts in each instance were not above background.

latent infection both in neurons in the trigeminal ganglion and in the brain. An analogous invasion of the CNS that probably occurs in man as well as herpes simplex virus DNA has been detected in brain tissue by *in situ* hybridization in dementia, one case of chronic schizophrenia,[18] and by blot hybridization in four cases of MS and three controls.[19]

CONCLUSIONS AND PROSPECTUS

The picture that begins to emerge from these studies is that during common viral infections virus genes may be deposited quite frequently in the human CNS. The implications for disease are far less clear, but some simple hypotheses can be discarded. First of all, both MS cases and controls exhibit the same phenomena, and secondly, in MS there is no tendency for covert infection of oligodendrocytes or for cells in the plaque. We therefore cannot attribute the pathology in MS to a unique tropism of a virus, and we cannot invoke an unusual susceptibility in MS patients to neurological involvement during virus infection.

This is not to say that the genetic residuum of infection has no role in disease; it is quite conceivable that virus genetic information in the nervous system may be expressed at very low levels that we cannot detect as yet, but sufficient to provoke an immunopathological demyelinating process in the individual destined to be afflicted with MS. For this part of the story we must turn to our colleagues in immunology. For our part we intend to continue to use these exceptionally sensitive hybridization methods to enlarge our vision of the viral flora in man, with the hope of illuminating some aspect of chronic disease by the discovery of virus infection in unexpected places.

ACKNOWLEDGMENT

We thank R. Frautschi for prepartion of the manuscript.

REFERENCES

1. BRAHIC, M.T. & A.T. HAASE. 1981. Lentiviriniae: Maedi/visna virus group of infections. Comparative aspects and diagnosis. *In* Comparative Diagnosis of Viral Disease, vol 4., part B. E. Kurstak & C. Kurstak, Eds.: 619. Academic Press. New York.
2. HAASE, A.T. 1975. The slow infection caused by visna virus. Curr. Top. Microbiol. Immunol. **72:** 101–156.
3. GEORGSSON, G., J.R. MARTIN, J. KLEIN, P.A. PALSSON, N. NATHANSON & G. PETURSSON. 1982. Primary demyelination in visna: An ultrastructural study of Icelandic sheep with clinical signs following experimental infection. Acta Neuropathol. (Berlin) **57:** 171–178.
4. HAASE, A.T., L.S. STOWRING, O. NARAYAN, D. GRIFFIN & D. PRICE. 1977. The slow persistent infection caused by virna virus: Role of host restriction. Science **195:** 175–177.
5. BRAHIC, M., L. STOWRING, P. VENTURA & A.T. HAASE. 1981. Gene expression in visna virus infection. Nature **292:** 240.
6. HAASE, A.T., L. STOWRING, J.D. HARRIS, B. TRAYNOR, P. VENTURA, R. PELUSO & M. BRAHIC. 1982. Visna DNA synthesis and the tempo of infection *in vitro.* Virology **119:** 399–410.
7. HAASE, A.T., P. VENTURA, C.J., GIBBS & W.W. TOURTELLOTTE. 1981. Measles virus nucleotide sequences: Detection by hybridization *in situ.* Science **212:** 672–675.
8. BLUM, H.E., A.T. HAASE, J.D. HARRIS, D. WALKER & G.N. VYAS. 1983. Detection of hepatitis B virus DNA in hepatocytes, bile duct epithelium, and vascular elements by *in situ* hybridization. Proc. Nat. Acad. Sci. U.S.A. **80:** 6685–6688.
9. HAASE, A.T., P. SWOVELAND, L. STOWRING, P. VENTURA, K.P. JOHNSON, E. NORRBY & C.J. GIBBS, JR. 1981. Measles virus genome in infections of the central nervous system. J. Infect. Dis. **144:** 154–160.
10. HALL, W.W. & P.W. CHOPPIN. 1981. Measles-virus proteins in the brain tissue of patients with subacute sclerosing panencephalitis: Absence of the M protein. N. Eng. J. Med. **304:** 1154.
11. NORRBY, E. 1978. Viral antibodies in multiple sclerosis. Prog. Med. Virol. **24:** 1–39.
12. HALL, W.W. & P.W. CHOPPIN. 1982. Failure to detect measles virus proteins in brain tissue of patients with multiple sclerosis. Lancet (April 24). pp. 957–958.
13. FRASER, K.B., I.V. ALLEN, M.A. ARMSTRONG, S.E. DERMOTT, M. HAIRE, J.H.D. MILLAR, P.V. SHIRODARIA & H.V. THORNE. 1982. Failure to detect replicating viruses in brain and other tissues from multiple sclerosis patients. Lancet (May 22). pp. 1185–1186.
14. ARNOLD, A.P. 1981. Quantitative analysis of steroid autoradiograms. J. Histochem. Cytochem. **29**(1A):207–211.
15. KOHNE, D.E., C.J. GIBBS, L. WHITE, S.M. TRACY, W. MEINKE & R.A. SMITH. 1981. Virus detection by nucleic acid hybridization: Examination of normal and ALS tissues for the presence of poliovirus. J. Gen. Virol. **56:** 223–233.
16. CARBRERA, C.V., C. WOHLENBERG, H. OPENSHAW, M. REY-MENDEZ, A. PUGA & A.L. NOTKINS. 1980. Herpes simples virus DNA sequences in the CNS of latently infected mice. Nature **288:** 288–290.
17. ROCK, D.L. & N.W. FRASER. 1983. Detection of HSV-1 genome in central nervous system of latently infected mice. Nature **302**(5908): 523–525.
18. SEQUIERA, L.W., L.H. CARRASCO, A. CURRY, L.C. JENNINGS, M.A. LORD & R.N.P. SUTTON. 1979. Detection of herpes-simplex viral genome in brain tissue. Lancet (Sept. 22). pp. 609–612.
19. FRASER, N.W., W.C. LAWRENCE, A. WROBLEWSKA, D.H. GILDEN & H. KOPROWSKI. 1981. Herpes simplex type 1 DNA in human brain tissue. Proc. Nat. Acad. Sci. U.S.A. **78**(10): 6461–6465.

Multiple Sclerosis: Epidemiology and HLA Associations

W. I. McDONALD

Institute of Neurology
National Hospital
Queen Square
London WC1N 3BG, United Kingdom

The three preceding papers have dealt with mechanisms by which viruses can damage the central nervous system. It is now appropriate to consider the reasons for thinking that such a discussion is relevant to multiple sclerosis (MS). They derive from the study of the epidemiology of the disease, and of the frequency of certain normal characteristics — in particular the human leukocyte-associated (HLA) antigens — in different racial and patient groups.

EPIDEMIOLOGY OF MULTIPLE SCLEROSIS

The first clue that the risk of developing MS was related to where an individual lives came from Davenport's survey[1] (published in 1922) of illness among drafted men, although as far back as 1903 Bramwell[2] had suggested that there might be a difference between the frequency of multiple sclerosis in Scotland and the northeastern United States. Davenport noted that MS was relatively more common in drafted men from the northern states. Nearly 30 years later, Limburg[3] provided evidence for this trend from mortality data, and Kurland's prevalence studies[4] in 1952 soon confirmed it.

This approach was quickly taken up elsewhere, and within a few years it was clear that for people of northern European origin the risk of developing MS increases with increasing latitude in both the northern and southern hemispheres. The evidence from mortality and morbidity data was consistent[5] but all epidemiological studies are subject to error from misdiagnosis and underreporting. The latter can be shown to account for much of the apparent increase in prevalence when a given region is resurveyed. This is well illustrated in Scotland. A survey by Sutherland[6] in 1956 showed an overall prevalence of 60 per 100,000 with 108 per 100,000 in the Orkney Islands. Resurveys in the Aberdeen region by Downie and his colleagues[7,8] showed a prevalence of 127 per 100,000 in 1970 and 144 per 100,000 in 1973, most of the additional cases in 1973 being found to have had evidence of the disease in 1970. The latest survey, which has not yet been published, shows a prevalence of 178 per 100,000 (Downie and Phadke, personal communication). In the meantime Poskanzer *et al.*[8] had resurveyed the Orkneys and found a prevalence of 309 per 100,000.

Prevalence studies in many countries have led to the conclusion that with certain exceptions (see below) there is a high risk (prevalence $\geq$40 per 100,000) above latitude 40° in both the northern and the southern hemispheres.[10] There is a medium risk (20–39 per 100,000) between this latitude and the Tropics of Capricorn and Cancer, and a low risk ($\leq$19 per 100,000) between the Tropics themselves. Whether there is a sharp transition between zones, or a smoother gradient, is unknown. It is of course true that the high- and low-risk zones also correspond with high and low doctor/patient ratios, raising the possibility of underrecognition of the disease in low latitudes. The influence of migration on prevalence of the disease however suggests that the observations reflect a true differential.

Migration Studies

It has been known for more than 30 years that in South Africa the risk of developing multiple sclerosis was higher in northern Europeans who had migrated there in adult life than those of the same stock who were born there, or who migrated in childhood.[10,11] Kurtzke *et al.*[12] found a prevalence of 12.8 per 100,000 among 29,287 individuals aged 0–14 at migration from the United Kingdom (four cases) compared with 62.2 per 100,000 among 9,968 individuals migrating between ages 15 and 19 (seven cases). Comparable figures were obtained from migrants for northern Europe as a whole. Thus there is between a 5:1 and a 6:1 greater risk of developing MS in those who migrated after childhood. Similar data were obtained from a study of migration to Hawaii.[13,14] The prevalence of multiple sclerosis among migrants from the north and west of the United States (where the prevalence is approximately 40 per 100,000) was 37.6 per 100,000 for those who migrated after the age of 15 but 3.7 for those who migrated before this age. The total numbers are smaller than in the South African investigation, there being only 34 cases in all. Recent evidence suggests that there is a similar trend within the United States.[16]

What of migration from low-risk to high-risk zones? The evidence is less satisfactory because the populations at risk are even smaller. But as far as they go, they support the notion of a regional differential in risk. In Israel, the adjusted annual incidence rate was higher (2.0 per 100,000) in immigrants from Africa and Asia who had migrated before the age of 15 than in those who had migrated after that age (0.4 per 100,000).[15] Kurtzke and Bui-Quoc-Huong[17] surveyed 3,451 half-Vietnamese migrants to Paris and found three cases of MS, corresponding to a crude prevalence rate of 89 per 100,000. Cases of MS are seen in the Indian and West Indian populations in the United Kingdom; Dean[18] has them under surveillance but it is too early to draw reliable conclusions.

In summary, the epidemiological data are broadly consistent and suggest the operation of an environmental factor in the etiology of the disease. The influence of age at migration on risk further suggests that the factor is more potent in childhood, although the observations by Detels *et al.*[19] indicate that it remains significant in later decades.

Clusters

The third general conclusion from epidemiological studies is that the environmental factor may be infective in nature. The notion of an infective origin for MS is venerable, having been argued strongly by Pierre Marie[20] in the last decade of the nineteenth century. Poskanzer *et al.*[21] noted a similarity in the geographical distribution of polio and MS and suggested that the latter too might have a viral origin. Liebowitz and Alter,[15] noting a higher standard of hygiene in the parental home of patients than controls in Israel, thought that the infection might be enteric in nature.

The occurrence of clusters of cases in restricted regions has been recognized for many years but interpreting their significance has been difficult because clustering can occur as a statistical effect, without biological significance. A remarkable example has been reported recently.[22] In a careful survey of the Faroe Islands, Kurtzke and Hyllestedt found that there had been no cases of MS recognized prior to the Second World War. Between 1943 and 1960, 24 cases appeared and there has been only one further case since. This clustering of cases in space and time strongly suggests that an environmental factor was operating and they argued cogently for its being infective, and possibly related to the advent of the British army just before the epidemic began.

If the environmental agent in multiple sclerosis is infective, what is its nature? Cook *et al.*[23] found an association between contact with small pets and MS and suggested a role for the distemper virus. Others have failed to find such a connection,[24] although an alleged outbreak of distemper on the Faroes in the early 1940s gave added interest to the hypothesis. The problem is unresolved.

Genetic Factors

The fourth thing that epidemiology has told us about multiple sclerosis is that there is probably a genetic influence on susceptibility to it. MS is rare or absent in certain racial groups (*e.g.* the Bantu) including some, such as Orientals and Gypsies, who may share a common environment with European Caucasoids in whom the disease is relatively common.

The scale of the difference in prevalence between Orientals and European Caucasoids living at comparable latitudes is indicated by the figures for Sapporo, Japan (43° north — two per 100,000) and Boston, Massachusetts (42° north — 41 per 100,000).[5] Similar differences (though in a small population) exist in Hawaii[13,14] and on the west coast of the United States where the populations at risk are larger. Detels *et al.*[19] compared mortality data in California and Washington State. They found that the annual age- and sex-adjusted death rate was consistently lower in the Japanese (and Chinese), both native-born and foreign-born, than in the whites. Again the numbers are small but the conclusions are supported by a more recent prevalence study that showed a lower rate in the Japanese than in the Europeans, and that the north/south gradient, which was so striking in the Europeans, was absent.[58] This strongly suggests the existence of a genetic factor.

In Hungary there are two racially distinct populations — the European Caucasoids and the Gypsies (who migrated from northern India to the Balkans in the second century A.D. and thence to the rest of Europe about 500 years ago).[25] Their language retains affinities with North Indian tongues. They number about 110,000 in the trans-Danubian counties. The prevalence has been determined in a hospital-based study, which is not ideal, but the differences are striking. In the Caucasoids the prevalence is about what one might expect — 37 per 100,000 — whereas in the Gypsies only two cases have been identified.[26]

Summary

The study of the disease in different populations has provided good evidence that there is an environmental factor involved in its etiology. It is probably more potent in childhood than in adult life and it is probably infective in nature. Certain populations are relatively insusceptible, probably for genetic reasons. More compelling evidence for a genetic factor comes from twin studies that are reviewed elsewhere in this volume.

GENETIC ASSOCIATIONS

I now wish to review what has been learned about the nature of the genetic element in the etiology of MS from the study of certain normal characteristics in different populations.

HLA System

Weak associations with HLA-A3 and HLA-B7 were first reported in European Caucasoids in the early 1970s.[27,28] Similar associations were subsequently found in Iranians,[29] but not in Arabs[30] and Israelis.[31] The evidence from India is conflicting.[32,33] By the mid 1970s it was becoming clear that there are stronger associations with gene products of the D and DR loci. The position can be summarized as follows:

North European Caucasoids. There is a strong association with DW2 and/or DR2 for most northern European Caucasoids wherever they live, although the association is somewhat weaker in North America than in northern Europe itself, Scandinavia and Australia.[34,35,36] Our United Kingdom figures[37] are representative of the northern European data: DR2 is found in 19% of controls and in 55% of patients with MS. An association with DW2 has also been found in the North American Negro.[38] The exception to this general rule appears to be the Orkney and Shetland Islands where no D/DR association was found.[39] This result is rather surprising since strong associations with DR2 are found in both Scandinavia and Britain, and the Islanders have racial ties to both places. The explanation is not clear. Technical factors may contribute: Poskanzer *et al.*[39] included atypical cases (22% of their total series of 91 patients), whereas the other data are based on findings on typical cases. The investigation also depended on the use of frozen cells with which some laboratories have had difficulty. However, Poskanzer *et al.* did observe the usual linkage between A3, B7 and DW2 in controls, suggesting that the observed lack of association between MS and DW2 in that series was real. Finally, Compston[40] has pointed out that the frequency of B7, DW2 and DR2 in patients from the Orkney and Shetland Islands is not significantly different from that found in other northern European patients with multiple sclerosis, the lack of an association arising from the fact that the frequency of these antigens in the healthy Islanders is significantly higher than in healthy controls in England, Northern Europe and the United States.

Investigations in Germany,[41] France,[42] and the United Kingdom (J.R. Batchelor, unpublished observations) have shown a significant association with DR3 as well as DR2. In the French study DR2 and DR3 were found in 13.8% of the MS group compared with 2.6% of controls. The combination was particularly associated with the progressive form of the disease.

Mediterranean Populations. In both the Jordanian Arabs[30] and the Italians[34] there is an association with DR4.[a] In the former, DR4 was found in 15/43 controls and 28/32 cases of MS.

Japanese. No HLA association has been found in the Japanese, the earlier weak association with DRW6[34] not having been confirmed on a larger sample.[43]

Hungarians. The results in Hungary[26] are of special interest. The frequency of DR2 in the Caucasoid population is in keeping with the results from elsewhere in Europe (19.5% in the controls and 42.7% in the patients with MS). In the Gypsies, however, DR2 is present in 56.5% of the controls (and both the patients) and yet the disease is rare in this ethnic group.

What are we to make of the HLA data with its apparent contradictions? We

[a]The association actually demonstrated was with a locally defined antigen (BT102) that is largely equivalent to DR4.

cannot ignore the rather strong association usually seen in Caucasoids. However, the first observations, that specifically different associations are seen with northern Europeans on the one hand and southern Europeans and Arabs on the other, secondly that no HLA association is seen in the Japanese, and thirdly that the disease is very rare in a population in which the incidence of HLA-DR2 is high, indicate that the presence of HLA-DR2 alone is neither sufficient nor necessary for the development of the disease. This interpretation is consistent with the family data that shows less than the expected sharing of HLA haplotypes.[44,45] It is strongly supported by the NIH twin data[46] which showed that in the two pairs of dizygotic twins concordant for multiple sclerosis only one of each pair was DW2 positive.

If we accept that the HLA association has some relevance, what explanation might there be for the apparent discrepancies? There are several possibilities, not all mutually exclusive. The first is that susceptibility is conferred by HLA-DR2 or HLA-DR4 in the northern European Caucasoid and Mediterranean groups respectively and that the environmental agent is different in different regions. The absence of an association in the Japanese and Indians is not necessarily against this explanation. There are many other possible associations still to be explored since the HLA region is complex and still incompletely characterized. It is, however, difficult to account for the Hungarian observations on this basis alone. A second possibility is that DR2 and DR4 are acting as markers for a single hitherto unidentified susceptibility gene in the HLA region.[47,48] A third possibility is that more than one genetic factor is involved in the etiology of the disease. Recent work has demonstrated that there are indeed other significant associations with multiple sclerosis on the sixth chromosome, and on the fourteenth.

Properdin, one of the components of the alternative complement pathway, exists in a number of different forms. This polymorphism is coded for at a locus within the HLA region on the sixth chromosome known as Bf. Two laboratories, Stewart's in Sydney[49] and Batchelor's in London[37] have demonstrated a significant association of the Bf system with MS. There was a negative association with one of the two common alleles, BfF. In our own data,[37] BfF was present in 36% of the controls but only 14% of the patients with MS. There was a corresponding increase in the frequency of the other common allele BfS. This association was not seen with isolated optic neuritis, although the association with DR2 was. The observations suggest that the Bf system may influence dissemination of lesions, or the rate at which they accumulate, a hypothesis which we are testing at present in collaboration with Downie and his colleagues in the large group of patients in Aberdeen.

Recently it has been reported that a particular haplotype (C4A*4) concerned with the control of the protein C4 in the classical complement pathway is associated with multiple sclerosis.[50] Confirmation of this observation is awaited.

There have been two independent reports of an association between MS and the Gm system[51,52] which is encoded on the fourteenth chromosome.[53] Stewart and Kirk[51] found an increase of the phenotype 1, 17, 21, 26 ($p < 0.01$) in a well-studied group of patients in Sydney, Australia but the difference was of borderline significance when other, admittedly less well investigated cases were included. The finding may however be significant, since Pandey *et al.*[52] also found a significant excess of the phenotype 1, 17, 21 in patients with multiple sclerosis ($p = 0.02$).

In summary, MS in most, but not all ethnic groups is associated with certain genetic characteristics. The best documented are those coded for in the HLA region of the sixth chromosome, in particular the HLA antigens themselves. Less well documented associations implicate both the classical and alternative complement pathways and the control of antibody structure.

CONCLUSION

At present any attempt to synthesize the data that I have reviewed must be heavy with speculation. It is noteworthy that the genetic associations so far identified relate to the regulation of the immune system and antigen-antibody interactions. It is also known that the HLA profile of an individual influences not only the pattern of response to bacterial antigens[54] but susceptibility to certain autoimmune diseases of the liver[55] and thyroid.[56] There is evidence that in the mouse, the counterpart of the HLA gene products is involved in the recognition of exogenous antigens by sensitized T lymphocytes.[57] The same is probably true for man. Although it seems likely that the development of MS depends upon an interaction between an environmental agent (or agents) and the immune response to it, the nature of the interaction and the mechanism of damage to the nervous system has still to be elucidated. This will require an understanding of the nature of the environmental factor and a more complete characterization of the genetic background and immunological disorder in MS.

Finally, it is important to remember that our ideas about etiology have been formulated on the basis of conclusions sometimes drawn from the study of small numbers of patients. It is appropriate to conclude with a remark of Professor E. D. Acheson (personal communication): "In the study of multiple sclerosis the epidemiological method as employed up to the present has been operating at the limits of its power. I would not like to see any good idea about the etiology of multiple sclerosis fail to be followed up because it did not seem to fit with the conclusions which have been drawn from epidemiological studies."

REFERENCES

1. Davenport, C. D. 1922. Multiple sclerosis from the standpoint of geographic distribution and race. Arch. Neurol. Psychiatry (Chicago) **8:** 51–58.
2. Bramwell, B. 1903. On the relative frequency of disseminated sclerosis in this country (Scotland and the North of England) and in America. Rev. Neurol. Psychiatry (Edinburgh) **1:** 12–17.
3. Limburg, C. C. 1950. The geographic distribution of multiple sclerosis and its estimated prevalence in the US. Proceedings of the Association for Research in Nervous and Mental Disease. **28:** 15–24.
4. Kurland, L. T. 1952. The frequency and geographic distribution of multiple sclerosis as indicated by mortality statistics and morbidity surveys in the United States and Canada. Am. J. Hygiene **55:** 457.
5. Acheson, E. D. 1972. The epidemiology of multiple sclerosis. *In* Multiple sclerosis: A Reappraisal. D. McAlpine, C. E. Lumsden & E. D. Acheson, Eds. Churchill Livingstone. London.
6. Sutherland, J. 1956. Observations on the prevalence of multiple sclerosis in northern Scotland. Brain **79:** 635–654.
7. Sheperd, D. I. & A. W. Downie. 1978. Prevalence of multiple sclerosis in North-East Scotland. Br. Med. J. **2:** 314–316.
8. Sheperd, D. I. & A. W. Downie. 1980. A further prevalance study of multiple sclerosis in North-East Scotland. J. Neurol. Neurosurg. Psychiatry **43:** 310–315.
9. Poskanzer, D. C., L. B. Prenney, J. L. Sheridan & J. Y. Kondy. 1980. Multiple sclerosis in the Orkney and Shetland Islands. 1. Epidemiology, clinical factors and methodology. Journal of Epidemiology and Community Health **34:** 229–239.
10. Acheson, E. D. 1977. Epidemiology of multiple sclerosis. Br. Med. Bull. **33:** 9–14.
11. Dean, G. 1949. Disseminated sclerosis in South Africa. Br. Med. J. **1:** 842–845.
12. Kurtzke, J. F., G. Dean. & D. P. J. Botha. 1970. A method for estimating the age at

immigration of white immigrants to South Africa with an example of MS importance. S. Afr. Med. J. **44:** 663–669.
13. Alter, M., M. Okihiro, W. Rowley & T. Morris. 1971. Multiple sclerosis among Orientals and Caucasians in Hawaii. Neurology **21:** 122–130.
14. Alter, M. & M. Okihiro. 1971. When is multiple sclerosis acquired? Neurology **21:** 1030–1036.
15. Liebowitz, U. & M. Alter. 1973. Multiple Sclerosis: Clues to Its Cause. North Holland. Amsterdam.
16. Kurtzke, J. F., G.W. Beebe & J. E. Norman. 1979. Migration and multiple sclerosis in the United States. Neurology **29:** 579.
17. Kurtzke, J. F. & Bui-Quoc-Huong. 1980. Multiple sclerosis in a migrant population. 2. Half-orientals immigrating in childhood. Ann. Neurol. **8:** 256–260.
18. Dean, G., R. Brady, H. McLoughlin, M. Elian & A. M. Adelstein. 1977. Motor neurone disease and multiple sclerosis among immigrants to Britain. Br. J. Prev. Soc. Med. **31:** 141–147.
19. Detels, R., J. A. Brody & A. H. Edgar. 1972. Multiple sclerosis among American, Japanese and Chinese migrants to California and Washington. J. Chronic Dis. **25:** 3–10.
20. Marie, P. 1895. Lectures on diseases of the spinal cord. Translated by M. Lubbock. The New Sydenham Society. London.
21. Poskanzer, D. C., K. Schapiro & H. Miller. 1963. Multiple sclerosis and poliomyelitis. Lancet **2:** 917–921.
22. Kurtzke, J. F. & K. Hyllested. 1979. Multiple sclerosis in the Faroe Islands. I. Clinical and epidemiological features. Ann. Neurol. **5:** 6–21.
23. Cook, S. D., B. H. Natelson, B. E. Levin, P. S. Chavis & P. C. Dowling. 1978. Further evidence of a possible association between house dogs and multiple sclerosis. Ann. Neurol. **3:** 141–143.
24. Kurland, L. & D. Brian. 1978. Multiple sclerosis in canine pets. Ann. Neurol. **3:** 97–100.
25. Gyódi, E., T. Tauszik, Gy. Petrányi, Á. Kotvász, Gy. Pálffy, I. Takács, P. Nemák & S. R. Hollán. 1981. The HLA antigen distribution in the gypsy population in Hungary. Tissue Antigens **18:** 1–12.
26. Pálffy, Gy. 1982. MS in Hungary, including the gypsy population. *In* Multiple Sclerosis East and West. Y. Kuroiwa & L.T. Kurland, Eds.: 149–157. Karger. Basel.
27. Naito, S., N. Namerow, M. R. Mickey & P. Terasaki. 1972. Multiple sclerosis: Association with HL-A3. Tissue Antigens **2:** 1–4.
28. Jersild, C., A. Svejgaard & T. Fog.1972. HL-A antigens and multiple sclerosis. Lancet **1:** 1240–1241.
29. Lotfi, J., I. Derakhshan, Gh. Hassiri & B. Nikbin. Unpublished observations.
30. Kurdi, A., I. Ayesh, A. Abdallat *et al.* 1977. Different B-lymphocyte alloantigens associated with multiple sclerosis in Arabs and North Europeans. Lancet **1:** 1123–1125.
31. Brautbar, C., I. Cohen, E. Kahana, M. Alter, F. Jørgensen & L. Lamb. 1977. Histocompatibility determinants in Israeli Jewish patients with multiple sclerosis. Tissue Antigens **10:** 291.
32. Wadia, N. H., V. S. Trikannad & P. R. Krishnaswamy. 1981. HLA antigens in multiple sclerosis amongst Indians. J. Neurol. Neurosurg. Psychiatry **44:** 849–851.
33. Singhal, B. S. 1982. Clinical profile and HLA-studies in Indian multiple sclerosis patients from the Bombay region. *In* Multiple Sclerosis East and West. Y. Kuroiwa & L. T. Kurland, Eds.: 123–134. Karger. Basel.
34. Bodmer, W. F., J. R. Batchelor, J. G. Bodmer, H. Festenstein & P. J. Morris. 1978. Histocompatibility Testing 1977. Report of the 7th International Histocompatibility Workshop and Conference, Oxford. Munksgaard. Copenhagen.
35. Batchelor, J. R., D. A. S. Compston & W. I. McDonald 1978. The significance of the association between HLA and multiple sclerosis. Br. Med. Bull. **34:** 279–284.
36. Stewart, G. J. 1980. The HLA system and multiple sclerosis. Ph.D. thesis. University of Sydney.
37. Fielder, A. H. L., J. R. Batchelor, B. Nason Vakarelis, D. A. S. Compston & W. I.

McDonald. 1981. Optic neuritis and multiple sclerosis: Do factor B alleles influence progression of disease? Lancet **2:** 1246–1248.
38. Dupont, B., R. P. Lisak, C. Jersild *et al.* 1977. HLA antigens in black American patients with multiple sclerosis. Transplant. Proc. Suppl. **1:** 181–185.
39. Poskanzer, D. C., P. I. Terasaki, L. B. Prenney, J. L. Sheridan & M. S. Park. 1980. Multiple sclerosis in the Orkney and Shetland Islands. III. Histocompatibility determinants. Journal of Epidemiology and Community Health **34:** 253–257.
40. Compston, D. A. S. 1982. Multiple sclerosis in the Orkneys. Lancet **2:** 98.
41. Grosse-Wilde, H., J. Bertrams, W. Schuppien, B. Netzel, W. Kuppelt & E. Kuwert. 1977. HL-A-D typing in 111 MS patients: Distribution of four HL-A-D alleles. Immunogenetics **4:** 481–488.
42. Madigand, M., J. J-F. Oger, R. Fauchet, O. Sabouraud & B. Genetet. 1982. HLA profiles in multiple sclerosis suggests two forms of disease and the existence of protective haplotypes. J. Neurol. Sci. **53:** 519–529.
43. Naito, S., T. Tabira & Y. Kuroiwa. 1982. HLA studies of multiple sclerosis in Japan. *In* Multiple Sclerosis East and West. Y. Kuroiwa & L. T. Kurland, Eds.: 215–222. Karger. Basel.
44. Ebers, G. C., D. W. Paty, C. R. Stiller, R. F. Nelson, T. P. Seland & B. Larsen. 1982. HLA-typing in multiple sclerosis sibling pairs. Lancet **2:** 88–90.
45. Compston, A. & S. Howard. 1982. HLA typing in multiple sclerosis. Lancet **2:** 661.
46. Williams, A., R. Eldridge, H. McFarland, S. Houff, H. Krebs & D. McFarlin. 1980. Multiple sclerosis in twins. Neurology **30:** 1139–1147.
47. Terasaki, P. I. & M. R. Mickey. 1976. A single mutation hypothesis for multiple sclerosis based on the HLA system. Neurology **26** (6, Part 2): 56–58.
48. Stewart, G. J., J. G. McLeod, A. Basten & H. V. Bashir. 1981. HLA family studies and multiple sclerosis: A common gene dominantly expressed. Hum. Immunol. **3:** 13–29.
49. Stewart, G. J., A Basten & R. L. Kirk. 1979. Strong linkage disequilibrium between HLA-DW2 and BfS in multiple sclerosis and in the normal population. Tissue Antigens **14:** 86–97.
50. Schroder, R., H. Zander, A. Andreas & G. Mauff. 1983. Multiple sclerosis: Immunogenetic analyses of sib-pair double case families. II. Studies on the association of multiple sclerosis with C2, C4, Bf, C3, C6, and GLO polymorphisms. Immunobiology **164:** 160–170.
51. Stewart, G. J. & R. L. Kirk. 1982. The genetics of multiple sclerosis. *In* Multiple Sclerosis. J. Hallpike, C. Adams & W. Tourtellotte, Eds.: 97–128 Chapman and Hall. London.
52. Pandey, J. P., J-M. Goust, J-P. Salier & H. H. Fudenberg. 1981. Immunoglobulin G heavy chain (Gm) allotypes in multiple sclerosis. J. Clin. Invest. **67:** 1797–1800.
53. Croce, C. C., M. Shander, J. Martinis *et al.* 1979. Chromosomal location of the genes for human immunoglobulin heavy chains. Proc. Nat. Acad. Sci. U.S.A. **76:** 3416–3419.
54. Whittingham, S., J. D. Mathews, M. S. Schanfield *et al.* 1980. Interactive effect of Gm allotypes and HLA B locus antigens on the human antibody response to a bacterial antigen. Clin. Exp. Immunol. **40:** 8–15.
55. Whittingham, S., J. D. Mathews, M. S. Schanfield, B. D. Tait & I. R. Mackay. 1981. Interaction of HLA and Gm in autoimmune chronic active hepatitis. Clin. Exper. Immunol. **43:** 80–86.
56. Uno, H., T. Sasazuki, H. Tomai & H. Matsumoto. 1981. Two major genes, linked to HLA and Gm, control susceptibility to Graves' disease. Nature **292:** 768–770.
57. Zinkernagel, R. M. & P. C. Doherty. 1974. Immunological surveillance against altered self components by sensitized T lymphocytes in lymphocytic choreomeningitis. Nature **251:** 547–548.
58. Detels, R., B. Visscher, R. Malmgren & J. Dudley. 1982. Frequency and patterns of multiple sclerosis among Japanese-Americans. *In* Multiple Sclerosis East and West. Y. Kuroiwa & L. T. Kurland, Eds.: 171–175. Karger. Basel.

DISCUSSION OF THE PAPER

B. G. Arnason (*University of Chicago*): DR2 and DW2 are closely linked in Caucasians but are distinct and there are populations, for example blacks in Africa, who have a substantial proportion of DR2 but no DW2, and in whom MS is unknown and one could ask whether DW2 is a better marker than DR2 and whether the DR2 marker in Caucasians is a happenstance. My question therefore is, in the gypsies, did anyone look at DW2?

I. McDonald (*National Hospital, London*): No, nobody has looked at DW2 in gypsies, so far as I know.

Family and Twin Studies in Multiple Sclerosis

HENRY F. McFARLAND,[a] JEFFREY GREENSTEIN,[a]
DALE E. McFARLIN,[a] ROSWELL ELDRIDGE,[b]
XIAN-HAU XU,[a] AND HELEN KREBS[a]

[a]*Neuroimmunology Branch*
[b]*Neurogenetics Branch*
Intramural Research Program
National Institutes of Neurological and Communicative Disorders and Stroke
National Institutes of Health
Bethesda, Maryland 20205

A genetic influence in multiple sclerosis (MS) was initially suggested by the increased incidence of the disease in some families. The demonstration from population studies of an overrepresentation of HLA B7 and DR2 determinants among MS patients has provided further evidence for a genetic influence on the etiology of MS. These findings have led to the hypothesis that the genes coding for these HLA determinants may be closely associated with or in linkage dysequilibrium with genes that determine susceptibility to MS.

FAMILY STUDIES

Over the past years a number of families with two or more affected members have been reported. Most of these reports have described ten or fewer families and have examined the segregation of HLA haplotypes in the affected and unaffected members. Affected members have been found to share a haplotype in a majority of the families. Many families exist, however, in which the affected members do not share a haplotype. This is particularly true when affected members are in different branches or in different generations of the family. Consequently the interpretations of these family studies have been varied, concluding either that linkage can or cannot be demonstrated.

In order to define better this genetic influence, studies of linkage analysis and sibling pair analysis have been undertaken, largely using pooled pedigrees from previously published families. The linkage analysis studies have addressed a number of questions relating to the existence of an MS susceptibility gene including the mode of inheritance (dominant or recessive) and the "tightness" of the linkage to HLA or the recombination distance. These have used a number of mathematical models.

An analysis of pooled pedigrees by Tiwari *et al.* supported linkage to the HLA complex[1] and a study of 40 families by Haile *et al.* yielded similar results.[2] In each case loose linkage was postulated, indicating a gene that was a moderately large number of recombination units from the HLA complex. This would seem inconsistent with the strong association with B7 and DR2 found in population studies. A reanalysis of the original data and of pedigrees from the eighth HLA workshop indicated that tight linkage to HLA may exist in a majority of the families but that no linkage existed in the remaining families.[3,4] A more recent analysis has been published using 161 previously reported multiplex families.[5] The results of this study were interpreted as consistent with two determinants, one tightly linked to HLA and the other unlinked. The possibility remained that the unlinked element was an environmental factor. The evidence presented suggests an interaction between the linked and unlinked determinants. In pedigrees lacking B7 or DR2, linkage of susceptibility to HLA could not be established. These findings were interpreted as indicating disease or etiological heterogeneity. Also, the results from this study indicated a dominant form of inheritance in families in which linkage to HLA was thought to be established. The relatively high number of unaffected homozygotes in these families would argue, therefore, for a strong environmental influence.

Analysis of the genetic influence in MS has also been studied using sibling pair analysis, the analysis of shared haplotypes between pairs of affected sibling. Since this approach does not consider unaffected individuals, it should not be influenced by factors such as age of onset, subclinical disease or reduced penetrance. Stewart *et al.* have recently reported on 100 sibling pairs.[6] All but nine of these pairs were derived from the literature, the same data used in the studies discussed above. In these 100 pairs, 37 shared two haplotypes (expected: 25), 50 shared one haplotype (expected: 50), and 13 did not share a haplotype (expected: 25). Unequivocal typing (identifying the parental derivation of a haplotype that may be shared by both parents) was reported in 35 pairs. Of the 35 pairs, 14 shared two haplotypes (expected: 35/4), 17 shared one haplotype (expected: 35/2), and four failed to share a haplotype (expected: 35/4). These findings were interpreted as supporting linkage of an MS susceptibility gene to HLA with a dominant mode of inheritance.

A similar analysis has been employed by Ebers *et al.* in a study of 40 sibling pairs obtained from a population-based patient survey.[7] All were unequivocally typed. Of these 40 pairs, 12 shared two haplotypes (expected: 10), 18 shared one haplotype (expected: 20), and 10 did not share a haplotype (expected: 10). These findings did not differ significantly from the expected distribution, and therefore, did not support linkage to the HLA complex. Since linkage-analysis studies indicated linkage was more readily demonstrated in DR2 families, it is important to evaluate separately the sibling pair data for the DR2 pairs. Thirty-two pairs were typed for DR and 19 were DR2. Of the 32 pairs, 11 shared two haplotypes (four of 19 DR2 pairs), 13 shared one haplotype (nine of 19 DR2 pairs), and eight did not share a haplotype (six of 19 DR2). These results do not indicate that the incidence of shared haplotypes is greater in the DR2 pairs than the non-DR2 pairs or greater than the expected frequency.

It is difficult to reconcile these results with those discussed previously. Since a vast majority of these analytical studies have been done using, in part, the same pooled data extracted from the literature, it is understandable that errors in that data could account for some of the present inconsistencies. Errors could involve inclusion of non-MS families. Disease heterogeneity with data weighted more towards an HLA-linked form of disease might also account for these differences.

TWIN STUDIES

The study of twins has provided another approach to the examination of genetic influence on susceptibility to MS. A significant influence should be reflected by a substantially greater concordance rate among monozygotic (MZ) twins as compared to dizygotic (DZ) twins. If the genetic influence were sufficient for disease, 100 percent concordance would be expected in the MZ twins. If the genetic influence were a necessary part of a multifactoral process the concordance rate should be greater in the MZ twins as compared to the DZ twins but would be expected to be less than 100 percent. Because environmental factors should be similar in both MZ and DZ twins, an absence of genetic influence would be expected to result in a similar concordance rate in both types of twins, with the likelihood of a slight increase in MZ sets. Despite the attractiveness of this approach, ascertainment represents a major weakness inherent in most studies of twins. Concordant sets are more likely to be identified and MZ twins may be recruited more readily than DZ twins. These difficulties can be overcome only by using a population-based study. Despite these flaws, useful information can be gained from twin studies.

A study of twins was undertaken by the Neuroimmunology Branch (NIB) of the National Institutes of Health (NIH) six years ago.[8] The goals of this study were to identify a large number of MZ and like-sex DZ twins either concordant or discordant for MS. These twins were to be evaluated with detailed clinical examinations, determination of HLA makeup, CSF findings and immunological studies. The results of the initial phase of this study were reported in 1980.

Twins were ascertained through advertisement in the *MS Messenger* and by direct referral from physicians. A total of 94 sets of twins were initially identified. Medical records were reviewed in order to identify sets in which there was a high probability that at least one twin had MS. From these, 30 sets were identified that were willing to come to NIH for evaluation.

Following admission each twin was evaluated clinically by three neurologists and classified as clinically definite, probable, possible or not MS. In addition, an uncertain category was added for patients with neurological signs but without a history of neurological dysfunction and without a satisfactory explanation. Also in this group were individuals with an inconclusive history or with an alternative diagnosis. Twins were considered concordant if one twin had a diagnosis of definite or probable MS and the other twin a diagnosis of definite, probable or possible MS. Twins were not considered discordant unless the second twin was classified as not having MS.

In the initial study of thirty sets, 16 were monozygotic and 14 were dizygotic. The 14 DZ sets consisted of eight female sets and six male sets. One MZ set was thought not to have MS. An additional three MZ and two DZ sets were placed in the uncertain group. In these sets this classification was based on abnormal neurological findings (three sets) or a history of possible episodic disease (one set). All four co-twins had definite or probable MS.

The concordance for the remaining 12 MZ and 12 DZ sets is shown in TABLE 1. This resulted in a concordance rate of 50% for the MZ twins and 17% for the DZ twins. At the time of the initial report, however, only one of the MZ and two of the DZ discordant twins were over 50 years of age. In addition, as shown in TABLE 2, a number of the discordant twins were found to have CSF abnormalities consisting of either elevations in IgG or IgM levels or oligoclonal bands on agarose electrophoresis.[8] Consequently it was felt that the most valuable information to be gained from this study would be obtained on longitudinal follow-up of these twins.

Over the past year a majority of the twins have been reevaluated at NIH. Particular emphasis has been placed on twins originally classified as discordant or uncertain. Five of six MZ discordant and all of the MZ uncertain twins were reevaluated (excluding the set in which the probands are classified as not MS). Six of 10 DZ discordant sets were evaluated at NIH and two additional sets were contacted by phone. Two sets were lost to follow-up. The two DZ uncertain sets were evaluated at NIH (TABLE 1).

During the five years since the initial study, two of the original discordant sets have become concordant. Both of these have been MZ twins (sets 8 and 10). None of the discordant DZ twins have become concordant. In both of those twins previously considered unaffected the onset of disease was characterized by a relapsing-remitting course. None of the twins classified as uncertain have developed further evidence of disease. With the two additional MZ concordant sets, the concordance rate was increased to 67% in the MZ twins.

Over the past two years three additional sets of twins have been referred to the Neuroimmunology Branch. All were monozygotic. One set (#31) was classified as discordant when initially seen. One year later the unaffected twin had the onset of neurological disease consistent with clinically definite MS. The next set (#32) was concordant when seen. The third twin set (#33) was classified as uncertain on the basis of an unexplained transient hemiparesis in the supposedly unaffected twin. The addition of these sets establishes the concordance in MZ twins at 10 out of 14.

TABLE 1. Clinical Classification of Twins

	1979		
Monozygotic	16		
Concordant	6		
Discordant	6		
Unclassified	3		
Not MS	1		
Dizygotic	14		
Concordant	2		
Discordant[a]	10		
Unclassified	2		
	1983		
	Original	New	Total
Monozygotic	16	3	19
Concordant	8	2	10
Discordant	4	0	4
Unclassified	3	1	4
Not MS	1	0	1
Dizygotic	14	0	14
Concordant	2	0	2
Discordant[b]	10	0	10
Unclassified	2	0	2

[a]Three sets examined; one set contacted by phone.
[b]Six sets examined; two sets contacted by phone; two sets lost to follow-up.

The significance of the dramatically higher concordance rate in the MZ twins is uncertain. This could reflect an important genetic influence on susceptibility. Further, the disparity between these findings and those obtained by analysis of sibling pairs may suggest a genetic influence not linked to HLA. This would be supported by the finding that neither of the DZ concordant sets shares an HLA haplotype. A relative influence of multiple genes, some of which are not linked to HLA, could also be consistent with these results. However, the possible ascertainment bias favoring concordant sets and probably MZ sets makes interpretation difficult. It is also likely that female sets may be more readily identified. It is unknown if this bias could account for these findings. The development of concordance in two of the original six discordant MZ sets compared to none of the ten DZ sets supports observed differences.

A more extensive epidemiological study has been performed using a larger twin sample taken from the 94 twin pairs from which our sample was selected.[9] This study

TABLE 2. Relationship of Shared Haplotypes and CSF Abnormalities to Concordance

Set	Sex	Age	Shared Haplotype	IgG	IgM	CSF Bands	IEF
			DIZYGOTIC Concordant				
13A	F	39	0	−	−	−	8
B				−	−	−	13
14A	F	45	0	−	+	−	21
B				−	−	+	9
			Discordant				
15A	F	55	2	−	+	M	12
B				−	−	M	8
16A	F	62	1	−	−	M	24
B				−	−	+	1
17A	F	39	1	−	+	+	18
B				−	−	+	6
18A	F	49	2	−	−	M	1
B				−	−	+	5
19A	F	47	0	+	−	+	22
B				−	−	M	13
20A	F	38	1	−	+	M	13
B				−	+	+	20
21A	M	36	2	−	+	+	20
B				−	−	+	3
22A	F	42	2	+	−	+	NT
B				NT	NT	NT	NT
23A	M	42	0	−	−	+	21
B				−	−	M	10
24A	M	32	0	−	+	+	26
B				−	−	M	11
			MONOZYGOTIC Concordant				
Set[a]	Sex	Age[b]	Shared Haplotype	IgG[c]	IgM[d]	CSF Bands[e]	IEF
1A	F	56	2	+	−	M[h]	3
B				−	+	+	14
2A	F	35	2	+	−	M	12
B				−	+	+	13
3A	F	53	2	+	−	+	22
B				+	+	+	6
4A	F	51	2	+	−	+	14
B				+	+	+	6
5A	F	44	2	−	+	M	26
B				−	−	−	15
6A	F	67	2	+	−	+	4
B				−	−	−	15
8A[f]	F	34	2	+	+	+	4
B				−	−	−	3
10A[f]	F	34	2	−	+	−	9
B				−	+	−	1
31A[g]	M	32	2	−	−	+	NT
B				−	−	+	NT
32A[g]	F	36	2	NT	NT	+	NT
B				NT	NT	+	NT
			Discordant[i]				
7A	M	60	2	−	−	+	11
B				−	−	M	4
9A	F	47	2	+	−	+	21
B				−	−	−	9
11A	F	36	2	+	−	+	20
B				−	−	M	7
12A	F	49	2	−	−	M	4
B				−	−	−	1

[a] Set numbers correspond to those used in initial report.
[b] Age in 1983.
[c] IgG determined by RIA upper limits of normal of ratio to albumin 0.25.
[d] IgM determined by RIA upper limits of normal of ratio to albumin $1.98 \times 10^{-3.5}$.
[e] Determined using electrophoresis in agarose gel.[8]
[f] Discordant at time of initial report.
[g] Net sets.
[h] Monoclonal band.
[i] In each discordant set the "A" twin is affected.

included the patients that were evaluated by the NIB and, in addition, sets that met the selection criteria but were unable to come to NIH. Unlike-sex DZ twins were also included. This resulted in an additional 27 sets, for a total of 51. Of the 22 MZ sets, eight were concordant (36%). In contrast, three of the 26 DZ twin sets were concordant (12%).

The larger study of Mackay and Myrianthopoulos found only a slightly higher concordance rate in MZ as compared to DZ twins.[10] After five years of follow-up and the addition of some new sets, 39 MZ and 29 DZ sets were identified using ascertainment similar to that in the NIB study. Of these sets six MZ and three DZ sets were considered definitely concordant. Although the concordance rate is slightly higher in the MZ twins, it is far lower than the rate identified in the NIB study. This may be explained by the greater number of twins in this previous study or by differences in ascertainment with a greater bias towards concordant sets in our study. This critical question can only be resolved in a population-based twin study.

One effort has been made to perform such a study using twins identified from a registry of twins who were veterans of military service.[11] This study identified 16,000 sets of male twins. Of these, 23 sets were thought to have one or both members affected with MS. Eleven of these were rejected after further review and three sets refused participation. The nine remaining sets consisted of five MZ and four DZ sets. One MZ set was definitely concordant and one additional set was possibly concordant based on one episode of retrobulbar neuritis. None of the DZ twin sets was concordant. Although the number of sets analyzed is small, the concordance rate was substantially greater in the MZ sets as compared to the DZ twins.

Even a concordance rate of 40% or 50% in MZ twins would not necessarily suggest a particularly strong genetic influence, especially since the environmental similarities may be greater in MZ twins. The relatively large number of twins classified as uncertain on the basis of subtle abnormalities on exam or by history could indicate a high incidence of subclinical disease in this population. The existence of subclinical disease in unaffected MZ twins could mark a significant genetic influence on susceptibility and it would be impossible to establish the actual magnitude of this influence without identifying subclinically affected individuals.

The possibility of subclinical disease was further suggested by the cerebrospinal fluid (CSF) findings in the initial study.[8] Five of the discordant DZ twins had oligoclonal bands. Monoclonal bands were found in two MZ and four DZ unaffected twins.

These findings have been further analyzed using isoelectric focusing with silver staining or transblotting and immunoperoxidase staining to identify oligoclonal bands.[12] Two or more bands were found in 12 of the 15 unaffected twins. Two of those with less than two bands were MZ, including one of the twins who has subsequently developed MS. These findings have been discussed in detail elsewhere.[12] No correlation between bands and the presence of shared HLA haplotypes was observed and bands were found in the three DZ twins who did not share a haplotype with their affected twin. Two interpretations of these findings seem most reasonable. First, these CSF changes could reflect a high incidence of subclinical disease in both the MZ and DZ twins. This would at least argue against any substantial genetic influence or susceptibility linked to HLA. It would support a strong environmental influence. The possibility that clinical expression of disease is genetically influenced cannot be excluded. Since concordance is not greater in DZ twins sharing both HLA haplotypes, it would seem more likely that this influence is determined by genes outside the major histocompatibility complex (MHC) linkage group.

A second interpretation is that these CSF abnormalities reflect an environmental factor that does not necessarily correlate with the presence or absence of disease. This environmental factor could be important or necessary for disease. Disease, however, would be dependent on the genetically determined susceptibility of the individual. Also, the results of this study suggest that this genetic influence would most likely be either polygeneic or not HLA-linked. It seems unlikely that even a population-based twin study free of ascertainment bias will be able to resolve these questions, since the possibility of subclinical disease will remain. Separation of these hypotheses will require definitive identification of affected individuals. There seems little question that multiple factors are related to the cause of MS. This discussion has dealt only with studies of families and twins that relate to a genetic influence on disease. Twin studies also provide a powerful tool for identification of other possible etiological factors. Environmental differences may be identified in epidemiological studies of MZ and DZ discordant twins.[9,11] Detailed immunological studies of discordant twins may allow identification of differences in exposure to infectious agents or in immunoregulatory mechanisms.[13] Again, the possibility of subclinical disease is a critical consideration in this approach. We are presently beginning a study in which discordant twins will be evaluated by nuclear magnetic resonance in an effort to establish the extent of subclinical disease. Hopefully, these studies of twins will lead to a better understanding of the importance of genetic and environmental factors in multiple sclerosis.

REFERENCES

1. Tiwari, J. C., S. E. Hodge, P. I. Terasaki & M. A. Spence. 1980. HLA and the inheritance of multiple sclerosis: Linkage analysis of 72 pedigrees. Am. J. Hum. Genet. **32:** 103–111.
2. Haile, R. W., W. E. Hodge, B. R. Visscher *et al.* 1980. Genetic susceptibility to multiple sclerosis: A linkage analysis with age of onset correction. Clin. Genet. **18:** 160–167.
3. Haile, R. W., L. Iselius, S. E. Hodge, N. E. Moston & R. Detels. 1981. Segregation and linkage analysis of 40 multiplex multiple sclerosis families. Hum. Hered. **31:** 252-258.
4. Tiwari, J. L., N. E. Morton, J. M. Lalovel, H. Zander, B. R. Hawkins & Y. W. Cho. 1980. Multiple sclerosis. *In* Histocompatibility Testing. P. I. Terasaki, Ed.: 687–692. Munksgaard. Copenhagen.
5. Ho, H., J. L. Tiwari, R. W. Haile, P. I. Terasaki & N. E. Morton. 1982. HLA-linked and unlinked determinants of multiple sclerosis. Immunogenetics **15:** 509–517.
6. Stewart, G. J., J. G. McLeod, A. Basten & H. V. Bashir. 1981. HLA family studies and multiple sclerosis: A common gene, dominantly expressed. Hum. Immunol. **3:** 13–29.
7. Ebers, G. C., D. W. Paty, C. R. Stiller, R. F. Nelson, T. P. Seland & B. Larsen. 1982. HLA-typing in multiple sclerosis sibling pairs. Lancet **1:** 88–90.
8. Williams, A., R. Eldridge, H. McFarland, S. Houff, H. Krebs. & D. McFarlin. 1980. Multiple sclerosis in twins. Neurology **30:** 1139–1147.
9. Currier, R. D. & R. Eldridge. 1982. Possible risk factors in multiple sclerosis as found in a national twin study. Arch. Neurol. **39:** 140–144.
10. Mackay, R. P. & N. C. Myrianthopoulos. 1966. Multiple sclerosis in twins and their relatives. Arch. Neurol. **15:** 449–462.
11. Bobowick, A. R., J. F. Kurtzke, J. A. Brody, Z. Grubec & M. Gillespie. 1978. Twin study of multiple sclerosis: An epidemiologic inquiry. Neurology **28:** 978–984.
12. Xu, X. & D. E. McFarlin. 1984. Oligoclonal bands in cerebrospinal fluid: Twins with multiple sclerosis. Neurology **34:** 769–774.
13. Greenstein, J. & H. McFarland. 1982. Immunological responses to viruses in multiple sclerosis: Cell-mediated immunity. Clinics in Immunology and Allergy, vol. 2. pp. 371–383.
14. Lersild, C., G. S. Hansen, A. Sveygarrd, J. Fog, M. Thomsen & B. Dupont. 1973. Histocompatibility determinants in multiple sclerosis with special reference to clinical course. Lancet **2:** 1221–1225.

Pathogenetic Mechanisms in Multiple Sclerosis

A Summary

BYRON H. WAKSMAN

National Multiple Sclerosis Society
New York, New York 10017

Among the many subjects treated in detail in this section, I wish to select two for comment. One concerns the relationship between multiple sclerosis (MS) and other demyelinative diseases in man and experimental animals. The other has to do with the complexity of the MS lesion and its relation to functional change as experienced by the patient. Part of this discussion has appeared in earlier reviews.[1-4]

In TABLE 1 are listed the principal demyelinative diseases. All have in common the fact that they are (or begin as) primarily perivascular, inflammatory lesions, limited to myelinated tissue and accompanied by parenchymal damage, which in turn may range from simple demyelination to total necrosis. They differ with respect to lesion distribution and time course. One group is limited to the central nervous system (CNS) and another to the peripheral nervous system (PNS). One group is expressed as a monophasic illness whereas another, of which MS is the prototype, is prolonged in time. Certain cases are clearly related to antecedent viral infection and others appear not to be.

Virtually every variation among the human diseases is duplicated today in reproducible animal models that are easily studied and manipulated. If one starts with the working hypothesis that all the lesions observed are autoimmune, *i.e.,* based on an immune response to one or more myelin antigens, even when initiated by viral infections, the various cases fall neatly into place. Let us consider them individually.

Central and peripheral myelin differ significantly in antigenic makeup. It is quite clear from experimental work both with crude CNS and PNS myelin and with purified antigens, such as myelin basic protein (MBP) and P2, that the distribution of lesions between CNS and PNS is determined by the distribution of antigen(s) to which the immunized individual is responding. From this standpoint, it is highly probable that MS is attributable to an immune response to CNS myelin components.

On the other hand variations in lesion distribution within the CNS may depend on strictly local factors such as the nature of the local vascular bed and the blood-tissue barrier. The disease experimental autoimmune encephalomyelitis (EAE) differs markedly in distribution in different strains of animals within a single species and can give pathologic pictures resembling transverse myelitis, "sporadic" encephalitis, optic neuritis, or neuromyelitis optica.

The difference between acute monophasic illness and chronic relapsing or progressive disease is linked straightforwardly, in animal experiments, to one or more genes in the immune response (I) region of the major histocompatibility complex (MHC). In most animal strains, EAE is monophasic and is shut off, more or less permanently, by a suppressor T cell response. The SJL mouse strain, in which a chronic relapsing or progressive form of disease (REAE) is readily produced by immunization with myelin and an entirely similar chronic disease by various neurotropic viral infections, is characterized by early loss of normal suppressor T cell function, resistance to induction and maintenance of specific immune tolerance, and consequently exaggerated and prolonged autoimmune phenomena. This regulatory abnormality has been mapped to the I region of the MHC. MS susceptibility appears linked similarly to genes in the D(DR) region of the MHC, in which the T cell-mediated regulation of immune responses is encoded. It is therefore appropriate to speculate that the chronic character of MS results from a genetically determined abnormality of regulatory T cell function or, in simpler terms, from the failure of suppressor T cells to turn off the immune response that causes MS completely or permanently. The critical difference between MS and other demyelinative disease of the CNS would then be its *chronic character, determined by faulty immune regulation.*

Now let us turn to the question of viral infection. Many investigators have hesitated to accept EAE as a model for either acute monophasic demyelinative disease or MS since, as they rightly point out, these are not preceded by a purposeful immunization

TABLE 1. Demyelinative Diseases of Central and Peripheral Nervous System

Human Diseases	Animal Models[a]
Acute Monophasic Diseases	
Acute disseminated encephalomyelitis	SFV-encephalitis?
Postinfectious encephalomyelitis	
Postrabies vaccinal encephalomyelitis	EAE
"Sporadic" encephalitis	
Hemorrhagic necrotizing leukoencephalitis	
Optic neuritis	
Transverse myelitis	
Neuromyelitis optica (Devic's disease)	
Guillain-Barré polyneuritis	MDV-polyneuritis EAN
Chronic Relapsing or Progressive Diseases	
Multiple sclerosis Balo's concentric encephalitis	REAE and REAE-like disease induced by Theiler's and other viruses
Chronic relapsing polyneuropathy	REAN

[a]EAE: experimental autoimmune encephalomyelitis; EAN: experimental autoimmune neuritis; MDV: Marek's disease virus; REAE and REAN: chronic relapsing or progressive EAE and EAN; SFV: Semliki forest virus. (Reprinted with modifications from ref. 1, with permission of the publishers.)

with myelin, except in the case of rabies vaccination. However several new findings permit the unequivocal statement that viral infection can and does lead to autoimmunization against myelin antigens in favorable cases. In mice, in particular of the SJL strain, Theiler's murine encephalitis virus produces a chronic demyelinative disease resembling REAE associated with sensitization to myelin antigens and transferable by simple lymphocyte transfer (without transfer of virus) to normal syngeneic recipients. A number of other neurotropic viruses produce similar chronic demyelinative disease in SJL mice. In a study of human subjects infected with measles, rubella, or varicella, lymphocytic sensitization to MBP was shown to occur and, when the infection was followed by encephalitis, such sensitization could be demonstrated in over half the cases.

In MS, inferences concerning antecedent viral infection rest for the present on three types of evidence. Retrospective studies of monozygotic twins discordant for MS show a very much larger number of early viral infections in the affected twin of each pair. Also, in an established MS population, exacerbations were shown to occur more frequently in the period immediately following episodes of upper respiratory or gastrointestinal infection (childbirth, however, was also shown in independent studies to be sometimes followed by MS or to trigger exacerbations of preexisting MS). Finally, the epidemic of MS in the Faroe Islands following the arrival of British troops in 1940 and the less sharply defined MS epidemics in Iceland, associated with the coming of foreign troops in the two world wars, carry the same implication.

The failure hitherto to find clear-cut lymphocytic sensitization to CNS myelin antigens in MS neither strengthens nor weakens this argument. In EAE, where we can say with some confidence that the disease process is the direct consequence of the action of immune T lymphocytes specific for MBP or other myelin antigens, such lymphocytes can be found in significant numbers in the peripheral circulation only transiently, during a peak period of output from lymph nodes draining an immunization site.

What are we to say of cases of monophasic or prolonged demyelinative disease where no antecedent virus infection is apparent clinically? We must not lose sight of the fact, established for example in detailed studies of influenza epidemics, that many individuals who show no clinical sign of infection nevertheless show serological conversion or a rise in antibody titer to the virus. The implication is that these are people with preexisting immunity in whom the virus replicates to a limited degree yet enough to stimulate T cell help and a secondary response of effector cells (B cells in this case). If the role of a virus in autoimmunity is just that, to stimulate helper T cells and a secondary response of effector cells specific for myelin antigen(s), such clinically inapparent infection with influenza or other enveloped viruses (myxo- or paramyxoviruses, poxviruses, herpesviruses) may be quite enough to trigger an episode of autoimmune demyelinating disease. This picture is more persuasive than the alternative of persistent viral genome, *e.g.*, of herpes or EB virus, with reactivation in response to conventional inductive stimuli. In such a case it should become possible to find complete infectious virus in the CNS, yet no such virus has ever been found.

Let us turn now to the question of complexity in the evaluation of the MS lesion. The elements of the MS lesion have been fully described, in anatomic terms, by many careful investigators. Yet it is not possible, with present knowledge, to relate individual features unequivocally to known immunologic mechanisms: *e.g.*, the vascular lesion and edema to antigen-antibody complexes and/or complement activation; the infiltrating inflammatory cells to a T cell-mediated reaction; or the demyelination to "innocent bystander" damage, to antibody-dependent cell-mediated cytotoxicity, or to complement-mediated lysis. Our ignorance of the physiologic-pharmacologic events taking place at the site of acute or chronic lesion formation is even more profound. One can do little more than speculate about macromolecular lymphokines and enzymes that may be released from the activated T and B lymphocytes and macrophages in the lesion, the vasoactive amines, prostaglandins, leukotrienes, and neurotransmitter substances released from these and other cells at the site, and their secondary effects on vascular endothelium, on the infiltrating cell populations, and on conduction in nerve fibers passing through the area.

Similarly one cannot relate the patient's neurologic defect at any one time to any one or more of the known anatomic or physiologic changes. Traditionally demyelination was held responsible for loss of function. Yet this clearly can not be the explanation for the rapidly reversible symptomatology of the acute MS attack, which is now thought to depend more on edema. Even the late glial scar may interrupt conduction to some degree. It follows that, if one wishes to assess a patient's disease thoroughly, as in a clinical trial of a new agent, the traditional Kurtzke or other scores based on neurologic examination alone cannot provide us with a complete account of what is happening at the site of the lesion. Rather one must attempt to evaluate each individual feature of the disease process separately, as suggested in TABLE 2.[a] Surely this table will require extensive revision in the coming years.

The lymphocytic studies published over the last several years have shown changes in the levels of suppressor T cells (bearing the T5 and T8 markers, discernible with monoclonal antibodies of the OKT series) and natural killer (NK) cells in the blood and CSF. These promised much, in the way of understanding the immunoregulatory defect in MS, and promised as well to be of diagnostic or prognostic value. At present there is a suggestion that they may be a consequence of cell-surface modulation by prostaglandins released from the activated monocytes (macrophages) found in the circulation and CSF, perhaps as a spillover from the site of actual lesion formation. If

TABLE 2. Parameters Measuring Extent and Activity of Demyelinative Disease[a]

Impairment of Function
Subjective blindness
Visual acuity, visual fields
Visual evoked potentials
Number and Size of Lesions
Ophthalmoscopy
Nuclear magnetic resonance scan
Postmortem histology
Disease "Activity"[b]
Vascular lesion and edema: enhanced CT scan
Blood and CSF macrophage activation: lysosomal enzymes, prostaglandin production
Demyelination: MBP, CNPase in CSF; new NMR applications
Lymphocytic studies in blood and CSF
Scarring (Gliosis)
Activation of astrocytes: GFAP in CSF

[a]Visual system used as representative "sample" of central nervous system.

[b]CNPase: cyclic nucleotide phosphorylase; CSF: cerebrospinal fluid; CT: computerized axial tomography; GFAP: glial fibrillary acidic protein; MBP: myelin basic protein; NMR: nuclear magnetic resonance scan.

that proves to be true, they would have little use as an index of underlying mechanisms. This does not detract from their possible importance in disturbed immune regulation that may determine the protacted nature of the disease process in MS.

TABLE 2 carries us as far as "blindness." It does not address questions of cognitive deficit, handicap, and adjustment in the socioeconomic sphere that must be evaluated by other means to be considered later in this volume. In a clinical trial of a new therapeutic modality, the scientist would wish to follow the tests listed in TABLE 2, in order to know its effect on the actual disease process, whereas the patient and his physician might well pay more attention to these "other means" that deal with the quality of life.

[a]My choice of the visual system as a particularly illustrative sample of the CNS was prompted by a suggestion of Prof. W. I. McDonald.

REFERENCES

1. WAKSMAN, B. H. 1983. Immunity and the nervous system: Basic tenets. Ann. Neurol. **13:** 587–591.
2. WAKSMAN, B. H., T. YONEZAWA & H. LASSMAN, Eds. 1983, Inflammation and Demyelination in the Central Nervous System. Springer-Verlag. Berlin.
3. WAKSMAN. B. H. 1983. Viruses and immune events in the pathogenesis of multiple sclerosis. *In* Viruses and Demyelinating Diseases. C. Mims, M. L. Cuzner & R. E. Kelly, Eds. Academic Press. New York.
4. WAKSMAN, B. H. & W. E. REYNOLDS. 1984. Minireview: Multiple sclerosis as a disease of immune regulation. Proc. Soc. Exp. Biol. Med. **175:** 282–294.

GENERAL DISCUSSION

G. C. EBERS (*University of Western Ontario, London, Ontario*): Dr. McFarland, there are a couple of assumptions that are made in most linkage analyses of HLA data; one of them is that there has been time for panmixia, which is to say that the population is mixed randomly, and in fact this may be an unwarranted assumption for a couple of reasons. The first of these is that it's been shown in mice, for example, that mice preferentially mate by HLA type.

The second factor is that for most of man's history we have actually lived rather isolated in small groups and it's only been recently, in the last 200 years, that the opportunity for what Genesis called panmixia has really existed, so the assumptions in those analyses may not be true. The second is that the susceptibility which is HLA-linked is in fact a single gene and that is a single HLA-linked gene. If one looks at experimental immunization situations, and in fact there are a number of different HLA or H2 determinants that can be associated with a specific immune response, so many different H2s can be associated with a high level of response to a given single simple antigen.

R. T. JOHNSON (*Johns Hopkins University, Baltimore, MD*): Dr. McFarland, would you like to comment on that? Particularly the part about being more likely to breed with similar HLA.

H. MCFARLAND (*NINCDS, Bethesda, MD*): I don't have any experience with that but I agree with what the speaker says. I think the possibility of multiple genes, HLA genes, is certainly viable. There is one comment I'd like to make to Dr. Waksman's remarks. We actually have typed some of our patients for SB: we now have typed 30 of our patients. We find no association with SB. This is curious because this is the same population that does seem to have a fairly high frequency of DR2 and I think what that's saying is that the SB reagents are probably so poor at this point and that these determinants are so polymorphic that we don't yet have the proper reagents. Right now we find no association with SB.

J. N. WHITAKER (*Memphis VA Medical Center*): Dr. ter Meulen, in the transfer after *in vitro* exposure, do you look to see what part of the basic protein is responsible or have you done that with intact basic protein up to now?

V. TER MEULEN (*University of Würzburg, Würzburg, FRG*): It was only done with intact basic myelin protein preparation, not with peptides.

JOHNSON: In your article showing the passive transfer, you took cells from animals with the relapsing disease and stimulated them *in vitro* with killed JHM and then transferred as well? It wasn't on your chart in the *Nature* article though I thought you'd done it.

TER MEULEN: No, this was another paper that you have seen. With relapses, we have not done any transfers.

JOHNSON: You haven't tried? You didn't use that as a control for your transfer?

TER MEULEN: What we are trying right now is to separate the JHM-stimulated from the basic myelin protein-stimulated cells and then transfer with cloned cells and see what happens. That would eliminate the possibility that you carry something over.

L. SCHEINBERG (*Albert Einstein College of Medicine, Bronx, NY*): Dr. Waksman, would you be a little bit more cautious in your statement that immunosuppression arrests all demyelinating diseases?

B. WAKSMAN (*National Multiple Sclerosis Society, New York*): You simply want me to say yes, I think.

SCHEINBERG: I think there's no evidence whatsoever that you've disseminated the encephalomyelitis.

WAKSMAN: Dr. Scheinberg has raised this question with me on other occasions. It seems to me that that result qualifies as a good experiment and you have to say that it suggests strongly that immunosuppression suppresses at least temporarily the progress of that disease.

I. McDonald (*National Hospital, London, England*): I wonder whether Dr. Prineas might say a little more about the acute case that he mentioned this morning and I think it was the acute case of 1976, in which if my understanding is right there was but a single episode with a history of three months. Now I'd be interested to know whether there was other evidence pathologically of more chronic lesions in those patients? I think looking at it from the clinical end, as opposed to the pathological end, clinicians would not be able to accept into the clinically definite category of multiple sclerosis a patient with a single episode with a single sign.

J. W. Prineas (*University of Medicine and Dentistry of New Jersey, Newark*): The circumstances that would allow you to accept a case with a single sign and a single episode would be an autopsy case with numerous typical lesions. I think that's correct, isn't it?

McDonald: I would only accept it if there was evidence of lesions of different ages. The point I'm getting at is that whereas any observation of an acute demyelinating process is clearly of great importance in understanding mechanisms of demyelinating disease generally, I think one can't assume that the monophasic illness with one lesion of a single age or multiple lesions of the same age as judged morphologically is the same thing as multiple sclerosis. It might be the first episode of that disease but it doesn't fulfill the ordinary criteria that one requires in clinical studies.

Prineas: Well, this group of so-called fulminating acute MS is really an extraordinarily interesting disease from the point of view of the pathologist who wants to see the early lesion and the question is really, is this MS or not? It's obviously different from ordinary MS but from a pathological point of view you cannot distinguish the lesions in these acute cases from the freshest lesions observed in typical chronic relapsing cases. The 1976 case with a three-month history was a woman who had typical lesions virtually everywhere. She died of lesions that were mostly in the brain stem but she had large periventricular plaques. The 41-day case is the case that provided the lesion with the perivascular accumulation of IgG, and also was the case that had multiple classical MS lesions. One of the most important things in thinking about multiple sclerosis in the last couple of years has been the development of chronic models. The EAE model has been a substantial help in bringing the two diseases together. What has happened is that people have examined chronic EAE and noticed that with time, the lesions in these rodents become larger and look more and more like MS lesions. What hasn't been done formally is to go in the opposite direction in multiple sclerosis and look at the earliest lesions in MS and see whether they approximate increasingly towards the picture that one sees in acute EAE and, I might add, acute disseminated encephalomyelitis.

I have now a series of 16 patients with a duration to death from first symptom of less than 18 months, and this is a series that has been put together since 1967. The interesting thing that's emerged from this series is that the earliest lesions that one sees do not look anything like the lesions that one sees in acute disseminated encephalomyelitis. The lesions do not get smaller, they do not become more and more microscopic or more and more diffuse. The distinctive characteristic feature of the acute MS plaques in the chronic relapsing case is that all of its characteristics are retained, all the way back into the very acute phase of the disease. So acute multiple sclerosis is a real entity, its only relation in terms of morphology is chronic relapsing multiple sclerosis and there's really very little relationship to acute disseminated encephalomyelitis.

M. B. Bornstein (*Albert Einstein College of Medicine, Bronx, NY*): Dr. Prineas, I think that there's a great deal of evidence suggesting that multiple sclerosis begins before the age of 15, but may become clinically apparent much later. There are a number of instances of routine postmortem examinations that have demonstrated marked involvement with so-called multiple sclerosis in patients who had never had symptoms at all. Isn't it quite possible that the earliest lesions that you may be seeing may still represent many years of development, which is different from what one sees in either ADE or the acute EAE?

PRINEAS: I'm aware of course of the subclinical lesions. This is not just a verbal description; you've seen the lesions that I recited this morning. How long does it take a macrophage to digest myelin once it has ingested it? It's probably a few hours. It takes months and months for all the lipid to disappear but if you see a macrophage containing recognizable myelin and undigested myelin basic protein, how long does myelin basic protein retain its immunological identity in a phagosome surrounded by hydrolytic enzymes? I'm sure I could ask Norton that and he mentioned this morning that it's extraordinarily susceptible to proteolytic enzymes so we know that those macrophages have acquired that myelin probably within a few hours of death. I don't think the problem of the long-standing lesion really is an issue in trying to decide the identity of the acute fulminating MS case. The literature contains numerous examples of so-called fulminating MS where at autopsy, in addition to fresh lesions, old lesions were present as well.

JOHNSON: I think the idea of having disease before age 15, from the epidemiological data, or having infection or exposure does not necessarily mean disease. Those two things have to be kept very clearly separated. The disease process can be fulminating much later. Any time anybody talks about incubation period and disease and infection I'm always reminded of Alan Dickinson's somewhat perverse experiment in which he took a very low-grade strain of scrapie and put it in a very genetically resistant strain of mice, in which case he could show titer going up with age of the animal but because of the genetic combinations he'd chosen, the animal died of senescence before developing symptoms or pathological lesions. Now that doesn't make it not infected, it certainly got the disease. It just had an incubation period that was longer than possible survival.

A. VANDENBARK (*Portland VA Hospital, Portland, ORE*): A question for Dr. ter Meulen. Were there any discernable immunologic differences in susceptible *versus* nonsusceptible strains of rats to the coronavirus?

TER MEULEN: We have put JHM virus into BN rat (BN rats normally are resistant to EAE) and we do not get any clinically recognizable disease in these rats despite the fact that we see some demyelination. The neuropathologists tell us that these lesions are a little different from those we see in Lewis rats and they're probably the result of the oligodendroglial infection and destruction and subsequent demyelination. Interestingly, we get an immune response towards the virus but when we check for sensitization of lymphocytes against myelin basic protein, it's negative. It is the same as what we see in EAE in Lewis rat *versus* BN rats. Obviously the genetic makeup is important in the Lewis rat for providing the proper conditions for transfer.

Immunoregulation in Multiple Sclerosis[a]

BARRY G. W. ARNASON, JACK P. ANTEL, AND
ANTHONY T. REDER

Department of Neurology and the Brain Research Institute
University of Chicago
Chicago, Illinois 60637

Over the past several years, studies emanating from many different laboratories have documented that something is awry with immune regulation in multiple sclerosis (MS). Since most current thinking holds that multiple sclerosis will likely prove to be an autoimmune process, possibly triggered by an infectious event, a careful exploration of immune regulation in multiple sclerosis may be directly relevant to the pathogenesis of the disease. In keeping with the past history of multiple sclerosis research, there remains a substantial disagreement as to the nature, magnitude, and underlying significance of aberrancies in immune regulation in multiple sclerosis. The discussion that follows attempts to consider these matters in a general way, but it should be recognized that some of the opinions to be expressed are those of the authors and may not be generally agreed upon by workers in the field.

EARLY OBSERVATIONS

Abnormalities of peripheral blood lymphocytes in MS were first documented in 1975. T lymphocytes at that time were identified by their capacity to form rosettes with sheep red blood cells (SRBC), the number of rosettes formed giving a count of T cells present. The method was crude, but it was possible to discern T cell subsets within the overall T cell population on the basis of the avidity of the rosettes that were formed (*i.e.*, by the number of SRBC adherent to each cell) as well as by the speed with which the rosettes were formed (T active). Oger *et al.*[1] found the number of avid T cells (>10 SRBC bound to each T cell) to be reduced in the circulation in multiple sclerosis. Subsequently Kately and Bazzell[2] reported that T-active cell numbers (rapidly formed rosettes) were reduced in multiple sclerosis, although Goust *et al.*[3] found T-active cell numbers to be normal. It is still unclear whether T-avid and T-active cells comprise identical, similar, or different populations. No correlation between these abnormalities and disease activity, as assessed clinically, has been detected to the present.

Though it is evident that avidity must reflect some surface property of T cells, the basis for it remains unknown. It is perhaps germane to note that evidence has been brought forward recently to suggest that the density of SRBC receptors is greater on T suppressor cells than on other T cells.[4] Thus, were the surface properties of T suppressor cells aberrant in multiple sclerosis, a point to which we shall return, the decline in avidity of T cells for SRBC might find a logical explanation.

The avidity of T cells for SRBC can be manipulated experimentally. Administration of aspirin (a prostaglandin synthetase inhibitor) to multiple sclerosis patients restores avid T cell numbers to normal, whereas exposure of T cells from normal donors

[a]This work was supported by grants from the National Multiple Sclerosis Society and the Kroc Foundation.

to prostaglandin E_1 reduces avid T cell numbers down to levels found in multiple sclerosis.[5] It is known that prostaglandins are released by activated macrophages and that activated macrophages abound in multiple sclerosis lesions. Thus, T cells in multiple sclerosis may have their surface properties modulated by released prostaglandins, and this may be the basis for the changes observed. Regardless of mechanism, it is evident that the surface properties of T cells are not immutable and, in fact, can be rapidly altered both in health and disease. For this reason alone, a cautious interpretation should be given, in terms of biological significance, to abnormalities found in circulating lymphocytes in multiple sclerosis.

There is additional evidence for surface membrane alterations of lymphocytes in multiple sclerosis. Levy *et al.*[6] reported that up to 50% of peripheral blood lymphocytes from MS patients adhered to measles-virus-infected Hep-2 cells. This value was 2–3 times greater than that obtained with lymphocytes from controls. In the initial study, multiple sclerosis and control groups did not overlap, but subsequent experience has revealed considerable overlap even though it confirms the validity of the core observation. Avid T cell number varies inversely with Hep-2 cell binding number. Aspirin treatment of multiple sclerosis patients drops Hep-2 binding down to control level. Conversely, prostaglandin E_1 treatment of control cells increases their Hep-2 binding capacity.[5] There is no consensus as to whether T cells alone bind to Hep-2 cells or whether B cells bind as well. Dore-Duffy (cited in ref. 7) finds a further abnormality in lymphocyte adherence in multiple sclerosis. She reports that T cells from multiple sclerosis patients stick better to fresh human white matter than do T cells from controls with other neurological diseases. The overall sense that we obtain from this earlier work is that the surface properties of T cells are not normal in multiple sclerosis, but of course work of the sort just outlined begs the question as to whether an abnormality in T cell function follows or accompanies these changes.

SUPPRESSOR CELLS IN MULTIPLE SCLEROSIS

When mononuclear cells are driven to proliferate by exposure in tissue culture to the lectin concanavalin A (Con A), suppressor cells are activated. When these activated suppressor cells are blocked with mitomycin (this maneuver prevents their further replication) and then mixed with fresh cells from the same donor, the capacity of the preactivated, but blocked, cells to blunt the proliferative response of the fresh autologous cells to Con A provides a measure of suppressor-cell activity. This suppressor activity is mediated at least in part by T cells bearing the $T8^+$ antigen (see below), although other cell subpopulations, including monocytes, may contribute to the overall suppressor effect. Antel *et al.*[8] employed this assay system to study suppressor-cell function in multiple sclerosis. It was found that suppressor-cell activity fell to low and sometimes unmeasurable levels during attacks of disease. As an attack ended, suppressor activity rebounded to high normal levels. In patients with clinically stable disease, some showed normal suppressor function whereas others had reduced function. In patients with progressive disease, T suppressor cell function is also subnormal.[9]

The assay described above is two-armed—either a failure in release of suppressor factors or an inability to respond to them could account for a blunted response. When the suppressive effects of supernatants from Con A-activated cells are tested on proliferating cell lines the rate of proliferation is decreased, indicating that suppressor-factor generation is impaired in multiple sclerosis. Studies by Goust *et al.* in a different suppressor-cell assay indicate that refractoriness of responder cells to suppressor factors may also occur.[10] Several other assays of suppressor function have been developed and applied to the study of multiple sclerosis.[11-13] There would appear to be general agreement that suppressor function is profoundly depressed during multiple sclerosis attacks but rebounds as attacks end.

Functional assays of suppressor-cell function are cumbersome, tedious, and difficult to perform. Given the earlier demonstration that surface components on T cells were not normal in multiple sclerosis, attention turned to a more detailed study of surface properties. Huddlestone and Oldstone[14] reported that, during attacks of multiple sclerosis, cells of a T cell subset known as T_G cells were reduced in number, whereas during remissions of multiple sclerosis, T_G subset cell numbers were increased above expected values (see also ref. 15). T_G cells bear a receptor for the Fc portion of IgG and can be detected by their capacity to form rosettes with ox RBC that have been coated with a subagglutinating quantity of anti-ox RBC IgG. The T_G cell subset normally comprises about 15% of circulating T cells and there is firm evidence that some but not all T_G cells are suppressor cells. Thus, the data obtained with T_G cell enumeration and those obtained with functional assays reinforced each other in indicating that something was awry with T suppressor cells during attacks of multiple sclerosis. Note that the T_G cell subset does not coincide with the T suppressor subset defined by the monoclonal antibody, OKT8, subsequently discussed.

Even more recently, monoclonal antibody markers that distinguish between T cell subsets have become available and have been employed in the study of multiple sclerosis. The current status of this work is reviewed in detail elsewhere in this volume. In brief, total T cell number as measured with the pan-T cell monoclonal antibody marker known as OKT3 is modestly but significantly reduced in multiple sclerosis; T suppressor cell number, as measured with the OKT8 antibody, is somewhat reduced in progressive disease (there is general agreement on this point) and may or may not be reduced during attacks, different laboratories obtaining different results. During attacks, when suppressor-cell function is clearly compromised, the counting techniques reveal at best a modest decline in T suppressor-cell number. With a second monoclonal marker for T suppressor cells known as OKT5, a more profound fall in countable suppressor cells has been reported in multiple sclerosis cases with active disease. This antibody, however, is not generally available. The data outlined above suggest that changes in function may or may not be tied to surface properties depending on the surface property being studied. Reduced suppressor function without apparent reduction in T suppressor number is characteristic of the aging process and is reported to occur in chronic active hepatitis.[16,17]

In an attempt to reconcile differences in enumeration studies of T cell subsets, Reder *et al.*[18] measured density of the T8 antigen on suppressor cells using the fluorescence intensity of the second antibody in an indirect immunofluorescence assay as the indicator in multiple sclerosis patients and in controls. It was found that the quantity of OKT8 bound by T cells in multiple sclerosis was reduced whenever disease was active, even though sufficient antibody might still be bound so that OKT8 positive cells would be counted and called positive, particularly when fluorescence microscopy rather than a fluorescence-activated cell sorter (FACS) was used for counting purposes. It was suggested that the differences between laboratories in counts of OKT8 positive cells might well depend primarily on technical considerations, particularly when a fluorescence-activated cell sorter was used to count cells.

Antel *et al.*[19] deliberately modulated the T8 antigen off T cells by exposing them to OKT8 monoclonal antibody in tissue culture. Under these circumstances, T8-OKT8 complexes are pinocytosed or shed, thus effectively stripping the cell of the T8 antigen. Modulated cells showed depressed suppressor function *in vitro*, indicating that down-regulation of T suppressor-cell surface markers can compromise function. This having been stated, it must be pointed out that there appear to be considerable discrepancies in individual cases between the number of suppressor cells that can be counted and the suppressive activity exerted on fresh autologous T cells that can be generated.

T suppressor cells act on B cells as well as on T cells, and, in fact, the initial demonstration that OKT8-binding cells exerted suppressive activity was shown by means of an assay in which the capacity of B cells to generate IgG (in the presence of T helper cells) under the influence of the lectin pokeweed mitogen (PWM) was measured directly with and without the addition of $OKT8^+$ cells. Using this assay,[20] it was possible to show that, in the aggregate, T regulator-cell control of B cell responses was aberrant in multiple sclerosis. Possible defects reported have included reduced T suppressor function, augmented T helper activity, and B cell resistance to T cell regulatory influences. Our data indicate that the magnitude of B cell response in this culture system is mainly dependent on the functional activity of T suppressor cells ($T8^+$ cells) rather than on T suppressor counts. However, as the number of T suppressor cells added to a B cell plus T helper-cell culture system was increased, there came a point, even with T suppressor cells from multiple sclerosis patients with defective suppression, where suppression became clearly evident. Overall the data indicate that counting T suppressor cells gives a very imperfect sense of their function, and that mere counting of cells, and this point is reiterated elsewhere in this volume, is not at the present time of value in predicting presence or absence of disease activity in any individual patient. What is clear is that the marker abnormalities and the functional abnormalities detected to date are only very tenuously linked one to the other, if at all. There is an obvious need to attempt to find better markers that will correlate with function.

Some effort has been directed to the study of T helper-cell function and helper-cell counts in multiple sclerosis. No abnormalities have been detected up to the present. Likewise there is evidence (reviewed elsewhere in this volume) that natural killer cell and killer-cell function may be abnormal in multiple sclerosis.

B CELLS IN MULTIPLE SCLEROSIS

An increased IgG content in the spinal fluid is characteristic of multiple sclerosis, and it has been amply documented that the bulk of the spinal fluid IgG found in spinal fluid from multiple sclerosis patients is synthesized in brain. Not surprisingly, given this result, B cell infiltrates within brain are prominent in multiple sclerosis. When IgG in the spinal fluid is analyzed electrophoretically it resolves into a series of so-called oligoclonal bands. Demonstration of such bands has found widespread use as a test helpful in the diagnosis of multiple sclerosis.

Oligoclonal bands in spinal fluid are also seen in chronic infections of the central nervous system. The prototype here is subacute sclerosing panencephalitis (SSPE), a chronic measles virus infection of the brain. Oligoclonal bands in SSPE spinal fluid can be absorbed out with measles virus preparations, indicating that the monoclonal IgG in the spinal fluid is antibody to measles virus. Innumerable attempts have been made to absorb out IgG bands from multiple sclerosis spinal fluid with viruses and with brain fractions, but without success. These failures may mean no more than that the correct virus has not been chosen for study or that the multiple sclerosis-relevant tissue antigen is elusive. When spinal fluid from multiple sclerosis patients is electrophoresed, it becomes evident that the oligoclonal bands stand out against a diffuse smear of background IgG. This polyclonal, or multi-multi-minor oligoclonal, background IgG is also synthesized in brain, for the most part.

The question can be posed: What drives the B cells in brain in multiple sclerosis to synthesize immunoglobulins? Continuing contact with the multiple sclerosis antigen is of course one and, perhaps, the leading possibility. Mattson *et al.*[21] employed a sensitive isoelectric focusing technique to analyze the IgG eluted from individual MS plaques obtained at autopsy. They found that oligoclonal bands differed between plaques from the same patient. B cells taken from the circulation can be driven to make immunoglobulin in tissue culture by exposing them to the lectin pokeweed mitogen in the presence of T helper cells. If the IgG produced is analyzed by isoelectric focusing techniques, regardless of whether the B cells come from MS patients or from controls, oligoclonal bands are found.[22] This finding indicates that certain clones of the vast B cell repertoire are preferentially represented within the circulating B cell pool at any given point in time. From this result it follows that were B cells drawn from the circulation into plaques by some nonspecific means during an attack of MS, a restricted heterogeneity in their response would be expected. Since different plaques develop at different times, it might be anticipated that different restricted heterogeneities would be expressed within different plaques, as is found.

Antiviral antibodies are present in multiple sclerosis spinal fluid and these antibodies have been shown to be synthesized in brain. Many multiple sclerosis patients have anti-measles antibodies in their spinal fluid, many have anti-rubella antibodies, anti-herpes antibodies, *etc.*, and a substantial proportion of patients have antibodies to several viruses at the same time. Although it could be argued that any given virus might be the cause of MS, they cannot all be. It follows that much, perhaps all, of the antibody found in the spinal fluid in multiple sclerosis is "nonsense antibody" in terms of the pathogenesis of the disease. The question then becomes the following: If antigen does not drive the B cells, what does? No answer to this question can be given. Clearly, B cells in brain could have escaped normal regulator influences and be self-driven. This seems improbable since isolated B cells do not drive spontaneously *in vitro.* Alternatively, a B cell activator may be present in MS brain. Candidates here would be factors released by T cells, or by macrophages, or some breakdown product of myelin.

As documented elsewhere in this volume, several immunosuppressive treatments are under trial in multiple sclerosis. Azathioprine, which is undergoing clinical trial, does reduce systemic B cell response in multiple sclerosis to normal levels.[23] If B cell response is critical in multiple sclerosis, then azathioprine might prove to be an effective remedy; if B cell hyperresponse is an epiphenomenon, then azathioprine treatment may well fail. The issue remains unresolved.

SPINAL FLUID CELLS IN MULTIPLE SCLEROSIS

Study of cells in spinal fluid is difficult in multiple sclerosis because so few of them are available. Spinal fluid in multiple sclerosis contains an insufficient number of cells for most immunological assays in current use.

Noronha *et al.*[24] employed the methodology of flow cytometry to study spinal fluid cells in multiple sclerosis. In this technique, cells are treated with the dye acridine orange (AO) and passed single file past a laser beam of light. Acridine orange binds both to DNA and RNA. When struck by light, the AO bound to DNA fluoresces green, whereas that bound to RNA fluoresces red. The fluorescence emitted can be detected by photomultiplier tubes and a measure of the DNA and RNA content of each and every cell that passes the laser beam can be obtained.

Normal lymphocytes are in the resting, or G_0, stage of the cell cycle. Activation of lymphocytes proceeds in an orderly sequence through G_1 (increased RNA), S (increased DNA), G_2 (further increase in RNA, but with doubled DNA), and finally mitosis. Noronha *et al.*[24] found that the proportion of activated cells (G_1) was increased in multiple sclerosis, even in patients in remission. The activated cells bind the OKT4 monoclonal antibody, a marker for T helper cells. During frank attacks, additional activation (more cells in S and G_2) was seen. The data suggested that some immunocyte activity is ongoing at all times in multiple sclerosis, even though this activity may not be reflected in any change in the clinical presentation. The point is of potential importance, in our view, for treatment strategies. If a therapy for multiple sclerosis can be developed it would seem unwise to restrict its use to times of frank attack.

Enumeration of spinal fluid cells in multiple sclerosis using monoclonal antibodies has revealed that T cells predominate at all times and that the proportion of T cells rises during attacks, approaching 90–95% of the total.[25] T suppressor-cell representation falls during attacks and T helper-cell (OKT4+ve) representation increases.[26,27] B cells are rare in spinal fluid at all times despite their presence within the brain in substantial numbers. Response of spinal fluid cells to lectin is defective in multiple sclerosis.[28] This may reflect the fact, as mentioned above, that many cells are preactivated. With the development of methods employing T cell growth factor to expand spinal fluid T cell populations in tissue culture, rapid progress in the analysis of spinal fluid cells in multiple sclerosis is to be anticipated.

REFERENCES

1. OGER, J. J-F., B. G. W. ARNASON, S. H. WRAY & J. P. KISTLER. 1975. A study of B and T cells in multiple sclerosis. Neurology **25:** 444–447.
2. KATELY, J. R. & S. J. BAZZELL. 1979. Immunological dysfunction in multiple sclerosis. I. Diminution of "active" thymus-derived lymphocytes and presence of immunomodulating serum factors. Clin. Exp. Immunol. **35:** 218–226.
3. GOUST, J. M., P. M. HOFFMAN, J. PRYJMA, E. L. HOGAN & H. H. FUDENBERG. 1979. Defective immunoregulation in multiple sclerosis. Ann. Neurol. **6:** 150.
4. HOWARD, F., J. A. LEDBETTER, J. WONG, C. P. BIEBER, E. B. STINSON & L. A. HERZENBERG. 1981. A human T lymphocyte differentiation marker defined by monoclonal antibodies that block E rosette formation. J. Immunol. **126:** 2117–2122.
5. DORE-DUFFY, P. & R. B. ZURIER. 1979. E-rosette formation in normals and patients with multiple sclerosis: Effect of prostaglandin and aspirin. Clin. Immunol. Immunopathol. **13:** 261–268.
6. LEVY, N. L., P. S. AUERBACH & E. C. HAYES. 1976. A blood test for multiple sclerosis based on adherence of lymphocytes to measles infected cells. N. Engl. J. Med. **294:** 1423–1427.
7. ARNASON, B. G. W. & B. H. WAKSMAN. 1980. Immunoregulation in multiple sclerosis. Ann. Neurol. **8:** 237–240.
8. ANTEL, J. P., B. G. W. ARNASON & M. E. MEDOF. 1979. Suppressor cell function in multiple sclerosis: Correlation with clinical disease activity. Ann. Neurol. **5:** 338–342.
9. PATY, D. W., L. F. KASTRUKOFF & L. HIOB. 1981. Chronic progressive multiple sclerosis has low suppressor cell levels. Trans. Am. Neurol. Assoc. **106:** 276–279.
10. GOUST, J. M., E. L. HOGAN & P. ARNAUD. 1982. Abnormal regulation of IgG production in multiple sclerosis. Neurology **32:** 228–234.
11. GONZALEZ, R. L., P. C. DAU & L. E. SPITLER. 1979. Altered regulation of mitogen responsiveness by suppressor cells in multiple sclerosis. Clin. Exp. Immunol. **36:** 78–84.
12. WICHER, V., W. OLSZEWSKI & F. MILGROM. 1979. Dual response of lymphocytes from multiple sclerosis patients to myelin basic protein. Clin. Exp. Immunol. **37:** 114–119.
13. NEIGHBOR, P. A. & B. R. BLOOM. 1979. Absence of virus-induced lymphocyte suppression and interferon production in multiple sclerosis. Proc. Nat. Acad. Sci. **76:** 476–480.

14. HUDDLESTONE, J. R. & M. B. A. OLDSTONE. 1979. Levels of T suppressor (T_G) lymphocytes are reduced during attacks of multiple sclerosis (MS). Fed. Proc. **38:** 1420.
15. SANTOLI, D., L. MORETTA, R. LISAK, D. GILDEN & H. KOPROWSKI. 1978. Imbalances in T-cell subpopulations in multiple sclerosis patients. J. Immunol. **120:** 1369–1371.
16. ANTEL, J. P. & B. G. W. ARNASON. 1979. Suppressor cell function in man: Evidence for altered sensitivity of responder cells with age. Clin. Immunol. Immunopathol. **13:** 119–124.
17. ALEXANDER, G. J. M., A. L. EDDLESTON, K. T. NOURI-ARIA & R. WILLIAMS. 1983. Contrasting relations between suppressor-cell function and suppressor-cell number in chronic liver disease. Lancet **1:** 1291–1293.
18. REDER, A. T., J. P. ANTEL, J. J-F. OGER, T. A. MCFARLAND, M. ROSENKOETTER & B. G. W. ARNASON. 1984. Low T8 antigen density on lymphocytes in active multiple sclerosis. Ann. Neurol. **16:** 242–249.
19. ANTEL, J. E., J. J-F. OGER, S. JACKEVICIUS, H. W. KUO & B. G. W. ARNASON. 1982. Modulation of T lymphocyte differentiation antigens: Potential relevance for multiple sclerosis. Proc. Nat. Acad. Sci. U.S.A. **79:** 3330–3334.
20. ANTEL, J. P., M. ROSENKOETTER, A. REDER, J. J-F. OGER & B. G. W. ARNASON. Correlation of *in vitro* IgG secretion with T suppressor cell number and function in multiple sclerosis. Neurology. In press.
21. MATTSON, D. J., R. P. ROOS & B. G. W. ARNASON. 1980. Isoelectric focusing of IgG eluted from multiple sclerosis and subacute sclerosing panencephalitis brains. Nature **287:** 335–337.
22. OGER, J. J-F., J. P. ANTEL, S. MARIOTTI & B. G. W. ARNASON. 1980. In vitro IgG secretion by lymphocytes of multiple sclerosis patients and controls in response to pokeweed mitogen stimulation. Neurology **30:** 448.
23. OGER, J. J-F., J. P. ANTEL, S. JACKEVICIUS, A. B. C. NORONHA & B. G. W. ARNASON. 1982. Influence of azathioprine (Imuran) on in vitro immune function in multiple sclerosis. Ann. Neurol. **11:** 177–181.
24. NORONHA, A. B. C., D. P. RICHMAN & B. G. W. ARNASON. 1980. Detection of in vivo stimulated cerebrospinal fluid lymphocytes by flow cytometry in patients with multiple sclerosis. N. Engl. J. Med. **303:** 713–717.
25. NAESS, A. & H. NYLAND. 1978. Multiple sclerosis-T lymphocytes in cerebrospinal fluid and blood. Eur. Neurol. **17:** 61–66.
26. CASHMAN, N. R., C. MARTIN, J-F. EIZENBAUM, J-D. DEGOS & M-A. BACH. 1982. Monoclonal antibody defined immunoregulatory cells in multiple sclerosis cerebrospinal fluid. J. Clin. Invest. **70:** 387–392.
27. OGER, J. J-F., J. P. ANTEL, S. JACKEVICIUS, A. B. C. NORONHA & B. G. W. ARNASON. 1981. Increased CSF T helper cell population in active MS. Excerpta Med. **548:** 177.
28. KAM-HANSEN, S., H. LINK, A. FRYDEN & E. MÖLLER. 1979. Reduced in vitro response of CSF lymphocytes to mitogen stimulation in multiple sclerosis. Scand. J. Immunol. **10:** 161–169.

Indicators of Disease Activity in Multiple Sclerosis

Studies of Myelin Basic Protein-like Materials[a]

JOHN N. WHITAKER

Research and Neurology Services
Memphis VA Medical Center
and
Departments of Neurology and Anatomy
University of Tennessee Center for the Health Sciences
Memphis, Tennessee 38104

The availability of a laboratory method for ascertaining the status of disease activity in multiple sclerosis (MS) is of major importance because of the unpredictable course of the disease,[1] the apparent multiple phases of tissue injury and repair,[2] and the large number of subclinical lesions in the central nervous system (CNS) in MS.[3-6] As a result of these features, the patient's history and clinical findings may reflect neither the presence, timing or site of CNS myelin injury in MS. This situation makes it difficult or impossible, even with detailed and quantitative examinations, to distinguish clinically therapeutic responses from spontaneous changes or to detect episodic worsenings in an MS patient whose course is progressive.

There is an evident need for an objective and quantitative index of disease activity in MS which, optimally, would also be feasible and readily applicable to patient care. Measurements of evoked potentials in MS patients may show changes paralleling disability but have not demonstrated a good correlation between electrophysiologic abnormalities and clinical activity.[7-9] CNS imaging by nuclear magnetic resonance, which is remarkable in the detection of tissue lesions in MS,[5] currently seems unlikely to provide a feasible means for frequent assessment. The number[10] and immunoregulatory effects[11] of peripheral blood lymphocyte subsets may show alterations as the activity of disease changes, but the consistency of these changes is uncertain.[12] The presence of a quantitative increase and oligoclonal characteristics of cerebrospinal fluid (CSF) immunoglobulin G increases the confidence of the clinical diagnosis of MS,[13] but change in either is absent or minimal as clinical activity in MS changes.[14]

Another approach that has the potential attributes of objectivity, quantitation and feasibility for monitoring disease activity is measuring the levels of released myelin constitutents in body fluids. The morphological demonstration[15] of myelin debris in the CSF of persons with acute MS and other diseases of CNS myelin established that myelin components should appear in CSF after myelin injury. This, in turn, implied that certain proteins, lipids or enzymes characteristic of CNS myelin[16] might serve as quantifiable markers of myelin damage. At the present time the quantitation of basic protein (BP) or BP peptides in CSF is the most reliable laboratory method for determining disease activity in MS.[17] Although the measurement of other myelin proteins or components may also prove useful in monitoring different phases of disease

[a]This work was supported by the Research Program of the Veterans Administration and the National Multiple Sclerosis Society (grant no. RG 1111–C–5).

activity in MS,[18] the use of BP for this purpose has been demonstrated the most clearly.

Basic protein has been extensively studied because of its ability to induce experimental allergic encephalomyelitis.[19] BP accounts for 30% of CNS myelin proteins.[16] In the human, BP occurs with a monomeric molecular weight of 18,500 and is composed of approximately 169[b] amino acids.[20] The amino acid sequence of human BP has been reported.[20] Knowledge of the primary structure of BP has permitted investigation of the molecular sites responsible for its disease-inducing, antigenic and nonimmunological biological properties.[21] It is relevant to the measurement of BP or BP peptides by immunoassay that BP has multiple independent determinants spread throughout the molecule.[22–25]

A number of independent investigations have shown that in association with active CNS demyelination, BP, or fragments thereof, can be detected in CSF. Different types of radioimmunoassay (RIA) methods have been utilized in which intact BP[26–31] or a BP peptide[32–34] serves as the radiolabeled antigen permitting a sensitivity of one nanogram or less per assay tube. The assay that we have utilized consists of an antibody to BP reacting with a radioligand of human BP peptide 43–88 in a four-day nonequilibrium RIA with a second antibody used in the separation step.[32,33] Of critical importance in this and other immunoassays of BP or its peptides is the inclusion of a cationic protein, in this instance, methylated bovine serum albumin, to reduce nonspecific binding of the radioligand to the test tube.[32] In the assay we have used, values equal to or higher than two ng per ml of CSF are considered elevated.[32] Most of the assays have been validated by the standard criteria used for establishing a RIA, but the identification of the material immunologically measured as BP has not yet been documented by an independent test of biological activity. For this reason, the material being detected must be cautiously viewed at present as cross-reactive with BP or immunoreactive with antibodies to BP. Although there are minor differences among reports on BP-like material in CSF, each has shown that such material appears in human CSF during active demyelination or when myelin breakdown occurs as part of more generalized CNS tissue damage. Thus, patients with MS in an active phase have detectable or elevated levels of BP-like material, but CSF specimens from MS patients not in active phases are negative and CSF from patients with other types of acute CNS myelin injury may be positive. The presence of BP-like material in CSF is not disease-specific. Multiple sclerosis patients with chronic progressive cases may have low levels of BP-like material in CSF[28] but frequently have none.[32,33] The BP-like material in CSF is unrelated to the level of total protein or immunoglobulin G[32] and rapidly decreases or becomes undetectable after CNS myelin injury. Whether this is due to degradation, binding or efflux from CNS of BP-like material is not clear.

The amount of BP released from damaged CNS myelin is unknown. The amounts of BP-like material detected in CSF by immunoassay are stated in terms of equivalents or inhibition produced by BP or BP peptide, and, until the form of the BP antigenic material in CSF is known, its molar concentration will remain uncertain. Also, the typical values of 10–20 ng of BP-like material per ml of CSF represent the level in lumbar subarachnoid space after dilution in the CSF compartment which is replaced three times in 24 hours.[35] Therefore, BP-like material can be detected in CSF in the presence of these dilutional and distributional factors without considering the impact of the amount of BP or its peptide entering blood directly without passage through the CSF.

[b]The numbering of residues in human BP is based on the sequence of bovine BP.[66,67] Peptide 43–88 is the fragment of BP formed by the cleavage of the two phenylalanyl phenylalanine bonds.

It is obviously highly desirable that blood or urine be substituted for CSF as the body fluid to be frequently sampled in assessing CNS demyelination. The detection of BP in the circulation has been problematic, in part because of the presence of proteinases,[36] binding proteins[37–39] and other interfering substances.[30] Efforts to quantitate BP-like material in urine revealed that the apparent presence of BP peptide was, in fact, the result of proteolytic degradation of the radioligand.[40] Basic protein-like material in CSF is not the artifactitious result of degradation of the radioligand BP peptide 43–88.[40]

Attempts to measure BP peptides in body fluids must address a number of potential problems occurring at various steps from release of the antigenic material from the CNS to quantitation by immunoassay. The form of the material released from CNS, its passage in CSF, blood, extraneural tissue and urine, the processes of collection and storage and the immunoassay itself may each include one or more variables influencing the detection of the antigen. Binding or further degradation of peptide may occur at any of these steps, and dilution of the peptide(s) entering blood or urine is expected. Drugs, hormones or electrolyte changes may also influence the way the body clears BP peptides. The choice of collection vials and the presence of inhibitors, anticoagulants, *etc.*, may allow adherence to the surface of a storage vessel or permit further changes by degradation or binding. Although these problems seem enormous, similar obstacles have been overcome in assays of peptide hormones like ACTH[41] when the chemical identity or biological actvity of the peptide was known.

It is presumed that the accurate detection of BP-like material in blood or urine necessitates the correct identification of the BP peptide(s) present. More precise identification of the BP peptide(s) present should permit more sensitive immunoassays and may also influence the preparation of a radioligand that would be less readily degraded. Hence, our own investigations have been focused on the identity of the BP peptide released, its clearance and catabolism and the immunochemical features of small peptides of BP. Four observations form the background to our approach: (1) the BP antigenic material in CSF contains at least the carboxyl portion of peptide 43–88[32,42]; (2) the kidney is a major organ for the clearance[43] and degradation[44,45] of BP peptide 43–88; (3) small fragments from human BP peptide 43–88 may have neoantigenic determinants that are not shared by large BP peptides or the intact BP molecule[46–48]; and (4) previous errors in the sequence of amino acid residues in BP peptide 43–88 have now been corrected[49] but had a marked influence on immunochemical studies of small fragments derived from this region of the BP molecule.

FEATURES OF BP-LIKE MATERIAL IN CSF

The BP-like activity in CSF has been interpreted to be BP molecule itself of 18,500 molecular weight, because it displaced radioiodinated BP in an RIA,[26] or as large as 50,000 molecular weight because of its features on electrophoresis.[27] Further studies have disclosed that BP-like activity in CSF may exist in a range of sizes.[50] Larger forms predominate in patients with cerebral infarction and necrotic brain damage, whereas smaller sizes predominate in patients with acute MS.[50,51] The BP-like material in CSF of patients with strokes also follows a less predictable time course than in MS in both appearance and disappearance.[33] The difference in sizes plus the differences in temporal appearance of CSF BP-like material in acute MS and cerebral infarctions suggest differences in the mechanisms of production or disposal of BP-like material in these two conditions. Antibody to BP has been found in the CSF of many,[50,52] but not of all,[53,54] persons with MS. It is also not disease-specific but may exist in complexed or aggregated form to reduce the amount of BP-like material detected.[50] The frequency and specificity of the CSF antibody to BP are unknown.

Detailed immunochemical studies of the nature of the BP-like material in CSF have been limited in number. Most of the antisera that have been used in immunoassays of BP-like material in CSF have been produced in animals receiving whole BP or mixtures of BP and other brain components. As a result, antibodies against different determinants of BP are formed. An antiserum to whole BP that also detects BP-like material in CSF may react with different fragments of BP,[28] but this does not identify which fragment or fragments are present. Other studies[32,42] indicate that an epitope in BP peptide 43–88, particularly near its carboxyl end, shared with intact human BP, is the critical determinant of the antigen form of BP present in CSF after CNS myelin injury. This antigenic form appears to be present in both small and large molecular weight material released in different types of brain injury.[50]

The BP-like material in CSF has been demonstrated to cross-react with BP peptide 43–88 but not with BP peptide 1–42 and 89–169.[42] Based on these findings,[33] attention has been directed at the region of BP containing residues 43 through 88 for detecting small fragments of BP in blood and urine. However, these findings have been interpreted cautiously because antisera reactive with BP peptide 43–88 show wide variation in their detection of BP-like material in CSF.[42] It is possible, therefore, that portions or conformations of either BP peptide 1–42 or BP peptide 89–169 might exist in CSF but not be detected by the antisera tested.

Using the Na_2SO_4 assay,[55] the detection of BP-like material in CSF cross-reactive with bovine BP peptide 89–169 has been reported.[34] Because the form of BP in CSF followed CNS myelin injury would presumably serve as the substrate for the formation of small fragments of BP in the circulation, the possible presence of BP-like material cross-reactive with BP peptide 89–169 in CSF was reexamined. A rabbit antiserum used for detection of BP 89–169[34] was kindly provided by Dr. K. Hempel, and this antiserum and eight other antisera from the author's laboratory were tested by double antibody-RIA (DA-RIA) having sensitivities 0.1–1.0 ng per assay tube for the detection of BP peptide 89–169. With none of these nine antisera or the one previously tested[42] could any material in CSF specimens (known to contain high levels of material cross-reactive with BP peptide 43–88) be detected in the immunoassays. The reasons for this discrepancy between our findings and those of others[34] are unclear but might possibly result from differences in the RIAs used. At present, the emphasis on BP peptide 43–88 as the major BP peptide to consider in identifying what small fragments of BP may appear in blood or urine seems still to be warranted.

CLEARANCE AND DEGRADATION OF BP

Information on the metabolic fate of BP or its fragments subsequent to their release from CNS in the human is unavailable. In the rabbit, infused human BP peptide 43–88 is rapidly cleared (half-life of 50–60 minutes) from the blood and catabolized by the kidney with no material that cross-reacts with BP peptide 43–88 entering urine.[43] The kidney contains proteinases capable of degrading BP peptide 43–88 into small fragments,[44–46] and the proteinases present in human kidney are different from those in rat, dog, guinea pig and rabbit kidney.[56] Two separate neutral proteinases in the human renal extract degrade human BP peptide 43–88. One has an apparent molecular weight of 550,000 and is inhibited by leupeptin but not by EDTA and *N*-ethylmaleimide. The second has an estimated molecular weight of 210,000 and is inhibited by EDTA and *N*-ethylmaleimide but not by leupeptin.

Consideration has been given as to whether small fragments of BP would appear in urine because of the endopeptidases and exopeptidases present in blood, various tissues (especially the kidney) and urine which might effect such extensive degradation that no immunoreactive material would remain. The facts that BP-like material can be detected in CSF in conditions in which increased CSF proteolytic activity is also present[57,58] and that BP-like material can be detected in the blood of animals after conditions for collection of blood and radioligand have been correctly chosen[43,59] suggest that degradation is limited and that the degradation products may still be large enough, *i.e.*, peptides of five to seven amino acid residues, for immunochemical detection. In the rabbit virtually all of the clearance and degradation of infused BP peptide 43–88 occurs in the kidney with none of this peptide detected in urine,[43] but treatment of animals with maleic acid, a toxin for renal proximal convoluted tubular epithelium where membrane-bound proteinases are present, results in the passage of BP peptide 43–88 from blood into urine of rabbits in an immunoreactive form.[60] Renal clearance and degradation of released BP peptides are presumed to occur in humans so that the identification of the small fragments of BP created by human renal proteinases should permit their detection. The degradation of human radioiodinated BP peptide 43–88 by human renal proteinases results in both small and intermediate size radiolabeled fragments,[45] some of which should be immunochemically detectable.

IMMUNOCHEMICAL FEATURES OF FRAGMENTS OF BP PEPTIDE 43–88

Three[55] or four[61] antigenic determinants have been estimated to exist in the whole BP molecule. However, there appear to be numerous potential determinants, especially when BP peptides are used as immunogens or radioligands.[40,47,62,63] For the clearer identification of the BP-like material in CSF and for the detection and quantitation of small peptides of BP in blood and urine, different antisera and radioligands were selected for use in immunoassays. In view of the cross-reaction of BP peptide 43–88 with the antigenic form of BP entering CSF,[32,42] emphasis was given to the antigenicity and detection of small fragments containing parts of human BP peptide 43–88.[46] Antisera raised against BP, BP peptide 43–88 or small fragments of BP peptide 43–88 were to be used in immunoassays with radioligands of BP, BP peptide 43–88 or fragments of BP peptide 43–88. Among species examined, the region of BP encompassing residues 43 through 88 shows more substitutions and variations in primary sequence than in other portions of the BP molecule.[20] Based on the published sequences for human BP peptide 43–88,[20,64] human BP peptides 51–67, 67–80, 74–84, 79–88 and 83–95 were synthesized, conjugated to ovalbumin to produce antibodies in rabbits or sheep and used as radioligands in DA-RIA.[46] The lengths of peptides 51–67 and 67–80 were selected because of the presence of tyrosine at position 67 that made it possible to radioiodinate each of these naturally occurring peptides. For peptides 74–84, 79–88, and 83–95, it was necessary to add tyrosine in order to be able to use lactoperoxidase-catalyzed radioiodination to prepare radioligands. The results of this approach demonstrated that cross-reactivities between small fragments of BP peptide 43–88 and either BP peptide 43–88 or intact BP were usually marginal or absent.[46] In each of these assays CSF was also tested. Except for the assays using antisera directed against the *C*-terminal portion of BP peptide 79–88 and radiolabeled BP peptide 43–88 (not BP peptide 79–88) as radioligand, immunoreactive material could not be detected.

Although a portion of BP peptide 79–88 appears to be shielded in the intact BP molecule or acquire a neoantigenic form when isolated,[47,48] the unexpected peptide-specificity or marked peptide-preference of the antibodies to the other fragments of BP

TABLE 1. Immunochemical Effect of Glycine-Histidine Inversion in Human BP Peptide 67–80

		Precipitation of Radioligand	
Animal	Immunogenic BP Peptide	BP Peptide 67–80 (His Gly 76–77)[a]	BP Peptide 67–80 (Gly His 76–77)[b]
Sheep 157	67–80 (Gly His 76–77)[b]	<1:200[c]	>1:50,000
Rabbit 221	67–80 (Gly His 76–77)[b]	<1:200	1:50,000
Rabbit 222	67–80 (Gly His 76–77)[b]	<1:200	>1:50,000

[a]Correct sequence.
[b]Incorrect sequence.
[c]Dilution of antiserum at which 5% net precipitation of radioligand occurs.

peptide 43–88[46] prompted a reexamination of the disputed primary sequence of human BP peptide 43–88.[20,64] Fast atom bombardment mass spectrometric analysis of tryptic fragments of human BP peptide 43–88 has been used to resolve the sequences in question.[49] The correct sequences are histidine-glycine[20] at residues 76–77 and glutamic acid-asparagine[64] at positions 82–83. Previous immunochemical studies[46] with human BP peptides 51–67 and 83–95 were conducted with peptides containing the correct sequence. However, all the work performed with human BP synthetic peptides 67–80, 74–84, and 79–88 involved peptides with the incorrect sequence.[46]

Polyclonal antisera, Rabbit (R) 221, R222 and Sheep (S) 157, previously raised against the incorrect sequence of human BP peptide 67–80 do not react with human BP peptide 67–80 containing the correct sequence (TABLE 1) nor with human BP peptide 43–88 or intact BP (see Table III in ref. 46). Polyclonal antisera (R301 and S213) raised against the correct sequence of human BP peptide 67–80 react with the correct sequence of human BP peptide 67–80, human peptide 43–88 and human BP but not with peptide 67–80 containing the incorrect sequence (TABLE 2). Thus, inversion of histidine and glycine at residues 76–77 has a marked influence on the generated antisera and on immunoassays in which BP peptide 67–80 is used as the radioligand. As measured by displacement of radioiodinated BP peptide 67–80 by BP, BP peptide 43–88 and BP peptide 67–80, there is still a preferential reaction with the small peptide

TABLE 2. Characteristics of Three Antisera Reacting with BP Peptide 67–80

Antiserum	R133	R301	S213
Immunogen	BP 43–88–OA	BP 67–80–OA	BP 67–80–OA
Dilution	1:4500	1:4500	1:4500
Radioligand	BP 67–80	BP 67–80	BP 67–80
% Bound	45	46	41
Inhibitor Peptides			
BP 67–80[a]	$>10^3$	$>10^3$	$>10^3$
BP 67–80[b]	1.0[c]	1.0	1.0
BP 43–88	0.5	2.6	6.6
BP (1–169)	1.0	2.6	9.0

[a]Incorrect sequence of glycine-histidine at residues 76–77.
[b]Correct sequence of histidine-glycine at residues 76–77.
[c]Molar ratio of amount relative to BP peptide 67–80 (correct sequence) to displace 50% of radioligand.

for antisera (R301 and R302) raised against it as compared to an antiserum (R133) raised against BP peptide 43–88 (TABLE 2).

Data obtained also indicate that the correction of sequence at residues 82 and 83 has a major impact on the immunochemical reactivity directed against bovine BP peptide 79–88, in particular its carboxyl portion (TABLE 3). For example, R276 was immunized against human BP peptide 83–95 conjugated to ovalbumin.[46] This antiserum was previously shown to react well with peptide 83–95, BP peptide 43–88 and intact BP but not peptide 79–88 (incorrect sequence) by direct binding (Table I in ref. 46). By displacement DA-RIA using radiolabeled BP peptide of Tyr 83–95 as the radioligand, neither BP peptide 43–88 nor intact BP reacted well (see Table III in ref. 46). Subsequent studies with this antiserum have shown that it reacts well with BP peptide 79–88 with the correct sequence at residues 82–83 and confirms the previous finding that it does not react at all with BP peptide 79–88 with the incorrect sequence. Other findings demonstrate that R276 antiserum reacts with BP peptide 83–88 and suggest that the asparagine at residue 83 (rather than at erroneous aspartic acid) is a critical part of the determinant. The importance of asparagine may also explain why the attachment of the amino terminal tyrosine to BP peptide 83–95 for purposes of radioiodination affected the cross-reactivity of BP peptide 43–88 and BP in the displacement DA-RIA (see Table III in ref. 46). R276 antiserum reacts with BP peptide 43–88 but not BP peptide 43 –87 (see below).

Human BP peptide 43–88 has been the main portion of BP used for immunochemical[42,46] and metabolic studies[43,44] related to the presence of material cross-reactive with this peptide in CSF and other body fluids. When studies with reverse-phase, high-performance liquid chromatography were begun, it became evident that preparations of human BP peptide 43–88 contained 70–80% BP peptide 43–88 and 20–30% BP peptide 43–87.[65] Since there are two phenylalanine residues in BP peptide 43–88, the partial reduction in the phenylalanine content in the amino acid analysis from the admixture of BP peptide 43–87 that lacks the *C*-terminal phenylalanine was not appreciated. The presence of peptide 43–87 was not considered to be important immunochemically; however, recent studies on the comparison of reactivities with BP

TABLE 3. Characteristics of Two Antisera Reacting with BP Peptide 79–88

Antiserum	R276	R131
Immunogen	BP 83–95–OA	BP 43–88–OA
Dilution	1:1000	1:1000
Radioligand	BP Peptide 79–88	BP Peptide 79–88
% Bound	34	46
Inhibitor Peptides		
BP 43–88	1.0[a]	1.0
BP 43–87	$>10^3$	$>10^3$
BP 79–88[b]	$>10^3$	68
BP 79–88[c]	1.2	3.7
BP 81–88	1.0	$>10^3$
BP 83–88	1.8	$>10^3$
BP (1–169)	$>10^3$	4.3

[a]Molar ratio of amount relative to BP peptide 43–88 required to displace 50% of radioligand from antibody.

[b]Incorrect sequence with glutamine-aspartic acid at residues 82–83.

[c]Correct sequence with glutamic acid-asparagine at residues 82–83.

TABLE 4. Characteristics of Two Antisera Detecting BP-like Material in CSF

Antiserum	R79	S45
Immunogen	HU BP-RSA	HU BP-OA
Dilution	1:800	1:8000
Radioligand	HU BP 43–88	HU BP 43–88
% Bound	36	42
Inhibitor Peptides		
HU BP 43–88	1.0[a]	1.0
HU BP 43–87	78.3	1.9
HU BP 79–88	1.1	$>10^3$
GP BP 79–88	4.9[b]	$>10^3$
BO BP 79–88	16.3	$>10^3$
HU BP 81–88	$>10^3$	$>10^3$
HU BP 81–86	$>10^3$	$>10^3$
HU BP 83–88	$>10^3$	$>10^3$
HU BP 79–84	$>10^3$	$>10^3$
HU BP 83–95	$>10^3$	$>10^3$
BP (1–169)	1.1	0.9
CSF-MS		
(1) inactive	0	0
(2) active	11.3 ng/ml	5.0 ng/ml
(3) active	5.0 ng/ml	3.0 ng/ml

[a] Molar ratio of amount relative to BP peptide 43–88 required to displace 50% of radioligand.
[b] The R79 serum used is from a different bleeding than previously reported[42] to react better with guinea pig BP peptide 79–88.

peptides 43–87 and 43–88 underscore again the influence of the *C*-terminal portion of BP peptide 43–88 on its immunochemical reactivity (TABLES 3 and 4).

As mentioned above, many antisera reacting with BP fail to detect BP-like material in CSF. The availability of an array of BP peptides of the correct sequence and a better appreciation of the number of epitopes in BP peptide 43–88 has permitted further characterization of what epitopes in BP peptide 43–88 are being recognized by antisera-detecting immunoreactive BP in CSF. Two antisera studied showed an equal reactivity with BP peptide 43–88 and intact BP but differed in other features (TABLE 4). Antisera directed at BP peptide 43–88 and that can detect BP-like material in CSF may show little or no reaction with BP peptide 43–87. One antiserum, R79, appears to detect differences among BP peptides 79–88 containing the human, guinea pig or bovine sequence (TABLE 4). These peptides differ only at residue 79.[64] Another antiserum, S45, which also detects BP-like material in CSF does not discriminate as much between BP peptides 43–87 and 43–88, but BP peptide 43–88 produces a slightly greater displacement than BP peptide 43–87 in DA-RIA (TABLE 4). Related to epitopes recognized in the *C*-terminal portion of BP peptide 43–88 or possibly to the affinity of the reaction, different amounts of BP-like material can be measured in CSF from acute phase MS patients (TABLE 4).

SUMMARY

Defining the immunochemical basis for the detection of BP peptides in body fluids has led to an appreciation of the complexity of the number and location of epitopes in

BP peptide 43–88. There appear to be roles for epitopes based on both sequence and conformation of these small peptides. Antisera to some of the fragments of BP peptide 43–88 may have restricted reactivity with BP peptide 43–88 and BP. The amount of BP-like material that enters CSF and cross-reacts with BP peptide 43–88 is related to the recognition of an epitope or epitopes in the *C*-terminal portion of this peptide. The immunochemical detection of BP peptides in body fluids is dependent on the precise identification of the BP peptides present.

REFERENCES

1. Lhermitte, F., R. Marteau, J. Gazengel, G. Dordain & D. Deloche. 1973. Z. Neurol. **205:** 47–59.
2. Prineas, J. 1975. Hum. Pathol. **6:** 531–554.
3. Chiappa, K. H. & A. H. Ropper. 1982. N. Engl. J. Med. **306:** 1140–1150, 1205–1211.
4. Sears, E. S., A. McCammon, R. Bigelow & A. Hayman. 1982. Neurology **32:** 815–820.
5. Young, I. R., A. S. Hall, C. A. Pallis, N. J. Legg, G. M. Bydder & R. E. Steiner. 1981. Lancet **2:** 1063–1066.
6. Namerow, N. S. & L. R. Thompson. 1969. Neurology **19:** 765–774.
7. Matthews, W. B. & D. G. Small. 1979. J. Neurol. Sci. **40:** 11–21.
8. Walsh, J. C., R. Garrick, J. Cameron & J. G. McLeod. 1982. J. Neurol. Neurosurg. Psychiat. **45:** 494–500.
9. Davis, S. L., M. J. Aminoff & H. L. Panitch. 1983. Ann. Neurol. **14:** 147.
10. Reinherz, E. L., H. L. Weiner, S. L. Hauser, J. A. Cohen, J. A. Distaso & S. F. Schlossmann. 1980. N. Engl. J. Med. **303:** 125–129.
11. Antel, J. P., B. G. W. Arnason & M. E. Medof. 1979. Ann. Neurol. **5:** 338–342.
12. Paty, D. W., L. Kastrukoff, N. Morgan & L. Hiob. 1983. Ann. Neurol. **14:** 445–449.
13. Walsh, M. J. & W. W. Tourtellotte. 1983. *In* Multiple Sclerosis. J. F. Hallpike, C. W. M. Adams & W. W. Tourtellotte, Eds.: 275–358. Williams and Wilkins. Baltimore.
14. Mattson, D. H., R. P. Roos & B. G. W. Arnason. 1981. Ann. Neurol. **9:** 34–41.
15. Herndon, R. M. & M. Johnson. 1970. J. Neuropathol. Exp. Neurol. **29:** 320–330.
16. Norton, W. T. 1981. *In* Basic Neurochemistry. 3d ed. G. J. Siegel, R. W. Albers, B. W. Agranoff & R. Katzman, Eds.: 63–92. Little, Brown. Boston.
17. Whitaker, J. N. & D. S. Snyder. 1982. Immunol. Allergy **2:** 469–482.
18. Trotter, J. L., C. L. Wegescheide & W. F. Garvey. 1983. Ann. Neurol. **14:** 554–558.
19. Hashim, G. A. 1978. Immunol. Rev. **39:** 60–107.
20. Carnegie, P. R. & W. J. Moore. 1980. *In* Proteins of the Nervous System. 2d ed. R. A. Bradshaw & D. M. Schneider, Eds.: 119–143. Raven. New York.
21. Whitaker, J. N. 1984. Antigenic determinants of myelin basic protein and its peptides. *In* Proceedings of the First International Congress of Neuroimmunology. F. Spreafico & P. O. Behan, Eds.:179–191. Raven Press. New York.
22. Driscoll, B. F., A. J. Kramer & M. W. Kies. 1974. Science **184:** 73–75.
23. Whitaker, J. N., C.-H. J. Chou, F. C.-H. Chou & R. F. Kibler. 1975. J. Biol. Chem. **250:** 9106–9111.
24. Randolph, D. H., R. F. Kibler & R. B. Fritz. 1977. J. Immunol. Methods. **18:** 215–224.
25. Whitaker, J. N., C.-H. J. Chou, F. C.-H. Chou & R. F. Kibler. 1979. Mol. Immunol. **16:** 495–501.
26. Cohen, S. R., R. M. Herndon & G. M. McKhann. 1976. N. Engl. J. Med. **295:** 1454–1457.
27. Carson, J. H., E. Barbarese, P. E. Braun & T. A. McPherson. 1978. Proc. Natl. Acad. Sci. U.S.A. **75:** 1976–1978.
28. Cohen, S. R., B. Jubelt, B. R. Brooks, R. M. Herndon & G. M. McKhann. 1980. Ann. Neurol. **8:** 25–31.

29. Ohta, M., F. Matsubara, T. Konishi & H. Nishitani. 1980. Life Sci. **27:** 1069–1074.
30. Delassalle, A., C. Jacque, J. Drovet, M. Raoul, J. C. Legrand & F. Cesselin. 1980. Biochimie **62:** 159–165.
31. Burgisser, P., J. M. Mattieu, N. de Tribolet & E. Gautier. 1982. Schiverz. Med. Wochenschr. **112:** 643–647.
32. Whitaker, J. N. 1977. Neurology **27:** 911–920.
33. Whitaker, J. N., R. P. Lisak, R. M. Bashir, O. H. Fitch, J. M. Seyer, R. Krance, J. A. Lawrence, L. T. Ch'ien & P. O'Sullivan. 1980. Ann. Neurol. **7:** 58–64.
34. Biber, A., D. Englert, D. Dommasch & K. Hempel. 1981. J. Neurol. **225:** 231–236.
35. Wood, J. H. 1981. *In* Neurobiology of Cerebrospinal Fluid, vol. 1. J. H. Wood, Ed.:1–16. Plenum. New York.
36. Pescovitz, M. D., P. Y. Paterson, J. Kelly & L. Lorand. 1978. Cell. Immunol. **39:** 355–365.
37. McPherson, T. A., J. J. Marchalonis & V. Lennon. 1970. Immunology **19:** 929–933.
38. Lennon, V. & I. R. MacKay. 1972. Clin. Exp. Immunol. **11:** 595–603.
39. Bernard, C. C. & G. Lamoureux. 1975. Intl. Arch. Allergy Immunol. **48:** 597–609.
40. Whitaker, J. N., M. A. Heinemann & O. F. Smith. 1982. Neurology **32:** A86.
41. Donald R. A. 1977. *In* Handbook of Radioimmunoassay. G. E. Abraham, Ed.: 319–390. Marcel Dekker. New York.
42. Whitaker, J. N., R. M. Bashir, C.-H. J. Chou & R. F. Kibler. 1980. J. Immunol. **124:** 1148–1153.
43. Bashir, R. M. & J. N. Whitaker. 1980. Neurology **30:** 1184–1192.
44. Whitaker, J. N., M. A. Heinemann & B. G. Uzman. 1982. Biochem. J. **201:** 543–553.
45. Whitaker, J. N. & M. A. Heinemann. 1983. Neurology **33:** 744–749.
46. Whitaker, J. N. 1982. J. Immunol. **129:** 2729–2733.
47. Fritz, R. B. & C.-H. J. Chou. 1983. J. Immunol. **130:** 2180–2182.
48. Whitaker, J. N., C.-H. J. Chou, F. C.-H. Chou & R. F. Kibler. 1977. J. Exp. Med. **146:** 317–331.
49. Gibson, B. W., R. D. Gilliom, J. N. Whitaker & K. Biemann. 1984. J. Biol. Chem. **259:** 5028–5031.
50. Bashir, R. M. & J. N. Whitaker. 1980. Ann. Neurol. **7:** 50–57.
51. Palfreyman, J. W., R. V. Johnston, J. G. Ratcliffe, D. G. T. Thomas & C. D. Forbes. 1979. Clin. Chim. Acta **92:** 403–409.
52. Panitch, H. S., C. J. Hooper & K. P. Johnson. 1980. Arch. Neurol. **37.** 206–209.
53. Gutstein, H. S. & S. R. Cohen. 1978. Science **199:** 301–303.
54. Chou, C.-H. J., W. W. Tourtellotte & R. F. Kibler. 1983. Neurology **33:** 24–28.
55. Day, E. D. & O. M. Pitts. 1974. Immunochemistry **11:** 651–659.
56. Whitaker, J. N. & M. A. Heinemann. 1983. Comp. Biochem. Physiol. **74B:** 445–448.
57. Cuzner, M. L., A. N. Davison & P. Rudge. 1978. Ann. Neurol. **4:** 337–344.
58. Alvord, E. C., S. Hruby & L. Sires. 1979. Ann. Neurol. **6:** 474–482.
59. Bashir, R. M. & J. N. Whitaker. 1983. J. Neuroimmunol. **4:** 91–104.
60. Whitaker, J. N. Unpublished observations.
61. Wallace, A. D., R. Shapira & R. B. Fritz. 1978. Immunochemistry **15:** 47–54.
62. Day, E. D. 1982. Clin. Immunol. Newsletter **3:** 53–59.
63. Lazarus, K. J., G. A. Hashim, V. A. Varitek, P. V. Paterson & E. D. Day. 1983. J. Immunol. **131:** 275–281.
64. Shapira, R., S. S. McKneally, F. Chou & R. F. Kibler. 1971. J. Biol. Chem. **246:** 4630–4640.
65. Gilliom, R. D., J. N. Whitaker & J. M. Seyer. 1983. J. Chromatogr. **254:** 211–218.
66. Eylar, E. H., S. Brostoff, G. Hashim, J. Caccam & P. Burnett. 1971. J. Biol. Chem. **246:** 5770–5784.
67. Brostoff, S. W., W. Reuter, M. Hichens & E. H. Eylar. 1974. J. Biol. Chem. **249:** 559–567.

DISCUSSION OF THE PAPER

G. HASHIM (*St Luke's Hospital, New York, NY*): The work you have described concentrated on peptide 44–89. Have you done any work with peptides from the *N*-terminus 40 residues and *C*-terminus 70 residues?

J. N. WHITAKER (*Memphis VA Medical Center*): We've not looked at those because in examining spinal fluid we don't find any material that cross-reacts with either BP peptide 1–42 or BP peptide 89–169. The amount of work that's required to look at these small peptides has been such that we focused on 44–88.

Characterization of Cerebrospinal Fluid Lymphocytes in Multiple Sclerosis[a]

JOHN R. RICHERT,[b,c] JOHN W. ROSE,[c] XIAN-HAU XU,[c]
JEFFREY I. GREENSTEIN,[c] HENRY F. McFARLAND,[c]
AND DALE E. McFARLIN[c]

[b]*Department of Neurology*
Georgetown University Medical Center
Washington, D.C. 20007

[c]*Neuroimmunology Branch*
National Institute of Neurological and
Communicative Disorders and Stroke
Bethesda, Maryland 20205

INTRODUCTION

The cerebrospinal fluid (CSF) frequently reflects pathological processes occurring within the central nervous system (CNS). Multiple sclerosis (MS) is commonly associated with characteristic immunoglobulin abnormalities and a mild CSF pleocytosis.[1] The antigenic target(s) of these CSF immunoglobulins and lymphocytes have not been delineated. Studies of antigenic reactivity of CSF T cells have been hampered by the small numbers of cells available. One approach has been to expand CSF T cells nonspecifically under conditions that might successfully maintain the antigenic reactivity of various lymphocyte populations.[2] Alternatively, we have attempted to select for and expand populations of T cells with predefined antigenic specificities.[3]

We have successfully derived five T cell lines and five T cell clones from the CSF of patients with MS. Two T cell lines and two clones are reactive with myelin basic protein (BP) and one line is specific for measles virus. Each cell line maintained significant mitogenic responsiveness. CSF absorption studies performed with one BP-reactive T cell line resulted in absorption of both polyclonal and oligoclonal IgG.

MATERIALS AND METHODS

Patient Populations

CSF for cell-surface phenotypic analysis was obtained by lumbar puncture from 12 MS patients and four patients with other neurologic disease (OND). Of the MS patients studied, six had chronic progressive disease and six were evaluated 1–3 weeks

[a]Dr. Richert is the recipient of an NINCDS Teacher Investigator Award. This work was supported in part by NIH grant no. 1 RO1 NS 18510–01A1, National Multiple Sclerosis Society grant no. RG 1529–A–1, and a Georgetown University Biomedical Research Support Grant. Dr. Xu is a visiting Chinese scholar supported by NMSS grant no. SG 603–A–1. Dr. Greenstein's current address is: Department of Neurology, Temple University Medical Center, Philadelphia, Pennsylvania.

after the onset of an acute exacerbation. No CSF samples were obtained within the first week of an exacerbation. Diagnoses in patients with OND included peripheral neuropathy, old poliomyelitis, chronic otitis media, and chronic optic neuritis.

CSF cells to be placed in long-term culture were obtained from an additional four patients with definite MS and one patient with possible MS. One patient (patient no. 4) was a known measles responder, as measured by the proliferative response of his peripheral blood mononuclear cells (PBM).

Culture Conditions

Cells were separated from CSF by centrifugation at 300 g for 10 minutes, then placed into culture in RPMI 1640 supplemented with antibiotics (gentamicin or penicillin/streptomycin), 2 mM L-glutamine, 1 mM sodium pyruvate, 25 mM Hepes buffer, 10% pooled A^+ plasma, 25 IU/ml heparin, irradiated (2500–6000 rads) autologous ficoll-hypaque purified PBM, and antigen, as previously described.[3] Antigen consisted of glutaraldehyde-fixed and sonicated measles virus-infected Vero cells,[4] rat BP (RBP, 50 μg/ml), or human BP (hBP, 1 μg/ml, generously provided by Mrs. Gladys Deibler and Dr. Marian Kies[5]). Interleukin 2 (IL-2, T cell growth factor, kindly provided by Dr. Phil Lake) was added for the first time either at the beginning of culture (cell lines from patients 1–3), after two days of culture (patient 4), or after five days of culture (cell line from patient 5) at a final concentration of 20%.[6] Growing cells were fed weekly with complete medium, fresh antigen, and irradiated feeders. Fresh IL-2 was added either simultaneously with each feeding (cells from patients 1–4) or on the following day (patient 5), and again 3–4 days later. After one month in culture in the presence of 1 μg/ml hBP, cells from patient 5 were cloned by limiting dilution at an average of 0.3 cells/well.[7] Growing clones were maintained as described above, with the exception that irradiated (2500 rads) feeders consisted of a mixture of autologous and allogeneic PBM.

Fluorescence Cell-Surface Analysis

Approximately 10^4 fresh CSF cells, 7×10^5 cultured CSF cells, and 10^6 fresh PBM were washed and incubated at 4° C for 90 min with each first-stage antibody. These included OKT-3, OKT-4, OKT-8, and OKM (Ortho),[8] as well as anti-HLA-DR framework antibody (New England Nuclear). The P3x63Ag8 mouse ascites fluid served as negative control. After the first-stage incubation the cells were washed and incubated at 4° C for 30 min with a fluorescein-labeled $F(ab')_2$ fragment of goat anti-mouse IgG. Labeled cells were analyzed manually or on a fluorescence-activated cell sorter (FACS-IV).

Proliferation Assays

One week after the previous full feeding and three days after the previous IL-2 supplement, 10^4 or 10^5 cells were removed from long-term culture, washed, and placed in each well of a 96-well microtiter plate in 0.2 ml medium (without IL-2), with 2.5×10^4 or 2.5×10^5 irradiated autologous PBM respectively. Soluble antigen or mitogen was added to the appropriate wells, and the cells were incubated at 37° C for 96 hrs. Assays for virus-specific proliferation were performed on monolayers of virus-infected or uninfected Vero cells.[9] Tritiated thymidine (^{3}H-TdR) was added at 1 μCi/well over the last 4 or 18 hrs of culture. The wells were harvested on a semiautomatic cell harvester (MASH-II).

Absorption of CSF IgG

Cultured BP-reactive CSF cells from patient 2, uncultured PBM from patient 2, and cloned BP-reactive CSF cells from patient 5 were each suspended in 0.3 ml phosphate-buffered saline (PBS) and mixed with 0.3 ml CSF from patient 2. Each suspension was incubated at room temperature for one hour, then kept at 4° C for 23 hrs. The cells were then removed by centrifugation at 1000 g for 15 minutes. Each absorbed sample was subsequently absorbed a second time with fresh cells over the next 24 hrs.

Analysis of CSF IgG and Albumin

Twenty μl samples from the absorbed and unabsorbed CSF specimens from patient 2 were applied to 5 × 10 mm sheets of filter paper and placed at the pH 5.7 region of an isoelectric focusing gel (ampholine polyacrylamide gel plates, pH 3.5–9.5, LKB).[10] The samples were focused for four hrs, then transferred to nitrocellulose paper by electrophoretic blotting. The transblotted samples were stained with an avidin-biotin-peroxidase system using a mouse anti-human IgG.[10] In brief, the nitrocellulose-bound protein was incubated with mouse anti-human IgG, then reacted with biotin-conjugated horse anti-mouse IgG. This in turn was exposed to an avidin:biotinylated horseradish peroxidase complex, and developed in substrate containing diaminobenzidine and hydrogen peroxidase. CSF albumin in each sample was quantitated with a commercially available radial immunodiffusion (RID) assay kit (Calbiochem-Behringer).

RESULTS

Cell-Surface Phenotypic Analysis of Fresh CSF Cells

Fresh CSF cells and PBM were examined by indirect immunofluorescence. The percentage of OKT-3$^+$ cells in the CSF averaged 88.8 ± 2.8 for the MS population and 94.5 ± 1.5 for OND subjects (TABLE 1). The percentage of OKT-8$^+$ CSF cells was diminished in the MS group (20.3 ± 1.9) as compared with the OND group (25.0 ± 4.7). A moderate degree of overlap was seen in these studies. The OKT-4/OKT-8 ratio was slightly higher in the MS CSF cell populations (3.85 ± 0.4 *versus* 3.08 ± 0.16). These differences were not statistically significant, however. In addition, no significant difference was seen in the profiles of PBM in the two groups. Subdividing the MS patients into those with chronic progressive disease and those 1–3 weeks postexacerbation did not uncover any further differences (data not shown).

Antigen-Specific Proliferation by Long-Term Cultured CSF Cells

CSF cells from four patients were expanded in the presence of antigen, IL-2 and autologous irradiated PBM. Cells from patients 1–3 were cultured with RBP. Because PBM from patient 4 had previously been found to proliferate in response to measles virus, CSF cells from this patient were cultured with measles antigen. After two months in culture the CSF cells were assayed for proliferation in response to RBP and a panel of virus-infected Vero cells.

Cultured cells from patients 1 and 2 demonstrated mild proliferative responses to RBP (TABLE 2), but no response to measles, mumps, or vaccinia viruses. Cells from patient 3, which had also been maintained in the presence of BP, failed to respond to either BP or measles antigen. CSF cells from patient 4 proliferated in response to measles virus but not to BP or to mumps or vaccinia viruses.

Mitogenic Responses of Cultured CSF Cells

After two months in culture the cell lines were assayed for their responses to the mitogens concanavalin A (Con A), phytohemagglutinin (PHA), and pokeweed mitogen (PWM), as well as to IL-2 (TABLE 3). Maximal responses in most instances

TABLE 1. Cell Surface Phenotypic Analysis of Fresh PBM and CSF Cells

Source of Cells	Percent of Total Cells				
	OKT-3	OKT-4	OKT-8	anti-DR	4:8 Ratio
CSF					
OND	94.5 ± 1.5	69.3 ± 0.8	25.0 ± 4.7	5.8 ± 0.8	3.08 ± 0.16
MS	88.8 ± 2.8	71.1 ± 3.3	20.3 ± 1.9	6.6 ± 1.8	3.85 ± 0.4
PBM					
OND	76.0 ± 4.7	57.0 ± 4.4	27.5 ± 1.7	12.0 ± 2.1	2.12 ± 0.27
MS	78.8 ± 3.2	58.4 ± 3.0	26.2 ± 1.8	10.3 ± 0.7	2.3 ± 0.16

Fresh PBM and CSF lymphocytes were incubated with mouse monoclonal antibodies directed against cell-surface antigens, then stained with $F(ab')_2$ fragments of fluorescein-labeled goat anti-mouse IgG. Results are expressed as the percentage of the total number of cells that reacted with each antibody.

were observed at 96 hrs. All cell lines maintained their responsiveness to both mitogenic stimulation and to IL-2.

Role of Irradiated Feeder Cells in the Mitogenic Response of Cultured CSF Cells

The mitogenic responses shown in TABLE 3 were obtained in the presence of irradiated autologous PBM that served as "feeder" cells in culture. In previous work reported by Burns *et al.*[2] CSF cells maintained in culture for approximately one month in the absence of irradiated feeders failed to respond to mitogenic stimulation. Therefore the role of irradiated PBM was examined (FIG. 1).

After four months in culture CSF cells from patient 1 were assayed with and without additional irradiated autologous PBM. Cerebrospinal fluid cells alone responded vigorously to Con A, PHA, PWM, and IL-2, whereas the irradiated PBM alone produced minimal responses. Significant augmentation of the proliferative responses was seen when irradiated PBM were added to the long-term cultured CSF cells. The degree of augmentation was more pronounced in the response to mitogens than in the response to IL-2.

TABLE 2. Proliferation of Cultured CSF Lymphocytes in Response to Antigens

		^{3}H-TdR Incorporation (cpm) Antigen in Assay				
Patient	Antigen in Long-Term Culture	Vero Cells	BP	Measles	Mumps	Vaccinia
1	BP	379 ± 20	*1,017 ± 9*	424 ± 63	313 ± 32	219 ± 6
2	BP	2,664 ± 200	*7,196 ± 506*	3,084 ± 244	ND	ND
3	BP	196 ± 42	260 ± 5	149 ± 11	ND	ND
4	measles virus	23,042 ± 2,514	21,758 ± 1,896	*100,403 ± 5,653*	25,316 ± 2,285	23,560 ± 1,766

After two months in culture CSF cells were assayed for antigen-specific proliferation. 10^4 BP-cultured cells or 10^5 cells that had been cultured with measles antigen were placed in 96-well trays with antigen and 2.5×10^4 or 2.5×10^5 irradiated autologous PBM respectively. Cells were incubated for 96 hours and pulsed with 1 μCi ^{3}H-TdR. Results are expressed as mean cpm ± SE.

Cell-Surface Phenotypes of Fresh vs. Cultured Cells

Fluorescent cell-surface phenotypic analysis of the cultured CSF cells was performed and compared with the profiles observed with fresh CSF cells and PBM obtained at the time of initiation of culture. Cultured cells were studied after two months *in vitro.*

The majority of fresh CSF cells were T lymphocytes, as evidenced by the high percentage of OKT-3$^+$ cells detected (TABLE 4). The percentage of OKT-3$^+$ cells was further augmented after long-term culture. The percentage of OKT-8$^+$ cells in the cultured populations was variable. Interestingly, the cell line that best maintained its rate of growth after a year *in vitro* was the one demonstrating the lowest percentage of OKT-8$^+$ cells (from patient 2, 0.4%). The most strikingly consistent change in the profile of long-term cultured cells concerned the percentage of DR$^+$ cells, which increased approximately twofold or more in every instance. The majority of these DR$^+$ cells were T lymphocytes, as evidenced by the high percentage of OKT-3$^+$ cells, suggesting that long-term culture had selected for populations of activated T cells.

TABLE 3. Proliferation of Cultured CSF Lymphocytes in Response to Mitogens

	^{3}H-TdR Incorporation (cpm) Mitogen in Culture				
Patient	None	Con A	PHA	PWM	IL-2
1	415 ± 4	24,427 ± 1,434	64,579 ± 4,019	20,491 ± 356	35,712 ± 1,019
2	3,909 ± 221	10,444 ± 671	82,192 ± 5,257	30,155 ± 2,929	32,326 ± 2,268
3	320 ± 39	32,385 ± 2,418	56,265 ± 1,137	23,193 ± 486	19,798 ± 214
4	4,549 ± 508	55,327 ± 3,724	50,504 ± 1,928	31,410 ± 1,892	20,104 ± 1,490

After two months in culture 10^4 CSF cells were incubated for 96 hrs with mitogen (5 μg/ml Con A, 1 μg/ml PHA, 1:500 PWM) or 20% IL-2 in the presence of 2.5×10^4 irradiated autologous PBM. After 96 hrs each well was pulsed with 1 μCi ^{3}H-TdR. Results are expressed as mean cpm ± SE.

Cloned BP-reactive CSF T Cells

Subsequently fresh CSF cells were obtained from a patient with possible MS (two episodes, five years apart, of transient posterior column dysfunction with a spinal level of L_{2-3}, with a mild CSF pleocytosis and eight oligoclonal IgG bands, without clinical, electrophysiologic or radiologic evidence of disease elsewhere in the CNS) and placed into culture with 1 μg/ml hBP. The cell line grew slowly and demonstrated only a minimal, if any, proliferative response to hBP (TABLE 5). After one month in culture the cells were cloned by limiting dilution in the presence of hBP. Five clones were isolated, two of which demonstrated mild proliferative responses to hBP (TABLE 5). Clone 3 stained positively with OKT-3 and OKT-4 and negatively with OKT-8, whereas clone 5 stained only with OKT-3 (98.3%) but not with OKT-4, OKT-8, Leu 2a, or Leu 3a (data not shown).

CSF Absorption Studies

In order to determine if CSF oligoclonal IgG might be absorbed by the cultured CSF cells, CSF from patient 2 was, on two successive days, incubated with the

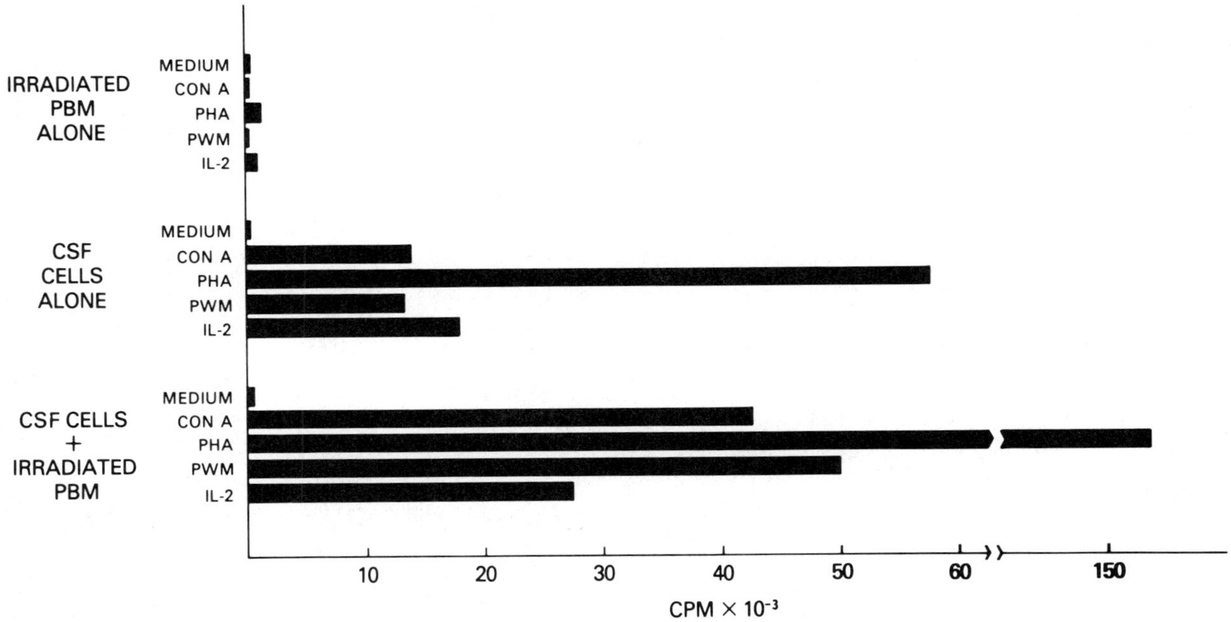

FIGURE 1. After four months in culture CSF cells from patient 1 were washed and placed in microtiter plates at 10^4/well. Irradiated (6,000 rads) autologous PBM were either added to the cultured cells or were placed in separate wells at 2.5×10^4/well. Mitogens and IL-2 were added to the appropriate wells, and the cells were incubated for 96 hrs. ^{3}H-TdR (1 μCi) was added to each well over the last 18 hrs of culture.

TABLE 4. Cell Surface Phenotypes of Fresh and Cultured Cells

	Percentage of Cells Stained with Fluorescent Antibody											
	Patient 1			Patient 2			Patient 3			Patient 4		
Antibody	PBM	CSF	CCSF	PBM	CSF	CCSF	PBM	CSF	CCSF	PBM	CSF	CCSF
OKT-3	72	83	90	68	ND	76	75	63	88	63	ND	92
OKT-4	41	56	52	47	ND	81	51	55	90	50	ND	67
OKT-8	31	18	34	16	ND	0.4	27	14	6.7	13	ND	24
Anti-DR	19	19	78	21	28	53	25	24	54	23	7.9	20
OKM	7.0	5.0	2.3	12	ND	0	12	ND	0	15	ND	0

Fresh PBM, fresh CSF cells, or cultured CSF cells (CCSF) underwent FACS analysis as in TABLE 1. Results are expressed as the percentage of the total number of cells that stained with the fluorescent antibody. (ND = not determined.)

TABLE 5. BP-reactive T Cell Clones

Cells	Concentration of hBP in Assay (μg/ml) 0	0.01	0.1	1.0	10.0
Cell line	66 ± 36	ND	182 ± 48	191 ± 17	190 ± 44
Clone 3					
Experiment 1	49 ± 1	140 ± 32	247 ± 65	1,655 ± 249	154 ± 2
Experiment 2	35 ± 3	26 ± 6	804 ± 108	453 ± 47	79 ± 15
Clone 5					
Experiment 1	37 ± 7	8 ± 6	251 ± 63	525 ± 78	45 ± 10
Experiment 2	233 ± 34	ND	1,150 ± 258	1,037 ± 50	175 ± 29

CSF cells from patient 5 were cultured for one month in the presence of 1 μg/ml hBP, then cloned by limiting dilution. Ninety-six-hour proliferation assays were performed on the cell line after three weeks of culture and on the cloned populations after three and four months *in vitro*. Results are expressed as mean cpm ± SE.

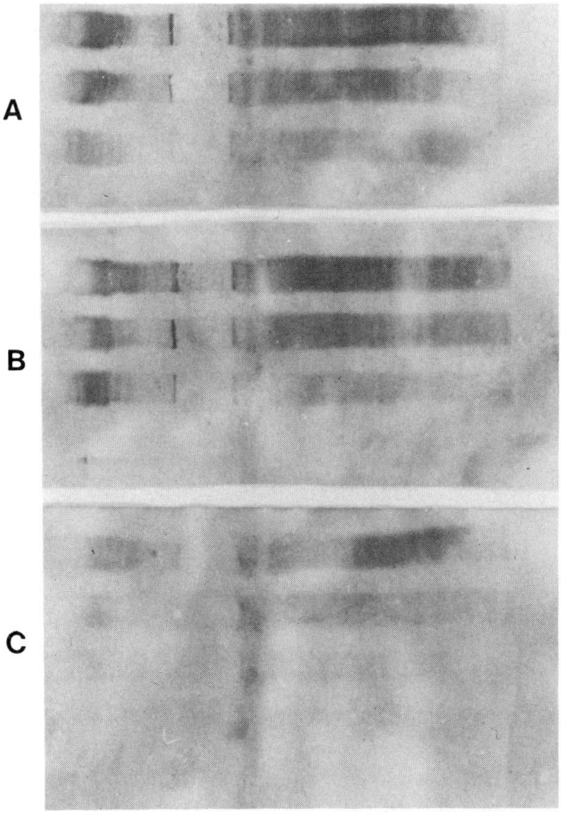

FIGURE 2. Unabsorbed CSF from patient 2 (**A**), CSF absorbed with autologous PBM (**B**), or CSF absorbed with the autologous BP-reactive CSF T cell line (**C**), each at final dilutions of 1:2, 1:4, and 1:8 (from top to bottom within each group), were isoelectro-focused, then transferred to nitrocellulose paper by electrophoretic blotting, and stained with the avidin-biotin-peroxidase system as described in "Materials and Methods."

autologous CSF cell line for one hour at room temperature, followed by 23 hrs at 4° C. The results are shown in FIG. 2. Both oligoclonal and polyclonal IgG were absorbed by the cells. In contrast, little, if any, CSF IgG from patient 2 was absorbed by autologous uncultured PBM. This experiment was repeated, this time using cloned BP-reactive CSF T cells from patient 5 (clone no. 5) as a control absorbent (FIG. 3). Again, CSF IgG was absorbed only by the autologous CSF cell line. The albumin concentrations were nearly identical in these three samples: 27.1 mg per dl in CSF absorbed by the autologous cell line, 28.0 mg per dl in CSF absorbed by autologous PBM, and 28.3 mg per dl in CSF absorbed by the allogeneic BP-reactive T cell clone.

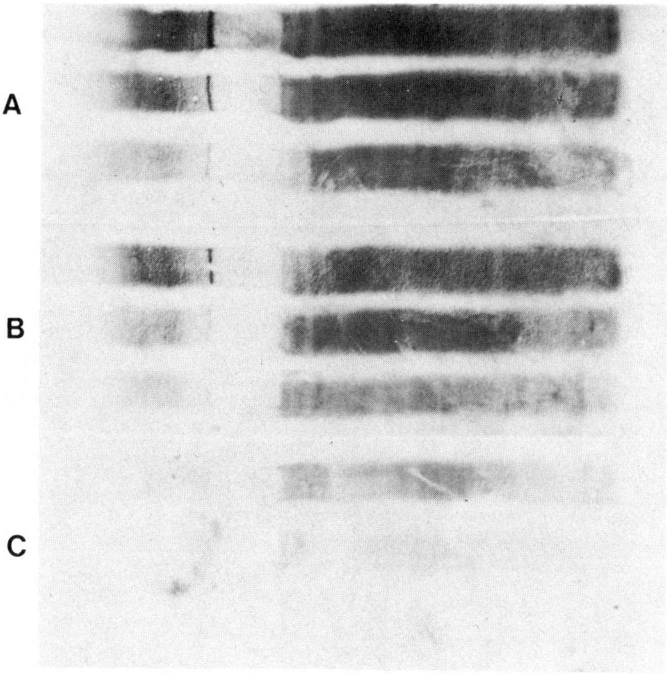

FIGURE 3. Unabsorbed CSF from patient 2 (**A**), CSF absorbed with an allogeneic BP-reactive CSF T cell clone (**B**), or CSF absorbed with the autologous BP-reactive CSF T cell line (**C**) were analyzed exactly as described in FIGURE 2. Each sample was run at final dilutions of 1:2, 1:4, and 1:8 (from top to bottom within each group).

DISCUSSION

The presence of perivenular mononuclear cell infiltrates as well as the frequent occurrence of a mild CSF pleocytosis in MS suggest that the study of CSF lymphocytes may yield clues as to the pathogenetic mechanisms involved in this disease. T cells express effector or suppressor function or may provide help in the generation of antibody or cytotoxic T cell responses. The expansion of CSF T lymphocytes *in vitro* permits the detailed analysis of cells potentially involved in the development of demyelinating lesions.

Others have studied the cell-surface phenotypic characteristics of MS cerebrospinal fluid T cells and have variably reported either no change[11] or alterations[12] in the numbers of helper or cytotoxic/suppressor phenotypes during different stages of the disease. Our limited evaluation to date of patients with chronic progressive disease or those who were seen relatively late after the onset of an acute exacerbation suggests that these subjects may exhibit mild alterations in the constitution of their CSF T lymphocytes. Although these patients demonstrated only a mildly diminished percentage of OKT-8^+ cells and a slightly higher T4/T8 ratio than subjects with OND, both groups exhibited higher T4/T8 ratios than the baseline values previously reported.[11,12] For the OND group, this may reflect the inclusion of patients with chronic inflammatory disease. Whether this might indicate modulation of suppressor cell or cytotoxic T cell populations cannot be determined from these data.

In order to select for and expand specific T cell populations reactive with antigens of potential pathogenetic relevance in MS, we maintained CSF cells from four patients in long-term culture with either BP or measles virus antigen. Cell lines from patients 1 and 2 demonstrated mild degrees of proliferation to BP. The cell line from patient 4, who had previously been identified as a measles responder as measured by the proliferative response of his PBM, proliferated specifically to measles virus antigen. The cell line from patient 3 responded to neither BP nor measles virus. Vigorous proliferative responses were maintained to all mitogens tested, and these were further augmented by the presence of irradiated autologous feeder cells. Previous attempts by ourselves and others[2] to maintain CSF cells in culture in the presence of mitogens or IL-2 but without irradiated feeders met with limited success. The presence of these feeders appears necessary for both the maintenance of the cell lines over an extended period of time *in vitro* as well as for generating maximal mitogenic responses.

The relatively small increments in proliferation seen in the presence of BP or measles virus suggested that either significant sensitization to these antigens had not occurred *in vivo* in the CNS or that optimal culture conditions had not been achieved, perhaps in part because of potential inhibitory influences present in culture. Cell-surface phenotypic analysis demonstrated the persistence of OKT-8^+ cells in most of the long-term cultured cell lines. This suggested the possibility that suppressor T cells may have played an inhibitory role in the antigen-specific proliferation of the cultured cells.

Subsequently a fifth CSF cell line was established, this one cultured in the presence of hBP. After three weeks in culture it demonstrated minimal, if any, antigen-induced proliferation. Lymphocytes from this cell line were then cloned by limiting dilution. Two T cell clones were isolated that proliferated in response to BP. Dose-response studies showed maximal responses with 0.1–1.0 μg/ml hBP. Clone 3 is OKT-3^+ 4^+ 8^- whereas clone 5 is OKT-3^+ 4^- 8^- Leu $2a^-$ Leu $3a^-$. Further analysis of these clones is currently underway.

We have begun to use the cell lines and clones in an attempt to analyze CSF oligoclonal bands of IgG. To date the antigen binding specificities of the oligoclonal IgG found in MS CSF are unknown.[1] We have considered the possibility that this IgG might be anti-idiotypic. To test this hypothesis we attempted to absorb oligoclonal IgG with an autologous long-term cultured BP-reactive CSF cell line. This resulted in a more generalized absorption of both oligoclonal and polyclonal IgG. Significant amounts of IgG were neither absorbed by autologous fresh PBM nor by an allogeneic long-term cultured BP-reactive T cell clone. Albumin levels in CSF absorbed by these three groups of cells were comparable. Attempts to block binding via Fc receptors on the cell line by preincubating the cell line with human serum are now in progress. At the moment CSF is not available from patient 5, from whom the BP-reactive clones were derived. The question of whether the observed absorption of CSF IgG by the autologous CSF cell line will prove to be an isolated finding or whether it will be demonstrated to be of more general significance must await the development of additional cell lines from patients whose CSF is also available. Should oligoclonal IgG subsequently be shown to be anti-idiotypic, reacting with cells of restricted antigenic specificity, this method has the potential for indirectly identifying an antigen of pathogenetic consequence in MS.

ACKNOWLEDGMENTS

The authors wish to thank Cynthia Burnside, Laura Muehl, and Marjorie Flerlage for technical assistance, Elizabeth Mingioli for performing the FACS analyses, and Heidi Hartt-Crum for typing the manuscript.

REFERENCES

1. McFarlin, D. E. & H. F. McFarland. 1982. N. Engl. J. Med. **307:** 1183–1188, 1246–1251.
2. Burns, J. B., B. Zweiman & R. P. Lisak. 1981. J. Clin. Immunol. **1:** 195–200.
3. Richert, J. R., D. E. McFarlin, J. W. Rose, H. F. McFarland & J. I. Greenstein. 1983. J. Neuroimmunol. **5:** 317–324.
4. Bellini, W. J., D. E. McFarlin, G. D. Silver, E. S. Mingioli & H. F. McFarland. 1981. Infect. Immunity **32:** 1051–1057.
5. Deibler, G. E., R. E. Martenson & M. W. Kies. 1972. Prep. Biochem. **2:** 139–165.
6. Lamb, J. R., D. D. Eckels, P. Lake, A. H. Johnson, R. J. Hartzman & J. N. Woody. 1982. J. Immunol. **128:** 233–238.
7. Richert, J. R., H. F. McFarland, D. E. McFarlin, W. J. Bellini & P. Lake. 1983. Proc. Natl. Acad. Sci. U.S.A. **80:** 555–559.
8. Reinherz, E. L., P. C. Kung, G. Goldstein & S. F. Schlossman. 1979. Proc. Natl. Acad. Sci. U.S.A. **76:** 4061–4065.
9. McFarland, H. F. & D. E. McFarlin. 1979. Ann. Neurol. **6:** 101–106.
10. Xu, X.-h. & D. E. McFarlin. 1983. Neurology **34:** 769–774.
11. Hauser, S. L., E. L. Reinherz, C. J. Hoban, S. F. Schlossman & H. L. Weiner. 1983. Neurology **33:** 575–579.
12. Panitch, H. S. & G. S. Francis. 1982. N. Engl. J. Med. **307:** 560–561.

DISCUSSION OF THE PAPER

V. ter Meulen (*University of Würzburg, Würzburg, FRG*): Did you try to use CSF as the antigen for stimulation of your T cell clones?

J. R. Richert (*Georgetown University Medical Center, Washington, D.C.*): No, we haven't used either CSF or immunoglobulin to stimulate the clones as yet.

Further Lymphocyte Characterization in the Central Nervous System in Multiple Sclerosis[a]

UTE TRAUGOTT AND CEDRIC S. RAINE

Departments of Neuropathology, Neurology and Neuroscience
and
The Rose F. Kennedy Center for Research in Mental Retardation and Human Development
Albert Einstein College of Medicine
Bronx, New York 10461

INTRODUCTION

Whereas the clinical and pathological picture of multiple sclerosis (MS) has been known for more than a century, the pathogenetic mechanisms underlying this primary demyelinating disease still remain a mystery.[1-4] Though a viral etiology is implicated initially, autoimmune phenomena are believed to play an essential role in the expression of the CNS disease. The viral theory has been supported by the frequently observed increases in antibody titers against measles and other viruses in serum and cerebrospinal fluid (CSF).[5-8] On the other hand, abnormalities of the cellular and humoral immune system, as well as extensive studies on experimental allergic encephalomyelitis (EAE), the major animal model for MS, support the concept that MS might be an autoimmune disease.[9-12] In the CSF, IgG is frequently elevated and oligoclonal bands are detectable in most cases.[13-16] Furthermore, sensitization of the cellular and humoral immune system against myelin antigens has been documented.[10,17-22] However, none of the above phenomena are specific for MS and can also be found in other neurological conditions in which white matter destruction has occurred and might therefore represent epiphenomena. Quantitative evaluation of lymphocyte subsets in the blood has revealed decreases in circulating T cell subsets, some of which (T_G cells and $T8^+$ cells)[10,18,23,24] correlated with exacerbations. Similar changes could sometimes also be observed in the CSF, which might reflect CNS pathology somewhat better than the blood.[25] Though $T8^+$ cells display significant quantitative changes, only $T4^+$ cells (helper/inducer T cells) in the CSF have been demonstrated to become activated during exacerbations.[26] This indicates blastogenic transformation and might suggest a significant role of $T4^+$ cells in the disease process. In addition, natural killer cells and killer cells have been shown to be decreased in the circulation and to display a reduced response to interferon.[27,28] All these findings suggest a dysregulation of the immune system in MS patients. Although considerable information on immunologic abnormalities in blood and CSF has accumulated over the last few years, knowledge of immunopathogenetic mechanisms occurring at the level of the target organ, the CNS, is still limited. By routine morphologic criteria, certain types of MS lesions have been defined using the degree of inflammation, consisting of

[a]This work was supported in part by NMSS grant no. RG–1001–D–4, and USPHS grant nos. NS 08952, NS 11920, and NIHR–G008200046.

lymphocytes, macrophages and some plasma cells, and the presence of myelin degradation products as indicators for disease activity.[12,29,30] However, until recently, a more detailed analysis of inflammatory cells in MS lesions *in situ* was not possible because of the unavailability of specific markers. By immunocytochemistry, plasma cells and IgG deposits have been demonstrated in MS plaques[31-33] but information on the localization of T cells was restricted to crude technology such as the application of rosette formation *in situ* and the use of heterologous antisera.[34,35] With the introduction of highly specific monoclonal antibodies against certain differentiation antigens on pan T cells, T cell subsets and other hematogenous cells,[36,37] it became possible to characterize in detail inflammatory cells within MS lesions. The following results are an extension of recent work[38] and might provide a better understanding of lesion pathogenesis in MS.

TABLE 1. Material Used for Localization of Lymphocytes

Patient	Age	Sex	Duration of Disease	Clinical Diagnosis	Lesion Activity	No. of Blocks Studied
Multiple Sclerosis						
1. G.I.	42	F	4 mo	acute	acute	23
2. J.B.	54	F	5 mo	acute	acute active chronic	10
3. T.B.	44	F	1 y	remitting	acute subacute	4
4. H.E.	26	F	10 y	remitting	acute subacute	16
5. B.J.	38	M	13 y	remitting	chronic active	6
6. C.M.	43	F	2 y	remitting	chronic silent	3
7. Y.I.	50	F	10 y	chronic progressive	chronic active	10
8. L.A.	32	M	4 y	chronic progressive	chronic silent	8
9. C.R.	40	M	7 y	chronic stable	chronic silent	23
Subacute Sclerosing Panencephalitis						
1. F.W.	12	F	8 mo	SSPE	subacute	8
2. M.R.	14	M	5 mo	SSPE	subacute	4
Controls						
1. B.S.	34	M	6 mo	leukemia	none	2
2. T.K.	38	F	4 y	SLE	none	2
3. A.L.	64	M	8 mo	cancer of lung	none	1

MATERIALS AND METHODS

Monoclonal antibodies were used in combination with the peroxidase-anti-peroxidase (PAP)[38,39] or avidin-biotin peroxidase complex (ABC-40) method for the *in situ* localization of inflammatory cells. For this, brain tissue from nine MS cases (two acute, four remitting, two chronic progressive and one chronic stable MS) was available. These tissue samples contained acute, subacute, active chronic and silent chronic lesions (TABLE 1). To compare the results obtained in MS with those of a viral inflammatory disease, CNS tissue was studied from two cases of subacute sclerosing panencephalitis (SSPE). Brain material from patients with leukemia, systemic lupus erythematosus (SLE) and carcinoma of the lung was used as normal control.

For the modified four-step PAP technique,[38] frozen sections were fixed with acetone and then incubated with 0.1% H_2O_2 and 3% normal swine serum in Tris/saline. This was followed by the consecutive exposure to monoclonal antibodies (mAb) at the appropriate dilutions, rabbit anti-mouse Ig, swine anti-rabbit Ig and rabbit PAP. Pan (total) T cells were labeled with anti-T11 and anti-T3 mAb, helper/inducer T cells with anti-T4 mAb, suppressor/cytotoxic T cells with anti-T8 mAb and cytotoxic $T4^+$ cells with anti-TQ_1 mAb. These monoclonal antibodies were kindly provided by Dr. Ellis L. Reinherz (Harvard Medical School, Boston, Massachusetts). Natural killer (NK) and killer (K) cells were characterized by anti-Leu-7 mAb (Becton Dickinson) and Ia-bearing cells (B cells, macrophages and activated T cells) by an anti-Ia mAb (New England Nuclear, New Jersey). For labeling of B cells, acetone-fixed frozen sections were stained by the three-step PAP technique with the IgG fraction of rabbit anti-human Ig (IgG + IgA + IgM), followed by sheep anti-rabbit Ig and rabbit PAP.[39] A brown reaction product was obtained after incubation with PAP by exposure to diaminobenzidine (DAB). One of the sections, processed in duplicate, was then counterstained with hematoxylin to facilitate pathologic evaluation. In some experiments, 4-chloro-1-naphthol (CN) was used to obtain a blue color on reactive cells. In double-labeling studies, $T8^+$ cells were stained with DAB and oligodendrocytes with an anti-galactocerebroside (GC) antiserum in combination with CN.[41] The working dilution for the monoclonal and conventional antibodies used was established on normal human lymph node or spleen tissue. The specificity of each monoclonal antibody for hematogenous cells was tested on normal brain sections and was indicated by the absence of reactivity with CNS elements. As has been reported previously, the application of anti-Leu 7 to frozen sections of lymph nodes resulted in labeling of some cells within the follicles only and $T8^+$ cells did not react.[42] From all blocks, sections were also stained with H+E for the determination of lesion activity. In selected blocks, degradation products of myelin were demonstrated by oil-red-0 staining.

RESULTS

H+E stained sections revealed that one of the acute MS cases contained acute lesions only, whereas in the other case, acute, active chronic and concentric Balo-type lesions were found. The CNS tissue from patients with clinically remitting or chronic progressive MS showed both active and silent chronic lesions, and in the one case with clinically inactive chronic MS, only silent chronic lesions were seen (TABLE 1).

Acute MS Lesion

By routine morphology, the acute MS lesion is characterized by a diffuse margin and extensive parenchymal and perivascular infiltrates, which consist mainly of small and large mononuclear cells (lymphocytes and macrophages; see FIG. 1).

Throughout this type of lesion, dense infiltrates of $T11^+$ cells (pan T cells) were found (FIG. 2) distributed within the parenchyma as well as in perivascular cuffs. $T11^+$ cells showed the highest denisty in the lesion center; the density tapered off towards the lesion edge and virtually no infiltrating T cells could be detected within the unaffected white matter. $T4^+$ cells (helper/inducer T cells) and $T8^+$ cells (suppressor/cytotoxic T cells) displayed a similar distribution pattern to $T11^+$ cells (TABLE 2)[43,44] and both T cell subsets were absent from normal white matter. Whereas $TQ1^+$ cells (cytotoxic

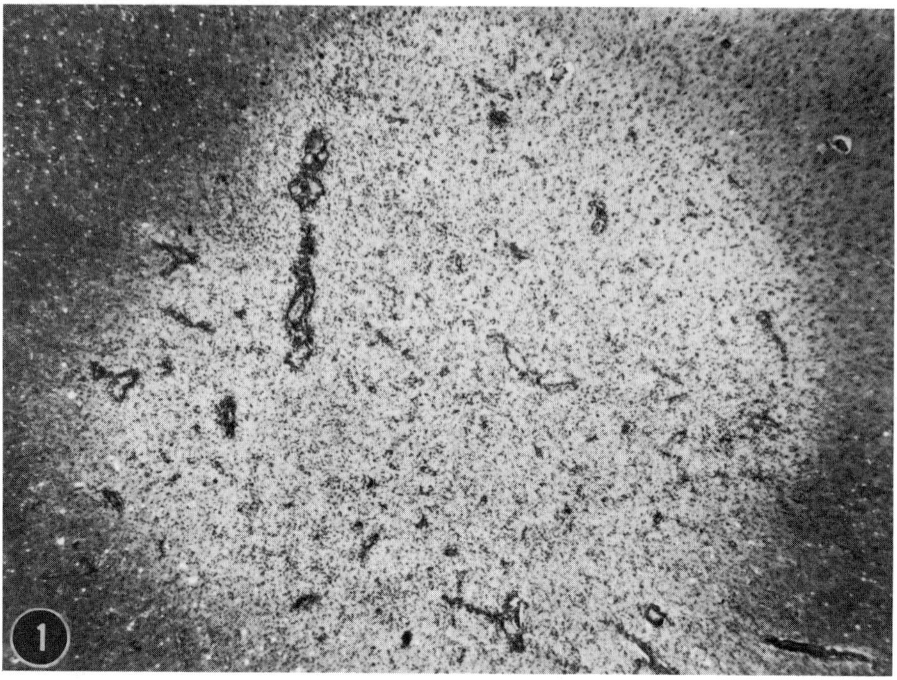

FIGURE 1. Acute MS, H+E: a small lesion with a diffuse margin and extensive infiltrates is shown (×100).

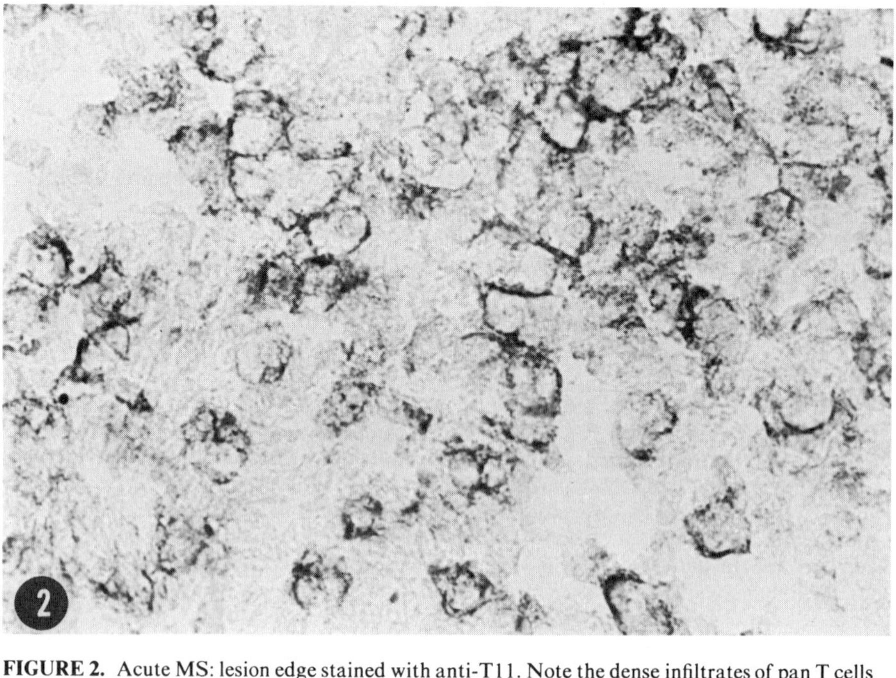

FIGURE 2. Acute MS: lesion edge stained with anti-T11. Note the dense infiltrates of pan T cells (×640).

$T4^+$ cells) were found in considerable numbers, Leu 7^+ cells (NK and K cells) were rare.

As judged by morphologic criteria from counterstained sections, most Ia^+ cells within acute MS lesions were homogeneously staining macrophages (FIG. 3). Foamy macrophages were less common and small Ia^+ cells (B cells and activated T cells) were rare. Ia^+ macrophages were so tightly packed within the center of the lesion that normal white matter could not be discerned. The denisty of large Ia^+ infiltrating cells, which were sometimes seen in close association with small mononuclear cells, decreased towards the edge of the lesion where CNS tissue elements became apparent between inflammatory cells. No Ia^+ macrophages were detectable outside the lesion proper. At the lesion edge, Ia^+ endothelial cells, to which Ia^+ macrophages were frequently attached, could be found in moderate numbers. In acute MS, infiltrating T cells and Ia^+ macrophages were virtually absent from normal white matter, but Ia^+ endothelial cells were occasionally seen (FIG. 4). The presence of Ia^+ endothelial cells in the center of the lesion, although highly likely, could not be demonstrated unequivocally because of the dense cellular infiltrates.

TABLE 2. Quantitative Evaluation of $T11^+$, $T4^+$, $T8^+$ and Ia^+ Cells in MS Lesions of Different Ages

Cell Type	$T11^+$	$T4^+$	$T8^+$	Ia^+
Acute MS Lesion				
Center	179.1 ± 66.0	114.5 ± 17.5	172.9 ± 28.3	167.1 ± 40.1
Edge	91.8 ± 15.4	73.3 ± 20.4	81.6 ± 24.4	70.9 ± 6.0
Active Chronic MS Lesion				
Center	17.9 ± 2.1	8.1 ± 4.9	6.0 ± 3.5	124.1 ± 9.1
Edge	57.9 ± 20.9	42.1 ± 17.0	31.6 ± 24.4	78.4 ± 7.1
Normal WM	24.4 ± 12.6	49.1 ± 18.8	24.1 ± 6.9	32.1 ± 11.6
Silent Chronic MS Lesion				
Center	1.3 ± 1.5	0.6 ± 1.0	0.4 ± 0.6	3.1 ± 2.8
Edge	5.0 ± 6.1	2.3 ± 2.8	1.6 ± 1.9	17.9 ± 3.6

Numbers given represent the mean values ± 1 SD of the cell numbers present in selected representative areas of 0.1 mm^2.

Sections reacted with anti-Ig showed a staining pattern of cells reminiscent of that obtained with anti-Ia mAb which stained B cells and macrophages. The latter became demonstable with anti-Ig, since IgG is known to attach nonspecifically to the Fc receptors, present in increased numbers on activated macrophages. In addition, IgG precipitates could be demonstrated throughout the lesion.

Thus, in acute MS, large numbers of $T11^+$, $T4^+$, $T8^+$, $TQ1^+$ and Ia^+ cells were randomly distributed throughout the lesion. Infiltrating cells displayed the highest density in the lesion center, decreased in numbers towards the lesion edge and were virtually absent from normal white matter. By immunocytochemistry, a relatively sharp outline of acute MS lesions was seen which differed significantly from the classical diffuse lesion margin of H+E stained sections.

Active Chronic MS Lesions

In H+E sections, active chronic MS lesions are characterized by a sharply demarcated edge with a variable intensity of inflammation, consisting of lymphocytes,

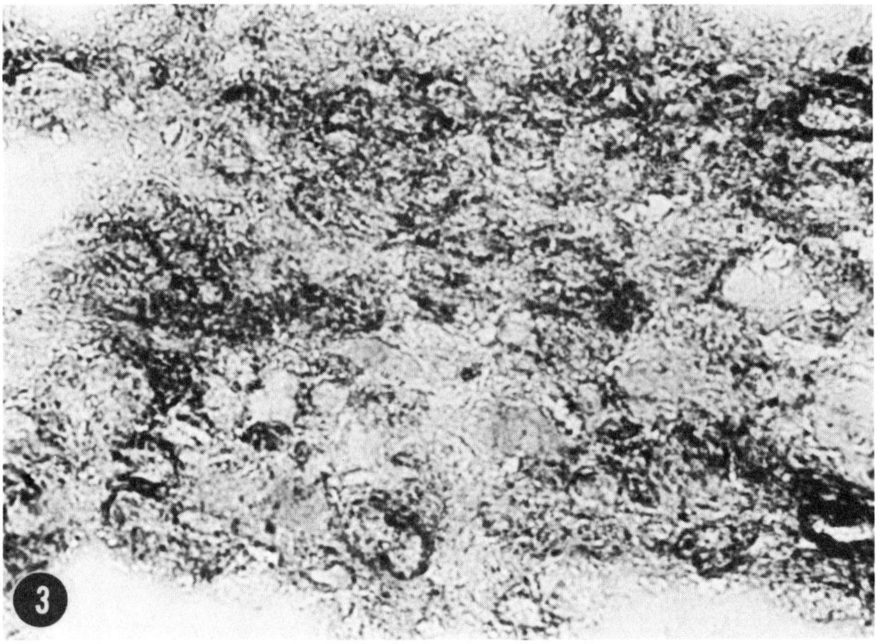

FIGURE 3. Acute MS: center of lesion stained with anti-Ia. Large numbers of Ia-positive macrophages are seen ($\times 640$).

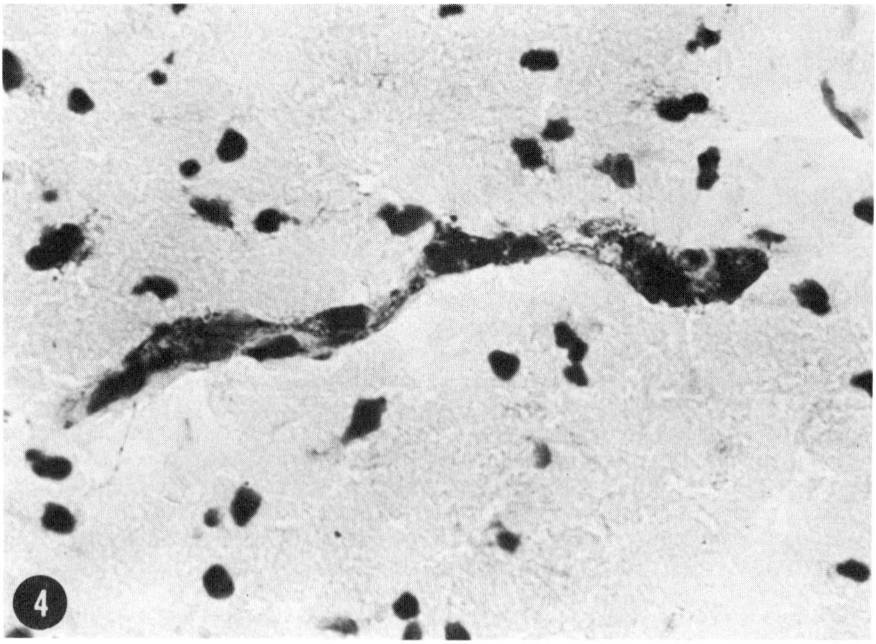

FIGURE 4. Acute MS: lesion edge stained with anti-Ia. Some Ia^+ macrophages are seen adjacent to Ia^+ endothelial cells ($\times 640$).

macrophages and some plasma cells. The old lesion center, made up of a dense astrocytic scar tissue, is largely depleted of myelin and oligodendrocytes whereas many axons are spared. Some foamy cells are frequently present in the old lesion center. However, in more recent and active lesions, foamy cells containing myelin debris are numerous in or close to the lesion center. Between these latter two extremes of lesion activity, the active chronic MS lesion covers a large spectrum of pathologic changes, ranging from a mildly active plaque made up of astrocytic scar tissue at the center, and a narrow zone of some hypercellularity consisting mainly of foamy cells at the edge, to the highly active areas. In the latter, tightly packed, myelin debris-laden macrophages predominate in the lesion center and dense mononuclear infiltrates are detectable at the lesion edge. According to these differences in lesion activity, the immunocytochemical findings varied greatly from lesion to lesion. A variability in activity could also be seen within a single plaque, indicating that lesion progression does not always radiate uniformly but might be restricted to certain areas.

The immunocytochemical changes described herein are those of a very active chronic MS lesion with a broad zone of inflammatory cells at the sharply demarcated lesion edge (FIG. 5). In the lesion center, $T11^+$ cells (pan T cells) were found only in small numbers but macrophages were numerous. The density of $T11^+$ cells increased continuously from the center towards the edge of the lesion where they reached their highest numbers and were found both in the parenchyma and in perivascular areas (FIG. 6). Moderate numbers of $T11^+$ cells were also detectable in the normal-appearing white matter adjacent to the lesion. $T4^+$ cells (helper/inducer T cells) showed a distribution pattern similar to that of $T11^+$ cells. They were least numerous in the center and showed increasing numbers towards the edge of the lesion, from where they also extended in considerable numbers deeply into the adjacent normal-appearing white matter. In contrast to the uniform presence of $T11^+$ cells, $T4^+$ cells showed a marked predilection for the white matter parenchyma (FIG. 7). The observed large size of $T4^+$ cells might be suggestive of recent blastogenic transformation. In addition, Ia antigen was demonstrable on some $T4^+$ cells, indicating activation. $T8^+$ cells also showed a lower density in the center of the plaque and the highest numbers at the edge of the lesion and in a narrow zone of the adjacent normal-appearing white matter (FIG. 8). In contrast to $T4^+$ cells, which were predominantly localized within the parenchyma, $T8^+$ cells showed a predilection for perivascular cuffs. Whereas in the present acute MS case no inflammatory cells could be detected within the normal CNS parenchyma, small numbers of T cells and T cell subsets were present within the normal white and gray matter parenchyma close by and remote from active chronic lesions. A few Leu 7^+ cells (NK and K cells) and $TQ1^+$ cells (cytotoxic $T4^+$ cells) were found at the edge of active chronic MS lesions and were rare within the lesion proper and in the normal white matter.

The distribution pattern of Ia^+ cells was the reverse of that of T cells, in that they were most numerous in the lesion center and decreased consistently towards the lesion edge. Most Ia^+ cells in active chronic MS lesions were macrophages, as seen in counterstained sections (FIG. 9). In the lesion center, Ia^+ macrophages frequently showed a vacuolated cytoplasm reminiscent of foamy cells. Nearer the lesion edge, the cytoplasm of macrophages stained more homogeneously and the cells were sometimes tightly packed within perivascular areas with only a few Ia^+ cells in the adjacent white matter parenchyma. These dense perivascular infiltrates might have represented monocytes that have just entered the CNS.

At the lesion edge, and less frequently within normal white and gray matter parenchyma, Ia antigen could occasionally be found on endothelial cells, similar to acute MS lesions. Interestingly, not all but only selected Ia^+ endothelial cells along some vessels could be detected throughout the gray and white matter parenchyma.

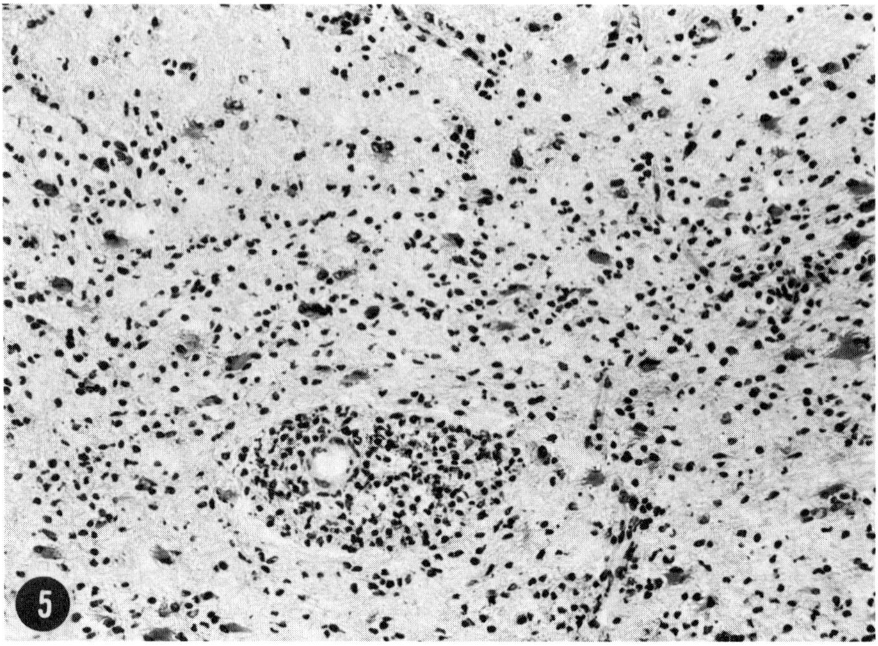

FIGURE 5. Active chronic MS, H + E: sharply demarcated lesion edge with dense parenchymal and perivascular infiltrates. Some hypertrophic astrocytes can also be seen (×160).

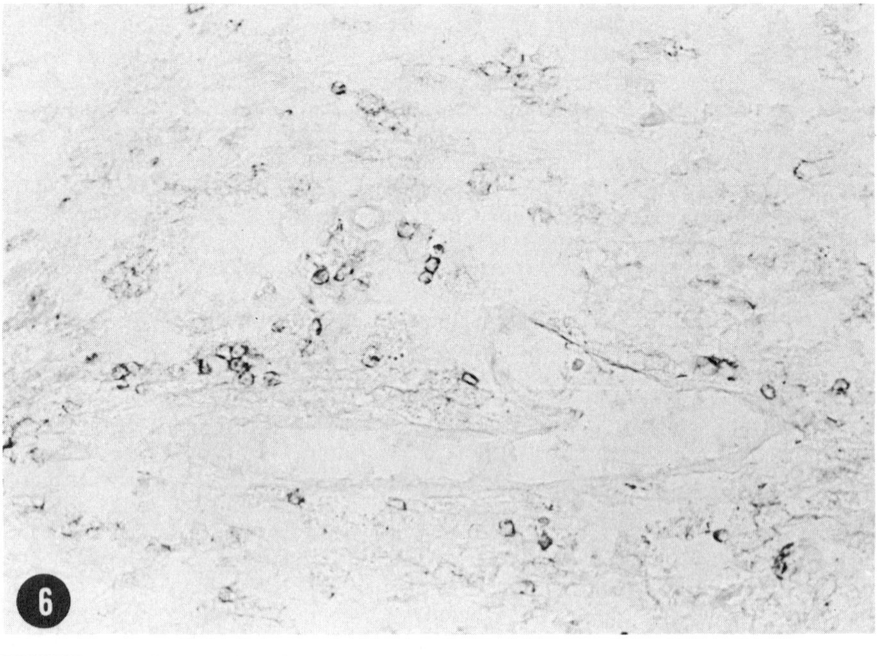

FIGURE 6. Active chronic MS: lesion edge stained with anti-T11. Pan T cells are present in a perivascular area and in the parenchyma (×260).

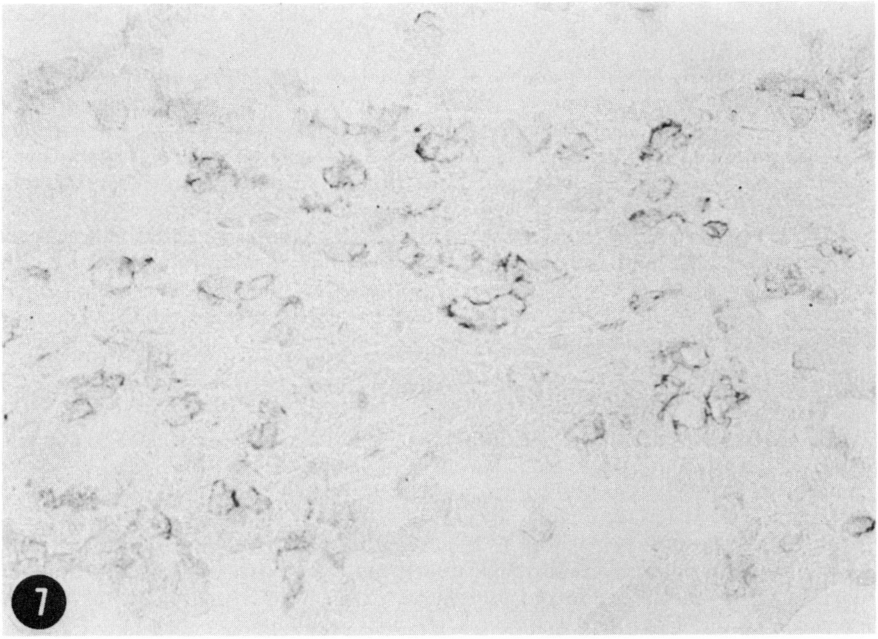

FIGURE 7. Active chronic MS: normal white matter adjacent to lesion edge, stained with anti-T4. Helper/inducer T cells are detectable (×400).

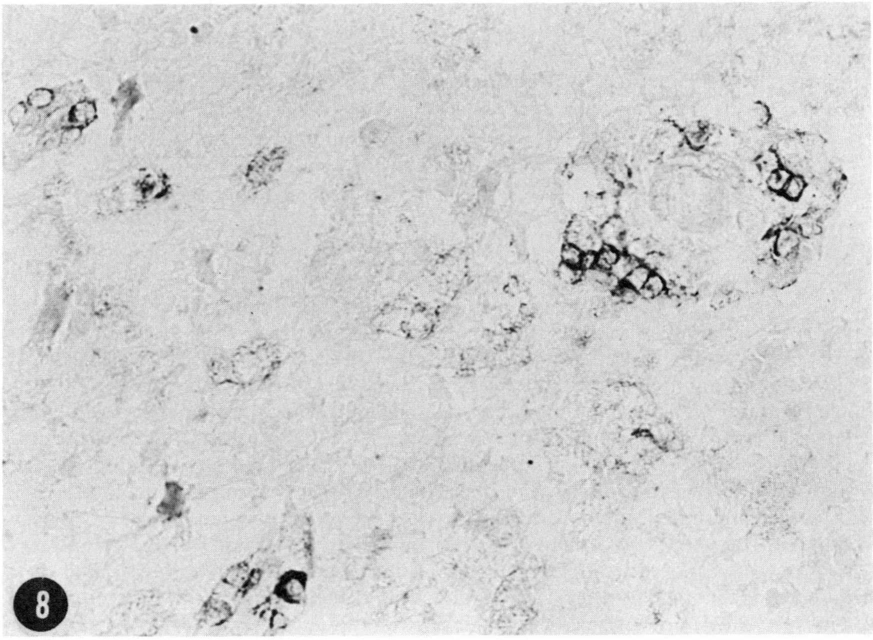

FIGURE 8. Active chronic MS: lesion edge stained with anti-T8. Suppressor/cytotoxic T cells are found in perivascular cuffs (×400).

Similar to acute MS, the presence of Ia^+ endothelial cells in the lesion center could not be established with certainty because of the density of the infiltrates and the frequent close association between Ia^+ macrophages and endothelial cells. Throughout active chronic MS lesions, close contact between Ia^+ macrophages and lymphocytes could be detected in counterstained material. In serial sections, some of these could be demonstrated to be $T4^+$ or $T8^+$ cells. This close association between T cells and accessory cells of the immune system (Ia^+ macrophages) might be indicative of antigen presentation and/or cell-to-cell interaction. The distribution pattern of B cells and Ig-containing macrophages, as seen by staining with anti-Ig antibody, was similar to that of Ia^+ cells. In addition, Ig deposits that showed some higher density at the lesion edge could be demonstrated.

Silent Chronic MS Lesions

In contrast to active MS plaques, silent chronic MS lesions lack significant hypercellularity but display a center containing astrocytic scar tissue and a sharply demarcated edge. However, a few lipid-laden macrophages can also be found without being indicative of active disease.

Small numbers of $T11^+$ and $T4^+$ cells could be demonstrated within this type of lesion, as well as within normal CNS parenchyma. Whereas some $T8^+$ cells could be detected in the normal white and gray matter, they were virtually absent from the lesion center. Similar to active chronic MS lesions, small numbers of $T11^+$, $T4^+$, $T8^+$ cells and Ia^+ macrophages could be seen throughout the CNS but Ia^+ endothelial cells were rare. $TQ1^+$ cells (cytotoxic $T4^+$ cells) were rarely found in silent chronic lesions and Leu 7^+ cells (NK and K cells) showed sometimes a focus-like accumulation in normal white matter. Ia^+ macrophages were found less frequently in silent than in active chronic MS lesions. The denisty of infiltrates was usually low in the lesion center and some accumulation could occasionally be found at the lesion edge (FIG. 10). The majority of the foamy cells within silent chronic MS lesions was Ia-negative and the frequency of Ia positivity increased somewhat towards the lesion edge.

Some Ig deposits could be demonstrated throughout the lesion and Ig was detectable on most macrophages.

DISCUSSION

The pathology of MS lesions has been studied in detail by routine morphology.[12,29,30] The predominantly mononuclear infiltrates and the close similarity of pathologic changes between active MS lesions and lesions in EAE[12] support the concept of autoimmune mechanisms. This aspect was further underlined by immunologic studies on circulating factors that have revealed sensitization of the cellular and humoral immune system against myelin antigens.[9,10,13–28] However, the relevance of the immunologic abnormalities in the blood and CSF for lesion activity has not yet been established. The insight into pathogenesis obtained from routine morphologic evaluation of CNS tissue is limited. More information on the immunopathologic mechanisms leading to tissue destruction at the level of the target organ, the CNS, might be provided by a more detailed analysis of inflammatory cells within lesions using immunocytochemical methods. The results might yield a montage of immunopathologic events during lesion formation in MS and in the future, might provide a rationale for a highly selective therapeutic manipulation of the immune system to arrest the disease process.

Previous immunocytochemical studies have focused mainly on the localization of IgG and plasma cells within MS lesions.[31–33] Investigations on T cells, the effector cells

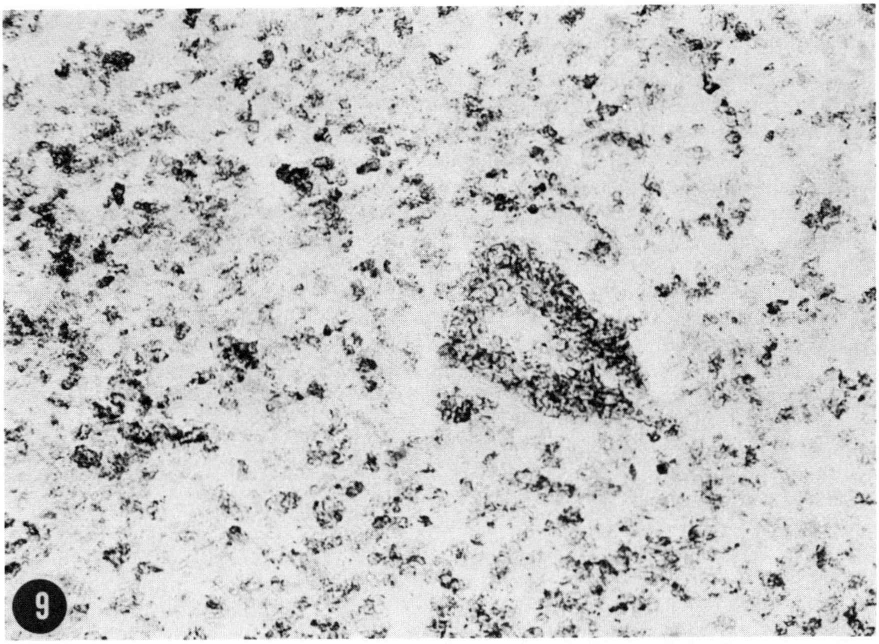

FIGURE 9. Active chronic MS: lesion center stained with anti-Ia. Dense infiltrates of large Ia^+ cells can be seen in the parenchyma and perivascular cuffs ($\times 260$).

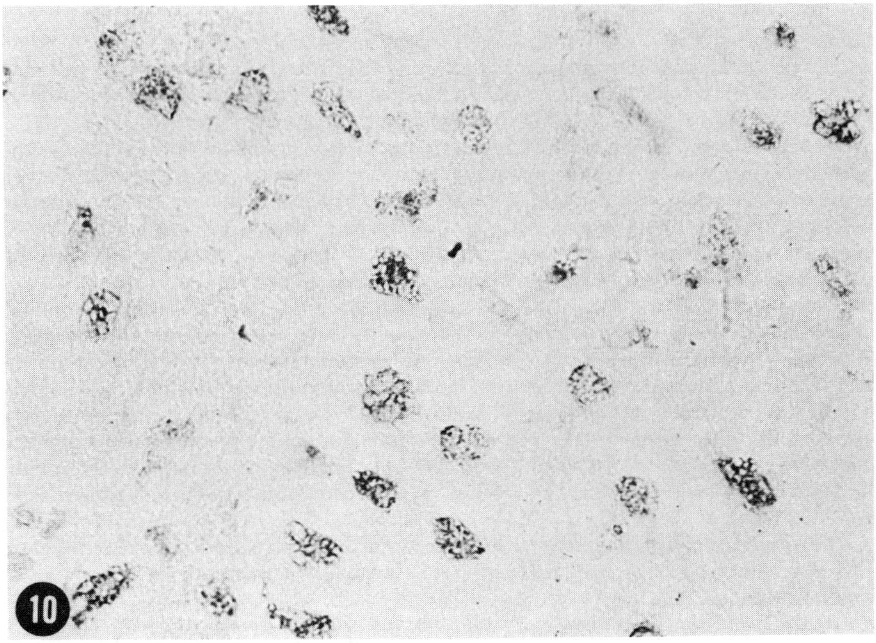

FIGURE 10. Silent chronic MS: lesion edge stained with anti-Ia. Some Ia^+ foamy cells are seen at the lesion edge ($\times 400$).

of the cell-mediated immune system, are rare.[34,35,38,43,44] This has mainly been due to the unavailability of highly specific markers suitable for application *in situ*. In one study, in which a heterologous antiserum against T cells was used on MS and SSPE material, T cells were reported to be present mainly in perivascular cuffs and rare in the parenchyma.[35] The application of rosette formation for the localization of T cells *in situ*, a less sophisticated technique, only allowed a general statement on the presence or absence of this cell type and did not facilitate a detailed morphologic evaluation and recognition of individual T cells.[34]

Studies on the localization of lymphocyte subsets within the human CNS are scarce but some basic work has been performed on EAE lesions in the guinea pig[45–47] and in the mouse.[48] In CNS lesions from guinea pigs, T and B cells were labeled by monoclonal and conventional antibodies, respectively, in combination with indirect immunofluorescence. In acute EAE, T cells were found to be the first inflammatory cells to appear within the CNS and to be localized mainly within the parenchyma. B cells and Ig-containing macrophages became demonstrable later and showed a predilection for meninges and perivascular cuffs. In chronic EAE lesions, a similar distribution pattern of T and B cells was detectable and relapses were accompanied by an increase in the density of T cell infiltrates within the parenchyma. These observations supported the previously described importance of T cells for the induction of EAE.[49]

In CNS lesions of mice with acute EAE, T cells, in particular Lyt 1^+ cells which are functionally equivalent to $T4^+$ cells, were found to outnumber B cells. Lyt 1^+ cells were mainly localized in meninges and perivascular cuffs and were rare in the parenchyma.[48]

These preliminary data encouraged similar investigations on MS lesions. For this, pan T cells ($T11^+$), T cell subsets, Ia^+ cells and Ig-bearing cells were localized in MS lesions of various ages using monoclonal and conventional antibodies in combination with the PAP and ABC technique. It was found that lesion progression in MS seemed to be associated with infiltrates of $T4^+$ cells, whereas active myelin breakdown depended upon the presence of Ia^+ macrophages.[38,41,42]

Whereas in one of our cases of acute MS only acute lesions were found by routine pathology, in the other, both acute and active chronic lesions were detectable. When analyzed by immunocytochemistry, each of the lesions displayed the distribution pattern of inflammatory cells described above. The observed random presence of all types of inflammatory cells throughout acute MS lesions is reminiscent of the distribution of infiltrating cells described in SSPE brain[50] and in skin lesions of lepromatous leprosy.[51] In the latter, the lack of a distinct organization of hematogenous cells has been suggested to reflect the incapability of a defective immune system to eliminate successfully the infectious agent (mycobacterium leprae). This defect seemed to be closely associated with the presence of undifferentiated macrophages. In SSPE, measles virus is known to persist within the CNS, leading to continuously elevated antibody titers. In the event that similar immunopathologic mechanisms are operative in MS, the persistent immunogen might not be an infectious agent but might be an endogeneous myelin antigen, such as myelin basic protein (MBP) or galactocerebroside (GC).

The absence of inflammatory cells from normal-appearing white matter in acute MS is in sharp contrast to their ubiquitous detectability in normal white and gray matter in chronic MS.

The distinct distribution pattern of infiltrating cells in active chronic MS lesions, in which T cells were most numerous at the edge of the lesion and in the adjacent normal white matter, and where Ia^+ macrophages predominated in the lesion center, is in sharp contrast to the findings on acute MS. The presence of considerable numbers of lymphocytes, $T4^+$ cells in particular, in the normal white matter close to an actively growing lesion could not have been established with certainty by routine pathologic evaluations because of the close morphologic similarities between glial elements such as oligodendrocytes and lymphocytes. $T4^+$ cells are known to be essential in the development of an immune response, interacting with both antigen-presenting cells (Ia^+ macrophages) and the various types of effector cells. Therefore, the detectability of considerable numbers of $T4^+$ cells in the white matter adjacent to an active lesion might imply an essential role of this T cell subset for lesion progression. This would also be supported by the presence of Ia antigen on some $T4^+$ cells, indicating activation of these cells (own observation), by the relatively large size of $T4^+$ cells, suggestive of blastogenic transformation, and by the presence of activated $T4^+$ cells within the CSF during exacerbations.[26]

Furthermore, $T4^+$ cells might also be operative at the level of the humoral immune response, enhancing antibody production by plasma cells. The low density of Leu 7^+ and $TQ1^+$ infiltrates in active chronic MS suggests no major importance of these cell types for the pathogenetic mechanisms in this type of lesion. Whether $TQ1^+$ cells might be essential for the development of acute MS lesions, in which they were found in large numbers (see above), has yet to be established. A larger spectrum of monoclonal antibodies will have to be applied to obtain more information on the relevance of cytotoxic T cells for lesion development in MS. The distribution of $T8^+$ cells, which appeared as a ring-like infiltrate along the lesion edge extending only slightly into the adjacent normal white matter, might reflect the attempt of $T8^+$ cells to limit lesion progression, perhaps by the release of a suppressor factor. It might also be indicative of a reduced migratory ability of $T8^+$ in comparison to $T4^+$ cells. A more detailed analysis in regard to the immunologic function of $T8^+$ cells is not possible to date because the T8 differentiation antigen is detectable on two functionally quite distinct T cell subsets, namely suppressor and cytotoxic T cells. The vacuolated cytoplasm of the majority of macrophages in the center of active chronic MS lesions indicated their long-lasting involvement in myelin breakdown. That immune-pathogenetic mechanisms were involved in demyelination was suggested by the presence of Ia antigen on most macrophages, which acted as effector cells. The increasing frequency of homogeneously staining large Ia-positive cells closer to the lesion edge might be suggestive of a more recent disease process, at which time not all macrophages have yet taken up and degraded myelin. The hematogenous origin of macrophages in MS lesions might be assumed from the tightly packed perivascular infiltrates of homogeneously staining macrophages at the lesion edge that were accompanied by only a few Ia^+ cells in the parenchyma.

As an early event during lesion development, the presentation of specific antigen to T cells in conjunction with Ia antigen is required to trigger a cell-mediated immune response. Though Ia^+ macrophages are known to be accessory cells of the immune system, they might not be essential for lesion initiation in MS since they are inaccessible to circulating lymphocytes. Thus, another cell type might be involved in antigen presentation in the CNS. As an interesting alternative for the latter, the recently reported presence and the inducibility of Ia antigen on endothelial cells by short contact with sensitized lymphocytes might be suggested.[54] In MS lesions, Ia antigen could only be detected on some endothelial cells. The higher frequency of Ia^+ endothelial cells in acute and active chronic MS, rather than in silent chronic MS lesions, parallels the degree of disease activity and supports the possible importance of Ia^+ endothelial cells for antigen presentation and lesion activity. The detectability of MBP and GC on endothelial cells of MS brain sections (own unpublished observation) is of interest in this regard. However, Ia and myelin antigen will have to be demonstrated simultaneously to allow the conclusion that antigen is presented on endothelial cells. Furthermore, the observed close contact between lymphocytes and Ia^+ macrophages in tissue from acute and active chronic MS might represent the morphologic equivalent *in situ* of cell-to-cell interactions required, according to *in vitro* studies, for the development of an immune response.

In the CNS tissue from one case of silent chronic MS, no (or only mild) hypercellularity was seen by routine morphology, and this consisted mainly of lipid-laden macrophages, whereas lymphocytes could not be detected. However, using immunocytochemical techniques, small numbers of lymphocytes could be demonstrated in the lesion area and normal CNS parenchyma. This observation underlines the necessity to apply highly sensitive methods for the analysis of pathologic changes for more detailed information. According to the present classification of MS lesions, the presence of inflammatory cells, in particular of lymphocytes, would be indicative of an active lesion activity. This observed discrepancy regarding the demonstrability of lymphocytes by routine pathology and by immunocytochemistry might require a reevaluation of the present lesion classification, concentrating more on the density of inflammation than on the presence of lymphocytes. The detectability of T cells and macrophages in normal MS tissue might be related to the chronicity of the disease process and might be essential for the development of new lesions but does not seem to be indicative of active disease.

Although the insult leading to the initial destruction of CNS white matter in MS remains unknown, later events during lesion formation might be reconstructed from the present study (and some additional speculations) as follows. Activated lymphocytes come in contact early on with some endothelial cells in the CNS and this exposure might trigger the expression of Ia antigen on endothelial cells. Should a myelin antigen, such as MBP or GC, be present simultaneously with the Ia antigen, the requirements for antigen presentation to T cells are given and a local immune response might be initiated. After a change in vascular permeability, T cells, in particular $T4^+$ cells, might then invade the white matter parenchyma in large numbers and recruit nonantigen-specific T cells. Contact of $T4^+$ cells with the appropriate antigen leads to blastogenic transformation and release of lymphokines. Possibly attracted by lymphokines, numerous activated macrophages displaying enhanced phagocytic activity appear within the normal white matter. Macrophages attack the myelin directly, leading to stripping of myelin lamellae, or induce demyelination by soluble products. As the lesion progresses, $T4^+$ cells continue to infiltrate the adjacent normal-appearing white matter in large numbers, whereas $T8^+$ cells remain, at least temporarily, localized at the lesion edge. This again is followed by increasing numbers of Ia-positive macrophages and demyelination. As lesion activity subsides, the numbers of infiltrating T cells and macrophages decrease and only a few inflammatory cells and Ia-positive endothelial cells persist throughout the lesion area and the normal white matter parenchyma, providing an essential requirement for further lesion development and progression of the disease. Further studies in combination with more specific markers will be required before more precise functional implication can be inferred.

ACKNOWLEDGMENT

We thank Drs. Labe C. Scheinberg, Murray B. Bornstein, James M. Powers, John W. Prineas and Dikran S. Horoupian for providing brain tissue, Dr. Ellis L. Reinherz for providing monoclonal antibodies, Patricia Kennedy for technical expertise and Nanci E. Legg for secretarial assistance.

REFERENCES

1. McAlpine, D., C. E. Lumdsen & E. D. Acheson. 1972. *In* Multiple Sclerosis: A Reappraisal. Williams and Wilkins. Baltimore.
2. Hallpike, J. F. 1983. Clinical aspects of multiple sclerosis. *In* Multiple Sclerosis. Pathology, Disease and Management. J. F. Hallpike, C. W. M. Adams & W. W. Tourtellotte, Eds.: 129–162. Williams and Wilkins. Baltimore.
3. Kurtzke, J. F. 1970. Clinical manifestations of multiple sclerosis. *In* Handbook of Clinical Neurology, vol. 9. P. J. Vinken & G. W. Bruyn, Eds.: 161–216. North-Holland. Amsterdam.
4. Poskanzer, D. & R. D. Adams. 1974. Multiple sclerosis and the demyelinating diseases. *In* Harrison's Principles of Internal Medicine. McGraw-Hill. New York. pp. 1815–1821.
5. Johnson, R. T. 1975. Adv. Neurol. **13:** 1–46.
6. Cook, S. D. & P. C. Dowling. 1980. Neurology **30**(2): 80–91
7. Cremer, N. E., K. P. Johnson, G. Fein & W. H. Litosky. 1980. Arch. Neurol. **37:** 610–615.
8. Norrby, E. 1978. Prog. Med. Virol. **24:** 1–39.
9. Leibowitz, S. 1983. The immunology of multiple sclerosis. *In* Multiple Sclerosis: Pathology, Disease and Management. J. F. Hallpike, C. W. M. Adams & W. W. Tourtellotte, Eds.: 379–412. Williams and Wilkins. Baltimore.
10. McFarlin, D. E. & H. F. McFarland. 1982. N. Engl. J. Med. **307:** 1183–1188, 1246–1251.
11. Raine, C. S. & S. H. Stone. 1977. N.Y. State J. Med. **77**(11): 1693–1695.
12. Raine, C. S. 1976. Experimental allergic encephalomyelitis and related conditions. *In* Progress in Neuropathology, vol. 3. H. M. Zimmerman, Ed.: 225–251. Grune and Stratton. New York.
13. Johnson, K. P. 1980. Neurology **30:** 106–109.
14. Tourtellotte, W. W. 1970. Cerebrospinal fluid in multiple sclerosis. *In* Handbook of Clinical Neurology, vol. 9. P. J. Vinken & G. W. Bruyn, Eds.: 324–382. North-Holland. Amsterdam.
15. Casey, B. R., S. T. Wong, A. J. Mason, R. Lee & H. C. Ford. 1981. Clin. Chim. Acta **114:** 187–194.
16. Link, H. & M. A. Laurenzi. 1979. Ann. Neurol. **6:** 107–110.
17. Lisak, R. P. 1980. Neurology **30:** 99–105.
18. Waksman, B. H. 1981. Immunol. Today **2:** 87–93.
19. Sheremata, W., D. D. Wood, A. A. Moscarello & J. B. R. Cosgrove. 1978. J. Neurol. Sci. **37:** 165–170.
20. Kennedy, P. G. E. & R. P. Lisak. 1979. J. Neurol. Sci. **44:** 125–133.
21. Panitch, H. S., C. J. Hooper & K. P. Johnson. 1980. Arch. Neurol. **37:** 206–209.
22. Traugott, U., D. S. Snyder & C. S. Raine. 1979. Ann. Neurol. **6:** 13–20.
23. Huddlestone, J. R. & M. B. A. Oldstone. 1979. J. Immunol. **123:** 1615–1618.
24. Reinherz, E. L., H. L. Weiner, S. L. Hauser, J. A. Cohen, J. A. Distaso & S. F. Schlossman. 1980. N. Engl. J. Med. **303:** 125–129.
25. Cashman, N., M.-A. Bach, C. Martin, J.-D. Degos & J. F. Bach. 1982. Neurology **32**(Part 2): A69.
26. Noronha, A. B. C., D. P. Richman & B. G. W. Arnason. 1980. N. Engl. J. Med. **303:** 713–717.
27. Merrill, J., M. Jondal, J. Seelen, M. Ullberg & A. Siden. 1982. Clin. Exp. Neurol. **47:** 419–430.
28. Neighbour, A. P., A. E. Miller & B. R. Bloom. 1981. Neurology **31:** 561–566.
29. Adams, C. W. M. 1975. J. Neurol. Sci. **25:** 165–182.
30. Greenfield, J. G. & R. M. Norman. 1971. Demyelinating diseases. *In* Greenfield's Neuropathology. W. Blackwood, W. H. McMenemey, A. Meyer, R. M. Norman & D. S. Russell, Eds.: 475–519. Arnold. London.
31. Esiri, M. J. 1980. Neuropathol. Appl. Neurology **6:** 9–21.
32. Prineas, J. W. & C. S. Raine. 1976. Neurology **6:** 29–32.

33. PRINEAS, J. W. & R. G. WRIGHT. 1978. Lab. Invest. **38:** 409–421.
34. NYLAND, H., S. MÖRK & R. MATRE. 1982. Neuropathol. Appl. Neurobiol. **8:** 403–411.
35. KRETH, H. W., R. DUNGER, H. RODT & R. MEYERMANN. 1982. J. Neuroimmunol. **2**(2): 177–183.
36. REINHERZ, E. L. & S. F. SCHLOSSMAN. 1980. Cell **19:** 821–827.
37. MEUER, S. C., S. F. SCHLOSSMAN & E. L. REINHERZ. 1982. Proc. Natl. Acad. Sci. U.S.A. **79:** 4395–4399.
38. TRAUGOTT, U., E. L. REINHERZ & C. S. RAINE. 1982. J. Neuroimmunol. **3:** 365–373.
39. STERNBERGER, L. A. 1979. The Unlabeled Antibody Peroxidase Antiperoxidase (PAP) Method. Wiley. New York. pp. 104–159.
40. HSU, S. & L. RAINE. 1981. J. Histochem. Cytochem. **29:** 1349–1353.
41. STERNBERGER, L. A. & S. A. JOSEPH. 1979. J. Histochem. Cytochem. **27:** 1424–1429.
42. SI, L. & T. WHITESIDE. 1983. J. Immunol. **130:** 2149–2155.
43. TRAUGOTT, U., E. L. REINHERZ & C. S. RAINE. 1983. Science **219:** 308–310.
44. TRAUGOTT, U., E. L. REINHERZ & C. S. RAINE. 1983. J. Neuroimmunol. **4:** 201–221.
45. TRAUGOTT, U., E. SHEVACH, J. CHIBA, S. H. STONE & C. S. RAINE. 1981. Science **214:** 1251–1253.
46. TRAUGOTT, U., E. SHEVACH, J. CHIBA, S. H. STONE & C. S. RAINE. 1982. Cell. Immunol. **68:** 261–275.
47. TRAUGOTT, U., E. SHEVACH, J. CHIBA, S. H. STONE & C. S. RAINE. 1982. Cell. Immunol. **70:** 345–356.
48. SRIRAM, S., D. SOLOMON, R. V. ROUSE & L. STEINMAN. 1982. J. Immunol. **129:** 1649–1651.
49. ORTIZ-ORTIZ, L., R. M. NAKAMURA & W. O. WEIGLE. 1976. J. Immunol. **117:** 576–579.
50. TRAUGOTT, U. 1983. Ann. Neurology **14:** 108.
51. MODLIN, R. L., F. M. HOFMAN, P. R. MEYER, O. P. SHARMA, C. R. TAYLOR & T. H. REA. 1983. Clin. Exp. Immunol. **51:** 430.
52. PETTINELLI, C. B. & D. E. MCFARLIN. 1981. J. Immunol. **127:** 1420–1423.
53. BERNARD, C. A. & I. R. MACHAY. 1983. J. Neuroimmunol. **4:** 61–65.
54. BURGER, D. R., D. FORD, R. M. VETTO, A. HAMBLIN, A. GOLDSTEIN, M. HUBBARD & D. C. DUMONDE. 1981. Hum. Immunol. **3:** 209–230.

DISCUSSION OF THE PAPER

J. MERRILL (*Reed Neurological Research Center, Los Angeles, CA*): A recent paper in the *Journal of Immunology* claimed that the T4 antigen may occur in the cytoplasm of normal monocytes or macrophages. I'd like to ask if you could exclude the possibility that any of the T4 positive cells you see in the normal-appearing white matter could be macrophages? Secondly, if you would comment on an observation made by Dr. John Roeder, that the Leu 7 or HNK 1 antibody may detect in myelin associated glycoprotein on the surface of an oligodendrocyte and if you're actually looking at some subset of oligodendrocytes in the normal-appearing white matter?

U. TRAUGOTT (*Albert Einstein College of Medicine, Bronx, NY*): As to whether I am able to determine that some of my T4 positive cells might be monocytes, I've done double labeling studies with anti-Ia and T4 antigen. Some populations do double stain—that could be either monocytes with T4 antigen, or T4 positive cells with Ia antigens which might be activated T4 positive cells and that question for these particular cells can only be determined if we use another marker for monocytes. But I also have a considerable number of T4 positive cells which do not double stain. As to the second question, I have of course stained normal brain with Leu 7 and if one monitors the technique carefully, there is no oligodendrocyte staining. I do have more background staining of myelin than with the other monoclonal antibodies. I also must say that T4 is a rather difficult monoclonal antibody because again, one has to be very careful to get clean staining.

D. E. McFarlin (*NINCDS, Bethesda, MD*): Before we enter the general discussion, I have given Dr. Weiner permission to present a couple of slides dealing with the subject we just heard from Dr. Traugott.

H. L. Weiner (*Harvard Medical School, Boston, MA*): We've recently had the opportunity to stain nine brains from patients with multiple sclerosis and one biopsy from an acute MS case that was felt to be a lymphoma. I'd like to share with you very briefly what we found and make one point. The major finding that struck us was the overrepresentation of T8 cells in the brains of these patients. We used identical staining techniques and the same antibodies that Traugott and Raine have used. Perivascular cuffs stained with T8 and showed infiltration of these cells into parenchyma. We didn't find as many T4 cells. In summary, what we found was that in perivascular cuffs, most prominently at the edge of active plaques, T8 positive cells, Ia-positive cells, various numbers of M1 positive cells and various numbers of T4 positive cells were present. But in all instances, the ratio of T8 to T4 was always either equal or there were dramatically increased numbers of T8 cells.

McFarlin: Dr. Traugott, would you like to comment on Dr. Weiner's findings?

Traugott: We have one finding in common and that is an extensive presence of infiltrates of Ia-positive macrophages in the lesion. With regard to the distribution of T4 and T8 positive cells, I know there is a very large variety in active chronic lesions and we had a case recently, the brain of which showed acute lesions, active chronic lesions and Balo-type lesions. If you check both lesions, you have the whole spectrum from acute MS lesions with a diffuse distribution of T8 cells as well as T4 in the parenchyma. If you check my last publication, in acute MS, slightly less T4 than T8 positive cells were in the parenchyma. In the established active chronic lesion with a predominance of T4, one has to classify carefully the lesions neuropathologically. In all our cases, we have performed the appropriate staining by routine pathology to age the lesion. In most cases of MS, one has the whole spectrum of lesion age and activity.

J. W. Prineas (*University of Medicine and Dentistry of New Jersey, Newark*): A comment for Drs. Traugott and Weiner. We are attempting to interpret the significance of the presence of various lymphocyte subsets on the basis of whether we think it's an active plaque or a healed plaque. The fact is that plaques are probably active only for a relatively short time on the basis of the clinical picture. That means that the plaque may be active for a few weeks or a month or two and then begin to resolve and it resolves over a long period and we know that there's lipid in those plaques for a year or two. That means that the majority of MS patients who have shown some clinical activity within a few years have plaques in which one finds lipid breakdown products and these are probably resolving lesions. That means that we should be presented with lymphocyte data for acute plaques, resolving plaques, chronically active plaques and for healed plaques. I think it's significant that both speakers who presented lymphocyte subset data have spoken about the acute plaque, the chronic active plaque, and the healed plaque but they haven't mentioned the most common plaque with myelin debris, the healing or resolving plaque.

J. Oger (*Vancouver, BC*): I want to congratulate Dr. Traugott for this nice work. I have two comments—one, that the reagents sold by some of the companies are called orthoclone and none of them pretends to be one clone. It should be known that there are at least three or four clones which have been called OKT-8 and the original description of the T suppressor cell count abnormality was done with OKT-5, a clone definitely different from OKT-8. Most of the time those monoclonal antibodies need to be titrated before being used and I have not heard any comments yet on how they are titrated. Those differences could explain some of the results which are still difficult to interpret, like the presence of OKT-8 on oligodendrocytes of ovine origin. The final comment would be also to really calculate, to try to have access to numbers in terms of the affinity of those monoclonal antibodies. We have done some preliminary experiments on that and very surprisingly the affinity of some of those commercially available monoclonal antibodies is far below what we would expect in terms of K binding.

D. HAFFORD (*Harvard University, Boston, MA*): Do you have a sense of what percent of the T4 positive cells are TQ1 positive? How many T4 class 2 restricted cells are in the parenchyma?

TRAUGOTT: I have not done any double labeling studies between T4 and TQ1 in brain but I have serial sections stained with T4 and the other one with TQ1 and the percentage of overlap would be about 10%, if at all.

J. BOOSS (*VA Medical Center, West Haven, CT*): We've also addressed the question of the subtype predominance in parenchyma and work done with Dr. Esiri of Oxford, quantitating both controls and patients with chronic noninflammatory neurologic diseases and patients with MS, has shown interesting things. Our findings showed T8 was unequivocally predominant within lesions and in normal-appearing white matter.

G. BIRNBAUM (*University of Minnesota, Minneapolis, MN*): Dr. Arnason suggested perhaps there is some antigenic sharing between CNS and circulating lymphocytes. I was wondering if there was any information as to the possibility of inducing a disease like chronic EAE after having injected animals with circulating lymphocytes?

TRAUGOTT: No.

A. VANDENBARK (*Portland VA Hospital, Portland, ORE*): This is directed to Dr. Traugott. I'm particularly interested in your observations about the Ia-positive endothelial cells that are in the region bordering the plaques. I wanted to ask if you'd seen in the center of any of the plaques whether the endothelial cells are Ia-positive and if not could you comment on the general condition of the endothelial cells at that point?

TRAUGOTT: The impression I have was that the presence of Ia-positive endothelials correlated somewhat with disease activity. The more active the disease, the higher the frequency and in those lesions, Ia-positive macrophages are so tightly-packed and in such close contact with the endothelial cells that I cannot be sure whether the endothelial cells are actually Ia-positive. At the lesion edge, where there are less Ia-positive macrophages as I have shown here, there are sometimes isolated Ia-positive endothelial cells and they are also detectable in normal white matter.

Studies of Interferon Production and Natural Killing by Lymphocytes from Multiple Sclerosis Patients

P. ANDREW NEIGHBOUR

Central Research and Development Department
E. I. du Pont de Nemours
Glenolden Laboratory
Glenolden, Pennsylvania 19036

INTRODUCTION

The immunological basis of multiple sclerosis (MS) has intrigued investigators for many years.[1] It is currently more or less accepted, but not yet proved, that an aberrant immune response might serve as an underlying primary factor responsible for the etiology or the pathogenesis of this chronic degenerative disease. Because of this suspicion, investigators have subjected peripheral blood mononuclear cells (PBMC) from MS patients to a plethora of immunological assays *in vitro*. As each new immunological phenomenon is described for healthy humans or experimental animals, it becomes applied to a group of MS patients for comparison with normal or other neurologically diseased individuals as controls. Over the past five years, one of the vogues in immunology has been the idea of nonspecific immunity. Numerous studies have been reported of nonspecific regulation (suppression or augmentation) and cytotoxicity mediated by MS patients' cells *in vitro*. In this review, I will describe and update some of the studies that have focused on two such nonspecific immune responses, namely interferon production and natural killer cell activity.

THE INTERFERON-NK CELL SYSTEM

Mononuclear leukocytes stimulated with viruses, antigens, mitogens and natural or synthetic double-stranded polynucleotides produce a variety of interferons.[2] Recent advances of molecular genetics have indicated that the interferons represent a complex family of molecular subspecies with distinct serological and chemical properties. The types of interferon produced in any given situation are determined by the nature of the interferon-inducing stimulus and the target cell being stimulated. Initially, interferons were described by their ability to induce an antiviral state in cells, thereby rendering them resistant to subsequent virus infection. Thus, for many years, it was believed that the sole physiological role of these molecules was to confer resistance to, and promote recovery from, virus infections. However, interferons were observed more recently to be capable of inducing numerous other changes of cell function.[3] Interferons have been shown to alter immune responses both positively and negatively. Now it is generally accepted that these molecules, which are members of a larger family of soluble biological response modifiers, function as regulators of both physiological (*e.g.*, fever inducing) and immunological processes.

One such immune function known to be regulated by interferons is that of the so-called natural killer (NK) cell. Natural killing is a term used to describe the spontaneous cytotoxicity of certain target cells that occurs without need for prior sensitization and is genetically unrestricted. This cytotoxicity is mediated by a heterogeneous population of effector cells that, to this day, remains only partially defined. Analysis of the effector cells involved in NK has so far failed to identify a unique phenotype shared only by NK effectors. Human NK cells appear to be contained within a population of lymphocyte-like cells with a large granular morphology and to be generally lacking in conventional T or B cell characteristics. A wide range of different cell types can serve as targets for NK, at least *in vitro*. Tumor cells from the same or different individual or species, certain virus-infected cells, and even some relatively undifferentiated hemopoietic cells can be spontaneously lysed by NK cells.

The relationship that exists between NK and the interferons has been established by numerous *in vivo* and *in vitro* experiments.[5] Whereas the short-term killing of NK-susceptible target cells by fresh PBMC (referred to here as endogenous NK) appears to be independent of interferons,[6] preincubation of effector cells with interferons or with interferon-inducing agents produces a significant and reproducible increase in cytolytic activity (augmented NK). Furthermore, interferons appear to be secreted by the PBMC following interaction with appropriate target cells.[7] However, though the interferon-producing cell in this instance is phenotypically indistinguishable from the cytotoxic NK cell, it has not yet been determined whether these two functions are mediated by the same cell.

The increase in cytolytic activity that results from interferon stimulation appears to be due to both the recruitment of previously nonfunctional NK cells and to the potentiation of cytolytic activity above the endogenous level.[8] This is seen as a shortening of the recycling time exhibited by each individual effector cell between lytic events. In addition, interferons can alter the expression of cell-surface components,[3] and so may alter the ability of the NK cells to recognize and bind via receptors to target cells.

The physiological role of this interferon-NK system has not been fully revealed despite intensive investigation in this area in recent years. Clearly, both interferons and NK can exert antiviral activities, and convincing data has been provided supporting the notion that NK cells play a significant role for certain mouse strains in resistance to, and recovery from, mouse cytomegalovirus infection.[9] Ablation of the interferon-NK system with specific anti-interferon or anti-NK cell antibodies has lent support to the hypothesis that it functions as a fundamental mechanism of immune surveillance against tumors and invading microorganisms.[4] However, there are numerous experimental exceptions that contradict this hypothesis. Furthermore, NK cells appear to be subject to regulation by several other biological response modifiers, such as interleukin-2,[10] suggesting that the interrelationship between the interferons and NK is not unique.

INTERFERON PRODUCTION BY MS PATIENTS

Several years ago, we described the observation that PBMC that had been stimulated with inactivated measles virus were capable of nonspecifically suppressing the mitogen responses of autochthonous responder lymphocytes.[11] Studies of 24 patients with either acute remitting or chronic progressive MS showed a significant decrease in their ability to exhibit this phenomenon. Additional experiments using cells from normal donors revealed that non-T, non-B null cells were the suppressive effector cells, and that acid stable alpha interferons (IFN-α) released into the culture supernates were implicated as the soluble mediators of this suppression.

When the culture supernates obtained from measles-stimulated PBMC from MS patients were titrated for interferon, they were found to contain significantly reduced antiviral activity.[11] In a larger study, we found that PBMC from 30% of MS patients tested *in vitro* produced significantly decreased levels of IFN-α when stimulated with measles, Newcastle disease virus or poly I:C.[12] Furthermore, gamma interferon (IFN-γ) production in response to concanavalin A stimulation was also significantly reduced in these patients. The observed defects were apparently unrelated to the severity or stage of disease.

Numerous studies have since been reported in which interferon production by MS patients' PBMC has been measured (TABLE 1). Although three studies have failed to observe any significant decrease in IFN-α or IFN-γ production *in vitro,*[13–15] reports from at least six other groups have seen these anomalies with a variety of interferon inducers.[16–23] None of these studies reported any significant correlation between the observed defects and clinical disease activity. However, two groups reported that the decreased interferon response resided largely among DRw-2$^+$ individuals,[19,20,23] an HLA antigen with high association for MS.

TABLE 1. Studies of Interferon Production in Multiple Sclerosis

Group	Year	Defective Production		Association with DRw-2	Ref.
		IFN-α	IFN-γ		
Neighbour *et al.*	1979	yes	yes	nd	11
Neighbour *et al.*	1981	yes	yes	nd	12
Benczur *et al.*	1981	yes	nd	no	16
Stoger *et al.*	1982	yes	nd	no	17
Khaletskaia *et al.*	1981	yes	nd	nd	18
Salonen *et al.*	1982	nd	yes	yes	19
Salonen *et al.*	1982	yes	nd	yes	20
Merrill *et al.*	1983	yes	nd	nd	21
Haahr *et al.*	1983	yes	nd	nd	22
Vervliet *et al.*	1983	no	yes	yes	23
Santoli *et al.*	1981	no	no	nd	13
Kaudewitz *et al.*	1983	no	no	no	14
Tovell *et al.*	1983	no	nd	nd	15

nd = not done

NATURAL KILLING BY MS PATIENTS

Because of the relationship between interferon and the NK cell system, we chose to study the NK activity of PBMC from MS patients.[24] Using a conventional 4-hour ^{51}Cr-release assay on K562 target cells, we observed that almost 30% of patients tested showed significantly reduced endogenous NK function. Decreased NK function has also been found by several, but not by all, of the groups studying this phenomenon in MS using a variety of different target cells and assay systems (TABLE 2).[13,14,16,22–31] In most of these studies, the responsiveness of MS patients' NK function to augmentation with exogenous interferons or interferon inducers has also been determined. As a general rule, those studies in which defective endogenous NK was observed also reported reduced augmented NK (TABLE 2). A common finding was that most MS patients responded to the augmenting stimulus, but the level of killing remained below that of augmented NK of normal donors. The majority of these reports also found a significant correlation between diminished NK activity and disease severity.

EXPLANATIONS FOR THESE OBSERVATIONS

After reviewing these varied reports, several fundamental questions arise. First, why are there so many conflicting and discrepant observations? Historically, there have always been conflicts and controversies surrounding *in vitro* studies of the immune response, particularly when these studies have utilized tissues and cells obtained from diseased humans. Indeed, this entire symposium exemplifies the diverse and contradictory nature of such studies in MS. However "definitive" the original report of an immunological aberration in MS, its publication is invariably followed by a multitude of additional "definitive" studies that alternately prove and disprove the original findings. Clearly, much of this is attributable to the heterogeneous nature of this disease. The pool of patients and controls enrolled in a particular study almost certainly varies between separate research centers. Some of the studies reviewed here, for example, observed that disease activity correlated with levels of endogenous and augmented NK.[24,26,30] Therefore, differences in the clinical status of the respective experimental subjects under study might yield conflicting data—no two MS clinics see a similar spectrum of patients. Three of the studies of interferon production found a possible genetic influence controlling this function, with DRw-2^{+} patient and control

TABLE 2. Studies of Natural Killing in MS

		Defects			
			Augmented NK		
Group	Year	Endogenous NK	IFN	IFN Inducers	Ref.
Benczur *et al.*	1980	yes	yes	nd	16
Gyodi *et al.*	1982	yes	yes	nd	25
Hauser *et al.*	1981	yes	nd	nd	26
Neighbour *et al.*	1982	yes	yes	yes	24
Merrill *et al.*	1982	yes	yes	nd	27
Merrill *et al.*	1982	yes	yes	nd	28
Uchida *et al.*	1982	yes	yes	nd	29
McGarry *et al.*	1982	yes	nd	nd	30
Mar	1980	no	nd	nd	31
Santoli *et al.*	1981	no	no	no	13
Kauderwitz *et al.*	1983	no	no	nd	14
Haahr *et al.*	1983	no	no	nd	22
Vervliet *et al.*	1983	no	no	no	23

nd = not done

donors responding less well than DRw-2^{-} individuals.[19,20,23] Although a genetic influence could not be confirmed in one additional study,[14] skewing of the major histocompatibility and associated genes between study populations might account for some of the differences seen in the results reported by different research groups. Finally, data are usually obtained from technically varied assay systems, in which the components of the assay and the methods of data collection and quantitation differ considerably. This variation could exaggerate or, conversely, suppress differences in these phenomena between donors. However, despite these inconsistencies, it appears that the peripheral interferon-NK system of a significant proportion of MS patients functions abnormally, at least *in vitro.*

A second aspect of these investigations, as yet completely unresolved, concerns the underlying basis of the observed defects. Two fundamental explanations have been proposed: (i) the effector cells responsible for these functions have become depleted from the peripheral circulation; or (ii) the effectors are present, but their activity is impaired. There have been a limited number of studies directed at resolving these two questions. The single cell cytolytic assay has enabled determination of the number of potentially active NK cells as well as measurement of their relative potency.[32] Using this method, Merrill *et al.*[27] have shown that many MS patients have reduced numbers of functional NK cells, because the number of cells capable of both binding and killing NK target cells was found to be significantly reduced. However, these results still do not answer the central question. Are the effector cells reduced in number, or is their activity impaired?

Another approach has been to attempt to measure the relative distributions of cells in the blood according to their expression of particular phenotypic markers. However, precise markers that are uniquely characteristic of NK and interferon-producing effector cells have yet to be defined. Depletion experiments have indicated that almost all of the major leukocyte subsets are capable of interferon synthesis when appropriately stimulated. Furthermore, cells that can engage in natural killing appear to express a wide range of overlapping phenotypic characteristics previously described as being typical of other defined subpopulations. For example, NK cells can bind sheep erythrocytes, a marker for T lymphocytes. However, they do not express a pan-T cell specific antigen termed T3. Moreover, the T8 antigen is held to be characteristic of cytotoxic/suppressor T cells. However, some T8^{+}, T3^{-} T cell lines can spontaneously lyse NK-susceptible target cells. NK effectors have been described morphologically as residing in the large granular lymphocyte (LGL) subpopulation. However, Merrill *et al.*[28] showed that the NK activity of PBMC and cerebrospinal fluid lymphocytes from MS patients could not be correlated with the relative numbers of LGL in these tissues. A monoclonal antibody specific for LGL, called HNK-1 or Leu-7, has also been used to enumerate the relative proportions of these cells in normal donors and MS patients.[33] In this study it was reported that a significant proportion of MS patients exhibited reduced numbers of HNK-1 cells in their circulation. Recently, however, we have experienced difficulty in correlating the numbers of HNK-1 or Leu-7 positive cells with NK function in normal donors. Furthermore, some NK activity appears to be mediated by cells that are not recognized by this antibody.[34] Recently, a new antibody called NK-15 or Leu-11, which appears to react with the Fc receptor for Ig on NK cells, has become available.[34] Cell sorting analysis has indicated that the most potent of NK cells reside in a Leu-11^{+}, Leu-7^{-} subpopulation of LGL. For these reasons, we have begun to analyze by flow cytometry the PBMC from MS patients for their reactivity to Leu-11 and other monoclonal lymphocyte subset-specific antibodies. FIGURE 1 shows the preliminary results obtained from the analysis of 24 active MS patients and 12 age-matched normal donor controls for a range of lymphocyte subset markers. As can be seen, there were no significant differences between groups in the relative numbers of PBMC exhibiting T and B cell markers. The mean number of Leu-11$^+$ cells in the MS patient group was lower than that of the normal donor group, but the difference was not significant ($p > 0.075$, Mann-Whitney Test, FIGURE 2). When the percentage of Leu-11-bearing cells was compared with the endogenous NK activity of a constant number of PBMC from some of these donors, no statistically significant correlation was seen (FIGURE 3). However, whereas most donors showed increased NK activity with increased Leu-11$^+$ cell number, a group of three MS patients with high numbers of Leu-11$^+$ cells exhibited extremely low NK. This result suggests that perhaps both explanations persist. Namely, in some donors, low NK is due to reduced numbers of effector cells whereas, in others, defective NK is due to functional impairment.

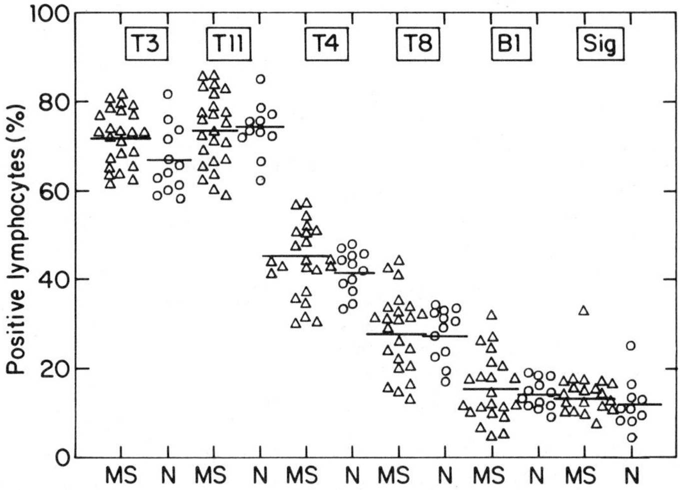

FIGURE 1. Scattergram of T and B lymphocyte subset distributions in 24 active MS patients (△) and 12 normal donors (○) as defined by monoclonal antibodies. Samples of anticoagulated whole blood were stained directly with FITC-conjugated monoclonal antilymphocyte antibodies and the lymphocytes were analyzed on an Ortho Spectrum III flow cytometer (Ortho Diagnostic Systems, Inc., Raritan, N.J.) after lysis of erythrocytes and electronic gating of monocytes and granulocytes. Horizontal lines represent the group means. No statistical differences between the groups were observed for each antibody when analyzed using the Mann-Whitney rank sum test ($p > 0.05$). Antibodies used were as follows: OKT3 and OKT11 (Ortho) for pan-T cells; OKT4 (Ortho) for helper/inducer T cells; OKT8 (Ortho) for suppressor/cytotoxic T cells; B1 (Coulter Immunology, Hialeah, Fla.) and SIg marker (Ortho) for B cells.

Conditions do exist in the circulation of MS patients that could lead to a selective loss of functional lymphocyte subsets. Antilymphocyte antibodies and immune complexes could alone or together bring about depletion of NK if they exhibited the appropriate anti-NK specificity. Studies to be presented at this conference have shown that some MS patients have antibodies to glycolipids in their serum,[35] and certain gangliosides have been described as characteristic markers of mouse NK cells.[36] The therapeutic administration of steroid and/or cytotoxic drugs might also be responsible for lowering NK function in the peripheral blood.[37] However, probably the most likely explanation for subset imbalance is that an active immune response leads to alterations

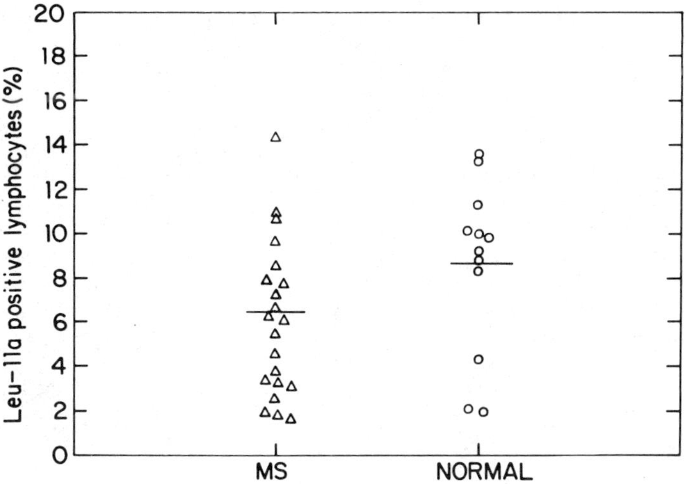

FIGURE 2. Scattergram showing the relative natural killer cell proportions in PBMC of 24 MS patients (△) and 12 normal donors (○) defined using the Leu-11a antibody (Becton Dickinson, Mountain View, Ca.) and stained as described in FIGURE 1.

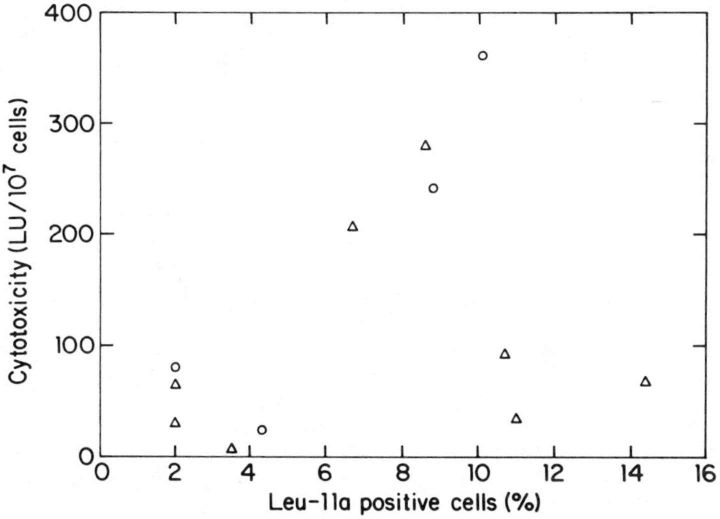

FIGURE 3. Relationship between endogenous NK activity and the proportion of Leu-11a positive NK cells in PBMC of eight MS patients (△) and four normal donors (○). NK activity was determined in a 4-hr ^{51}Cr-release assay against K562 cells by the method as described in ref. 24. Cytotoxic activity was calculated by exponential curve fitting of percent ^{51}Cr-release against effector:target cell ratio and expressed as lytic units (LU) per 10^7 cells, where 1 LU is defined as the number of effector cells to produce 30% specific lysis of 1×10^4 target cells.

in lymphocyte traffic which, in turn, results in an apparently selective loss of certain effector subpopulations from the circulation. The presumed target organ in MS would be the central nervous system (CNS). However, there is little evidence thus far that the cells infiltrating the CNS have NK ability.[27,28]

Impairment of cell function is another possibility. Antilymphocyte antibodies or immune complexes could block functional activity. Preactivation by circulating interferons or other biological response modifiers produced as part of an ongoing immune response might eventually reduce the levels of endogenous NK activity. It should be noted here, for example, that in trials of interferon and interleukin-2 therapy, and in patients in whom these lymphokines are to be found in the circulation, NK activity is frequently suppressed. Another possibility is that the NK effectors may be committed to the performance of other functions. For example, NK effectors are believed to be capable of antibody-dependent cell-mediated cytotoxicity, and this form of killing appears to be elevated in MS patients.[38]

Finally, prostaglandins are known to be capable of inhibiting NK cell function,[39] and MS patients' cells appear to synthesize increased levels of PGE_2,[40] which has been found to correlate with reduced NK activity.[21]

SIGNIFICANCE OF THESE OBSERVATIONS TO THE DISEASE

Although the precise explanations for the observed defects of interferon production and natural killing have yet to be determined, it is important to ask what we can learn from them about MS. First, it must be determined whether the abnormal responses described here are (i) primary defects of the disease associated with its etiology, or (ii) epiphenomena resulting from a generalized immunological assault. In the case of the latter, it is important to determine whether the defect is capable of affecting disease progression.

Two major unknowns interfere with our solution of this fundamental question. First, do *in vitro* immunological phenomena reflect *in vivo* immune processes and, second, do peripheral blood-derived cells reflect overall immune function? If altered lymphocyte traffic turns out to be the underlying basis for a loss of a particular functional activity, it would be erroneous to conclude that this function is defective systemically. Indeed, on the contrary, changes in traffic might indicate that those cells have moved to a tissue or organ site in order to perform their required function. Therefore, in order to understand the underlying immunological basis of multiple sclerosis, access to sites other than peripheral veins is required.

Another concern relates to the physiological appropriateness of the target cells used for study. The majority of NK studies are performed with tumor cells (K562 was derived from an erythroleukemia) and yet MS is clearly a non-neoplastic disease. NK effectors can lyse a variety of target cell types *in vitro,* but their ability to lyse these same cell types *in vivo* has not been fully established. Although a viral etiology for MS has also not been confirmed, virally infected target cells might be more appropriate for NK study. Hauser *et al.*[26] studied the NK activity of MS patients cells using measles-infected HeLa cells and found defective killing compared to normal donors.

In considering the significance of these defects to MS, it should be noted that MS patients exhibit many other apparently unrelated anomalies of immune function. Furthermore, defective interferon production and natural killing is seen in other chronic immunological diseases such as systemic lupus erythematosus and Sjögren's syndrome.[24,41]

CONCLUSIONS

Although the various investigations of the interferon-NK system in MS have not reached a general consensus, I believe that these studies do indeed indicate that there is a malfunction of this system in MS. The true extent of this malfunction, and its underlying basis, however, remain unclear at this time. For the reasons discussed above, it appears to me at the current time that the anomalies of interferon production and natural killing seen in the peripheral circulation are probably due to a generalized disturbance of systemic immune function and are not primary to the disease etiology. However, it should be noted that diminished immunocompetence occurring after disease onset might contribute to its progression, and could compromise the patient's well being. The ability to respond to an emerging latent or persistent virus infection at the beginning of a new exacerbation, for example, might be compromised. Clearly, carefully controlled horizontal studies with appropriate effector and target cells systems are required to determine whether malfunction of the interferon-NK system might precede clinical signs. Furthermore, therapies directed at correction of these defects, although not preventing the disease, might contribute to the control of disease progression.

SUMMARY

Peripheral blood lymphocytes from patients with multiple sclerosis (MS) have been shown by numerous investigators to function abnormally in a variety of immunological tests *in vitro*.

In this article, data concerning defective natural killer (NK) cell function and interferon production by MS patients' lymphocytes have been reviewed. Production of IFN-α and IFN-γ by appropriately stimulated lymphocytes has been shown to be significantly reduced in many patients with acute remitting or chronic progressive disease. Furthermore, a significant proportion of these patients has been found to exhibit reduced levels of endogenous and augmented NK cell activity. A likely explanation for these phenomena is that altered traffic occurring as a consequence of disease has led to a relative loss of NK and IFN-producing cells from the peripheral circulation. Flow cytometric data obtained using monoclonal antibodies that selectively label these effector populations were presented. Possible explanations for the observed defects and their significance relative to our understanding of the etiopathogenesis of MS were discussed.

ACKNOWLEDGMENTS

I am extremely grateful to Drs. B. R. Bloom, A. E. Miller, M. Bornstein and L. Scheinberg for their collaboration in the earlier studies, and to Dr. Celia Brosnan, Dr. Chuck Smith and Ms. Mona Litwak for the excellent assistance in recent investigations.

REFERENCES

1. WAKSMAN, B. H., Ed. 1983. Neuroimmunopathology. Clinics in Immunology and Allergy, vol. 2, no. 2. W. B. Saunders. London.

2. STEWART, W. E. 1979. The Interferon System. Springer-Verlag. New York.
3. STIEHM, E. R., L. H. KRONENBERG, H. M. ROSENBLATT, Y. BRYSON & T. C. MERIGAN. 1982. Interferon: Immunobiology and clinical significance. Ann. Int. Med. **96:** 80–93.
4. HERBERMAN, R. B., Ed. 1982. NK Cells and Other Natural Effector Cells. Academic Press. New York.
5. PERUSSIA, B., D. SANTOLI & G. TRINCHIERI. 1980. Interferon modulation of natural killer cell activity. Ann. N.Y. Acad. Sci. **350:** 55–62.
6. COPELAND, S. C., H. S. KOREN & P. J. JENSEN. 1981. Natural killing can be independent of interferon generated *in vitro*. Cell. Immunol. **62:** 220–225.
7. TRINCHIERI, G., D. SANTOLI, R. R. DEE & B. B. KNOWLES. 1978. Anti-viral activity induced by culturing lymphocytes with tumor-derived or virus-transformed cells. Identification of the anti-viral activity as interferon and characterization of the human effector lymphocyte subpopulation. J. Exp. Med. **147:** 1299–1313.
8. TARGAN, S. & F. DOREY. 1980. Interferon activation of 'pre-spontaneous killer' (pre-SK) cells and alteration in kinetics of lysis of both 'pre-SK' and active SK cells. J. Immunol. **124:** 2157-2161.
9. SHELLAM, G. R., J. E. ALLAN, J. M. PAPADIMITRIOU & G. J. BANCROFT. 1981. Increased susceptibility to cytomegalovirus infection in beige mutant mice. Proc. Natl. Acad. Sci. U.S.A. **78:** 5104–5108.
10. DOMZIG, W. & B. M. STADLER. 1982. The relation between human natural killer cells and interleukin 2. *In* NK Cells and Other Natural Effector Cells. R.B. Herberman, Ed.: 409–414. Academic Press. New York.
11. NEIGHBOUR, P. A. & B. R. BLOOM. 1979. Absence of virus-induced lymphocyte suppression and interferon production in multiple sclerosis. Proc. Natl. Acad. Sci. U.S.A. **76:** 476–480.
12. NEIGHBOUR, P. A., A. E. MILLER & B. R. BLOOM. 1981. Interferon responses of leukocytes in multiple sclerosis. Neurology **31:** 561–566.
13. SANTOLI, D., W. HALL, L. KASTROUKOFF, R. P. LISAK, B. PERUSSIA, G. TRINCHIERI & H. KOPROWSKI. 1978. Cytotoxic activity and interferon production by lymphocytes from patients with multiple sclerosis. J. Immunol. **126:** 1274–1278.
14. KAUDEWITZ, P., H. ZANDER, J. ABB, H. W. ZIEGLER-HEITBROCK & G. RIETHMULLER. 1983. Genetic influence on natural cytotoxicity and interferon production in multiple sclerosis in monozygotic discordant twins. Hum. Immunol. **7:** 51–58.
15. TOVELL, D. R., I. A. MCROBBIE, K. G. WARREN & D. L. TYRRELL. 1983. Interferon production by lymphocytes from multiple sclerosis and non-MS patients. Neurosci. Behav. Physiol. **33:** 640–643.
16. BENCZUR, M., G. PETRANYI, G. G. PALFFY, M. VARGA, M. TALAS, B. KOTSY, I. FOLDER & S. R. HOLLAN. 1980. Dysfunction of natural killer cells in multiple sclerosis, a possible pathogenic factor. Clin. Exp. Immunol. **39:** 657–662.
17. STOGER, I., M. TALAS, M. BENCZUR, E. GYODI, G. G. PETRANYI, G. PALFFY & B. KOTSY. 1982. Lack of correlation between impaired interferon production and natural killer activity of lymphocytes in multiple sclerosis. Arch. Virol. **71:** 259–265.
18. KHALETSKAIA, E. V., L. L. FADEEVA, A. I. SELEZNEVA, L. S. PRIIMIAGI & V. I. LUKA. 1981. Interferon production in multiple sclerosis. Vopr. Virusol. **2:** 218–221.
19. SALONEN, R., J. ILONEN, M. REUNANEN, J. NIKOLOSKELAINEN & A. SALMI. 1982. PPD-, PWM-, and PHA-induced interferon in stable multiple sclerosis: Association with HLA-Dw2 antigen and clinical variables. Ann. Neurol. **11:** 279–284.
20. SALONEN, R., J. ILONEN, M. REUNANEN & A. SALMI. 1982. Defective production of interferon-alpha associated with HLA-DW2 antigen in stable multiple sclerosis. J. Neurol. Sci. **55:** 197–206.
21. MERRILL, J. E., R. H. GERNER, L. W. MEYERS & G. W. ELLISON. 1983. Regulation of natural killer cell cytotoxicity by prostaglandin E in the peripheral blood and cerebrospinal fluid of patients with multiple sclerosis and other neurological diseases. Part I. Association between amount of prostaglandin produced, natural killer, and endogenous interferon. J. Neuroimmunol. **4:** 223–237.
22. HAAHR, S., A. MOLLER-LARSEN & E. PEDERSEN. 1983. Immunological parameters in

multiple sclerosis patients with special reference to the herpes virus group. Clin. Exp. Immunol. **51:** 197–206.

23. Vervliet, G., H. Claeys, H. Van Haver, H. Carton, C. Vermylen, E. Meulepas & A. Billiau. 1983. Interferon production and natural killer (NK) activity in leukocyte cultures from multiple sclerosis patients. J. Neurol. Sci. **60:** 137–150.
24. Neighbour, P. A., A. I. Grayzel & A. E. Miller. 1982. Endogenous and interferon-augmented natural killer cell activity of human peripheral blood mononuclear cells *in vitro.* Studies of patients with multiple sclerosis, systemic lupus erythematosus, or rheumatoid arthritis. Clin. Exp. Immunol. **49:** 11–21.
25. Gyodi, E., M. Benczur, G. Palffy, M. Talas, G. Petranyi, I. Foldes & S. R. Hollan. 1982. Association between HLA B7, DR2 and dysfunction of natural- and antibody-mediated cytotoxicity without connection with the deficient interferon production in multiple sclerosis. Hum. Immunol. **4:** 209–217.
26. Hauser, S. L., K. A. Ault, M. J. Levin, M. R. Garovoy & H. L. Weiner. 1981. Natural killer cell activity in multiple sclerosis. J. Immunol. **127:** 1114–1117.
27. Merrill, J. E., M. Jondal, J. Seeley, M. Ullberg & A. Siden. 1982. Decreased NK killing in patients with multiple sclerosis: An analysis on the level of the single effector cell in peripheral blood and cerebrospinal fluid in relation to the activity in the disease. Clin. Exp. Immunol. **47:** 419–430.
28. Merrill, J. E., A. Scott, L. Meyers & G. Ellison. 1982. Cytotoxic activity of peripheral blood and cerebrospinal fluid lymphocytes from patients with multiple sclerosis and other neurological diseases. Analysis at the single cell level using morphological and surface marker phenotype criteria. J. Neuroimmunol. **3:** 123–138.
29. Uchida, A., E. M. Maida, R. Lenzhofer & M. Micksche. 1982. Natural killer cell activity in patients with multiple sclerosis: Interferon and plasmapheresis. Immunobiology **160:** 392–402.
30. McGarry, R. C., J. Roder & D. Brunet. 1982. Mechanisms of natural killer cell depression in multiple sclerosis. *In* NK Cells and Other Natural Effector Cells. R. B. Herberman, Ed.: 1219–1225. Academic Press. New York.
31. Mar, P. 1980. Antibody-dependent cellular cytotoxicity in multiple sclerosis. J. Neurol. Sci. **47:** 285–303.
32. Ullberg, M. & M. Jondal. 1981. Recycling and target binding capacity of human natural killer cells. J. Exp. Med. **153:** 615–628.
33. Egan, M. L., S. L. Mendelsohn, T. Abo & C. M. Balch. 1983. Natural killer cells in systemic lupus erythematosus. Abnormal numbers and functional immaturity of HNK-1^+ cells. Arthritis Rheum. **26:** 623–629.
34. Lanier, L. L., A. M. Le, J. P. Phillips, N. L. Warner & G. F. Babcock. 1983. Subpopulations of human natural killer cells defined by expression of the Leu-7 (HNK-1) and Leu-11 (NK-15) antigens. J. Immunol. **131:** 1789–1796.
35. Endo, T., S. S. Stewart, S. K. Kundu, S. Osovitz & D. M. Marcus. 1984. Antibodies to glycosphingolipids in patients with multiple sclerosis. This volume.
36. Kasai, M., Y. Iwamori, Y. Nagai, K. Okumura & T. Tada. 1980. A glycolipid on the surface of mouse natural killer cells. Eur. J. Immunol. **10:** 175–180.
37. Ten Berge, R. J., H. K. Van Walbeek & P. T. Schellekens. 1982. Evaluation of the immunosuppressive effects of cyclophosphamide in patients with multiple sclerosis. Clin. Exp. Immunol. **50:** 495–502.
38. Merrill, J. E., B. Wahlin, A. Siden & P. Perlmann. 1982. Elevated direct and IgM enhanced ADCC activity in multiple sclerosis patients. J. Immunol. **128:** 1728–1735.
39. Droller, M. J., M. U. Schneider & P. Perlmann. 1978. A possible role of prostaglandins in the inhibition of natural and antibody-dependent cell-mediated cytotoxicity against tumor cells. Cell. Immunol. **39:** 165–177.
40. Dore-Duffy, P. & R. B. Zurier. 1981. Lymphocyte adherence in multiple sclerosis. Role of monocytes and increased sensitivity of MS lymphocytes to prostaglandin E. Clin. Immunol. Immunopathol. **19:** 303–313.
41. Miyasaka, N., W. Seaman, A. Bakshi, B. Sauvezie, V. Strand, R. Pope & N. Talal. 1983. Natural killing activity in Sjögren's syndrome. An analysis of defective mechanisms. Arthritis Rheum. **26:** 954–960.

Cytotoxic Cells in Peripheral Blood and Cerebrospinal Fluid of Multiple Sclerosis Patients

JEAN E. MERRILL, LAWRENCE W. MYERS, AND GEORGE W. ELLISON

Department of Neurology
UCLA School of Medicine
Los Angeles, California 90024

Because a persistent viral infection may stimulate an autoimmune-like response in multiple sclerosis (MS), we investigated natural killer (NK) cells and antibody-dependent cellular cytotoxicity (ADCC) in these patients. Patients with active disease had low NK whereas stable patients were normal. Patients in relapse had low numbers of NK cells. There were no functional NK cells in MS cerebrospinal fluid (CSF) though there were such cells in CSF of patients with acute CNS infection. In contrast, ADCC was normal or elevated in cells from MS blood and CSF. In normal people, NK activity is more sensitive than ADCC to prostaglandin (PGE) and interferon (IFN) which we thought might explain our findings in MS. Compared to controls, macrophages of MS patients make more PGE *in vitro* whereas MS CSF contains more endogenously produced PGE. There is an inverse correlation of NK activity and PGE production in MS patients. Compared to controls, MS NK activity is more sensitive to the effects of PGE, suggesting a possible *in vivo* mechanism for depressed NK activity and potential chronic virus persistence.

INTRODUCTION

Several research groups in addition to ours have found depressed NK activity in peripheral blood lymphocytes (PBL) of patients with multiple sclerosis.[1–5] We have further shown a lack of NK activity in CSF.[2] It has also been shown that MS patients produce lower levels of interferon,[6,7] and have an impaired response to exogenous IFN.[1,6] In contrast, MS patients may in fact have elevated ADCC activity.[3,8–10] Prostaglandin has been demonstrated to suppress spontaneous[11–13] and IFN-induced NK[14] though it has distinctively less of an effect on ADCC.[11,15] In an effort to investigate these abnormalities in the MS immune response further, we examined peripheral blood cell production of PGE *in vitro* as well as PGE levels in neat CSF in relationship to NK activity, quantitating amount produced, identifying cells producing it and the kinetics of production. We further examined the sensitivity of NK activity in MS to the effects of PGE to determine the step in the lytic process most susceptible to inhibition.

MATERIALS AND METHODS

Lymphocyte Donors

All multiple sclerosis patients and other neurological disease (OND) patients classified according to Schumacher *et al.*[16] were studied concomitantly with age- and sex-matched normal controls. None were on any medication, including aspirin, at the time of sampling nor had they been for at least one week prior to sampling. Peripheral blood samples were drawn in the morning and all cells handled at room temperature unless otherwise noted. In addition to fresh, neat (undiluted) MS and OND cerebrospinal fluids whose cells were removed, spinal fluids from 20 medication-free normal individuals and 35 psychiatric patients (16 schizophrenic, 6 manic, 13 depressed) who were medication-free for a week or more were assayed for PGE.

Cell Preparation

Peripheral blood was collected in heparinized tubes and the peripheral blood mononuclear cells separated from the red blood cells on ficoll-hypaque (FH, Pharmacia, Uppsala, Sweden).[17] For removal of macrophages and B cells, some samples were incubated on nylon wool columns for 30 min at 37°C.[18] The FH-treated cells are referred to as nylon wool passed (NWP) after treatment. Removal of adherent cells from nylon wool (NW Ad cells) was accomplished by placing the teased out nylon wool in a petri dish of cold Hanks' BSS without serum plus 0.1 mg/ml Versene (Microbiological Associates, Walkersville, MD) for 2 hr at 4°C. Mechanical agitation was used to loosen cells from the nylon wool.

MS spinal fluid was collected by lumbar puncture using a 22-gauge needle and OND CSF by a 20-gauge needle. The fluid was allowed to drip by gravity. CSF cells were spun down at 200 × g for 10 min in CSF to which 10% FCS had been added and immediately resuspended in RPMI 1640 plus 10% FCS. Aliquots of CSF without FCS were used to assay for PGE_1 and PGE_2. Esterase staining to determine monocytes/macrophages was according to Tucker *et al.*[19]

^{51}Cr Release Assay

The NK-sensitive target cell line used was MOLT 4. The ADCC-sensitive, NK-insensitive line used was a melanoma M14 with a 10^{-3} dil. Ab. The ^{51}Cr release assay was performed as previously described.[20] Target cells were labeled with ^{51}sodium chromate for 1 hr at 36°C. PBL were added in a twofold dilution titration for a final effector to a target cell ratio of 40:1 down to 2.5:1. Results on the effect of IFN and PGE_1 were comparable at 40:1, 20:1 and 10:1. Results at 20:1 are reported here. Labeled target cells, 10^4/well, were added to every well. The assays were harvested after a 3 hr incubation and results expressed as percentage of specific chromium released.[2]

Agarose Single Cell Cytotoxicity Assay

Nylon wool-passed peripheral blood mononuclear cells and CSF cells were tested for NK cell activity and ADCC using the agarose single cell cytotoxicity assay originally described by Grimm and Bonavida.[21] Briefly, effector and target cells were mixed and pelleted. The pellets were then incubated at 37°C for 10 min and resuspended by vigorous vortexing. To this was added 0.5% agarose (Pharmacia, Uppsala, Sweden) in RPMI 1640 and this mixture was then dropped onto petri dishes (NUNC, Roskilde, Denmark). Duplicates were incubated at 36°C for 3 hr and then harvested by staining with trypan blue for dead targets, followed by fixation.

Using an inverted microscope with a 32× objective, the proportion of lymphocytes bound to target cells was scored as a percent of the total lymphocyte population by counting 300 or 400 lymphocytes and the results expressed as percent target-binding cells (% TBC). Means were obtained by averaging these percents and standard deviations and errors were calculated as the product of % TBC times the percentage of dead conjugates, which yields the proportion of the total lymphocyte population that binds and kills sensitive targets. Data means were calculated as above. Target cells alone were greater than 95% viable after 3 hr. At time zero, targets conjugated to lymphocytes were also usually 98% viable, indicating very little lysis during the 10–15 min interval between conjugation at 37°C and the plating. Negative controls were normal rabbit serum plus lymphocytes and hyperimmune serum without lymphocytes for this assay and the ^{51}Cr release assay.

Measurement of PGE

NW Ad cells were plated at 5×10^5/well in triplicates in Falcon microtiter II plates in RMPI 1640 plus 10% FCS. Indomethacin (Sigma, St Louis, MO) was used at 3×10^{-8}M which had been found to be optimal for inhibition of PGE production (data not shown). Supernatants were harvested at 48 hr. Production of prostaglandin E_1 and E_2 (PGE_1 and PGE_2) by NW Ad cells *in vitro* as well as endogenous PGE_1 and PGE_2 in neat CSF was measured using an RIA kit (Clinical Assays, Cambridge, MA) according to Levine.[22] The RIA kit is sensitive to levels of PGE from 5 to 2000 pg total.

Treatment with Prostaglandin E_1 and Indomethacin

Prostaglandin E_1 and indomethacin (Sigma Chemical, St. Louis, MO) were dissolved in absolute ethanol to stock solutions of 0.028 M (10 mg/ml). PGE_1 was further diluted to between 10^{-6}M and to 10^{-11}M (final concentration) and indomethacin to 3×10^{-8}M (final) in RPMI 1640 with 10% FCS such that the ethanol was the same as or less than 0.01% at its final concentration in the cell suspension or assay. The ethanol control had no effect on the NK assay. The PGE_1 and indomethacin were added at time 0 of the assay and left in throughout the 3 hr time period.

Interferon Treatment

Those cells to be treated with human leukocyte interferon alpha (IFNα, a gift from Dr. Kari Cantell, Helsinki, Finland) were incubated for 60 minutes with 10^2 IU/ml IFN before starting the assay. Control cells without IFN were incubated in the same way. The IFN was left in the cell suspension during the 3 hr assay period.

Giemsa Staining to Determine Cell Morphology

Analysis of NWP peripheral blood lymphocytes and CSF lymphocytes alone or conjugated to either MOLT 4 or Chang liver cells was done as in Timonen *et al.*[23] Cell mixtures were cytocentrifuged onto an FCS-precoated microscope slide using a Cytospin Centrifuge (Shandon Elliot, Bewickly, PA). Cells were air dried, fixed 10 min in absolute methanol, rinsed and stained with 10% Giemsa in PBS for 20 min, followed by rinsing. Cells were examined under oil immersion.

The percentage of TBC was determined on the cell suspension prior to centrifugation and after staining. No disruption of conjugates was found to occur during the above procedure. Large granular lymphocytes (LGL) were identified as weakly basophilic, between 10 and 15 μm with azurophilic cytoplasmic granules.[24] For scoring LGL as percentage of the total NWP PBL population, at least 200 cells were counted.

RESULTS

Decreased NK Cell Numbers and Killing in MS Patients

The agarose cytoxicity assay measures a single lytic event because effectors are immobilized in agarose with one target, and allows for the calculation of the number of

TABLE 1. NK Activity in Peripheral Blood of MS and OND Patients

	Patients				Controls			
	TBC[a] (%)	Cytotoxic TBC[b] (%)	NK Cells[c] (%)	^{51}Cr Release[d] (%)	TBC (%)	Cytotoxic TBC (%)	NK Cells (%)	^{51}Cr Release (%)
13 acute relapsing	4.2 ($p < 0.02$)[e]	31 ($p < 0.05$)	1.5 ($p < 0.01$)	18.8 ($p < 0.02$)	7.2	54	3.8	43.2
18 chronic progressive	8.1 (ns)	47 (ns)	3.8 (ns)	28.8 ($p < 0.50$)	7.8	49	3.6	43.4
13 stable	8.6 (ns)	38 (ns)	3.2 (ns)	33.4 (ns)	7.3	40	3.1	33.7
12 OND	9.3 (ns)	55 (ns)	5.6 (ns)	44.5 ($p < 0.05$)	7.2	45	3.3	31.4

[a]The percentage of target-binding cells in the agarose single cell cytotoxicity assay as described in the Materials and Methods section.

[b]The percentage of conjugates showing target-cell killing.

[c]Calculated by multiplying the TBC percentage by the percentage conjugates showing a target-cell killing as described in the Materials and Methods section.

[d]^{51}Cr release calculated at an effector:target ratio of 20:1.

[e]Statistical significance between patient and control group calculated by the paired Student's *t* test.

NK cells (expressed as percentage of NK cells). This measurement is directly comparable betwen MS patients and controls because the total number of circulating PBL in MS patients is normal.[25,26] The ^{51}Cr-release assay measures the cumulative lytic events in a cell suspension where a single effector is free to kill one, detach from its target and kill again as has been shown by Ullberg and Jondal.[27] The data are summarized by mean values (TABLE 1).

Acute patients, on average, have fewer TBC and fewer of those that bind that can kill as reflected by the fact that they have only 40% of the percentage NK cells seen in the control group. As shown in TABLE 1, acute MS patients studied have lower NK activity as measured by the ^{51}Cr-release assay which may be a direct reflection of fewer NK cells. Chronic MS patients have the same number of TBC and these kill to the same extent as controls so there is no significant difference in percentage of NK cells in these patients compared with their controls. However, there is a statistically significant defect in NK activity as measured by ^{51}Cr release indicating that whereas a given MS effector cell bound to a target is just as effective in killing as a control effector cell, the mechanism for recycling of such effector cells to kill again may be impaired. Thus, the chronic patients may be distinguished from the acute patients in that they have normal numbers of NK cells but may have defective recycling.

Stable MS patients have normal numbers of NK cells (agarose assay) and activity (^{51}Cr assay). On average, OND patients have higher proportions of NK cells as the result of a higher percentage of TBC, a greater proportion of dead conjugates and also a higher NK activity by ^{51}Cr-released assay than their control group. This would indicate the possibility than an NK cell defect may not be a parameter of all neurological diseases but a particular feature in MS.

Variations in ^{51}Cr release of control groups are a reflection both of the daily variations in cell processing and assaying. The control-patient comparison is valid as these bloods were processed at the same time.

NK and ADCC Activity in Cerebrospinal Fluid

Data on NK cell activity in the lymphocyte population of the CSF are shown in TABLE 2. Stable MS patients usually have little or no CSF pleocytosis so they were not included in the CSF study. Whereas twenty out of 32 CSF samples from acute and chronic MS patients contained lymphocytes that would bind NK targets, there were only 15% as many TBC in acute CSF as acute PBL. Only 6 out of 32 CSF samples from MS patients had lymphocytes that could bind and kill NK targets and this killing was less than the lysis seen in the population of NK cells in the PBL. Thus there appear to be virtually no active spontaneous NK cells in the CSF of MS patients. Of the 19 OND patients studied in this context, six patients did not have central nervous system involvement (patients 5, 6, 7, 10, 12, and 18) and they had no lymphocytes in their CSF that could kill NK-sensitive targets. Patient 16 had a pseudotumor of the brain of unknown etiology but had no NK activity in the CSF lymphocyte population. However, patients 1, 4, 8, 13, 14, and 17 were experiencing acute-stage CNS viral meningitis and patients 15 and 19 had viral encephalitis, all with obvious CNS involvement. As mentioned previously, patients with CNS-involved viral infections had CSF lymphocytes that killed about the same proportion of conjugated targets as did their PBL, though in comparing percentage of NK cells they had fewer NK cells in the CSF than in the peripheral blood because of a lower proportion of target-binding cells (TABLE 2).

In contrast to the lack of NK activity in CSF is the presence of K cell activity or ADCC in this population of cells (TABLE 2). As in MS, OND patients' CSF lymphocytes are capable of mediating ADCC, though there are too few samples to know if this is greater than that in MS CSF.

Comparison of LGL Binding to NK and K Cell Targets with Proportions of NK and K Cells in NWP PBL and CSF As Measured in a Single Cell Assay

ADCC activity is elevated in MS patients both in K cell numbers (TABLE 3) and by ^{51}Cr release (data not shown).[3,10] It is thought that human NK and K cells have the morphology of a large granular lymphocyte, which is a low-avidity E rosette-forming cell.[28] No difference was found among the different groups of MS patients and controls in the number of LGL cells (TABLE 3). Chronic MS and OND have normal numbers of

TABLE 2. NK and ADCC Activity of CSF Lymphocytes from MS and OND Patients

	NK Activity[a]			ADCC Activity[a]		
	% TBC[b]	% Cytotoxic TBC[c]	% NK[b]	% TBC[b]	% Cytotoxic TBC[c]	% K[b]
			MS ACUTE RELAPSING			
1	0.9	0	0	7.1	50.5	3.6
2	0	0	0	8.0	46.8	3.7
3	0	0	0	11.5	30.5	3.5
4	0	0	0	nd[d]	—	—
5	0.8	0	0	—	—	—
6	1.3	16.3	0.2	—	—	
7	0.5	0	0	—	—	—
			MS CHRONIC PROGRESSIVE			
1	0.5	0	0	4.1	39.1	1.6
2	0	0	0	nd	—	—
3	0	0	0	2.1	0	0
4	1.5	41.7	0.6	3.2	57.1	1.8
5	0	0	0	12.0	25.0	3.0
6	0	0	0	15.3	60.0	9.2
7	1.0	0	0	3.8	50.0	1.9
8	1.4	0	0	2.7	0	0
9	3.8	9.5	0.4	4.5	13.3	0.6
10	3.8	50.0	1.9	22.4	30.0	6.7
11	1.7	0	0	9.6	16.7	1.6
12	3.3	25.0	0.8	1.5	0	0
13	1.4	0	0	7.7	75.0	5.8
14	1.5	0	0	2.9	46.2	1.3
15	1.3	0	0	5.0	50.0	2.5
16	1.2	0	0	10.3	14.3	1.5
17	0	0	0	2.6	0	0
18	0	0	0	3.7	50.0	1.8
19	—	—	—	7.8	21.1	1.6
20	—	—	—	6.3	38.5	2.4
21	1.0	0	0	nd	—	—
22	1.0	0	0	—	—	—
23	6.8	10.0	0.7	—	—	—
24	1.9	0	0	—	—	—
25	0	0	0	—	—	—
			OND			
1	5.5	42.6	2.3	3.7	45.2	1.7
2	—	—	—	25.0	33.3	8.3
3	1.0	0	0	—	—	—
4	2.1	66.7	1.4	4.7	23.5	1.1
5	4.0	0	0	6.0	16.5	1.0
6	16.3	0	0	8.2	0	0
7	11.1	0	0	—	—	—
8	3.5	100.0	3.5	—	—	—
9	15.4	0	0	33.3	33.3	11.1
10	0	0	0	nd	—	—
11	2.6	45.2	1.2	—	—	—
12	2.9	0	0	—	—	—
13	2.6	66.7	1.7	—	—	—
14	4.2	47.1	2.0	—	—	—
15	1.2	66.7	0.8	—	—	—
16	0.8	0	0	—	—	—
17	5.5	41.8	2.3	—	—	—
18	0	0	0	—	—	—
19	2.7	25.0	0.7	—	—	—

[a]Effector:target = 1:1 assayed in agarose. NK target: MOLT 4, all patients; ADCC target: Chang liver and M14.

[b]Percentage of total NWP population.

[c]Percentage of total TBC.

[d]Not done.

Note: OND patients include 4 Friedreich's ataxia, 2 pseudotumor, 1 neurosyphilis, 3 encephalitis, 1 conversion reaction, 1 cerebellar dysfunction, 1 peripheral neuropathy, 1 polyneuritis, 1 headache, 1 viral meningitis, 1 Guillain-Barré.

TABLE 3. A Comparison of LGL Conjugates to NK and K Cell Populations in MS and OND, NWP, PBL and CSF Cells

No. of Samples	Lymphocyte Source	LGL	LGL-MOLT 4 Conj.[a]	NK[c]	LGL Chang-Ab Conj.[a,b]	K[c]
		% Total NWP-PBL Population				
9	acute relapsing MS	7.7 ± 1.6	0.8 ± 0.3	2.7 ± 0.7	1.6 ± 0.4	3.3 ± 0.7
9	controls	7.9 ± 0.9	1.8 ± 0.5	4.0 ± 0.7	1.1 ± 0.3	1.8 ± 0.2
			($p < 0.02$)[d]	($p < 0.04$)	(ns)[e]	($p < 0.05$)
29	chronic progressive MS	7.4 ± 0.7	1.0 ± 0.1	3.2 ± 0.4	1.0 ± 0.1	2.8 ± 0.4
29	controls	7.7 ± 0.7	1.4 ± 0.2	3.2 ± 0.3	1.4 ± 0.4	1.6 ± 0.2
			(ns)	(ns)	(ns)	($p < 0.01$)
11	OND	9.8 ± 1.7	1.7 ± 0.4	3.9 ± 0.8	2.3 ± 0.4	2.5 ± 0.5
11	controls	10.0 ± 1.2	1.5 ± 0.07	3.2 ± 0.3	1.7 ± 0.3	1.7 ± 0.3
			(ns)	(ns)	(ns)	(ns)
		% Total CSF Lymphocyte Population				
18	MS CSF	3.8 ± 0.8	0.1 ± 0.05	0.2 ± 0.05	0.6 ± 0.2	2.5 ± 0.6
12	OND CSF	5.5 ± 1.2	0.9 ± 0.3	1.3 ± 0.7	0.5 ± 0.2	2.8 ± 1.8

[a] E:T ratio = 1:1. Results expressed as mean ±SE.
[b] Antiserum dilution is 10^{-3}.
[c] NK and ADCC is determined in agarose single cell cytotoxicity assay.
[d] p values: paired Student's t test comparing MS or OND patient and matched normal control.
[e] ns = not significant.

NK cells and normal numbers of LGL binding to MOLT 4. Compared to controls, active relapsing MS patients have lower numbers of NK as measured in the single cell assay and a reduced number of LGL that bind MOLT 4 (potential NK effectors).

There is no statistical difference between LGL binders to antibody-coated Chang or % K cells comparing OND patients and their matched controls. Relapse and progressive MS patients have more K cells in their NWP PBL than controls, but they do not have more LGL binders to the susceptible target than controls. Whereas in MS, % K cells is greater than % LGL-Chang conjugates, there is no significant difference among all three control groups of OND patients when comparing the % LGL-binders and % K cells to antibody-coated Chang cells. There is no ADCC activity or LGL binders to NK-resistant cell lines Chang liver and M14 melanoma in the absence of antibody (data not shown).

Both MS and OND CSF contain LGL though at proportions lower than in blood. There is no significant difference in % LGL in MS CSF compared to OND CSF. In parallel with the general lack of NK cells in MS CSF (TABLES 2 and 3) is the lack of LGL conjugates to MOLT 4 targets. The % NK activity in OND CSF can not be fully accounted for by LGL effectors as the % LGL binders is lower than % NK effectors. In the absence of antibody, no LGL bind to Chang liver cells (data not shown), whereas 0.5% of the total CSF population do bind when antibody is present. Because the average K cell proportion in MS and OND CSF is about 2.5%, the LGL is most likely not an effector cell in ADCC activity in the CSF.

The Effect of IFN and PGE_1 on ADCC and NK Activities

TABLE 4 shows the effect of interferon and prostaglandin E_1 on NK activity in normal individuals. Interferon does not enhance binding or killing in the single-cell assay against MOLT 4 but enhances ^{51}Cr release, indicating augmentation of recycling. Interferon inhibits the binding of TBC and, thus, indirectly the number of K cells (product of % TBC and % cytotoxic TBC) in the single cell assay at optimal antibody (Ab) concentrations (10^{-3}, Chang; 10^{-2}, M14), though it does not significantly alter the specific ^{51}Cr released.

NK effectors are sensitive to PGE_1 at a 100-fold lower concentration than their ADCC-effector counterparts. The magnitude of the PGE_1-induced inhibition of ADCC activity is less than that of NK activity at any given concentration above 10^{-8}M. At the single-cell level, ADCC activity is insensitive to 10^{-6}M PGE_1, whereas both % TBC and % cytotoxic TBC are reduced in NK cells (data not shown). While sensitive out to 10^{-9}M in the ^{51}Cr release assay, the NK activity is sensitive to 10^{-8} M in the single cell assay by virtue of the reduction in % TBC (data not shown).

In Vitro *or* in Vivo *Prostaglandin E Production vs. NK*

Activity of peripheral blood cells shows that there is a significant inverse relationship between PGE levels and functional NK as measured in the ^{51}Cr release assay. MS have higher *in vitro* PGE production and lower NK activity than normal or OND controls (TABLE 5). The coefficient of correlation of this association is −0.76 ($p < 0.03$) by Pearson correlation analysis. Although there are too few cells in the CSF to examine *in vitro* PGE synthesis, when we measured CSF PGE levels, we found higher circulating PGE and lower NK cell numbers in MS compared to OND CSF (TABLE 5). Pearson correlation analysis shows this high PGE is significantly correlated to the ability of TBC to kill (% cytotoxic TBC; $r = -0.57$, $p < 0.05$) and not to their ability to bind. There is a stronger association between high PGE and lower ^{51}Cr release (TABLE 5). MS patients had higher CSF levels of PGE than a wide panel of OND, psychiatric, or normal controls (TABLE 6). Storage of CSF at −70°C had no effect on PGE values (data not shown). Of the MS patients' CSF examined for PGE levels, 78% had cell counts 0–5/mm³, 4.85 of 6–10/mm³ and 7.45 greater than

TABLE 4. The Effect of Interferon and PGE_1 on NK and ADCC Activity[a]

Treatment	% NK Cell	% ^{51}Cr Release[b] NK Activity	% K Cell	% ^{51}Cr Release[b] K Cell Activity
IFN				
−	4.4 ± 0.4[e]	37.2 ± 3.4 (606)[c]	2.4 ± 0.4[e]	24.5 ± 2.1
+	4.7 ± 0.5	49.6 ± 3.5 (110.0)	1.5 ± 0.4	30.4 ± 2.7
p value	(ns)	(<0.02)	(<0.001)	(ns)
PGE[d]				
−	4.8 ± 1.9[e]	25.0 ± 4.1	4.6 ± 0.6[e]	36.3 ± 5.1
+	3.4 ± 0.9	15.0 ± 3.3	4.1 ± 0.2	33.1 ± 6.8
p value	(<0.01)	(<0.01)	(ns)	(ns)

[a]Effects are measured at the single cell level and with the ^{51}Cr release assay. Data are expressed as the means of nine NWP PBL samples ± SD. Paired Student's *t* test comparing results and PGE used to determine *p* values.

[b]E:T, 20:1.

[c]LU/10^7 cells, where 1 LU = the number of effector cells required to give 30% specific ^{51}Cr release.

[d]PGE at 10^{-8}M added at start of assay.

[e]NK:MOLT 4; 1:1 = E:T; ADCC M14 = 10^{-2}Ab, 1:1 = E:T.

TABLE 5. Relationship to NK of PGE Produced *in Vitro* by PBL or *in Vivo* in CSF of MS Patients and Controls

Subject[a]	n	PGE (ng/ml)	NK[c] (% ^{51}Cr Release[d])	% NK[n]
MS PBL[e]	17	1.38 ± 0.1[h,i,b]	21.7 ± 4.7 (41.7)	—
Control PBL	17	0.83 ± 0.2	37.5 ± 4.0 (62.5)	—
p value[g]		(<0.001)	(<0.01)	
OND PBL[f]	5	0.70 ± 0.3[i]	31.1 ± 9.2 (49.5)	—
Control PBL	5	0.58 ± 0.1	35.6 ± 5.7 (60.6)	—
p value[g]		(ns)	(ns)	
CSF				
MS in relapse[j]	5	0.38 ± 0.17[l,m]	—	0.3 ± 0.1
MS in progression	55	0.34 ± 0.08	—	0.3 ± 0.03
OND[k]	10	0.17 ± 0.02	—	1.7 ± 0.2
		(p < 0.001)[o]		(p < 0.005)

[a]NWP peripheral blood lymphocytes used for NK.
[b]From 48 hr, unstimulated, nylon wool adherent cell supernatants; per 10^6 cells.
[c]NK target; MOLT 4 at 20:1=E:T % ^{51}Cr release.
[d]Measured in LU (lytic units/10^7 cells); LU = no. of cells required to give 30% ^{51}Cr release.
[e]MS patients include 5 relapsing type patients (2 of which were experiencing exacerbations) and 12 patients in progression compared to age- and sex-matched controls.
[f]5 OND patients include 1 neurosyphilis, 2 stroke and 2 Friedreich's ataxia compared to age- and sex-matched controls.
[g]p value based on the Wilcoxon signed ranks test comparing patient and age- and sex-matched control.
[h]Mean ± SE.
[i]MS PGE levels were significantly greater than OND $p < 0.03$ using a separate variance t test, square root transformation.
[j]Relapsing type MS patients all experienced exacerbations at the time of study.
[k]OND patients included 1 encephalitis, 1 pseudotumor, 4 Friedreich's ataxia, 1 neurosyphilis, 2 stroke, 1 muscular dystrophy.
[l]Using neat CSF, centrifuged to remove cells.
[m]Mean ±SE.
[n]NK target: MOLT 4 in single cell assay in agarose as described in Materials and Methods section.
[o]Statistical evaluation using the separate variance t test, square root transformation comparing MS in progression and OND.

10/mm^3. The OND patients with 10/mm^3 were undergoing infections or inflammatory diseases of the central nervous system. On the average, MS CSF contained 1.74% macrophages by esterase staining,[19] whereas OND CSF contained 0.68%. Higher PGE levels in the CSF could not be correlated either with total cell counts or percentage of macrophages in either MS or OND CSF (data not shown) leading us to believe that circulating CSF macrophages alone may not be totally responsible for the PGE produced; brain tissue-associated macrophages may also contribute to the secreted PGE detected in the CSF.

The Effect of Indomethacin and PGE_1 on NK As Measured Both at the Single Cell Level and by ^{51}Cr Release

Peripheral blood lymphocyte NK activity in multiple sclerosis is more sensitive to PGE_1 than normal or OND control NK activity. This is seen both in the magnitude of inhibition at 10^{-6} and 10^{-9} M and the sensitivity of MS NWP cells to concentrations of PGE_1 as low as 10^{-9} M, whereas control NWP cells are sensitive only to 10^{-6} M (TABLE 7). We could see no difference in active disease between relapsing and chronic patients. Though indomethacin seems to have no effect on cells of OND and normal controls, it enhances NK activity in MS patients. As in the ^{51}Cr release assay, NK MS cells were more sensitive to PGE_1 than controls, inhibited both in percentage of TBC and in percentage of those TBC that could kill out to 10^{-9} M. OND and controls were equally sensitive out to 10^{-8} M (data not shown). Unlike the ^{51}Cr release assay, indomethacin did not boost MS NK activity at the single cell level (TABLE 7), suggesting that NK recycling (measured in ^{51}Cr release and not at the single cell level)[27] is the indomethacin-sensitive function of NK cells. In fact, the ^{51}Cr release NK activity is in general more susceptible to inhibition by PGE_1 out to more dilute concentrations than is the inhibition of the single cell level, suggesting that the effect of PGE is strongest against NK recycling and not target-cell recognition. Whereas MS and OND CSF cells have lower NK activity than in their homologous PBL, indomethacin did not enhance this activity (data not shown).

DISCUSSION

In previous reports we have shown that the majority of acute relapsing and chronic progressive patients have depressed NK activity[2-4,29] and elevated ADCC.[3,10] In trying to assess the reasons for the concomitant depression of one cytotoxic function and elevation of the other (which normally seem to parallel one another[24,30-32]) we have examined the relationship between the % NK and % K cells measured at the single cell

TABLE 6. PGE Measured in Neat CSF of MS and OND Patients and Normals

CSF Source	*n*	PGE (ng/ml)
MS in relapse[a]	5	0.33 ± 0.09[c]
MS in progression	71	0.38 ± 0.02
Total MS	76	0.375 ± 0.05[d]
Friedreich's ataxia	12	0.10 ± 0.02
Miscellaneous OND[b]	5	0.12 ± 0.02
Total OND	17	0.105 ± 0.01[d]
Schizophrenia	16	0.10 ± 0.02
Depression	13	0.05 ± 0.003
Mania	6	0.14 ± 0.05
Total psychiatric	35	0.087 ± 0.01[d]
Normal	20	0.065 ± 0.01[d]

[a]MS-relapse patients were experiencing exacerbation.
[b]Miscellaneous ONDs included 2 pseudotumor, 1 neurosyphilis, 1 encephalitis, 1 stroke.
[c]Mean ± SE.
[d]MS significantly elevated over OND, psychiatric patients and normals; $p < 0.0001$ by analysis of variance using the square root transformation of PGE level.

level and the percentage of large granular lymphocytes, which has been proposed to be the effector cell with NK-K function.[24,28] We have further examined the possibility that NK activity is depressed because of increased production of PGE *in vivo*[4,29] knowing that ADCC activity is much less sensitive to the suppressive effects of PGE.[15]

In contrast to the findings of Timonen *et al.*[24] that all NK and K cell activity must be confined to the LGL fraction, since the non-LGL fractions are devoid of such cytotoxic activity, we show indirectly that, at most, only 50% of the NK activity in normal and OND controls can be due to LGL. In acute relapse MS patients, not more than 30% of NK cells could be LGL (TABLE 3). This is a generous estimate because not all LGL-binders may actually be able to kill. Thus some NK cells do not have the LGL morphology. Despite the fact that MS patients have a normal % LGL in NWP PBL and that not all NK cells may be LGL, there probably is a correlation between percentage LGL binding NK target[3] and percentage NK, as acute relapse MS patients have a reduction of both in the PBL and the absence of both in the CSF (TABLE 3).

TABLE 7. Effect of PGE_1 and Indomethacin on PBL NK Activity as Measured at the Single Cell and by ^{51}Cr Release[a,e]

		Treatment	% TBC	% Cytotoxic TBC	% NK	% ^{51}Cr Release
10 MS[b]		0	7.0 ± 3.4	62.1 ± 15.8	4.1 ± 1.3[h,j]	18.1 ± 2.1
		indo[d]	4.7 ± 1.8	64.2 ± 19.5	3.0 ± 0.3[h,i]	28.1 ± 1.3[i]
	PGE_1	10^{-6} M	2.7 ± 3.0	44.4 ± 11.8	1.2 ± 0.1	4.1 ± 0.5
		10^{-9} M	5.7 ± 3.0[i]	42.9 ± 9.8[f]	2.4 ± 2.1[f,i]	13.5 ± 1.3[g]
		10^{-11} M	6.5 ± 1.8	49.9 ± 11.2[g,i]	3.2 ± 0.8[g,i]	21.5 ± 0.8
8 OND[b]		0	7.4 ± 2.0	65.0 ± 12.5	5.0 ± 2.0[h]	22.1 ± 1.5
		indo	5.2 ± 1.6	72.0 ± 2.0	4.0 ± 2.0	24.5 ± 0.39
	PGE_1	10^{-6} M	3.3 ± 1.5	38.0 ± 25.1	1.2 ± 1.4	5.1 ± 0.3
		10^{-9} M	8.4 ± 2.5	50.0 ± 10.9	4.2 ± 0.8[h]	23.5 ± 1.3[j]
		10^{-11} M	7.1 ± 2.1	88.0 ± 23.5	6.2 ± 0.8	26.4 ± 0.8
18 Control[c]		0	7.2 ± 2.8	50.0 ± 21.2	3.2 ± 1.0	26.1 ± 1.5
		indo	7.7 ± 5.5	57.2 ± 6.1	4.6 ± 3.8	29.5 ± 4.1[j]
	PGE_1	10^{-6} M	5.0 ± 2.2	37.0 ± 11.7	1.7 ± 0.5	6.5 ± 1.1
		10^{-9} M	5.8 ± 3.0	54.5 ± 10.9	3.2 ± 0.7	26.5 ± 0.5[j]
		10^{-11} M	8.1 ± 4.2	73.5 ± 23.2	6.0 ± 1.0	33.5 ± 1.1

[a]NK target: MOLT 4; single cell assay E:T = 1:1, % TBC and % NK = of total population, % cytotoxic TBC = of total TBC population, % NK = % TBC × % cytotoxic TBC; % ^{51}Cr release: E:T = 20:1.

[b]Ten MS patients: 1 acute relapsing type patient experiencing an exacerbation, 9 patients in progression. OND patients: 2 stroke, 1 polymyositis, 2 muscular dystrophy, 3 Friedreich's ataxia.

[c]Controls were age- and sex-matched. Data are pooled because individual control groups for MS and OND were not significantly different from each other.

[d]Indomethacin, 3×10^{-8} M.

[e]Mean ±SD.

[f]$p < 0.05$: statistical evaluation using Wilcoxon signed ranks test comparing patient and age- and sex-matched normal control.

[g]$p < 0.01$.

[h]Not significant.

[i]$p < 0.02$.

[j]ns, not significant; not significant if not specified.

If all LGL that bind antibody-coated Chang cells could kill, the LGL alone could account for the % K cells measured in the single cell assay in the NWP PBL of normals as well as OND patients (TABLE 3). In contrast, acute relapsing and chronic MS patients do not have lower proportions of LGL binding the K cell target, but they have an increased proportion of K cells compared with controls; thus, 50–55% of K cell activity in MS must be mediated by a non-LGL (TABLE 3). Similarly, in the CSF of MS and OND, despite detectable levels of LGL, very few of them bind to Chang cells, even in the presence of antibody. The proportion of LGL binding to Chang cells is far less than the % K cells measured by the single cell assay (TABLE 3). Together these data point to the existence of a non-LGL population capable of mediating NK in controls and NK and K cell-like activities in MS patients. Even though LGL are present in CSF, they do not appear to mediate NK or K activity, suggesting K cell activity in the CNS is normally mediated by a small mononuclear lymphocyte. It is known that lymph node NK cells may be distinguished from the blood NK cell[33]; the K cell may vary in its morphology from organ to organ, especially in a sequestered organ like the CNS.[34]

Unable to assign a defect in NK cell numbers directly to aberrations in LGL numbers, we examined the possibility of inhibition of NK by PGE. The fact that K cells are not as easily modulated by immunomodulators such as IFN and PGE_1 (TABLE 4),[15] and when they are, not to as dramatic a degree as NK cells, suggests an inherent homeostatic regulation of the cytotoxic machinery in these cells and may account for the discrepancy between normal or high ADCC and low NK in MS patients (TABLES 2 and 3). Thus the alternative explanation for the depressed NK activity seen in MS patients was hypothesized to be continuously increased concentration of immunosuppressive prostaglandin produced by activated monocytes/macrophages. Such activation could be mediated by immune complexes circulating in the peripheral blood[35] and in CSF.[35–37] Prostaglandins are known to increase intracellular levels of cyclic AMP rapidly, which leads to a turn off of NK cytotoxicity.[11,12] In normal individuals a subpopulation of monocytes has been shown to produce prostaglandins *in vitro* spontaneously.[38] In our earlier work we have also shown that co-cultivation *in vitro* of human NK cells and autologous monocytes results in rapid decrease of NK activity which most probably is prostaglandin-mediated as it is blocked by prostaglandin synthetase inhibitors.[13] Interestingly, the degree of NK suppression is related to the amount of prostaglandin exposure, as short-term exposure is reversible in character in contrast to long-term exposure. Thus, exposure of human NK cells to endogenously produced prostaglandin for 18 hr leads to an irreversible decrease in TBC, as well as in the fraction of active NK cells among TBC. This situation is thus comparable with what we find in peripheral blood in acute MS patients (TABLE 1) and is compatible with a role for prostaglandins as mediators of immunosuppression in MS. If depressed NK in MS CSF is due to PGE produced in the central nervous system, the PGE-producing cells may be tissue bound and, although CSF lymphocytes are removed from the circulating CSF PGE, the long-term effects of exposure to PGE may not be readily reversible.[39] In addition, our findings of elevated PGE production (TABLES 5 and 6)[29] and increased PGE sensitivity in NK of MS patients (TABLE 4) parallel similar findings in another system by Dore-Duffy and Zurier.[40,41] Furthermore, we hypothesize that the effect of PGE on IFN production[29] is partially due to its effect on NK cells in MS patients, both at the level of recycling[42] and at maturation of pre-NK to NK and IFN producers.[23] We have shown this by demonstrating an inverse relationship in activity or production and PGE production.[29]

This article has tried to demonstrate one probable reason for depressed NK activity in MS patients. MS mononuclear cells in the periphery and an as yet unidentified source in the CNS make levels of PGE that are capable of suppressing NK in both compartments. This suppression is a reflection of both higher than normal amounts of spontaneously produced PGE as well as increased sensitivity of the effector cells themselves. Continuous spontaneous production of elevated levels of PGE *in vivo* may result in the continuous expression of PGE receptors on NK cells and thus constant sensitivity. Investigation of the ability of PGE to maintain receptors on a cell's surface is an important next step to determine if its effect lies in preventing turnover and loss or stimulating replacement of these receptors. To understand increased sensitivity of MS cells to PGE we must try to discern if these patients have (i) more PGE receptor-positive cells, (ii) more receptors or higher affinity receptors/cells, or (iii) normal numbers of PGE-sensitive cells, but defective turnover of the PGE receptors compared to controls.

REFERENCES

1. Benczur, M., G. G. Y. Petranyi, B. Y. Palffy, M. Varga, M. Talas, B. Kotsky, I. Foldes & S. R. Hollan. 1980. Clin. Exp. Immunol. **39:** 657–662.
2. Merrill, J. E., M. Jondal, J. Seeley, M. Ullberg & A. Siden. 1982. Clin. Exp. Immunol. **47:** 419–430.
3. Merrill, J. E., A. Scott, L. Myers & G. Ellison. 1982. J. Neuroimmunol. **3:** 123–138.
4. Merrill, J. E., L. W. Myers & G. W. Ellison. 1983. J. Neuroimmunol. **4:** 239–257.
5. Hauser, S. J., K. A. Ault, M. J. Levin, M. R. Garovoy & H. L. Weiner. 1981. J. Immunol. **127:** 1114–1117.
6. Neighbour, P. A. & B. R. Bloom. 1979. Proc. Nat. Acad. Sci. U.S.A. **76:** 467–480.
7. Neighbour, P. A., A. E. Miller & B. R. Bloom. 1981. Neurology (Minneap.) **31:** 561–566.
8. Frick, E. & H. Stickl. 1980. J. Neurol. Sci. **46:** 187–197.
9. Mar, P. 1980. J. Neurol. Sci. **47:** 285–303.
10. Merrill, J. E., B. Wahlin, A. Siden & P. Perlmann. 1982. J. Immunol. **128:** 1728–1735.
11. Droller, M. J., M. N. Schneider & P. Perlmann. 1978. Cell. Immunol. **39:** 165–177.
12. Brunda, M. J., R. B. Herberman & H. T. Holden. 1980. J. Immunol. **124:** 2682–2687.
13. Jondal, M., J. Merrill & M. Ullberg. 1981. J. Immunol. **14:** 555–563.
14. Kendall, R. A. & S. Targan. 1980. J. Immunol. **125:** 2770–2777.
15. Merrill, J. E. 1983. J. Clin. Immunol. **3:** 42–50.
16. Schumacher, G. A., G. Beebe, R. F. Kibler, L. T. Kurland, J. F. Kurtzke, F. McDowell, B. Nagler, W. A. Sibley, W. W. Tourtellotte & T. L. Willman. 1965. Ann. N.Y. Acad. Sci. **122:** 552–570.
17. Boyum, A. 1976. Scand. J. Immunol. **5:** 9–12.
18. Julius, M. H., E. Simpson & L. A. Herzenberg. 1973. Eur. J. Immunol. **3:** 645–649.
19. Tucker, S. B., R. V. Pierre & R. E. Jordan. 1977. J. Immunol. Methods **14:** 267–269.
20. Jondal, M. & H. F. Pross. 1975. Int. J. Cancer **15:** 596–605.
21. Grimm, E. & B. Bonavida. 1979. J. Immunol. **124:** 2861–2869.
22. Levine, L., R. M. G. Cernosek & H. V. Vunakis. 1971. J. Biol. Chem. **246:** 6782–6785.
23. Timonen, T., E. Saksela, I. Virtanen & K. Cantell. 1980. Eur. J. Immunol. **10:** 422–427.
24. Timonen, T., J. R. Ortaldo & R. Herberman. 1981. J. Exp. Med. **153:** 569–582.
25. Huddlestone, J. & M. B. A. Oldstone. 1979. J. Immunol. **123:** 1615.
26. Merrill, J. E., G. Biberfield, G. Kolmodin, S. Landin & E. Norrby. 1980a. J. Immunol. **124:** 2758.
27. Ullberg, M. & M. Jondal. 1981. J. Exp. Med. **153:** 615.
28. Ault, K. A. & H. L. Weiner. 1978. Clin. Immunol. Immunopath. **11:** 60–76.
29. Merrill, J. E., R. E. Gerner. L. W. Myers & G. W. Ellison. 1983. J. Neuroimmunol. **4:** 223–237.
30. Kay, H. D., G. D. Bonnard, W. H. West & R. B. Herberman. 1977. J. Immunol. **118:** 2058–2066.

31. PERLMANN P. & J. C. CEROTTINI. 1979. *In* The Antigens. M. Sela, Ed.: 173–281. Academic Press. New York.
32. JENSEN, P. J. & H. S. KOREM. 1980. J. Immunol. **124:** 395–398.
33. EREMIN, O., J. ASHBY & J. P. STEVENS. 1978. Int. J. Cancer **31:** 35–41.
34. SCHLIEP, G. & K. FELGENHAUER. 1978. J. Neurol. **218:** 77–96.
35. DEICHER, H. H., M. Z. SCHWABEDISSEN, W. LIMAN, B. BARUTH, U. PATZOLD & P. HALLER. 1980. *In* Progress in Multiple Sclerosis Research. H. J. Bauer, S. Poser & G. Ritter, Eds.: 200–206. Springer-Verlag. Berlin, New York.
36. COYLE, P. K., B. R. BROOKS, R. L. HIRSCH, S. R. COHEN, P. O'DONNELL, R. T. JOHNSON & J. S. WOLINSKY. 1980. Lancet **ii:** 229–231.
37. GLIKMAN, G., S.-E. SVEHAG, E. HANSEN, O. HANSEN, S. HUSBY, H. NIELSON & C. FARRELLS. 1980. Acta Neurol. Scand. **61:** 333–347.
38. PICKER, L. J., H. H. RAFF, M. E. GOLDYNE & J. D. STOBO. 1980. J. Immunol. **124:** 2557.
39. KOREN, H. S., S. J. ANDERSON, D. G. FISCHER, C. S. COPELAND & P. J. JENSEN. 1981. J. Immunol. **27:** 2007–2013.
40. DORE-DUFFY, P. & R. B. ZURIER. 1979. J. Clin. Invest. **63:** 154–159.
41. DORE-DUFFY, P. & R. B. ZURIER. 1981. Clin. Immunol. Immunopath. **19:** 303–313.
42. ULLBERG, M., J. MERRILL & M. JONDAL. 1981. Scand. J. Immunol. **14:** 285–292.

Oligoclonal Banding in MS[a]

GEORGE C. EBERS

Department of Clinical Neurological Sciences
University Hospital
London, Ontario, Canada N6A 5A5

One of the most characteristic features of multiple sclerosis (MS) is the presence of oligoclonal IgG bands in the cerebrospinal fluid (CSF). It has now been some four decades since Kabat originally described the elevation of this immunoglobulin in CSF of MS patients.[1] Lowenthal subsequently showed the IgG was oligoclonal with a restricted heterogeneity seen on electrophoresis.[2] The banding pattern resembled that found in serum after repeated immunization[3] and in this context immunoglobulins in MS CSF have several features usually characterizing specific as opposed to nonspecific responses. In addition to the electrophoretic heterogeneity, there is an altered kappa/lambda light chain ratio[4] and a relative IgG subclass restriction.[5] The demonstration that cultured CSF cells produce the same oligoclonal pattern present in homologous CSF proves that the antibodies are locally produced.[6] It has been well established that these antibodies are of special use in diagnosis. Our initial experience with CSF electrophoresis has been previously reported,[7,8] and now covers over 2,000 patients examined with cellulose acetate or agarose electrophoresis (EP). The results for clinically definite MS patients are seen in TABLE 1. As can be seen from the table some 90% of MS patients showed an oligoclonal pattern. TABLE 2 demonstrates the results of patients with "possible MS" as previously defined.[9] The frequency of banding in this group approaches 40%. These results demonstrate, as have numerous others, that agarose electrophoresis is an effective and discriminating method of use in MS diagnosis.

A small number of MS patients appear never to develop oligoclonal banding throughout their course despite having autopsy-proved disease. We have shown that this correlates with the relative or absolute absence of plasma cells in plaques.[10] Of 13 cases with autopsy-proved MS three failed to show the banding pattern. The tissue sections from the three patients with negative banding were compared by blinded observers with sections from three patients showing a clear-cut banding pattern. A marked difference in the plasma cell numbers was evident, confirmed by using peroxidase-conjugated anti-immunoglobulin reagents.

As seen in TABLE 3 approximately 8% of patients undergoing CSF electrophoresis from a general neurology and neurological service have oligoclonal banding. These can be divided into two roughly equal groups. The first group consists of disorders in which there is local immune response in the nervous system or bands in the serum (see TABLE 4). These disorders include meningitis, encephalitis, paraneoplastic syndromes, neurosyphilis and others. The second group consists of a variety of disorders in which there is no obvious cause for oligoclonal banding. These are listed in TABLE 5—the most common of them being stroke. Actually in very few of these disorders was the presence of banding associated with diagnostic confusion. Previous data have also shown that oligoclonal banding in MS is relatively specific and we have previously shown how favorably this compared with diagnostic tests in other areas of medicine.[11]

It could be argued that the frequency of oligoclonal banding in patients with clinically definite MS has little practical value in diagnosis. In fact the patient posing more of a problem is the one with monosymptomatic demyelination. Heretofore it has

[a]This work was supported by research grants from the Multiple Sclerosis Society of Canada.

TABLE 1. Clinically Definite MS: Results of CSF Electrophoresis in 2150 Patients

	O.B.[a] Pos.	O.B. Neg.	Suspicious for O.B.	n
Agarose electrophoresis	212 (86.8%)	20 (8.2%)	12 (5%)	244
Cellulose acetate	250 (90.2%)	19 (6.9%)	8 (2.9%)	277
Total	462 (88.7%)	39 (7.5%)	20 (3.8%)	521

[a]Oligoclonal banding.

been difficult to prognosticate in such patients. However, recent studies carried out in our center demonstrate that the presence of banding is of considerable practical value. We followed 183 patients with monosymptomatic demyelination over a mean follow-up period of over three years. It was found that those patients having banding are much more likely to develop clinical dissemination over this follow-up period than those without it.[9] In addition to patients in whom the clinical diagnosis of MS is not possible, electrophoresis is also of value in patients with atypical presentations. A group of patients in whom the presence of oligoclonal banding has been particularly valuable is the 9% of our patient population who present it after 50 years of age.[12] The clinical syndrome in most of these patients consists of chronic myelopathy, however some 80% have oligoclonal banding in their CSF.

The method in most common use in North America for CSF electrophoresis is the Panagel system (Millipore Corporation). Agarose is bound to a cellulose backing and such gels are conveniently run, fixed, stained, and preserved. Although this technique provides satisfactory results some variability in the quality of these gels has been a problem. The technique of isoelectric focusing is capable of much higher resolution than agarose electrophoresis and has been used successfully in MS by Delmotte and others.[13,14] This technique resolves single antibodies into numerous bands differing only by post-translational differences. We have preparatively separated the sub-bands seen on electrofocusing from a single monoclonal serum band in a patient with MS and have shown that each sub-band bore the same idiotype.[15] This indicates that electrophoretic differences do not necessarily mean different antibodies. It is possible by using this sensitive technique to demonstrate bands in the serum of about 30% of MS patients that correspond to the densest bands seen in CSF.[8]

A curious feature of the oligoclonal banding pattern is that it tends to remain relatively constant over time in most patients, although small changes do occur. In rare instances patients with negative OB appear to develop it and we have documented this evolution in some 10 patients. The relative infrequency of this finding and the fact that the frequency of oligoclonal banding increases only slightly with disease duration might reflect the fact that in most patients the first clinical symptom may result from a plaque which is not the initial one—if indeed banding is a consequence of plaque development.

Using electrofocusing, one group has demonstrated subtle changes in banding pattern over time in the same patient and that Ig eluted from different plaques from

TABLE 2. Possible MS: Results of CSF Electrophoresis in 2150 Patients

	O.B. Pos.	O.B. Neg.	Suspicious for O.B.	n
Agarose electrophoresis	153 (34.4%)	274 (61.6%)	18 (4%)	445
Cellulose acetate	102 (33.6%)	187 (61.5%)	15 (4.9%)	304
Total	255 (34%)	461 (61.6%)	33 (4.4%)	749

TABLE 3. Non-MS: Results of CSF Electrophoresis in 2150 Patients

	O.B. Pos.	O.B. Neg.	Suspicious for O.B.	*n*
Agarose electrophoresis	34 (8.3%)	364 (89.2%)	10 (2.5%)	408
Cellulose acetate	29 (6.1%)	437 (92.6%)	6 (1.3%)	472
Total	63 (7.2%)	801 (91%)	16 (1.8%)	880

the same autopsied patient may differ in its electrofocusing pattern. From these data they suggested that the antibodies were irrelevant to the disease process.[16] Although this of course may be true, there are several problems with their argument. In the first place, these authors' apparent conviction that repeated immunization with the same antigen should lead to production of the same antibody pattern is clearly incorrect. The banding pattern (clonotype) in experimental immunization with the same simple antigen in a given animal changes over time.[17,18] There are numerous examples of the transitory nature of idiotype production during such prolonged immunizations. Specific clones appear to ascend and decline for reasons that are not entirely clear. If the immunological response in MS were to the same antigen, changes in banding pattern would not be unexpected. In fact, our experience is that in a majority of patients the banding pattern stays remarkably constant although small changes may occur. This has been confirmed by the use of anti-idiotypic sera to monitor levels of individual antibody bands.[19,20]

The demonstration of changes in banding pattern may have interpretations other than that of the activation of additional clones, although that possibility remains reasonable. Certainly post-translational differences may account for different electrophoretic mobilities of single antibodies. In addition a variety of proteolytic enzymes are present in plaques, and whereas IgG is relatively resistant to degradation, electrofocusing is so sensitive that minor changes might occur on this basis. It is certainly possible to produce multiple new bands from purified myeloma proteins with brief plasmin digestion (unpublished). The presence of free light chains in MS CSF provides another possible reason for altered banding patterns.

TABLE 4. Diagnoses[a] in Non-MS Patients Positive[b] for Oligoclonal Banding

G.B. syndrome	9
Viral meningitis	9
Viral encephalitis	8
Arachnoiditis	3
Polyneuropathy	3
Paraneoplastic cerebellar syndrome	3
Myelitis	2
Cryptococcal meningitis	1
Neurosyphilis	1
Chronic hepatitis	1
Polycythemia	1
Sarcoidosis	1
Lymphomatoid granulomatosis	1
Postepidural paraplegia	1
Focal encephalitis	1
Possible polymyositis	1
Diabetic neuropathy + monoclonal gammopathy	1
	Total = 47

[a]Disorders associated with local immune response or serum bands.
[b]Includes suspicious for O.B.

Since in primary immunization most of the newly synthesized antibody is nonreactive with the immunogen[21] it is possible that a number of irrelevant specificities are present in MS CSF or in plaques. Since a similar oligoclonal response is commonly seen in synovial fluid, especially in seronegative joint disease, the possibility that the oligoclonal response is secondary to the activation of a relatively few cells or reflects escape from immunoregulation in a restricted area outside the serum compartment warrants consideration.

A final point concerns what a band actually is. Ampholines establish pH gradients that are not completely linear and accordingly prolonged electrofocusing can lead to the production of artifactual bands. These are mostly clearly identified when normal serum and serum from other species are run parallel to one another. After several hours a clear-cut oligoclonal banding pattern develops but the fact that the bands have the

TABLE 5. Diagnoses[a] in Non-MS Patients Positive[b] for Oligoclonal Banding

Stroke	5
Psychosis	4
Headache	2
Dizzy spells, ? etiology	2
Disc	2
? ALS	1
C. spondylosis	1
Vertigo, ? etiology	1
Arnold-Chiari	1
Supranuclear palsy	1
CNS leukemia	1
Syncope	1
TIAs	1
Amyotrophy, ? cause	1
Spinal stenosis	1
Medulloblastoma	1
Acoustic neuroma	1
Reticular cell sarcoma	1
? Brain tumor	1
Possible metabolic myopathy	1
Spinocerebellar degeneration	1
Spondylitic myelopathy	1
	Total = 32

[a]Disorders not associated with local immune response or serum bands.
[b]Includes suspicious for O.B.

identical isoelectric points in all samples indicates their artifactual nature. These bands may be seen in some reported work.

We have compared agarose electrophoresis using commercial plates with laboratory-made agarose isoelectric focusing gels. Four hundred thirty consecutive neurological patients in whom CSF was available for electrophoresis were compared using these two methods (Voulters *et al.*, in preparation). The results are seen in FIGURE 1. A higher yield of positive results is found in both the clinically definite and possible groups using isoelectric focusing (IEF). The frequency in non-MS patients is higher with IEF than by electrophoresis although when patients with indefinite banding are added to those which are positive the results are not very different. The high frequency of the indefinite results with agarose electrophoresis reflects to a large extent the variability in the commercial agarose plates and better results can be obtained if these are excluded.

One approach to the study of CSF bands has been to produce antibodies that are anti-idiotypic to the CSF bands. Using the techniques of preparative electrofocusing and electrophoresis we have isolated bands from several MS patients and used them to generate antisera.[19,20] These antisera have proved useful in the study of MS CSF bands. A number of issues were examined using these antisera.

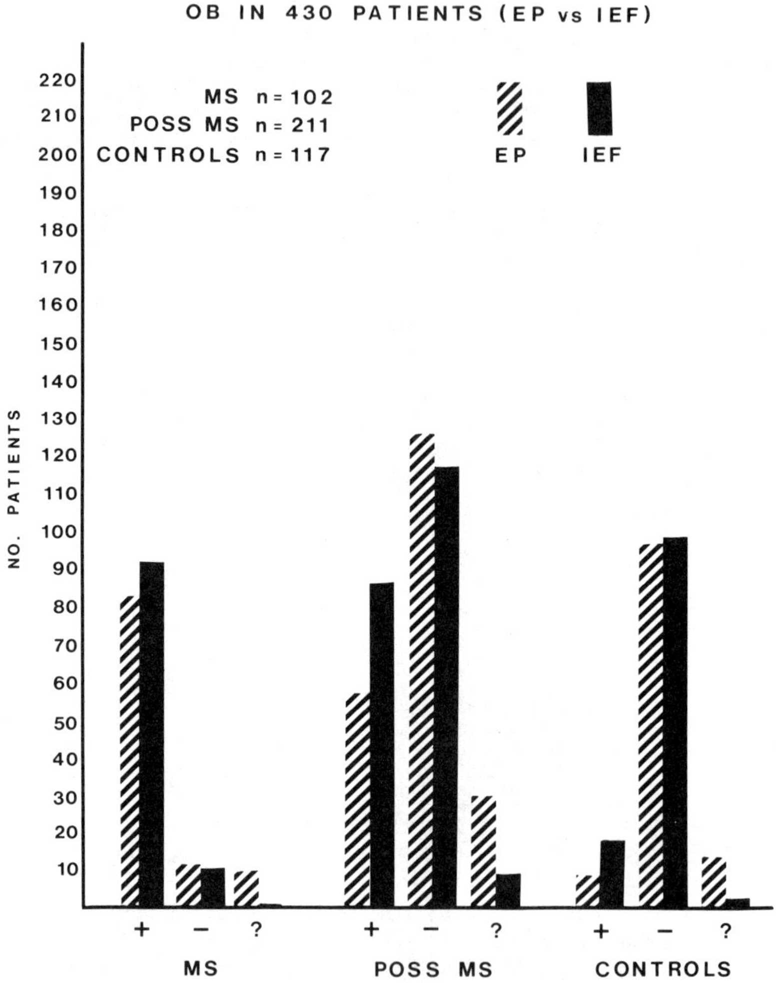

FIGURE 1. Comparison of oligoclonal banding results by agarose electrophoresis (EP) and isoelectric focusing (IEF); positive oligoclonal banding (+); negative oligoclonal banding (−); indefinite oligoclonal banding (?).

The first of these concerns the possibility of cross-idiotypic specificities. Using several different antisera no cross-idiotypic specificities have been identified. Such a specificity would suggest shared variable region determinants and in addition would imply that the idiotypes were produced against the same antigen (being coded for by common V-region genes). Other workers have subsequently found similar results.[22,23]

Since the anti-idiotype is almost always a specific marker for a given antibody it permits for the first time the measurement of the relative amounts of a specific antibody in serum and CSF. It has been rather surprising that the absolute amount of idiotype was actually higher in the serum than in the CSF in all cases. In only one instance were they almost equal. Although there is marked selective concentration of the idiotype in the CSF, given the relative amounts of IgG in the two compartments this finding was rather unexpected. If all the antibodies were synthesized in the nervous system, the relative ratios would presumably depend on the rate of degradation in the CNS and in the serum compartment. In addition, the relative rates of egress of the antibodies, (with bulk CSF flow) and ingress (limited by blood-CSF barrier) would play a role. The possibility for a relative sink effect is present such that antibodies will enter the serum compartment more easily than they leave it to enter the CSF. It is more likely that oligoclonal antibodies are synthesized both inside and outside the nervous system and the ratios raise suspicion that the B cells underwent their initial clonal expansion outside the nervous system.

Serial studies in two patients show that the level of idiotype remains relatively constant over two years of observation. Studies in an autopsied patient showed similar idiotype levels in IgG eluted from several different plaques.

We have previously shown that the interaction of anti-idiotype with idiotype can be used as a screen for antigen using antimeasles antibodies in SSPE because this interaction could be blocked by measles antigen.[19] Similar studies were carried out with anti-idiotype–idiotype in MS. Specifically, we have attempted to inhibit the interaction between anti-idiotype and idiotype using brain extracts, but without success. Furthermore, cellular activity to anti-idiotype could not be demonstrated in the patients in whom the idiotype was obtained. We have discussed some possible therapeutic implications from the study of antibody idiotype.[20]

To summarize, oligoclonal banding is useful in MS diagnosis and in the prognosis of monosymptomatic disease. We now use agarose electrofocusing as our routine method but the somewhat higher frequency of banding in non-MS must be taken into account. A suitable compromise would reserve agarose electrofocusing to resolve the indefinite patterns on agarose electrophoresis. Serum should be routinely run in parallel with CSF[7,24] and the amount of IgG should be kept constant for optimal results. However, good results may be obtained without attention to this latter detail. The significance of oligoclonal bands remains unclear. The possibility that at least some of the antibodies are relevant to pathogenesis has not been excluded although it would be expected from what is known that much of the antibody is the result of nonspecific activation. The study of the idiotypes of oligoclonal bands holds some promise for further understanding the significance of the banding phenomenon. Many investigators continue to feel that a relevant specificity is present somewhere in the oligoclonal response so commonly present in MS.

ACKNOWLEDGMENTS

We thank Holly Armstrong, Brenda Bass and Carole Sutherland for excellent technical assistance and for preparation of the manuscript.

REFERENCES

1. Kabat, E. A., D. H. Moore & H. Landow. 1942. An electrophoretic study of the protein components in the cerebrospinal fluid and their relationship to serum proteins. J. Clin. Invest. **21:** 571–577.

2. Lowenthal, A., M. Vansande & D. Karcher. 1960. The differential diagnosis of neurological disease by fractionating electrophoretically the CSF-globulins. J. Neurochem. **6:** 51–60.
3. Osterland, C. K., E. J. Miller, W. W. Karakawa & R. M. Krause. 1966. Characteristics of streptococcal group-specific antibody isolated from hyperimmune rabbits. J. Exp. Med. **123:** 599–614.
4. Link, H. & H. Zettervall. 1970. Multiple sclerosis: Disturbed kappa/lambda chain ratio of immunoglobulin G in cerebrospinal fluid. Clin. Exp. Immunol. **6:** 435–439.
5. Vandvik, B., J. B. Natvig & D. Wiger. 1976. IgG1 subclass restriction of oligoclonal IgG from cerebrospinal fluids and brain extracts in patients with multiple sclerosis and subacute encephalides. Scand. J. Immunol. **5:** 427–436.
6. Sandberg-Wollheim, M. 1974. Immunoglobulin synthesis in vitro by cerebrospinal fluid cells in patients with multiple sclerosis. Scand. J. Immunol. **3:** 717–730.
7. Ebers, G. C. & D. W. Paty. 1979. CSF electrophoresis in one thousand patients. Can. J. Neurol. Sci. **7:** 275–280.
8. Ebers, G. C. & D. W. Paty. 1979. Alkaline isoelectric focusing in polyacrylamide gel of cerebrospinal fluid in multiple sclerosis. Trans. Am. Neurol. Assoc. **104:** 230–233.
9. Moulin, D., D. W. Paty & G. C. Ebers. 1983. The predictive value of CSF electrophoresis in "possible" MS. Brain **106:** 809–816.
10. Ebers, G. C., M. Farrell & J. C. Kaufmann. 1983. Oligoclonal bands in MS-clinical pathological correlation. Neurology **33**(Supp. 2): 141.
11. Ebers, G. C. 1984. CSF in the diagnosis of MS. *In* The Diagnosis of MS. C. M. Poser *et al.*, Eds. Thieme-Stratton. New York. In press.
12. Noseworthy, J., T. Wonnacott, D. W. Paty, T. E. Feasby & G. C. Ebers. 1983. Multiple sclerosis after age 50. Neurology **33**(12)1537–1544.
13. Delmotte, P. & R. Gonsette. 1977. Biochemical findings in multiple sclerosis IV. Isoelectric focusing of the CSF gamma globulins in multiple sclerosis (262 cases) and other neurological diseases (272 cases). J. Neurol. **215:** 27–37.
14. Laurenzi, M. A. & H. Link. 1978. Comparison between agarose gel electrophoresis and isoelectric focusing of CSF for demonstration of oligoclonal immunoglobulin bands in neurological disorders. Acta Neurol. Scand. **15:** 148–156.
15. Ebers, G. C., G. P. Rice & H. Armstrong. 1980. Preparative isoelectric focusing in agarose. J. Immunol. Meth. **37:** 315–323.
16. Mattson, D. H., R. P. Roos & B. W. Arnason. 1980. Isoelectric focusing of IgG eluted from multiple sclerosis and subacute sclerosing panencephalitis brains. Nature **287:** 335–337.
17. Macario, A. J. L. & E. de Macario. 1975. Sequential changes in the persistence of antibody molecules during immune response with special reference to the binding properties of the antigen-combining site. Immunochem. **12:** 249–262.
18. Montgomery, P. C. & J. H. Pincus. 1973. Molecular restriction of anti-DNP antibodies induced by dinitrophenylated type II Pneumococcus. J. Immunol. **111:** 42–51.
19. Ebers, G. C., J. B. Zabriskie & H. G. Kunkel. 1979. Oligoclonal immunoglobulins in subacute sclerosing panencephalitis and multiple sclerosis: A study of idiotypic determinants. Clin. Exp. Immunol. **35:** 67–75.
20. Ebers, G. C. 1982. A study of CSF idiotypes in MS. Scand. J. Immunol. **16:** 151–162.
21. Askonas, B. A. & J. H. Humphrey. 1958. Formation of specific antibodies and γ-globulin in vitro. A study of the synthetic ability of various tissues from rabbits immunized by different methods. Biochem. J. **68:** 252–261.
22. Baird, L. G., T. G. Tachovsky, M. Sandberg-Wollheim, H. Koprowski & A. Nisonoff. 1980. Identification of an unique idiotype in cerebrospinal fluid and serum of a patient with multiple sclerosis. J. Immunol. **124:** 2324–2328.
23. Nagelkerken, L. M., R. C. Aalberse, H. K. Van Walbeek & T. A. Out. 1980. Preparation of antisera directed against the idiotype(s) of immunoglobulin G from the cerebrospinal fluid of patients with multiple sclerosis. J. Immunol. **125:** 384–389.
24. Walsh, M. J. & W. W. Tourtellotte. 1983. The cerebrospinal fluid in multiple sclerosis. *In* Multiple Sclerosis. J. F. Hallpike, C. W. Adams & W. W. Tourtellotte, Eds.: 275–359. Williams and Wilkins. Baltimore.

Antibodies to Glycosphingolipids in Patients with Multiple Sclerosis[a]

TAMAO ENDO,[b] S. SCOTT STEWART,[c]
SAMAR K. KUNDU,[b] SUSAN OSOVITZ,[b] AND
DONALD M. MARCUS[b,d]

[b]*Department of Medicine*
[c]*Department of Neurology*
[d]*Department of Microbiology and Immunology*
Baylor College of Medicine
Houston, Texas 77030

INTRODUCTION

Although antibodies to glycosphingolipids (GSLs) have been detected in the sera of patients with multiple sclerosis (MS), there is conflicting evidence concerning their frequency, specificity, and occurrence in other diseases.[1–5] Antibodies to asialo G_{M1} (TABLE 1) have been reported to occur in patients with systemic lupus erythematosus (SLE) with neurological involvement, but not in other patients with active SLE or in patients with other neurological diseases.[6] The long-term objectives of this study are to analyze the specificity of human anti-GSL antibodies, to determine their incidence in immunological and nonimmunological diseases that affect the nervous system, and to examine temporal fluctuations of antibody levels in relation to disease activity. In this report we present data on the frequent occurrence of antibodies to G_{M1} and asialo G_{M1} in the sera of patients with MS, SLE, and in individuals who have sustained traumatic or ischemic brain damage.

MATERIALS AND METHODS

Sphingomyelin, cholesterol and dicetylphosphate were purchased from Sigma Chemical Co. (St. Louis, MO); 4-methyl umbelliferylphosphate (UmP) was purchased from Polysciences, Inc. (Warrington, PA). Gangliosides and neutral glycolipids were prepared and characterized as described previously.[7,8] Ganglioside G_{M4} was a gift from Dr. Robert Yu, and G_{M1}, G_{D1a}, G_{D1b} and G_{Q1b} were provided by Fidia Research Laboratories (Abano Terme, Italy). Guinea pig serum was purchased from Flow Labs (McLean, VA).

Sera

Sera were obtained from hospitalized patients with definite MS, from patients with SLE who fulfilled the preliminary ARA criteria for diagnosis of this disease,[9] from

[a]This work was supported by research grant nos. AI 17712 from the United States Public Health Service and RG 1488 A–1 from the National Multiple Sclerosis Society.

TABLE 1. Structures of Glycosphingolipids[a]

Galactosylceramide	Gal-Cer
G_{M4}	NeuAc(α2–3)Gal-Cer
G_{D3}	NeuAc(α2–8)NeuAc(α2–3)Gal(β1–4)Glc-Cer
AsG_{M1}	Gal(β1–3)GalNAc(β1–4)Gal(β1–4)Glc-Cer
G_{M1}	Gal(β1–3)GalNAc(β1–4)Gal(β1–4)Glc-Cer | (α2–3) NeuAc
G_{D1a}	Gal(β1–3)GalNAc(β1–4)Gal(β1–4)Glc-Cer | (α2–3) |(α2–3) NeuAc NeuAc

[a]Nomenclature of Svennerholm.[16] Abbreviations: Gal, D-galactose; Glc, D-glucose; GalNAc, *N*-acetyl-D-galactosamine; NeuAc, *N*-acetyl neuraminic acid; Cer, ceramide (*N*-acylsphingosine).

comatose patients who were hospitalized in the Neurosurgical Intensive Care Unit following cranial trauma, and from patients with major cerebrovascular accidents. Control sera were obtained from healthy volunteers. The sera were stored at −20°C, and before testing the thawed specimens were inactivated by heating at 56° for 30 min and then centrifuged at 80,000 rpm for 15 minutes in an Airfuge (Beckman Instruments, Palo Alto, CA).

Preparation of Liposomes

A solution of sphingomyelin (1 μmol), dicetylphosphate (0.1 μmol), cholesterol (1 μmol) and glycolipids (20 μg) was dried in a rotary evaporator, stored for at least 1 hr *in vacuo*, and then the lipid film was swollen in 200 μl of 100 mM UmP solution at 60° by vigorous vortexing for 1 min. The preparation was then centrifuged twice at

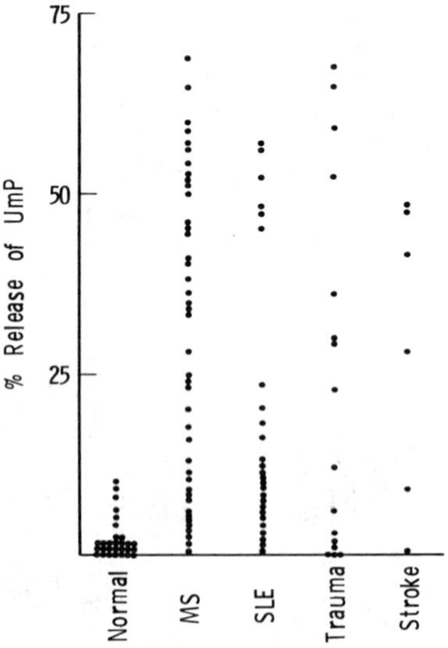

FIGURE 1. The percentage of UmP marker released from G_{M1} liposomes by sera of normal individuals and patients.

10,000 rpm for 10 min to remove untrapped UmP. The liposome lysis assay was performed by the method of Six *et al.*[10] The total reaction mixture of 1 ml contained 10 μl of liposomes, 5 μl of *E. coli* alkaline phosphatase (Sigma Chemical Co.), 30 μl of guinea pig serum, 15 μl of human serum and 20 mM Tris-HCI (pH 8.0) containing 150 mM NaCl, 0.15 mM Ca^{++} and 0.5 mM Mg^{++}. After incubation for 1 hr at room temperature the quantity of UmP released from the liposomes was determined with a Farrand Ratio Fluorometer-2 (Farrand Optical Co., Inc., Valhalla, NY).

Determination of Immunoglobulin Class

Samples of 0.1 ml of human sera diluted with 0.4 ml of Tris buffer (20 mM Tris-HCI, pH 7.4, 150 mM NaCl) were incubated with 0.2 ml of either Sepharose 4B, concanavalin A-Sepharose 4B or protein A Sepharose CL 4B (Pharmacia Fine Chemicals, Piscataway, NJ) with gentle rocking for 1 hr at 4°C.[11] After centrifugation at 500 rpm for 30 s, aliquots of 0.025 ml, 0.05 ml, 0.1 ml and 0.15 ml of the supernatant were assayed by the lipsome lysis technique.

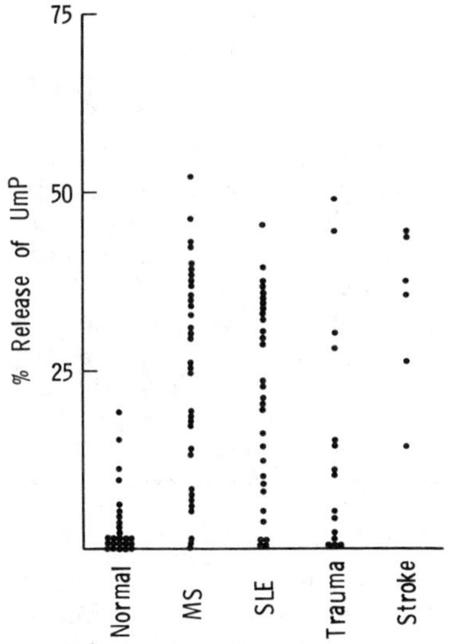

FIGURE 2. The percentage of UmP marker released from asialo G_{M1} liposomes by sera of normal individuals and patients.

RESULTS

Specificity of Lysis Assay

Most normal sera released less than 10% of the marker from liposomes that contained GSLs (FIGS. 1 and 2), and the sera that released more than this amount were considered to be positive. No significant lysis occurred if the GSL was omitted from the liposome or if the complement was inactivated by heating. To demonstrate that the lytic factor was an immunoglobulin, aliquots of six positive sera were passed over an

TABLE 2. Incidence of Antibodies to GSLs

Disease	No. of Samples	No. of Pos.[a]	Glycolipid in Liposome				
			G_{M1}	AsG_{M1}	Gal-Cer	G_{D1a}	G_{M4}
MS	81	60	48	41	1	2	3
SLE	42	24	13	21	4	3	6
Trauma	11	8	5	5	0	0	1
Stroke	6	6	4	6	1	0	2

[a]Release of greater than 10% of the marker from liposomes constitutes a positive test. Positive sera contain antibodies to one or more glycolipids.

immunoadsorbent column that contained affinity-purified goat antibodies to human immunoglobulins, or over a control column that contained normal goat IgG. The lytic activity was completely removed by the antihuman immunoglobulin column and was unaffected by the control column (data not shown).

Incidence of Antibodies

The sera of approximately 74% of the MS patients and 57% of the SLE patients contained antibodies to one or more GSLs (TABLE 2), as did most of the patients who had extensive head trauma or large cerebrovascular accidents. Antibodies against G_{M1} and asialo G_{M1} were detected most frequently in all categories of patients. Data on the frequency with which antibodies to G_{M1} and asialo G_{M1} occurred in the same sera or separately are presented in TABLE 3. Among patients who had antibodies to GSLs, antibodies to asialo G_{M1} only were found in 14/59 paients with MS and 1/22 patients with SLE, a significant difference ($p = 0.045$, Chi-square). Antibodies to asialo G_{M1} only occurred in 8/59 patients with MS and 9/22 patients with SLE ($p = 0.007$).

Immunoglobulin Class of the Antibodies

The immunoglobulin class of the antibodies was analyzed by preincubating sera with protein A-Sepharose to remove IgG and with Con A-Sepharose to remove IgM.[11] The Con A-Sepharose removed all antibodies to G_{M1} and asialo G_{M1} from ten sera, but no decrease in antibody titer resulted from preincubation with protein A-Sepharose or unsubstituted Sepharose (data not shown). These observations indicate that all of the lytic activity in these sera were present in the IgM class.

Temporal Variation in Antibody Titer

Initial studies of sera obtained from patients during a three-month period revealed no significant changes in antibodies to G_{M1} and asialo G_{M1} in 7/9 and 5/9 patients,

TABLE 3. Antibodies to G_{M1} and Asialo G_{M1}

Disease	No. of Samples	No. of Pos.[a]	Both Antibodies	G_{M1} Only	AsG_{M1} Only
MS	81	59	37	14	8
SLE	42	22	12	1	9

[a]Release of greater than 10% of the marker from the liposome constitutes a positive test.

respectively (FIG. 3). Changes in both antibodies were concordant in two patients, patient 82 developed antibodies against both GSLs, and antibodies against both disappeared in patient 92. Patients 85 and 93 had antibodies to asialo G_{M1} only when studied initially, and these antibodies disappeared three months later.

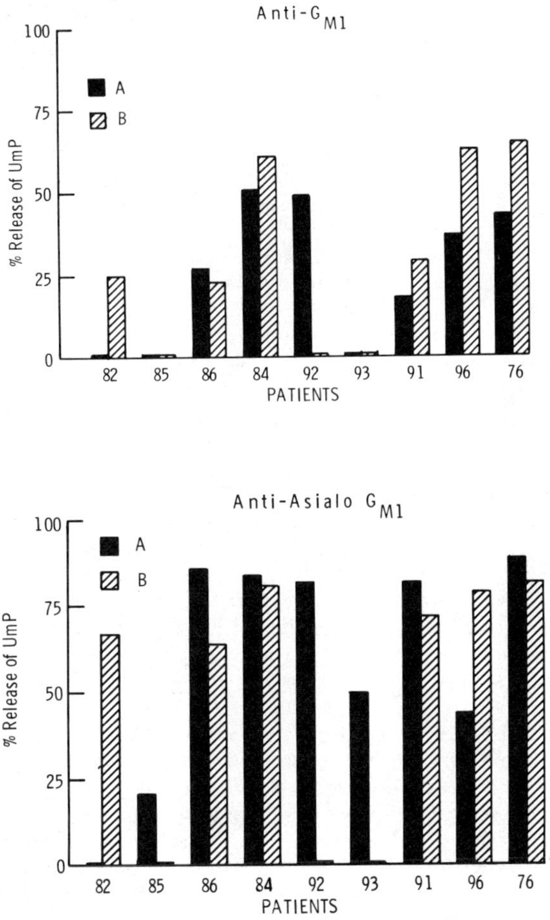

FIGURE 3. The release of marker from liposomes that contain G_{M1} (*upper panel*) or asialo G_{M1} (*lower panel*) by sera from nine patients with multiple sclerosis. The solid bars (*A*) represent the initial serum sample and the hatched bars (*B*) represent a sample obtained 3–4 months later.

DISCUSSION

These observations demonstrate that antibodies to G_{M1} and asialo G_{M1} are present in the majority of patients with MS. Although some patients had antibodies to only one of these GSLs, most patients had antibodies to both compounds. Our previous studies[12,13] of rabbit IgG antibodies raised against these glycolipids indicated that antiasialo G_{M1} antibodies were highly specific whereas anti-G_{M1} antibodies cross-reacted extensively with asialo G_{M1}, G_{D1b} and to a lesser extent with other glycolipids. We have analyzed four human sera that contained antibody to both glycolipids and found a similar pattern of specificity, namely, extensive cross-reaction of anti-G_{M1} antibodies with asialo G_{M1} but no reaction of antiasialo G_{M1} with G_{M1}.[14] These data indicate that sera which react with both GSLs contain a mixture of specific antibodies directed against asialo G_{M1} and antibodies that cross-react with both GSLs. A predominance of antibodies against these two compounds is also observed when rabbits are immunized with mixed brain gangliosides,[15] despite the fact that asialo G_{M1} is present only in trace amounts in brain tissue and G_{M1} is not the most abundant ganglioside. It is not clear whether the more abundant compounds, G_{D1a}, G_{D1b}, and G_{T1b}, are intrinsically less immunogenic or if they are hydrolyzed by neuraminidases that are present in inflammed tissues.

Our data differ from previous publications in several aspects. In contrast to Mullin *et al.*,[4] we did not observe significant release of trapped marker from liposomes in the absence of complement, nor did we find an extensive overlap of reactivity between normal and MS sera. We also observed more extensive release of marker than Arnon *et al.*,[5] most of whose positive sera released less than 20% of marker. We feel that certain technical aspects of liposome preparation and composition are crucial for obtaining stable liposomes that contain a large quantity of trapped marker. Liposomes that contain sphingomyelin exhibit less spontaneous release than those made with lecithin, and in forming the liposomes it is necessary to heat the suspension above the transition temperature of the lipids in order to trap a large amount of marker. We found no correlation between the presence of antibodies to asialo G_{M1} and neurological manifestations in patients with SLE, in contrast to a previous report.[6] Hirano *et al.* used a liposome agglutination technique that is much less sensitive than the liposome lysis assay that we used, but the apparent discrepancy between our reports cannot be attributed solely to this technical difference. We found comparable titers of antibodies to asialo G_{M1} and G_{M1} in patients with SLE, whereas no anti-G_{M1} antibodies were noted by Hirano *et al.* We did note, however, that the occurrence of antiasialo G_{M1} was significantly more frequent in patients with SLE than with MS.

We were unable to demonstrate the antibodies to these glycolipids by means of a solid phase enzyme-linked immunoadsorbent assay (ELISA). In our experience, the liposome lysis assay is more sensitive than the ELISA for measuring antibodies to GSLs, and some anti-GSL monoclonal antibodies give remarkably low titers in the ELISA assay. For example, we have compared the titers obtained in the liposome lysis and ELISA assays of three IgM monoclonal antibodies to glycolipids.[14] The titers obtained in the liposome lysis assay were five times, thirty times, and one thousand times higher than with the ELISA assay. The probable explanation for this observation is that many antibodies to carbohydrate determinants have relatively low association constants. Antibodies that have low association constants would be disassociated from antigen by the extensive washing procedure used in solid phase immunoassays. It is important to be aware of the possibility that the ELISA might not detect either polyclonal or monoclonal antibodies that could be detected by a liposome assay or by complement fixation.

Several factors might contribute to the appearance of these antibodies in our study population. The frequency of antibodies in the sera of patients who have experienced traumatic or ischemic injury to the CNS suggests that the antibodies can arise in response to inflammation and damage of neural tissues. Patients with MS or SLE do not generally have as extensive or severe damage to their nervous system as the trauma and stroke patients. A more appropriate control group would be patients with similar patchy lesions. A second possibility is that these antibodies are part of the polyclonal hypergammaglobulinemia. Finally, the antibodies may represent an autoimmune process that is responsible for some of the neuropathology associated with these diseases. A cellular immune response to gangliosides has been reported in patients with MS,[16,17] but highly purified gangliosides were not used in these studies, and the assay that was employed, formation of active E rosettes, is not widely used in studies of cellular immunity. At this time we are unable to evaluate the relative contributions of these factors in eliciting anti-GSL antibodies, nor can we determine whether these antibodies play a role in initiating or perpetuating the neural lesions of patients with MS or SLE. We are currently performing more longitudinal studies of patients to determine if the antibody titers fluctuate in relation to disease activity, and to ascertain if these antibodies can be demonstrated in cerebrospinal fluid.

SUMMARY

Antibodies to one or more glycosphingolipids were detected by means of a liposome lysis assay in the sera of 60/81 patients with multiple sclerosis, 24/42 patients with systemic lupus erythematosus and in the majority of patients with cranial trauma or cerebrovascular accidents. Antibodies against ganglioside G_{M1} and asialo G_{M1} were found most commonly and they were frequently present in the same sera. Among patients whose sera contained antibodies to glycolipids, anti-G_{M1} alone occurred more frequently in patients with multiple sclerosis (14/59) than in systemic lupus erythematosus (1/22; $p = 0.045$) and antiasialo G_{M1} alone was more common in patients with lupus (9/22) than in patients with multiple sclerosis (8/59, $p = 0.007$). In 10 sera analyzed, all of the antibodies against these two glycolipids were of the IgM class, and some fluctuation in antibody titers was noted over a three-month period. The role of these antibodies in the initiation or perpetuation of inflammatory diseases of the central nervous system remains to be determined.

ACKNOWLEDGMENTS

The authors thank Ms. Charlene Shackelford for assistance in the preparation of this manuscript, and Fidia Research Laboratories for their interest and support. Computational assistance was provided by the CLINFO Project, funded by the Division of Research Resources of the NIH under grant no. RR–00350.

REFERENCES

1. Yokoyama, M., E. G. Trams & R. O. Brady. 1962. Sphingolipid antibodies in sera of animals and patients with central nervous system lesions. Proc. Soc. Exp. Biol. Med. **11:** 350.
2. Hirsch, H. E. & M. E. Parks. 1976. Serological reactions against glycolipid-sensitized liposomes in multiple sclerosis. Nature **264:** 785.
3. Ryberg, B. 1978. Multiple specificities of antibrain antibodies in multiple sclerosis and chronic myelopathy. J. Neurol. Sci. **38:** 357.
4. Mullin, B. R., A. J. Montanaro, J. D. Reid & R. N. Nishimura. 1979. Interaction of multiple sclerosis serum with liposomes containing ganglioside G_{M1}. Ann. Neurol. **7:** 587.
5. Arnon, R., E. Crisp, R. Kelley, G. W. Ellison, L. W. Myers & W. W. Tourtellotte. 1980. Anti-ganglioside antibodies in multiple sclerosis. J. Neurol. Sci. **46:** 179.

6. Hirano, T., H. Hashimoto, Y. Shiokawa, M. Iwamori, Y. Nagai, M. Kasai, Y. Ochiai & K. Okumura. 1980. Anti-glycolipid autoantibody detected in the sera from systemic lupus erythematosus patients. J. Clin. Invest. **66:** 1437.
7. Kundu, S. K., A. Suzuki, B. Sabo, J. McCreary, E. Niver, R. Harman & D. M. Marcus. 1981. Erythrocyte glycosphingolipids of four siblings with the rare blood group p phenotype and their parents. J. Immunogenet. **8:** 357.
8. Kundu, S. K., M. A. Pleatman, W. A. Redwine, A. E. Boyd & D. M. Marcus. 1983. Binding of monoclonal antibody A2B5 to gangliosides. Biochem. Biophys. Res. Commun. **116:** 836.
9. Tan, E. M., A. S. Cohen, J. F. Fries, A. T. Masi, D. J. McShane, N. F. Rothfield, J. G. Schaller, N. Talal & R. Winchester. 1982. The revised 1982 criteria for the classification of systemic lupus erythematosus. Arthritis Rheum. **25:** 1271.
10. Six, H. R., W. W. Young, K. Uemura & S. C. Kinsky. 1974. Effect of antibody-complement on multiple vs. single compartment liposomes. Application of a fluorometric assay for following changes in liposomal permeability. Biochemistry **13:** 4050.
11. Boyle, M. D. P. & J. J. Langone. 1980. A simple procedure to use whole serum as a source of either IgG- or IgM-specific antibody. J. Immunol. Methods **32:** 51.
12. Naiki, M., D. M. Marcus & R. Ledeen. 1974. Properties of antisera to ganglioside G_{M1} and asialo G_{M1}. J. Immunol. **113:** 84.
13. Kundu, S. K., D. M. Marcus & R. W. Veh. 1980. Preparation and properties of antibodies to G_{D3} and G_{M1} gangliosides. J. Neurochem. **34:** 184.
14. Endo, T., D. D. Scott, S. S. Stewart, S. K. Kundu & D. M. Marcus. 1984. Antibodies to glycosphingolipids in patients with multiple sclerosis and SLE. J. Immunol. **132:** 1793.
15. Rapport, M. M., L. Graf, Y. L. Huang, W. Brunner & R. K. Yu. 1980. Antibodies to total brain gangliosides: Titer and specificity of antisera. *In* Structure and Function of Gangliosides. L. Svennerholm, H. Dreyfus & P. F. Urban, Eds.: 327–334. Plenum Press. New York.
16. Svennerholm, L. 1963. Chromatographic separation of human brain gangliosides. J. Neurochem. **10:** 613.

DISCUSSION OF THE PAPER

J. Oger (*Vancouver, BC*): I wanted to know if you had some differences in antibody levels between SLE with and without central nervous system involvement?

D. M. Marcus (*Baylor College of Medicine, Houston, TX*): Thank you for bringing that point up. One of our interests was that in a previous report from Japan several years ago antibodies to asialo G_{M1} were present only in patients with lupus and central nervous disease. That was not true in our studies. In the patients with lupus there was no correlation between clinical CNS activity and the presence or absence of antibodies. The previous report also said that anti-G_{M1} antibodies were not clearly evident in the lupus patients.

Oger: Have you sought a correlation between antilymphocyte antibodies and the presence of anti-G_{M1}?

Marcus: That's one of the things that we're trying to look at.

Immune Responses to Myelin Antigens in Multiple Sclerosis[a]

ROBERT P. LISAK, BURTON ZWEIMAN,[b]
JAMES B. BURNS, ABDOLMOHAMMAD ROSTAMI,
AND DONALD H. SILBERBERG

Department of Neurology
[b]Allergy and Immunology Section
Department of Medicine
University of Pennsylvania School of Medicine
Philadelphia, Pennsylvania 19104

The pathogenesis of multiple sclerosis (MS) has long been held to be autoimmune with inflammation and demyelination resulting from humoral or cell-mediated hypersensitivity to some component of myelin and/or oligodendrocytes. The evidence to date is indirect[1,2] and Witebsky's postulates have not been fulfilled. Both humoral and cell-mediated mechanisms have been investigated using many different immunologic techniques. Many different putative autoantigens have been studied and there have been attempts to delineate MS-specific antigens in the central nervous system (CNS). In addition, viral antigens have been considered as possible targets for humoral or cell-mediated reactions with tissue damage being the result of an innocent bystander effect.[3,4] For the sake of discussion, we will consider humoral reactivity separately from cell-mediated hypersensitivity. Evidence for and against an MS-specific CNS antigen will be considered separately. We apologize for our inability to cite all of the hundreds of original articles in this field in this brief review.

ANTIBODY TO STRUCTURAL CNS ANTIGENS

There have been innumerable studies of reactivity of serum from MS patients to one or several constituents of the CNS, especially components of myelin and/or oligodendrocytes (reviewed in refs. 1,2,5,6). One of the earliest and most promising lines of investigation related to the capacity of serum from some patients with MS to cause *in vitro* demyelination of myelinated rodent tissue cultures.[7] Serum and cerebrospinal fluid (CSF) of patients in acute exacerbation were reportedly more likely to have such activity.[7–9] This activity was said to be heat labile, complement dependent and found in the Ig (IgG and IgM) fraction of serum. In addition, serum of animals with experimental allergic encephalitis (EAE), an autoimmune disease induced by sensitization to CNS tissue and a useful model of MS, seemed to have parallel activity.[7,10,11]

However, there have been problems with these studies of MS sera. First, it has been clear from the beginning that serum from some normals and patients with other neurologic diseases, especially amyotrophic lateral sclerosis (ALS) in which loss of

[a]This work was supported in part by USPHS grant no. NS11037 and a Teacher Investigator Development Award (to Dr. Rostami), by National Multiple Sclerosis Society grant no. RG894D4, and by a Harry Weaver Young Neuroscientist Award (to Dr. Burns).

myelin is secondary, also causes *in vitro* demyelination in these rodent cultures.[7,11] Secondly, it has been recently reported that addition of fresh guinea pig serum as a source of complement fails to restore the heat-labile demyelinative activity.[12] Finally, the demyelinating activity can be demonstrated in MS sera in which Ig binding to live intact oligodendrocytes and myelin cannot be demonstrated.[12] As noted below, the situation in EAE is more clearly defined. Recent studies have shown that alternate[13] and classical[14] complement pathways can be activated in normal serum by contact with live myelinated CNS cultures and extracted myelin respectively.

There have been reports of *in vitro* bioelectric blocking activity in serum of patients with MS.[15–17] The nature of this factor and its specificity for MS have not been defined.[11,18,19]

Serum and CSF of MS patients is said to cause demyelination *in vivo* in the tadpole optic nerve.[20] In addition, it has recently been found that serum from patients with MS and some normals can cause *in vivo* demyelination after intraneural injection into the guinea pig optic nerve.[21] It is not as yet known whether: (a) there are quantitative differences between MS and controls; (b) this *in vivo* demyelinating effect has the same biologic characteristics in regard to heat lability as the *in vitro* factor; and, (c) the activity is in the Ig fraction. Such factors, even if not Ig and not restricted to MS patients, could be clinically important in causing demyelination if local factors such as deposition of immune complexes[22–24] or perivascular mononuclear cell infiltrate allowed the demyelinating factor access to myelin or oligodendrocytes.

It should also be mentioned that the relevance of the serum demyelinating factor in the pathogenesis of EAE is not clear.[18,25] The demyelinating factor seems to be Ig and much if not all of it is antigalactocerebroside (anti-GalC) and is not antibody to the acute EAE-inducing antigen myelin basic protein (MBP). In fact, serum from animals with MBP-induced acute EAE does not produce *in vitro* demyelination.[26] Whether antibodies to GalC or other CNS constituents are important in augmenting the acute EAE lesion or in the pathogenesis of recurrent or chronic EAE in the guinea pig[27] or mouse[28] is not yet clear.[25]

Immunofluorescence and immunoperoxidase techniques have been employed to look for antibodies to myelin in serum and CSF of patients with MS. Whereas some groups report binding by Ig of MS patients to frozen or fixed myelin,[29,30] there are many problems in the interpretation of such data. In most reports, binding is seen when normal serum is tested[29–32] although in many, but not all studies, binding by MS sera is of higher titer.[29,30] It is conceivable that some of the low-level binding of normal and MS serum Ig represents nonspecific (possibly Fc-mediated) binding to myelin[32] and that the greater binding by MS serum Ig seen in some studies is true antimyelin antibody. On the other hand, both the MS and normal serum Ig binding could be antibody to myelin; there are many instances of low-titer autoantibodies to other antigens in normal individuals (reviewed in ref. 33). A second problem relates to the demonstration that there is increased binding to CNS myelin of serum Ig of patients with Guillain-Barré syndrome, a peripheral nervous system demyelinative disorder, and perhaps more importantly with serum Ig of patients with ALS which is not a primary demyelinating disease.[30] Therefore, even if antibodies to myelin are found in the sera and CSF of patients with MS, it may be a consequence of demyelination rather than a cause. A third consideration is the lack of evidence of binding of Ig of MS patients to intact live myelin[12] noted earlier. If antibody to nonsurface components of myelin is present in MS sera or CSF, a prior attack on myelin would be required to allow the antibody to gain access to its target.

Several years ago we examined the binding of serum Ig to bovine oligodendrocytes in fresh suspension cultures and brain sections and detected what seemed to be relatively specific binding by MS serum Ig when compared to normals and patients with other diseases.[34] Subsequently, we[35,36] and others[37,38] have not been able to confirm such disease-specific increase in binding by Ig from serum or CSF of patients with MS to oligodendrocytes of several species in various culture systems. However, in some studies, a higher percentage of MS sera bound to oligodendrocytes in comparison to normals and some disease controls.[34,39,40] It is not clear if some[37,39] or all[41,42] of the binding noted is Fc mediated. The use of damaged oligodendrocytes or the presence of significant numbers of Fc receptor-bearing macrophage microglia[43,44] in culture systems can cause great difficulty in interpretation of binding unless the cell populations are unequivocally identified by their phenotypic markers.[45,46]

Many studies have examined the binding of serum and CSF of MS patients and controls to various components of CNS tissue and myelin using assays that range in sensitivity from precipitin reactions to complement fixation to radioimmunoassays (RIA) and enzyme-linked immunoadsorbant assays (ELISAs). Antigens tested have included: (a) crude extracts of brain,[47] (b) lipids, including mixed lipid extracts (reviewed in refs. 5,6), gangliosides[48,49] as well as other glycolipids including galactocerebroside,[6,50,51,52] and (c) proteins including MBP[5,53–58] and myelin proteolipid.[59] It is impossible to review these papers individually here, but we believe it is fair to say that as yet there is no incontrovertible evidence for increased antibody reactivity to any of these antigens that is specific for MS or related disorders such as acute disseminated encephalomyelitis (ADEM), acute hemorrhagic leukoencephalomyelitis (AHLE) or acute idiopathic optic neuritis (ON).

We have recently studied the binding of sera and CSF from patients with MS and controls to galactocerebroside (GalC), a major glycolipid of CNS and PNS myelin using several highly sensitive and specific assays. GalC is of special interest as a possible autoantigen in man since: (a) repeated sensitization to GalC in complete Freund's adjuvant results in a demyelinative neuropathy primarily affecting roots and dorsal root ganglia,[60] (b) antibodies to GalC bind to the surface of oligodendrocytes and Schwann cells and myelin *in vitro,* (c) antibodies to GalC cause complement-mediated demyelination and induce cytotoxic reactions in oligodendrocytes and Schwann cells *in vitro,* (d) antibodies to GalC cause inhibition of myelination and abnormalities of myelin formation *in vitro* in the absence of complement, and (e) antibodies to GalC cause *in vivo* complement-mediated demyelination of guinea pig optic nerve and rat sciatic nerve with intraneural injection (reviewed in ref. 25). We employed several sensitive and specific assays[61] including radioimmunoprecipitation of GalC containing liposomes,[62] complement-mediated release of ^{86}rubidium from GalC containing liposomes,[63] a solid-phase radioimmunoassay[64] and solid-phase ELISA.[61] We were unable to show significant differences in anti-GalC activity in serum of MS patients in comparison to that of normals or controls with any of these assays. We also found no difference between the CSF of MS patients and those with other neurological diseases that are also characterized by an increase in CSF Ig levels.[61]

T CELL-MEDIATED IMMUNITY TO CNS STRUCTURAL ANTIGENS

The similarities between lesions of MS and EAE have stimulated intensive efforts in patients with MS to demonstrate cell-mediated reactivity to myelin antigens, especially MBP, the antigen that induces acute EAE, a T cell-mediated hypersensitivity reaction. Although skin testing has been used, for ethical reasons most studies have employed various *in vitro* assays felt to correlate with *in vivo* cell-mediated immunity (reviewed in refs. 2,6,65,66).

Peripheral blood mononuclear (PBM) cells from patients with MS in various stages of disease and from control subjects have been studied for reactivity to CNS extracts, myelin, and MBP.[65–74] The majority of these studies describe some reactivity in normals and disease controls. Some investigators have found no reactivity in any subjects whereas others find increased reactivity in patients with MS, but the increased reactivity often failed to correlate with clinical disease activity. There have been few studies employing MBP fragments to determine reactivity in patients to the sequences of MBP responsible for EAE induction in various species.[75–77] In addition, we do not know which sequences of MBP might be encephalitogenic in man.

Peripheral blood mononuclear cells from patients with MS have been reported to induce *in vitro* cytotoxicity in rodent CNS cultures and such experiments have been taken to indicate T cell-mediated cytotoxicity to CNS.[78] We now know that such T cell cytotoxicity reactions are not likely to occur across histocompatibility barriers[79] so that such experiments may have in fact been studies of natural killer (NK) cell or antibody-determined cell cytotoxicity (ADCC) reactions. It is possible, however, that soluble antigen is released in these cultures and that cytotoxic T cells see and react to these autoantigens on antigen-presenting cells present within the PBM cell test population.

As noted, the low level of *in vitro* reactivity to MBP noted in various assays in control subjects, including normals, has confounded analysis of specificity of reactivity by blood lymphocytes of MS patients. It was not clear whether this was an artifact of the test systems or whether normal PBM contained autoreactive T cells. We have recently been able to derive MBP-specific T cell lines from the PBM of 6 to 9 normal individuals.[80] These cells, obtained by culture with guinea pig MBP and interleukin 2 (IL-2) exhibit cross-reactivity to human MBP and are $OKT3^+$, $OKT4^+$, $OKT8^-$. Thus, it can be shown that some normals have circulating autoreactive T cells. It is not as yet known whether PBM of patients with MS contain a higher frequency of MBP-reactive T cells or if MS patient MBP-reactive T cells are activated *in vivo* or react to different sequences of MBP than do peripheral blood T cells of normals.

Several years ago we developed techniques to allow us to culture the small number of cerebrospinal fluid lymphocytes (CSF-L) found in CSF samples of patients with MS.[81,82] We were subsequently able to demonstrate that CSF-L from patients with active CNS demyelinating diseases (acute exacerbations of MS, rapidly progressive MS and ADEM) had a greater *in vitro* response to MBP than CSF-L of patients with other inflammatory disorders of the CNS.[83,84] More importantly, paired *t* test analysis revealed greater reactivity to MBP of CSF-L when compared to PBM of the same active MS patients.[83] Patients with ADEM had increased *in vitro* MBP responses in both compartments, with PBM usually being more reactive than CSF-L. The small number of cells available precluded testing reactivity to other CNS antigens, viral antigens or standard soluble antigens. Others have subsequently found that CSF-L from patients with MS exhibit increased *in vitro* cellular reactivity to MBP[85] and viral antigens.[86]

We have been able to culture CSF-L of patients with MS and controls with mitogen and IL-2 to produce polyclonal expansion of CSF T cells.[87] These cells react in allogeneic mixed leukocyte reactions and, as would be expected with polyclonal mitogenic stimulation prior to culture with IL-2, both $OKT4^+$ and $OKT8^+$ cells can be demonstrated in these cultures.[88] We have been able to use our culture system to expand tetanus toxoid (TT)-reactive cell lines from MS CSF-L, an antigen which, unlike MBP or various viral antigens, would not be expected to be the target of an immunopathologic reaction within the CNS. These cells are TT-specific and bear the putative helper phenotype ($OKT3^+$, $OKT4^+$, $OKT8^-$). To date, we have been less successful in establishing MBP-reactive T cell lines from CSF-L.[88] Since there are T cells in the CSF that are reactive to nonpathogenic antigens, this will require demonstration of: (a) an increased frequency of MBP-reactive T cells, (b) a heightened state of *in vivo* reactivity of such cells, or (c) reactivity to a different sequence of MBP before we can begin to imply pathogenic significance to MBP-reactive T cells in the CSF of patients with MS. Pathogenic MBP-reactive T cells can be found with the CNS in EAE[89] and recently we have been able to expand MBP-reactive helper T cells isolated from the CNS of Lewis rats with actively induced EAE and successfully transfer disease with these CNS origin cells to naive recipients.[90]

OTHER CELL-MEDIATED REACTIONS TO CNS ANTIGENS

There are two other types of cell-mediated reactions of potential interest in MS. The first is NK cell cytotoxicity in which lymphocytes attach to and mediate cytotoxic reactions to various cell lines. To our knowledge, there is no evidence for MS-specific NK cell reactivity directed against normal human oligodendrocytes although glial tumors have been used as targets. The other type of cell-mediated immune reaction is the ADCC reaction. The specificity of these reactions is determined by antibody which reacts to antigen. Since the antigen binding involves the Fab portions of Ig, the Fc portion is available to interact with a cell (monocyte, null lymphocyte or perhaps a granulocyte) bearing an Fc receptor that can initiate a cytotoxic reaction. There have been studies of ADCC to MBP in multiple sclerosis.[91–93] In these studies MBP was bound to the surface of red blood cells which serve as indicator cells. The MBP-coated cells were subsequently reacted with MS or control sera and nonsensitized PBM. In this system increased cytotoxicity was reported to be mediated by MS sera. However, in these experiments MBP was artificially bound to the surface of a cell, although within the CNS MBP is not a surface constituent of oligodendrocytes or myelin.[43–45] ADCC reactivity mediated by MS and control serum and CSF are now being studied using oligodendrocytes[94] as targets. As noted, studies of interactions between MS lymphocytes and myelinated cultures are compatible with either an NK reaction or an ADCC reaction in which the PBM cells secrete antimyelin or antioligodendrocyte antibodies and cytotoxicity is caused by killer cells in the PBM.

BRAIN-SPECIFIC ANTIGENS IN MS

There have been studies designed to look for antigens present in the CNS of patients with MS that are specific for the disease. The identification of such an antigen, whether a neoantigen, viral antigen, or a genetically controlled mutation of a normal CNS constituent would be of immense importance. Although there have been reports of such MS-specific antigens,[95,96] others have not been able to demonstrate an MS-specific CNS antigen or a specific reaction between the immune system of patients with MS and an MS antigen.[97,98]

SUMMARY

Multiple sclerosis is considered to be a putative immunopathologic disease and there has been considerable effort over the years to prove an autoimmune etiology for it. To date, the evidence is all indirect and there is no proof of either antibody and/or cell-mediated hypersensitivity to any single identifiable CNS constituent whether a constituent of normal CNS or specific to the CNS of MS patients.

REFERENCES

1. Paterson, P. Y. 1977. Autoimmune neurological disease. *In* Autoimmunity. N. Talal, Ed.: 643–707. Academic Press. New York.
2. Lisak, R. P. 1980. Evidence for immunopathogenesis. Neurology **30**(2): 99–105.
3. Wisniewski, H. M. 1977. Immunopathology of demyelination in autoimmune disease and virus infections. Brit. Med. Bull. **33:** 54–59.
4. Fraser, K. B. 1977. Multiple sclerosis: A virus disease? Brit. Med. Bull. **33:** 34–39.
5. Lisak, R. P., R. G. Heinze, G. A. Falk & M. W. Kies. 1968. Search for antiencephalitogen antibodies in human demyelinative diseases. Neurology **14**(2): 122–128.
6. Leibowitz, S. 1983. The immunology of multiple sclerosis. *In* Multiple Sclerosis. J. F. Hallpike, C. W. M. Adams & W. W. Tourtellotte, Eds.: 379–412. Williams and Wilkins. Baltimore.
7. Bornstein, M. B. & S. H. Appel. 1965. Tissue culture studies of demyelination. Ann. N.Y. Acad. Sci. **122:** 280–286.
8. Kim, S. U., M. R. Muarry, W. W. Tourtellotte & J. A. Parker. 1970. Demonstration in tissue culture of myelinotoxic agents in cerebrospinal fluid and brain extracts from multiple sclerosis patients. J. Neuropathol. Exp. Neurol. **29:** 420–431.
9. Dowling, P. C., S. U. Kim, M. R. Muarry & S. D. Cook. 1968. Serum 19S and 7S demyelinating antibodies in multiple sclerosis. J. Immunol. **101:** 1101–1104.
10. Bornstein, M. B. & S. H. Appel. 1961. The application of tissue culture to the study of experimental "allergic" encephalomyelitis. I. Patterns of demyelination. J. Neuropathol. Exp. Neurol. **20:** 141–157.
11. Seil, F. J. 1977. Tissue culture studies of demyelinating disease: A critical review. Ann. Neurol. **2:** 345–355.
12. Johnson, A. B. & M. B. Bornstein. 1978. Myelin-binding antibodies in vitro: Immunoperoxidase studies with experimental allergic encephalomyelitis, anti-galactocerebroside and multiple sclerosis sera. Brain Res. **159:** 173–182.
13. Silberberg, D. H., M. C. Manning & A. D. Schreiber. 1982. Human serum demyelinates mouse cerebellum cultures. Neurology **32**(2): A84.
14. Vanguri, P., C. L. Koski, B. Silverman & M. L. Shin. 1982. Complement activation by isolated myelin. Activation of the classical pathway in the absence of myelin-specific antibody. Proc. Natl. Acad. Sci. U.S.A. **79:** 3290–3291.
15. Bornstein, M. B. & S. M. Crain. 1965. Functional studies of cultured brain tissues as related to "demyelinative" disorders. Science **148:** 1242–1244.
16. Cerf, J. A. & G. Carels. 1966. Multiple sclerosis: Serum factor producing reversible alterations in bioelectrical responses. Science **152:** 1066–1068.
17. Schauf, C. F. & F. A. Davis. 1978. The occurrence, specificity and role of serum neuroelectric blocking activity in multiple sclerosis. Neurology **28:** 426–430.
18. Seil, F. J., A. L. Leiman & J. M. Kelly. 1976. Neuroelectric blocking factors in multiple sclerosis and normal human sera. Arch. Neurol. **33:** 418–422.
19. Crain, S. M., M. B. Bornstein & V. A. Lennon. 1975. Depression of complex bioelectric discharges in cerebral tissue cultures by thermolabile complement-dependent serum factors. Exp. Neurol. **49:** 330–335.
20. Tabira, T., H. de F. Webster & S. H. Wray. 1976. Multiple sclerosis cerebrospinal fluid produces myelin lesions in tadpole optic nerves. N. Engl. J. Med. **295:** 644–649.
21. Sergott, R. C., M. J. Brown, R. M. DeGeorge, R. P. Lisak & D. H. Silberberg. 1983. Human serum can induce acute optic nerve demyelination. Neurology **33**(Suppl. 2): 141.
22. Tachovsky, T. G., R. P. Lisak, H. Koprowski, A. N. Theofelopoulos & F. J. Dixon. 1976. Circulating immune complexes in multiple sclerosis and other neurological diseases. Lancet **2:** 997–999.
23. Goust, J.-M., F. Chenais, J. E. Carnes, C. G. Hames, H. H. Fudenberg & E. L. Hogan. 1978. Abnormal T-cell subpopulations and circulating immune complexes in the Guillain-Barré syndrome and multiple sclerosis. Neurology **28:** 421–425.
24. Reik, L., Jr. 1980. Disseminated vasculomyelinopathy: An immune complex disease. Ann. Neurol. **7:** 291–296.

25. LISAK, R. P. 1984. Antibodies to galactocerebroside: Probes for the study of antibody-determined neurologic damage. *In* First International Congress of Neuroimmunology. P. O. Behan & F. Spreafico, Eds.:167–177. Raven Press. New York. In press.
26. SEIL, F. J., G. A. FALK, M. W. KIES & E. C. ALVORD, JR. 1968. The in vitro demyelinating activity of sera from guinea pigs sensitized with whole CNS and with purified encephalitogen. Exp. Neurol. **22:** 545–555.
27. RAINE, C. S., U. TRAUGOTT, M. FAROOQ, M. B. BORNSTEIN & W. T. NORTON. 1980. Helper antigens are needed for demyelination. J. Neuropathol. Exp. Neurol. **39:** 305.
28. LUBLIN, F. D. 1983. Adoptive transfer of murine delayed, relapsing experimental allergic encephalomyelitis: Role of programmed lymphocytes. Ann. Neurol. **14:** 114–115.
29. EDGINGTON, T. S. & D. J. D'ALESSIO. 1970. The assessment by immunofluorescence methods of humoral anti-myelin antibodies in man. J. Immunol. **105:** 248–255.
30. LISAK, R. P., B. ZWEIMAN & M. E. NORMAN. 1975. Anti-myelin antibodies in neurologic diseases: Immunofluorescent demonstration. Arch. Neurol. **32:** 163–167.
31. ALLERAND, D. & M. D. YOHR. 1964. Gammaglobulin affinity for normal human tissue of the central nervous system. Science **144:** 1141–1142.
32. AARLI, J. A., S. R. APARICIO, C. E. LUMSDEN & O. TONDER. 1975. Binding of normal human IgG to myelin sheaths, glia and neurons. Immunology **28:** 171–185.
33. ZWEIMAN, B. & R. P. LISAK. 1979. Autoimmunity and autoantibodies. *In* Clinical Diagnosis and Management by Laboratory Methods. J. H. Henry, Ed.: 1262–1300. W. B. Saunders. Philadelphia.
34. ABRAMSKY, O., R. P. LISAK, D. H. SILBERBERG & D. E. PLEASURE. 1977. Antibodies to oligodendroglia in patients with multiple sclerosis. N. Engl. J. Med. **297:** 1207–1211.
35. KENNEDY, P. G. E. & R. P. LISAK. 1979. A search for antibodies to glial cells in the serum and cerebrospinal fluid of patients with multiple sclerosis and Guillain-Barré syndrome. J. Neurol. Sci. **44:** 125–133.
36. KENNEDY, P. G. E. & R. P. LISAK. 1981. Do patients with demyelinating diseases have antibodies against human glial cells in their sera. J. Neurol. Neurosurg. Psychiat. **44:** 164–167.
37. TRAUGOTT, U., D. S. SYNDER & C. S. RAINE. 1979. Oligodendrocyte staining by multiple sclerosis serum is nonspecific. Ann. Neurol. **6:** 13–20.
38. STECK, A. & F. REGLI. 1980. Oligodendrocyte binding antibodies in multiple sclerosis: ^{125}I protein A studies. Neurology **30:** 540–542.
39. TRAUGOTT, U. & C. S. RAINE. 1981. Anti-oligodendrocyte antibodies in cerebrospinal fluid of multiple sclerosis and other neurologic diseases. Neurology **31:** 659–700.
40. GORNY, M. K., Z. WROBLEWSKA, D. PLEASURE, S. L. MILLER, A. WAJGT & H. KOPROWSKI. 1983. CSF antibodies to myelin basic protein and oligodendrocytes in multiple sclerosis and other neurological diseases. Acta Neurol. Scand. **67:** 338–347.
41. MA, B. I., B. S. JOSEPH, M. J. WALSH, A. R. POTVIN & W. W. TOURTELLOTTE. 1981. Immunoglobulin binding of multiple sclerosis serum and cerebrospinal fluid to Fc receptors of oligodendrocytes. Ann. Neurol. **9:** 371–377.
42. GOUST, J.-M., N. BANIK, A. BETHEA & L. M. SULLIVAN. 1981. Presence of Fc receptors (FcR) for IgG on oligodendrocytes (ODC). Neurology **31**(2): 146.
43. RAFF, M. C., K. L. FIELDS, S. HAKOMORI, R. MIRSKY, R. M. PRUSS & J. WINTER. 1979. Cell-type-specific markers for distinguishing and studying neurons and the major classes of glial cells in culture. Brain Res. **174:** 283–308.
44. KENNEDY, P. G. E., R. P. LISAK & M. C. RAFF. 1980. Cell-specific markers for human glial and neuronal cells in culture. Lab. Invest. **43:** 342–351.
45. KENNEDY, P. G. E. 1982. Neural cell markers and their applications to neurology. J. Neuroimmunol. **2:** 35–53.
46. LISAK, R. P., M. HIRAYAMA, D. KUCHMY, A. ROSENZWEIG, S. U. KIM, D. E. PLEASURE & D. H. SILBERBERG. 1983. Cultured human and rat oligodendrocytes and rat Schwann cells do not have immune response gene associated antigen (Ia) on their surface. Brain Res. **289:** 285–292.
47. RYBERG, B. 1978. Multiple specificities of anti-brain antibodies in multiple sclerosis and chronic myelopathy. J. Neurol. Sci. **38:** 357–382.
48. YOKOYAMA, M., E. J. TRAMS & R. O. BRADY. 1962. Sphingolipid antibodies in sera of

animals and patients with central nervous system lesions. Proc. Soc. Exp. Biol. Med. **111:** 350–352.

49. ARNON, R., E. CRISP, R. KELLY, G. W. ELLISON, L. W. MYERS & W. W. TOURTELLOTTE. 1980. Antiganglioside antibodies in multiple sclerosis. J. Neurol. Sci. **46:** 179–186.
50. HIRSCH, H. E. & M. E. PARKS. 1976. Serological reactions against glycolipid-sensitized liposome in multiple sclerosis. Nature **264:** 785–786.
51. RUUTIAINEN, J., M. REUNANEN & H. FREY. 1982. Galactocerebroside antibodies in multiple sclerosis. Acta Neurol. Scand. **65**(Suppl. 90): 260–261.
52. ENDO, T., S. S. STEWART, S. K. KUNDU, S. OSOVITZ & D. M. MARCUS. 1984. Antibodies to glycosphingolipids in patients with multiple sclerosis. This volume.
53. LENNON, V. & I. R. MACKAY. 1972. Binding of ^{125}I myelin basic protein by serum and cerebrospinal fluid. Clin. Exp. Immunol. **11:** 595–603.
54. BIGGINS, J. A., A. TAYLOR & E. A. CASPARY. 1978. Circulating antibody to myelin basic protein in relapsing-remitting multiple sclerosis? A comparative group and sequential study by radioimmunoassay. J. Neurol. Neurosurg. Psychiat. **41:** 1131–1134.
55. PANITCH, H. S., C. L. J. HOFFER & K. P. JOHNSON. 1980. CSF antibody to myelin basic protein. Measurements in patients with multiple sclerosis and subacute sclerosing panencephalitis. Arch. Neurol. **37:** 206–209.
56. GUTSTEIN, H. S. & S. R. COHEN. 1978. Spinal fluid differences in experimental allergic encephalomyelitis and multiple sclerosis. Science **199:** 301–303.
57. RUUTIAINEN, J., T. ARNADOTTIR, G. MOLNAR, A. SALMI & H. FREY. 1981. Myelin basic protein antibodies in the serum and CSF of multiple sclerosis and subacute sclerosing panencephalitis patients. Acta Neurol. Scand. **64:** 196–206.
58. SHORR, J., B. ROSTROM & H. LINK. 1981. Antibodies to viral and non-viral antigens in subacute sclerosing panencephalitis and multiple sclerosis demonstrated by thin layer polyacrylamide gel isoelectric focusing, antigen immunofixation and autoradiography. J. Neurol. Sci. **49:** 99–108.
59. TROTTER, J. L. 1983. Studies on the role of myelin proteolipid protein in chronic progressive experimental encephalomyelitis and multiple sclerosis. Ann. Neurol. **14:** 115.
60. SAIDA, T., K. SAIDA, S. H. DORFMAN, D. H. SILBERBERG, A. J. SUMNER, M. C. MANNING, R. P. LISAK & M. J. BROWN. 1979. Experimental allergic neuritis induced by sensitization with galactocerebroside. Science **204:** 1103–1106.
61. ROSTAMI, A., P. A. ECCLESTON, D. H. SILBERBERG, M. C. MANNING, J. B. BURNS & R. P. LISAK. 1983. Absence of antibodies to galactocerebroside in the sera and cerebrospinal fluid of human demyelinating disorders. Neurology **33**(Suppl. 2): 130.
62. FRY, J. M., R. P. LISAK, M. MANNING & D. H. SILBERBERG. 1976. Serologic techniques for detection of antibody to galactocerebroside. J. Immunol. Meth. **11:**185–193.
63. SLOVICK, D. I., T. SAIDA, R. P. LISAK & A. SCHREIBER. 1980. A new assay for lytic anti-galactocerebroside (GC) antibodies employing ^{86}rubidium release from GC-labelled liposomes. J. Immunol. Meth. **39:** 31–38.
64. ROSTAMI, A., P. A. ECCLESTON, D. H. SILBERBERG, M. HIRAYAMA, R. P. LISAK, D. E. PLEASURE & S. M. PHILLIPS. 1984. Generation and biological properties of a monoclonal antibody to galactocerebroside. Brain Res. **298:** 203–208.
65. KALLEN, B., O. NILSSON & C. THELIN. 1976. Effect of encephalitogenic protein on migration in agarose of leukocytes from patients with multiple sclerosis: Variable effect of the antigen in a large dose range with a literature review. Acta Neurol. Scand. **55:** 33–46.
66. LISAK, R. P., B. ZWEIMAN, D. WATERS, H. KOPROWSKI & D. E. PLEASURE. 1978. Cell-mediated immunity to measles, myelin basic protein and central nervous system extract in multiple sclerosis: A longitudinal study employing direct buffy coat migration assays. Neurology **28:** 798–803.
67. LISAK, R. P., P. O. BEHAN, B. ZWEIMAN & T. SHETTY. 1974. Cell-mediated immunity to myelin basic protein in acute disseminated encephalomyelitis. Neurology **24:** 560–564.
68. ROCKLIN, R. E., W. A. SHEREMATA, R. G. FELDMAN, M. W. KIES & J. R. DAVID. 1971. The Guillain-Barré syndrome and multiple sclerosis: In vitro cellular responses to nervous tissue antigens. N. Engl. J. Med. **284:** 803–808.

69. YOUNGCHAIYUD, U., A. S. COATES & S. WHITTINGHAM. 1974. Cellular immune response to myelin protein: Absence in multiple sclerosis and presence in cerebrovascular accidents. Aust. J. Med. **4:** 535–538.
70. VANDENBARK, A. A., J. V. HALLUM, R. L. SWANK, A. TONG & D. R. BURGER. 1979. Myelin basic protein binding cells in active MS. Ann. Neurol. **6:** 8–12.
71. TRAUGOTT, U., L. C. SCHEINBERG & C. S. RAINE. 1979. Multiple sclerosis: Circulating antigen reactive lymphocytes. Ann. Neurol. **6:** 425–429.
72. OFFNER, H., G. KONAT, N. E. RAUN & J. CLAUSEN. 1978. E-rosette forming lymphocytes in multiple sclerosis patients. Basic protein stimulation of rosette-forming cells. Acta Neurol. Scand. **57:** 380–384.
73. HUGHES, R., I. GRAY, R. CLIFFORD-JONES & M. STERN. 1979. Lymphocyte transformation in the presence of myelin basic protein in multiple sclerosis and control subjects. Acta Neurol. Scand. **60:** 65–75.
74. OFFNER, H., G. KONAT, N. J. LEGG, N. E. RAUN, H. WINTERBERG & J. CLAUSEN. 1980. Antigenic stimulation of active E-rosette forming lymphocytes in multiple sclerosis, systemic lupus erythematosus and rheumatoid arthritis. J. Clin. Immunol. Immunopathol. **16:** 367–373.
75. BERGSTRAND, H., B. KALLEN & O. NILSSON. 1974. Effect of basic encephalitogenic protein and some peptides derived from it on the migration in agarose gel of leukocytes from patients with multiple sclerosis and other neurological diseases or carcinoma. Acta Neurol. Scand. **50:** 227–247.
76. BERGSTRAND, H., B. KALLEN & O. NILSSON. 1975. Leukocyte migration in agarose, a study on multiple sclerosis: Evidence for qualitatively different responses to intact encephalitogenic protein and to peptides derived from it. Acta Allergol. **30:** 150–166.
77. COLBY-GERMINARO, S. P., W. SHEREMATA, B. BAIN & E. H. EYLAR. 1977. Studies of cellular sensitization to myelin antigens in multiple sclerosis. J. Neurol. Sci. **33:** 111–129.
78. BERG, O. & B. KALLEN. 1964. Effect of mononuclear blood cells from multiple sclerosis patients on neuroglia in tissue culture. J. Neuropath. Exp. Neurol. **23:** 550–559.
79. ZINKERNAGEL, R. M. 1977. H-2 restriction of cell-mediated virus specific immunity and immunopathology: Self-recognition, altered self, and autoaggression. *In* Autoimmunity: Genetic, Immunologic, Virologic and Clinical Aspects. N. Talal, Ed.: 363–384. Academic Press. New York.
80. BURNS, J. B., A. ROSENZWEIG, B. ZWEIMAN & R. P. LISAK. 1983. Isolation of myelin basic protein T-cell lines from normal human blood. Cell. Immunol. **81:** 435–440.
81. LEVINSON, A. I., R. P. LISAK & B. ZWEIMAN. 1974. A microtechnique for phytohemagglutinin transformation of 5,000 separated lymphocytes. Cell. Immunol. **14:** 321–326.
82. LEVINSON, A. I., R. P. LISAK & B. ZWEIMAN. 1976. Immunologic characterization of cerebrospinal fluid lymphocytes: Preliminary report. Neurology **26:** 693–695.
83. LISAK, R. P. & B. ZWEIMAN. 1977. In vitro cell-mediated immunity of cerebrospinal fluid lymphocytes to myelin basic protein in primary demyelinating diseases. N. Engl. J. Med. **297:** 850–853.
84. LISAK, R. P., B. ZWEIMAN & J. N. WHITAKER. 1981. Spinal fluid basic protein immunoreactive material and spinal fluid lymphocyte reactivity to basic protein. Neurology **31:** 180–182.
85. CZLONKOWSKA, A., M. POLTORAK, W. CENDROWSKI & J. KORLAK. 1982. Sensitization of cerebrospinal fluid and peripheral blood lymphocytes to myelin basic protein in multiple sclerosis. Acta Neurol. Scand. **66:** 121–129.
86. REUNANEN, M., A. SALMI, J. ILONEN & E. HERVA. 1980. Proliferation of multiple sclerosis cerebrospinal fluid lymphocytes after stimulation with measles virus antigens. Acta Neurol. Scand. **62:** 293–299.
87. BURNS, J. B., B. ZWEIMAN & R. P. LISAK. 1981. Long-term growth in vitro of human CSF T-lymphocytes. J. Clin. Immunol. **1:** 195–200.
88. BURNS, J. B., F. GUERRERO, B. ZWEIMAN & R. P. LISAK. 1983. Phenotype and antigen reactivity of cultured cerebrospinal fluid (CSF) T-cells. Ann. Neurol. **14:** 116.
89. NAPARSTEK, Y., A. BEN-NUN, J. HOLOSHITZ, R. TAMARA, A. FRENKEL, M. ROSENBERG &

I. R. COHEN. 1983. T lymphocyte lines producing or vaccinating against autoimmune encephalomyelitis (EAE). Functional activation induces peanut agglutinin receptors and accumulation in the brain and thymus of cell lines. Eur. J. Immunol. **13:** 418–423.

90. BURNS, J. B., A. ROSENZWEIG, B. ZWEIMAN, A. R. MOSKOVITZ & R. P. LISAK. 1983. Recovery of myelin-basic protein (MBP) reactive T-cells, capable of passive transfer of experimental allergic encephalomyelitis from rat spinal cord. Ann. Neurol. **14:** 115.

91. FRICK, E. & H. STICKL. 1980. Antibody dependent lymphocyte cytotoxicity against basic protein of myelin in multiple sclerosis. J. Neurol. Sci. **46:** 187–197.

92. EGGERS, A. E., L. TARNUN, C. R. PLANK & E. T. GAMBOA. 1981. Hyperreactivity to myelin basic protein in multiple sclerosis. J. Neurol. Sci. **52:** 385–390.

93. FRICK, E. & H. STICKL. 1982. Specificity of antibody-dependent lymphocyte cytotoxicity against cerebral tissue constituents in multiple sclerosis. Acta Neurol. Scand. **65:** 30–37.

94. MERRILL, J. E., L. W. MYERS & G. W. ELLISON. 1984. Cytotoxic cells in peripheral blood and cerebrospinal fluid of multiple sclerosis patients. This volume.

95. ROSTAGI, S. C., J. CLAUSEN, H. OFFNER, G. KONAT & T. FOG. 1979. Partial purification of multiple sclerosis brain-specific antigen. Acta Neurol. Scand. **59:** 281–296.

96. OFFNER, H., S. C. ROSTAGI, G. KONAT & J. CLAUSEN. 1979. Stimulation of active E-rosette forming lymphocytes by myelin basic protein and specific antigens from multiple sclerosis brains. J. Neurol. Sci. **42:** 349–355.

97. ROSTROM, B. 1981. Specificity of antibodies in oligoclonal bands in patients with multiple sclerosis and cerebrovascular disease. Acta Neurol. Scand. **63**(Suppl. 86): 1–84.

98. CHOU, C.-H. J., F. C.-H. CHOU, W. W. TOURTELLOTTE & R. F. KIBLER. 1983. Search for a multiple sclerosis specific brain antigen. Neurology **33:** 1300–1304.

GENERAL DISCUSSION

A. VANDENBARK (*VA Medical Center, Portland, ORE*): A question for Dr. Lisak. In view of the EAE model in which you can essentially condition cells *in vitro* with BP and then transfer clinical disease, in those cultures the BP response is very often also fairly minimal. When you measure the proliferation response of the BP responsive clones, it appears to be relatively minimal as you've seen, but still those cells mature and can differentiate to the effector cell stage to transfer clinical disease. My point is, is proliferation really the assay we should be looking at in terms of production of clinical effector cells?

R. P. LISAK (*University of Pennsylvania School of Medicine, Philadelphia, PA*): I agree that proliferation is but one type of assay. In man one can't do the transfer experiments. People have used other assays. What I'm saying is that even since you can get tetanus toxoid-reactive T cells out of the spinal fluid, in a disease in which no one has postulated that tetanus toxoid is the target antigen, one has to be very careful that you don't overinterpret the fact that you find BP reactive cells in MS CSF.

VANDENBARK: My comment is a plea for developing assays that measure differentiation rather than just proliferation.

J. N. WHITAKER (*Memphis VA Medical Center*): A question for Dr. Ebers. Can you comment again on the serial change in the oligoclonal bands, how long it takes to change and how close together do you have serial samples to see if they're really changing suddenly or if they're not changing at all? Does this monitor anything other than just progressive disability and progression of the disease?

G. C. EBERS (*University of Western Ontario, London, Ontario, Canada*): Well I didn't have time to get much in the way of figures about that but we've examined serial electrofocusing patterns in probably 25 or 30 patients up to five years and some small changes may occur but by and large, once the pattern is established, it tends to remain relatively constant.

As I mentioned there are difficulties in interpreting what small changes mean. Now they may mean that new clones have been activated but they also may have some trivial explanation. As far as significance, I really don't know. I think the cells remain active, they continue to produce immunoglobulin; we use our anti-idiotype reagents which is a different way of measuring specific antibody levels. We find that they tend to remain relatively the same over periods as long as three years.

WHITAKER: And what about the serial changes in the serum where you detect oligoclonal bands?

EBERS: In about 30% of MS patients who are examined by electrofocusing, one does demonstrate all of the clonal bands which correspond to the densest bands that one sees in the spinal fluid. But we haven't examined those serially.

A. COMPSTON (*University of Cardiff, Wales*): I should like to ask Dr. Weiner or Dr. Booss whether they think there are enough T8 cells infiltrating the CNS to account for the changes which are seen in peripheral blood?

H. WEINER (*Harvard Medical School, Boston, MA*): Yes.

D. M. MARCUS (*Baylor College of Medicine, Houston, TX*): Did Dr. Ebers look for the presence of the idiotype on the surface of lymphocytes, either in spinal fluid or blood?

EBERS: Yes we have and the cells appear to be, if they are indeed positive, so infrequent that it borders on what you get in the controls. So the answer is, no we have not conclusively demonstrated it.

P. DORE-DUFFY (*University of Connecticut School of Medicine, Farmington, CT*): A question for Dr. Merrill. Given the very small amounts of prostaglandin detectable in the CSF, did you attempt to correlate the amount of PGE you detected with the presence of Ia-positive cells in the cerobrospinal fluid, and I'm assuming you spun those out before the measurements? And secondly, did you check for the presence of red blood cells and leakage from the serum which could contribute to the PGE levels?

J. E. MERRILL (*Reed Neurological Research Center, Los Angeles, CA*): With regard to macrophages in CSF, we tried to eliminate all cells by spinning the CSF down and as you know there are very few esterase positive cells in CSF. We did try to make a correlation but were unable to. About the time we were doing this work a paper by Fontana *et al.* appeared which showed that activated astrocytes can make prostaglandin-E, so at this point we don't know whether CSF PGE is the result of the abundant macrophage population or a cell in the CNS. With regard to red blood cells, we had no contribution in the serum from the blood samples.

D. HAFFORD (*Harvard Medical School, Boston, MA*): A question for Dr. Merrill. Many of the NK cells appear to have T8 on the surface; have you had the opportunity to look at the number of T8 cells in the patients that had low NK activity?

MERRILL: We did not deliberately look at levels of T8 positive cells to try to relate to the natural killer selectivity but we did pan out T4 positive cells and T8 positive cells and asked if any of those cells could perform natural killing. The answer is yes and in fact it's elevated in MS patients. I would say that MS patients, in contrast to normal controls, have natural killer cells that are both T8 and T4. In fact T4 would be in greater abundance than T8.

HAFFORD: Certainly looking at the clonal level one sees a variety of different phenotypes on the NK-like cells.

Taxonomy and Diagnostic Parameters in Multiple Sclerosis

CHARLES M. POSER

Department of Neurology
Boston University School of Medicine
and
Harvard Medical School
Boston, Massachusetts

Veterans Administration Outpatient Clinic and Neurological Unit
Beth Israel Hospital
Boston, Massachusetts 02215

INTRODUCTION

Technical advances in diagnostic capabilities have given many physicians, including neurologists, a false sense of security in diagnosing multiple sclerosis (MS). The increasing dependency upon the results of these electrophysiological, immunological and tissue-imaging procedures has made doctors pay less attention to the history and the neurological examination. Although some enthusiasts claim the nuclear magnetic resonance (NMR) scan will render the clinical neurologist obsolete, the actual facts are quite different. Most if not all the specialized procedures that have been introduced are not specific for MS, many of them require careful interpretation, and some of them, despite their popularity, are irrelevant. The unfortunate result is that the number of patients with what should be called pseudo-MS appears to be growing.

Another area closely related to diagnosis is the question of introducing new and experimental therapeutic regimens. These must be tried only on MS patients whose diagnosis meets certain criteria, and very specific types of MS, known only from the history. Before initiating treatment both diagnostic criteria and nomenclatural definitions must be carefully considered. Conditions that are similar in one aspect or another to MS that create problems both in differential diagnosis and prognostication are a final consideration. Among those, of course, is hysteria. Almost a century ago, Farquhar Buzzard stated that "in its infancy the name given to MS is hysteria." The relationship of hysteria to MS is so well known that it will not be dealt with here. Among the other problems of the differential diagnosis is acute disseminated encephalomyelitis, more recently called disseminated vasculomyelinopathy.[2,3] When this occurs after a benign, unrecognized or subclinical infection it is hard to distinguish from the first attack of MS. Acute transverse myelitis, chronic progressive myelopathy, optic or retrobulbar neuritis and the spinocerebellar degenerations are among the classical differential diagnostic dilemmas.

DEFINITIONS

Devic's Disease

It has been common teaching for many years that Devic's disease should be considered simply as a variant of MS. Unfortunately, there is still much confusion regarding the use of the term. Though it originally was meant to indicate the coincidental occurrence in patients of optic neuritis and acute transverse myelitis, it has also been used to describe patients with these two lesions occurring at different times. The latter patients, however, probably have MS whereas the former are impossible to differentiate from patients with a postinfectious (or postvaccinal) encephalomyelitis clinically involving the optic nerve and the spinal cord. The term is a great favorite of Japanese writers on MS: *e.g.*, Kuroiwa *et al.*[4] use the phrase "neuromyelitis optica" (Devic) as one of the three classifications of MS ("acute bilateral optic neuritis and transverse myelitis within several weeks"). Such a condition may occur in a postinfectious encephalomyelitis and is almost impossible to differentiate from it. It is curious that this term should be retained when evoked potential studies have shown repeatedly that subclinical lesions in both the optic nerves and the spinal cord are the rule rather than the exception.[5] The reason why such a combination of clinically manifested lesions is more common among Orientals remains obscure. There seems to be no need to perpetuate the use of this very imprecise eponymic term.

Benign and Malignant MS

It is not difficult to characterize "benign" MS, although it may be of several types. The patient with very minor symptoms, or the one with neurological signs that persist but do not in any way interfere with function clearly belongs to that category. Such patients, of course, include those in whom MS is noted as retrospectively based on incidental autopsy findings. Another important group consists of those patients in whom paraclinical evidence of lesions forms an important basis of the diagnosis and whose symptomatic manifestations are relatively mild. There are many such patients whose disease hardly ever interferes with normal life activities. A subgroup of this are patients whose disease progresses to a certain point and then becomes completely arrested. Many MS patients have progressed to the point of being confined to a wheelchair, and then remain at the same level of disability without the occurrence of new signs or symptoms for many years. This is again more common than suspected.

On the other hand, there is no agreement about the definition of malignant MS. What is often confused with a malignant course is the rapid onset of significantly disabling symptoms. This almost invariably designates a young person who has become confined to a wheelchair within a couple of years or even of months. Such a patient often can overcome that aspect of disability and lead a productive life, the disease remaining quite stable for many years. That course is not malignant, it is simply bad luck that a single plaque occurred at a strategic level of the spinal cord. The truly malignant illness, most often seen in the very young patient, is multisystemic in its manifestations, often including an important cerebral component, in addition to severe motor, cerebellar, and brain-stem symptoms. The patient's disability is considerably more severe than paraplegia, because his or her mind, coordination, equilibrium, and vision are also affected soon. Relapses and remissions usually come in quick succession, the latter becoming shorter and shorter, the remissions less and less complete. The early appearance of cerebellar symptoms may be the augury of such a malignant course. Probably not more than 10% of MS patients are so afflicted.[6] Nothing in a patient's genetic or environmental background, or in the pathological appearance of the central nervous system, accounts for such a rapid and destructive course of illness.

Remitting-Relapsing and Chronic Progressive Course

The value of placing patients in such categories is questionable. These are, of course, based exclusively on the clinical manifestations of the disease. The usefulness of such classifications is doubtful, since the course of illness during the first few years does not seem to be predictive of outcome. Also, basing the evaluation of experimental treatment protocols on the changes induced in the course of illness seems simplistic. The CT scan has now provided increasing evidence that enhancing lesions, which may be the best index of disease activity at this time, can be observed in completely asymptomatic patients considered to be in remission. Similarly, new lesions may appear and disappear in various parts of the central nervous system while the patient continues to progress downhill clinically.[7,8]

Ebers *et al.*[9] have demonstrated by using the double-dose delayed contrast CT scan that enhancing lesions can be found in almost 10% of patients showing no clinical symptoms of disease activity, *i.e.*, in complete remission.

In general, the clinico-anatomical correlations between CT lesions and clinical signs and symptoms are poor.[10] It is no better between the appearance of enhancing lesions and clinical activity. Evidence for subclinical activity has also been provided in an interesting study by Likosky and Elmore,[11] who showed by means of various evoked response studies that changes took place without any corresponding clinical symptoms: evoked potential changes were found in 55% of clinical exacerbations and in 40% of clinically quiescent periods in 20 patients followed for a total of 209 patient months. There are also some old, but still convincing, pathological data showing that the appearance and removal of myelin Abbau proceeds almost continuously.[12] The demonstration of many silent lesions and the recognition of the fact that undiagnosed and unrecognized cases of MS exist,[13] coupled with the important contributions made by contrast CT scanning, suggest that MS is not, as it often appears, an intermittent disease. The complete unreliability of clinical symptoms as indices of disease activity needs to be emphasized both to physicians and patients.

DIAGNOSTIC CRITERIA

The recently proposed diagnostic criteria[14] were designed to be applied to research projects such as therapeutic trials and epidemiological studies. Strict criteria should also be used by clinicians in order to avoid the increasing problem of what can best be called the diagnosis of pseudo-MS. The new criteria are the first to incorporate the results of such procedures as evoked potential studies, which are actually extensions of the clinical examination. The laboratory-supported categories also include the results of examination of the cerebrospinal fluid for increased production of immunoglobulin G and the presence of IgG oligoclonal bands. No provision has been yet made for incorporating the observations of CT and nuclear magnetic resonance scanning. These two procedures will unquestionably enhance our diagnostic capability, but will also increase the risk of false positive diagnoses.

Even experienced clinicians vary considerably in their classification of MS into various categories. No set of criteria or guidelines can serve to classify adequately all cases of MS. The best hope lies in isolating a group of patients whose diagnosis of MS is unquestioned who can then be used for comparative purposes either for the evaluation of therapy or incidence and prevalence studies. A numerical scoring system designed to accomplish just that has been proposed by Poser *et al.*[15] and illustrates the variability of diagnostic classification. The system is based upon the frequency of signs and symptoms recorded in a large series of autopsy-proved cases of MS from the United States, England, and Norway.[16] When a series of patients from a German MS center was scored, 71% were called "definite" as opposed to only 57.5% called "definite" by the center's neurologists. Conversely, in a Canadian center 72% of patients had been called "definite," but only 63% of them fell into the "definite" category of the numerical scoring system.

PSEUDO-MULTIPLE SCLEROSIS

The occurrence of signs and symptoms indicating the possibility of multiple lesions in the central nervous system often suggests the diagnosis of MS to many physicians. A typical example is that of the 36-year-old man who over a period of a few weeks complained of blurring of vision in both eyes, persisting on the right, intermittent tremor of both hands, and numbness of the left thigh. His diagnosis of MS lasted for 10 years until he was found to have a diabetic retinopathy, familial essential tremor, and meralgia paresthetica.

One of the hallowed precepts that MS patients get worse, or have new symptoms with heat, may be deceptive. A 29-year-old man suddenly developed a left hemiplegia after climbing to the top of a mountain during a very hot day. He had been perfectly healthy until that time; when brought to a local emergency room, after having been in the air conditioned environment for about 30 minutes, the hemiplegia completely cleared. He was then admitted to a university hospital with the presumptive diagnosis of MS. However, he turned out to have had a completely asymptomatic total occlusion of the right internal carotid artery.

The practice of basing the diagnosis of MS essentially on laboratory data is hardly new, although there are now many more laboratory procedures to lead the clinician astray. For example, a 46-year-old woman with facial weakness, ptosis, diplopia, dysarthria, generalized weakness, and tingling of her hands and feet was diagnosed as having MS because her CSF colloidal gold curve was reported as 5555531100. Her history of repeated episodes of parotid swelling and suppuration, absence of tears, and decreased perspiration was ignored, and no attention was paid to the fact that her serum globulins amounted to over 7 g % and that serum electrophoresis revealed a gamma globulin of 27.5%. The correct diagnosis of Sjögren's disease was eventually made.[17] Another instance is the case of the young adult with some fluctuations of clinical signs and symptoms, with an enhancing CT lesion which disappeared and whose CSF IgG was 18% and showed two oligoclonal bands. The correct diagnosis of subacute sclerosing panencephalitis rather than MS was not suspected until oligoclonal bands were found in the serum. It is essential to establish that serum content of IgG and oligoclonal bands are normal for the correct interpretation of similar CSF findings.

The lack of specificity of CSF IgG and oligoclonal bands is well illustrated by the report by Link[18] who found these parameters to be abnormal in many other conditions, but most significantly in a relatively high proportion of conditions which may be confused with MS, such as postinfectious disseminated vasculomyelinopathy (TABLES 1 and 2). The higher number of conditions other than MS with CSF oligoclonal banding probably reflects the very high sensitivity of isoelectric focusing. Most neurologists, however, are not aware of the particular method used in demonstrating

TABLE 1. CSF Oligoclonal Bands[a]

Disease	Oligoclonal Bands on AIF[b] (%)	↑ IgG Index (%)	↑ IgG CNS Synthesis (%)
Multiple sclerosis (43)	95	72	47
Optic neuritis (10)	100	60	10
Aseptic meningoencephalitis (39)	44	26	16
Other neurological diseases (906)	14	4	3

[a]From Link (ref. 18).
[b]AIF: agarose isoelectric focusing.

TABLE 2. CSF Oligoclonal Bands in Other Neurological Diseases[a]

Paresthesia (68)	32%	Chronic myelopathy (17)	24%
Cerebral infarct (162)	12%	Transient ischemia (59)	7%
Epilepsy (22)	18%	Dementia (17)	29%
Parkinsonism (15)	13%	Amyotrophic lateral sclerosis (14)	14%
Radiculopathy (93)	5%	Polyneuropathy (53)	23%
Mononeuropathy (52)	4%	Guillain-Barré (14)	71%
Headache (106)	4%	Vertigo (68)	3%
Psychoneurosis (332)	2%		

[a]From Link (ref. 18).

CSF oligoclonal banding when they send CSF for that purpose. The CT scan can also lead the clinician astray. For example, a 33-year-old hypertensive alcoholic woman was involved in a minor automobile accident and suffered a fractured clavicle, a mild concussion, and scalp laceration. Within a few days she started complaining of fluctuating numbness of her right side. Two months later she developed right leg weakness that lessened and then recurred, followed a few weeks later by confusion, aphasia, right hemiparesis, and coma. The CT scan showed several lesions, including some contrast enhancement. The diagnosis of MS was made and then confirmed by two other neurologists. Subsequent CT scans, however, revealed destruction of brain tissue with strong evidence of the vascular nature of the illness, probably a progressive hypertensive encephalopathy.

ACUTE DISSEMINATED ENCEPHALOMYELITIS

It is difficult to distinguish between acute disseminated encephalomyelitis (ADEM) and the first attack of MS. The CT scan may help if classical periventricular lesions are present, just as they can differentiate MS from spinocerebellar degeneration. Examining the CSF for IgG and oligoclonal bands is of little value.[18] Although it is impossible to prognosticate in any individual case, the data provided by the studies of Thygesen[19] and van Bogaert[20] are of value. The former followed 29 cases of ADEM and noted that 24% had developed MS, whereas the latter noted the same in 26% of his 19 cases. These two independent studies suggest that only one out of four patients in the acute phase will later be diagnosed as having MS.

ACUTE TRANSVERSE MYELITIS

Many physicians believe that acute transverse myelitis (ATM) is a common presenting symptom of MS, although this is not true. Follow-up studies have shown that respectively 1.6%,[21] 3.4%,[22] 6%,[23] and 7.7%[24] of ATM patients develop MS (TABLE 3). Berman *et al.*[21] also have pointed out that none of their 747 MS patients had ATM as an initial symptom. Postinfectious vasculomyelinopathy and complications from various vaccinations are more common causes of ATM.[25,26] One extremely important way in which ATM is differentiated from MS is by subclinical involvement of spinal roots and peripheral nerves, the signs of which are somewhat masked by the myelopathy. Asymptomatic peripheral nerve involvement was demonstrated by means of electrodiagnostic studies in six out of nine patients with ATM after swine influenza vaccination.[27]

TABLE 3. Acute Transverse Myelitis and MS[a]

	n	MS (%)
Altrocchi (1963)[23]	67	6.0
Lipton & Teasdall (1973)[22]	29	3.4
Ropper & Poskanzer (1978)[24]	52	7.7
Berman *et al.*[a] (1981)[21]	62	1.6

[a]None of 747 MS patients presented with ATM.

Obtaining visual evoked responses in patients with ATM has become popular, since it is believed that demonstrating a lesion of the optic nerve helps fulfill the MS diagnostic criteria. It was pointed out by Poser *et al.*[14] that a period of at least one month must separate the two lesions. Thus, if at the time of ATM the visual evoked responses are normal but are abnormal two months later, they can be counted as paraclinical evidence in favor of MS. Both postinfectious and postvaccinal DVMP may, of course, involve the optic nerve[27–29] and the spinal cord at the same time.

Occasionally, visual evoked responses serve the unusual purpose of jogging the patient's memory. A 39-year-old woman admitted to the hospital with ATM had no recollection of any previous ocular involvement despite repeated questioning. Visual evoked studies revealed a marked delay in latency of the response in the left eye. When she was told this, she recalled an episode of complete loss of vision in the left eye nine years previously.

CHRONIC PROGRESSIVE MYELOPATHY

Deciding if patients with chronic progressive myelopathy (CPM) who have no clinical evidence of lesions elsewhere in the central nervous system do or do not have MS is difficult. In order to determine how many such patients will turn out to have MS, a number of follow-up studies are available. Depending to a large extent upon which patients are chosen as the basis for the study, the percentages vary widely, from 2.7%[30] (all myelopathies being considered regardless of cause, including tumors) to 37%. Only a single study, that of Marshall,[31] is completely reliable in that it is based on postmortem examinations: of 35 patients with intrinsic myelopathy, 34% proved to have MS (TABLE 4). The two series by Poser[32] are somewhat difficult to interpret: 45%

TABLE 4. Chronic Progressive Myelopathy and MS (Clinical)

	n	MS (%)
Marshall (1955)[31]	52	19
Marshall (1955)[31]	35	34 (autopsy)
Garde & Kjellin (1971)[58]	45	16
Hubbe & Dam (1973)[57]	24	25
Halliday & McDonald[36]	27	37
Ungar-Sargon *et al.* (1980)[30]	520	2.7
Ungar-Sargon *et al.* (1980)[30]	108	27.8 (DEF = 12.0)
Poser (1978)[32]	1271	45 (spastic paresis)[a]
Poser (1978)[32]	1271	8.6[b]

[a]All classes of MS.
[b]Spinal only for entire course.

of MS patients (possible, probable, and definite) had spastic paresis but only 8.6% of her 1271 MS patients developed no other signs or symptoms of the disease.

Additional laboratory procedures may not be very helpful (TABLE 5). The CT scan, and in particular the double-dose delayed CT scan, would be useful in demonstrating unequivocally that lesions are present within the brain. Paty *et al.*,[33] in their series of 72 patients with CPM, said nonspecific cerebral atrophy cannot be taken as confirmatory evidence. They observed only three cases in which cerebral lesions were actually demonstrated, a very low percentage of 4.2. This probably is a representative figure, in view of the number of cerebral lesions observed as incidental findings in patients at autopsy such as noted in the recent paper by Gilbert and Sadler.[13]

Visual evoked potential studies in patients with CPM have often shown a fairly high percentage of additional lesions: Bynke *et al.*[34] noted delayed visual evoked responses in 76% of their CPM patients, whereas Paty *et al.*[33] had 44%. Blink reflex latencies were abnormal in 40 patients (56%) in the group studied by Paty *et al.*[33] Of 27 patients with progressive spastic paraplegia who had normal optic discs, 13 had delayed responses.[36] Clinically definite MS could be diagnosed on other grounds in 10 patients and of these, 8 had delayed responses. No abnormality in the VEP was noted in 4 cases with spinal compression. Of the remaining 13, 5 had delayed responses. Blumhardt *et al.*[37] studied 131 patients with CPM and noted that 38 of them (29%) had abnormal visual evoked potentials (VEPs). The 100 patients with chronic disease

TABLE 5. Chronic Progressive Myelopathy and MS (Ancillary Tests)

	n	OB %	VEP %	Blink Reflex %	CT %
Link *et al.* (1976)[40]	73	66	—	—	—
Bynke *et al.* (1977)[34]	25	64	76		
Paty *et al.* (1979)[33]	72	44	44	56	4.2[a]
(BR + VEP = 27.8%)					

[a]Atrophy not included.

of duration longer than six months had a combined incidence of abnormalities of 35%. The relapsing cases had a slightly higher rate (36%) compared with the progressive ones (33%), but the difference was not significant. The chronic cases included 17 in which symptoms or signs could be attributed at least partly to cord compression. It is important that 15 of the 20 patients with abnormal myelograms had normal VEPs. In the five patients with abnormal VEPs and abnormal myelograms, three had cervical spondylosis of doubtful significance. Of these, two have subsequently developed signs and symptoms suggestive of MS. In the remaining two cases, there was unequivocal evidence of cord compression caused respectively by a prolapsed cervical and a thoracic disk. Blumhardt's group states that the proportion of the cases in the longer-duration group with optic nerve damage (33%) correlated closely with the available autopsy data, which suggests that about 34% of a similar patient population will have demyelinating disease.[31] In regard to brainstem auditory evoked potentials (BAEPs), Deltenre *et al.*[38] speculated that cervical spine disease may impair the vertebrobasilar circulation, which would explain abnormal BAEPs in this condition. They particularly stressed the relationship between MS and cervical spondylosis first noted by Brain and Wilkinson,[39] and they stated that on the basis of CSF or VEP abnormalities or follow-up data there was a possible correlation of the two conditions in six of their own cases. They cautioned about using the results of VEPs to exclude patients from myelography.

Deltenre *et al.*[38] also pointed out that although the occurrence of fully normal results of evoked response studies in genuine MS patients has been rare (1 out of 44, or 2.3% in their series), the reports of such results are much higher (34.7%) in a group of patients classified as "early probable" or "latent" and whose diagnosis is still unsettled. Thus, the occurrence of fully normal results for the entire battery described cannot eliminate the diagnosis of MS. The yield may not be high when these procedures are used to attempt to confirm a diagnosis of MS.

Blink reflex abnormalities were noted in 40 out of 72 patients (56%) by Paty *et al.*,[33] but no results on comparable series of patients with CPM given this test have been published.

In regard to CSF oligoclonal bands, Link *et al.*[40] noted such bands in 66% of 73 patients with CPM. Bynke *et al.*[34] saw them in 64% of 25 patients and Paty *et al.*[33] saw them in 44% of 72 patients. They considered the figure of 44% remarkably low as compared to the bands noted in 91% of 131 patients with clinically definite MS. It has been shown that oligoclonal bands can be demonstrated in other conditions, but in particular in postinfectious and postvaccinal encephalomyelitis. From a review of the available literature it is very difficult to determine how many patients with CPM actually have MS.

When the paper by Paty *et al.*[33] is considered carefully, it appears that evidence for two additional separate lesions revealed in the same patient by both abnormal visual evoked responses and blink reflexes occurred in only 20 patients (patients numbered 12 through 32), or 27.8%. Since it is not clear which patients are the ones with the CT scan lesions, assuming that these patients also had both abnormal VEPs and blink reflexes, this makes a total of 23 (31.9%). This is very close to the data published by Marshall[31] on the basis of autopsy studies.

In some parts of the country, the diagnosis of MS is said to be made only after a negative myelogram. McDonald and Halliday[41] published their policy in that regard as it applies to patients with CPM. They record the visual evoked responses, perform a CT scan, and examine the CSF, presumably for IgG and/or oligoclonal bands. If there is a characteristic delay in the VEP and normal size ventricles, and presumably no characteristic lesions and oligoclonal bands, they perform myelography only in the occasional patient in whom there remains a compelling reason for suspecting compression. They point out that they have recently seen a patient with progressive spastic paraplegia with atypical but gross abnormalities in the VEP who was seen to have enlarged ventricles on a CT scan and an Arnold-Chiari malformation and myelography in surgery.

In clinical practice, nontraumatic compressive lesions of the spinal cord are quite rare in the MS age group. Most of the time, it is sad to say, there is a tendency to ignore signs and symptoms that reflect a lesion above the foramen magnum in order to do a myelogram for no other reason but to avoid a potential law suit!

OPTIC AND RETROBULBAR NEURITIS

Most writers have said that the single most common cause of optic or retrobulbar neuritis (ON,RBN) is multiple sclerosis. How often ON or RBN represents the first (or only) episode of MS is still in question, however. Visual evoked response studies have amply documented the fact that involvement of the optic nerve in MS is considerably more common than suspected on the basis of clinical manifestations.[5]

TABLE 6. Optic Neuritis and MS (All Cases of MS)

Kuroiwa (1970)[59]	10%	Japan
Kito (1970)[60]	27%	Japan
Alter (1973)[61]	39%	Orientals
Alter (1973)[61]	29%	Caucasians
Nikoskelainen (1975)[62]	66%	Finland
Hutchinson (1976)[50]	78%	England[a]
Kahana *et al.* (1976)[63]	28%	Israel
Isayama *et al.* (1976)[64]	8.3%	Japan
Innis & Landy (1979)[49]	60%	Australia[b]
Link & Stendahl-Brodin (1983)[46]	33%	Sweden

[a]Actuarial prediction.
[b]Based on 53 replies from 109 ON patients.

Nonetheless, ON and RBN, as well as other lesions of the central nervous system, can occur as part of a disseminated encephalomyelitis,[2,3,20,25–29] which causes considerable difficulty in differential diagnosis.

Many studies have addressed this problem: Perkin[42] summarized 28 follow-up studies and noted that the percentage of ON patients who developed MS ranged from 0 to 85%. A review of 10 additional newer publications (TABLE 6) gives the range from 8.3% to 66%, with an actuarial prediction going up to 78%. None of these series differentiated between different classes of MS. However, four authors did provide data on how many ON patients developed what they called definite MS. The range is from 11.5% to 28% (TABLE 7). Decreased vision as one (not necessarily the only one) of the presenting symptoms of MS ranged from 20% to 43%. Nikoskelainen and Riekkinen[43] noted that ON was the first sign of MS in 67% of their patients. Some patients had suffered from mild neurological symptoms even before the outbreak of ON but they had not consulted their physician about them. In patients whose first symptom of MS was optic neuritis, the next symptoms appeared in 83% within five years, but in three patients the symptom-free period was more than 10 years. The initial attack in MS patients is usually unilateral, but in 16% to 22% it was bilateral. Optic neuritis was retrobulbar in only 48% of the cases.

Cohen *et al.*[44] prospectively studied 60 patients with uncomplicated ON for at least five years. Seventeen of these patients (28%) developed definite MS and four (7%) developed probable or possible MS. Six of the 17 who developed definite MS did so within the first year; 45% of the women, but only 11% of the men developed MS. Both sexes were at highest risk if the ON developed between 21 and 40 years, with 51% of patients in this age group progressing to MS whereas only 12% of the others developed the disease. There was an overall increased risk of MS with recurrent ON. In series in which a CSF oligoclonal IgG was measured, the frequency of abnormal values in patients with ON ranged from 17% to 51%.[42] Link *et al.*[45] noted that 21 of 40 patients with ON had oligoclonal IgG in their CSF as opposed to over 90% of their MS cases. On that basis, they suggested that at most 50% of the ON patients have MS, assuming

TABLE 7. Optic Neuritis and MS

	Definite (%)	Probable/Possible (%)
Kurland *et al.* (1966)[65]	11.5	1.6
Bradley & Whitty (1968)[66]	20	31
Compston *et al.* (1978)[48]	24.7	15.1
Cohen *et al.* (1979)[44]	28	7

that the presence or absence of CSF oligoclonal IgG is of prognostic value. The possible predictive value of CSF oligoclonal bands was strengthened by the report of Link and Stendhal-Brodin[46] that 9 out of 11 patients with ON who had such CSF oligoclonal bands subsequently developed MS, whereas only 1 of the 9 ON patients who did not later developed MS.

Histocompatibility antigen studies have also been carried out in order to study this problem. Stendahl *et al.*[47] noted that 36% of patients with ON had the DW2 determinant, as opposed to about 60% of MS patients. However, none of the 28 patients with ON had developed other signs of MS after 5 years.

Using an actuarial method, Compston *et al.*[48] delineated the factors influencing the chance of developing MS in patients with ON. One of the items studied was the prognostic significance of the histocompatibility antigen BT 101 (which is identical to DW2). In their series of 156 cases, 70% of the MS patients had this antigen as compared to 35% of 85 ON patients. The three factors which they considered significantly associated with the development of MS after ON were the presence of this antigen, recurrence of attacks of ON, and the occurrence of the initial attack in winter. Sixteen of 85 patients (19%) with ON only had recurrent attacks, compared with 27 out of 55 patients (49%) who had developed MS. In patients positive for BT 101, the prognostic significance of recurrent attacks is even more marked: 22 out of 47 patients (47%) who developed MS had recurrent attacks compared to only 5 out of 48 ON patients (10%). Innis and Landy[49] made the interesting observation that antigen BW4 showed a significant negative association with cases of ON progressing to MS since it was present in 17 of 23 patients with ON who did not develop MS as opposed to 8 of 30 who did. According to Hutchinson[50] recurrent ON does not appear to increase the risk of developing MS even when the recurrence is in the second eye. In adults, the risk of developing MS appears to be higher for 10 years after a simultaneous bilateral attack than after a unilateral attack, although the overall computed risk after 15 years is the same for both groups. It is surprising that so few investigators have attempted to establish the presence of asymptomatic lesions involving other parts of the nervous system in patients with optic neuritis. Nikoskelainen and Riekkinen[43] performed the hot bath test (they call it the Finnish sauna) on their ON patients and found that 43.4% developed weakness of the legs and blurring of vision. Matthews[51] measured somatosensory evoked potentials (SEPs) in 39 patients with unilateral acute RBN. Abnormalities were noted in only four patients (10%). In that series, the period of follow-up has been brief and information is incomplete, but of the four patients with abnormal SEPs, only one has developed signs of MS; of those with normal SEP, two have MS.

Only when more studies of this type have revealed what proportion of ON patients do not have other lesions will it be possible to determine reliably the prognostic significance of the first attack of ON. At this time, it seems that definite MS will develop in approximately one-third of patients with ON who have no historical, clinical, or paraclinical evidence of other lesions of the CNS.

VISUAL EVOKED POTENTIALS

The visual evoked potential test has become the single most commonly used confirmatory test for the diagnosis of MS. It is harmless and relatively easy to perform, the equipment is readily available, and it is relatively inexpensive. There are, however, many pitfalls in interpreting the data collected by this means.

Breen and Burde[52] called the VEP test "an experimental but not clinically significant tool." They pointed out that it is nonlocalizing anatomically, that universal standards for performing a VEP study do not yet exist, and that many technical and clinical factors can significantly affect the results. They concluded that "at this point in time, an abnormality in the VEP reflects dysfunction somewhere in the afferent visual system with no intrinsic localizing value. The test remains an interesting experimental tool, and with rare exceptions offers little information that is of value in the treatment of a specific patient." Eisen and Cracco[53] have also warned about the overuse of this test. Although these statements may be somewhat more pessimistic than warranted by actual clinical experience, the importance of emphasizing the nonspecific nature of the procedure cannot be overlooked. The lack of standardization is well illustrated by Kayed *et al.*[54] who listed no fewer than 14 sets of normative values, right-left differences, and delivery systems, from as many laboratories.

An informal survey of VEP experts throughout the world elicited replies from Paul Deltenre (Brussels), Andrew Eisen (Vancouver), Carl Ellenberger (Cleveland), Mark Hallett (Boston), Mogens Kjaer (Holstebro, Denmark), Ian McDonald (London, England), Saty Satya-Murti (Albany), and Arnold Starr (Irvine, California). They all commented on conditions that might affect the VEP. McDonald pointed out that the characteristic VEP abnormality in MS is a delay in the P100, with a well-preserved waveform; thus conditions in which the waveform is altered are not likely to be confusing when MS is being considered. Toxic amblyopias, vitamin B12 deficiency, and compression of the visual pathways (before the appearance of visual field changes) may cause problems in this regard. A central scotoma will abolish the P100, but the persistence of the paramacular P135 may cause an apparent delay. Ellenberger stated that "any condition (ocular or visual pathway) that reduces visual acuity, and most that impair the visual field, may cause an abnormality in the pattern-reversal evoked potential (PREP). The PREP is useful for the diagnosis of MS when the visual acuity is normal; then an abnormal delay of P100 is much more likely to relate specifically to conduction delay; when acuity is not normal, the PREP merely says that vision is not normal. There are better ways to measure visual abnormalities." In general, refractive error greater than 20/100 and age above 60 may alter the response. Nystagmus may be one of the few "false positives"; abnormalities of VEP are in reality caused by conditions other than MS and thus are not false positives. Among the conditions that have been reported or suspected of causing VEP alterations are glaucoma, migraine, drusen, most of the spinocerebellar degenerations, parkinsonism, and drugs causing the parkinsonian syndrome, chronic renal failure, amblyopia, hydrocephalus, drugs such as quinine and ethambutol, diabetes, optic neuropathies and retinopathies, lenticular opacities, and most lipidoses and leukodystrophies. Few of these, however, will need to be considered when testing the patient for MS, although inattention to the clinical features of the illness and overdependence upon the results of VEP may lead to the diagnosis of pseudo-MS.

CONCLUSION

Almost 20 years have elapsed since the Schumacher Committee proposed its diagnostic criteria for MS,[54] remarkably enough, also at a meeting sponsored by the New York Academy of Sciences. The development of new diagnostic techniques that can clearly demonstrate the presence of asymptomatic lesions and the advent of more accurate methods for measuring certain components of spinal fluid proteins have led to the publication of new, more rigid guidelines incorporating paraclinical evidence as well as the results of some of the spinal fluid examinations. The clinical history and the neurological examination continue to form the basis for the diagnosis of MS, particularly since most of the ancillary procedures available are but extensions of the clinical examination. Standards for the performance and the interpretation of these procedures are being prepared. Very soon radiologists and neurologists will have to devise strict criteria for evaluating the abnormalities detected by means of the CT and NMR scans. These procedures are already being overused and occasionally misinterpreted. The various tests that have become almost generally available with unexpected rapidity, so fast in fact that their full significance has not always been appreciated by the clinical neurologist, are often difficult to use and interpret. Incorporating paraclinical and laboratory data in the diagnostic criteria does not condone the apparent need of too many clinicians to initiate a diagnostic cascade of all possible technical procedures, from VEP to CT scan to spinal tap. In fact now more than ever the astute clinician has the opportunity to select the test or tests that best suit the patient's particular problem. Scheinberg's triad of "incontinence, impotence, and constipation"[56] in a 30-year-old man is more diagnostic of MS than evoked potentials and CT scans.

REFERENCES

1. BUZZARD, T. F. 1896. Lancet **1:** 1–5.
2. POSER, C. M. 1969. Acta Neurol. Scand. **45** (Suppl. 37): 1–44.
3. REIK, L. 1980. Ann. Neurol. **7:** 291–296.
4. KUROIWA, Y. 1982. *In* Multiple Sclerosis East and West. Y. Kuroiwa & L. T. Kurland, Eds.: 31–42. Kyushu University Press. Fukuoka, Japan.
5. POSER, C. M. 1980. Surv. Ophthalmol. **25:** 91–101.
6. PATY, D. W. & C. M. POSER. 1984. *In* The Diagnosis of Multiple Sclerosis. C. M. Poser *et al.,* Eds. Thieme-Stratton. New York.
7. AITA, J. F., D. R. BENNETT, R. E. ANDERSON *et al.* 1978. Neurology **28:** 251–255.
8. COLE, M. & R. J. ROSS. 1977. Neurology **27:** 890–891.
9. EBERS, G. C. & D. W. PATY. 1984. *In* The Diagnosis of Multiple Sclerosis. C. M. Poser *et al.,* Eds. Thieme-Stratton. New York.
10. LIKOSKY, W. & R. S. ELMORE. 1982. *In* Clinical Applications of Evoked Potentials in Neurology. J. Courjon *et al.,* Eds.: 535–540. Raven Press. New York.
11. POSER, C. M. 1980. Arch. Neurol. **37:** 471–474.
12. ROIZIN, L., M. HELFAND & J. MOORE. 1946. J. Nerv. Ment. Dis. **104:** 1–50.
13. GILBERT, J. J. & M. SADLER. 1983. Arch. Neurol. **40:** 533–536.
14. POSER, C. M., D. W. PATY, L. SCHEINBERG *et al.* 1983. Ann. Neurol. **13:** 227–231.
15. POSER, C. M., S. POSER & D. W. PATY. 1984. *In* The Diagnosis of Multiple Sclerosis. C. M. Poser *et al.,* Eds. Thieme-Stratton. New York. 1984.
16. POSER, C. M., J. PRESTHUS & O. HORSDAL. 1966. Neurology **16:** 791–798.
17. ATTWOOD, W. & C. M. POSER. 1961. Neurology **11:** 1034–1041.
18. LINK, H. 1982. *In* Multiple Sclerosis East and West. Y. Kuroiwa & L. T. Kurland, Eds.: 249–263. Kyushu University Press. Fukuoka, Japan.
19. THYGESEN, P. 1949. Arch. Neurol. Psychiat. **61:** 339–351.
20. VAN BOGAERT, L. 1950. J. Neuropathol. Exper. Neurol. **9:** 219–249.
21. BERMAN, M., S. FELDMAN, M. ALTER *et al.* 1981. Neurology **31:** 966–971.
22. LIPTON, H. L. & R. D. TEASDALL. 1973. Arch. Neurol. **28:** 252–257.
23. ALTROCCHI, P. 1963. Arch. Neurol. **9:** 111–119.
24. ROPPER, A. H. & D. C. POSKANZER. 1978. Ann. Neurol. **4:** 51–59.
25. REIK, L. 1982. Semin. Neurol. **2:** 106–114.
26. POSER, C. M. 1978. *In* Clinical Neurology. A. B. Baker & L. H. Baker, Eds.: **2**(25): 80–188. Harper & Row. New York.
27. POSER, C. M. 1982. Acta Neurol. Scand. **66:** 413–431.
28. KLINE, L. B., S. L. MARGULIES & S. J. OH. 1982. Arch. Neurol. **39:** 443–444.
29. SELBST, R. G., J. B. SELHORST, J. B. HARBISON *et al.* 1983. Arch. Neurol. **40:** 347–350.
30. UNGAR-SARGON, J. Y., R. E. LOVELACE & J. M. BRUST. 1980. J. Neurol. Sci. **46:** 1–12.

31. MARSHALL, J. 1955. Lancet **1:** 643–646.
32. POSER, S. 1978. Multiple Sclerosis. Springer-Verlag. Berlin.
33. PATY, D. W., W. T. BLUME, W. F. BROWN *et al.* 1979. Ann. Neurol. **6:** 419–424.
34. BYNKE, H., J. OLSSON & I. ROSEN. 1977. Acta Neurol. Scand. **26:** 55–69.
35. POSER, C. M., G. ROMAN & E. S. EMERY. 1978. Arch. Neurol. **35:** 166–170.
36. HALLIDAY, A. M., W. I. MCDONALD & J. MUSHIN. 1974. Neurology **24:** 360–361.
37. BLUMHARDT, L. D., G. BARRETT & A. M. HALLIDAY. 1982. *In* Clinical Applications of Evoked Potentials in Neurology. J. Courjon *et al.*, Eds.: 463–471. Raven Press. New York.
38. DELTENRE, P., O. VAN NECHEL, A. VERCRUYSSE *et al.* 1982. *In* Clinical Applications of Evoked Potentials in Neurology. Raven Press. New York. pp. 473–479.
39. BRAIN, W. R. & M. WILKINSON. 1957. Brain **80:** 456–478.
40. LINK, H., E. NORRBY & J. OLSSON. 1976. Arch. Neurol. **33:** 26–32.
41. MCDONALD, W. I. & A. M. HALLIDAY. 1977. Brit. Med. Bull. **33:** 4–8.
42. PERKIN, G. D. 1979. *In* Clinical Neuroimmunology. F. C. Rose, Ed.: 312–328. Blackwell. Oxford.
43. NIKOSKELAINEN, E. & P. RIEKKINEN. 1974. Acta Neurol. Scand. **50:** 690–718.
44. COHEN, M. M., S. LESSELL & P. A. WOLF. 1979. Neurology **29:** 208–213.
45. LINK, H., E. NORRBY & J. OLSSON. 1973. N. Engl. J. Med. **289:** 1103–1107.
46. LINK, H. & L. STENDAHL-BRODIN. 1983. N. Engl. J. Med. **308:** 1294–1295.
47. STENDAHL, L., H. LINK, E. MOLLER *et al.* 1976. J. Neurol. Sci. **27:** 93–98.
48. COMPSTON, D. A., J. R. BATCHELOR, C. J. EARL *et al.* 1978. Brain **101:** 495–511.
49. INNIS, M. & P. LANDY. 1979. Lancet **2:** 52.
50. HUTCHINSON, W. M. 1976. J. Neurol. Neurosurg. Psychiat. **39:** 283–289.
51. MATTHEWS, W. 1978. Lancet **1:** 443.
52. BREEN, L. A. & R. M. BURDE. 1981. J. Clin. Neuro-ophthalmol. **1:** 277–278.
53. EISEN, A. & R. CRACCO. 1983. Neurology **33:** 618–621.
54. KAYED, K., O. ROSJO & B. KASS. 1978. Acta Neurol. Scand. **57:** 317–324.
55. SCHUMACHER, G. A., G. BEEBE, R. KIBLER *et al.* 1965. Ann. N.Y. Acad. Sci. **122:** 552–568.
56. SCHEINBERG, L. 1983. Personal communication.
57. HUBBE, P. & A. DAM. 1973. Acta Neurol. Scand. **49:** 536–542.
58. GARDE, A. & K. G. KJELLIN. 1971. Acta Neurol. Scan. **47:** 555–568.
59. KUROIWA, Y., H. SHIBASAKI, N. INOUE *et al.* 1970. Adv. Neurol. Sci. **14:** 607–614.
60. KITO, S. 1970. Jap. J. Clin. Med. **28:** 2264–2272.
61. ALTER, M., J. GOOD & M. OKIHIRO. 1973. Neurology **23:** 631–639.
62. NIKOSKELAINEN, E. 1975. Optic Neuritis. Academic dissertation. University of Turku. Turku, Finland. pp. 7–41.
63. KAHANA, E., M. ALTER & S. FELDMAN. 1976. J. Neurol. **213:** 87–95.
64. ISAYAMA, Y., T. TAKAHASHI, T. SHIMOYOMA *et al.* 1982. Neurology **32:** 73–76.
65. KURLAND, L. T., G. E. BEEBE, J. F. KURTZKE *et al.* 1966. Acta Neurol. Scand., **42** (Suppl. 19): 157–176.
66. BRADLEY, W. G. & C. W. WHITTY. 1968. J. Neurol. Neurosurg. Psychiat. **31:** 10–18.

DISCUSSION OF THE PAPER

D. BARRIOS (*Caracas, Venezuela*): What will be the prognosis in the case with difficult optical neuritis but with oligoclonal bands in CSF?

C. M. POSER (*Boston University, Boston, MA*): I pointed out that one can get oligoclonal bands in optic neuritis, which is clearly the result of a postinfectious or postvaccination complication. I think that Dr. Link has published a number of such cases. Compston in England has a rather extensive series to which I'd be happy to give you the reference. He feels that one can predict on the basis of oligoclonal bands and in fact also the HLA BT101 which is the same as DW2. I must say I have some reservations about the value of this.

R. T. SCHAPIRO (*University of Minneapolis, Minneapolis, MN*): I guess I feel a need to represent the clinicians a little bit. I appreciate where Dr. Poser is coming from clinically but the day that hypertensive encephalopathy and MS consistently look alike I think it will be the time to pack it in. The other comment that I think I need to make is that most clinicians realize that evoked potentials have different normative values depending on the laboratory where they've been used; they would never take a random value and use that as the value to base the diagnosis upon.

POSER: The only thing I can say to answer your question Dr. Schapiro, is first of all I must respectfully disagree with you that most clinicians know about hypertensive encephalopathy, I didn't make this up. This is a real case, three neurologists missed this case.

T Regulator Cell Surface Antigens in Multiple Sclerosis[a]

ANTHONY T. REDER, JACK P. ANTEL, AND
BARRY G. W. ARNASON

Department of Neurology
and
Brain Research Institute
University of Chicago
Chicago, Illinois 60637

INTRODUCTION

The proportion of various cell subsets within the overall mononuclear cell population of peripheral blood is reported to differ in MS patients compared to age- and sex-matched controls. The differences are usually most apparent in those patients with active (progressive or relapsing) disease. Using monoclonal antibodies (mAbs) which recognize mononuclear cell surface proteins, the most consistently demonstrated changes have been found in the number of T suppressor (T_s) cells ($T8^+$, $T5^+$, Leu $2a^+$), although differences from controls have also been found in other cell subsets including total T cells ($T3^+$) and monocytes ($M1^+$). The extent to which the numbers of the above cell subsets in MS patients differ from non-MS individuals has, however, varied markedly from study to study.

In our study, we have analyzed some of the properties of T_s ($T8^+$) cells from MS patients that may contribute to the discrepancies existent among enumeration studies of T_s cells in MS and may be associated with the aberrant suppressor-cell function that has been rather consistently observed in MS patients.[1-3] Our data indicate that the density of $T8^+$ antigen on cells from MS patients with active disease is reduced.[4,5] Using immune modulation with OKT8 as a model of reduced T8 antigen density, we can demonstrate that distinguishing cells with low antigen density from nonfluorescent cells can be difficult, a factor that in turn increases the variability of results in T_s cell enumeration studies in MS. In addition, OKT8-modulated mononuclear cells exhibit reduced functional suppressor activity.

DONORS

The MS patients included in this study were clinically rated as having either active or stable disease. The active group was comprised of patients with gradually but continually increasing disability in the preceding one year (progressive MS) or with an exacerbation in the prior week (MS relapse). Stable patients had no clinically apparent change in function over the preceding year. In all assays, MS patients' cells were studied together with cells from an age (± 10 years)- and sex-matched control.

[a]This work was supported by grants from the National Multiple Sclerosis Society and the Kroc Foundation.

METHODS

Isolation and mAb Labeling of Mononuclear Cells

Peripheral blood mononuclear cells (PBM) were separated on ficoll-hypaque (Pharmacia) density gradients and washed ×3 in Hanks' Balanced Salt Solution (HBSS: GIBCO, Grand Island, NY) at 4°C. Cells ($n = 1 \times 10^6$) were pelleted in 2 ml Eppendorf tubes and incubated on ice for 30 minutes with mAbs recognizing peripheral T cells (OKT3), helper cells (OKT4), or suppressor/cytotoxic cells (OKT8, Ortho Pharmaceuticals, Raritan, NJ). Stock solutions of mAbs containing 0.1% Na azide were suspended in HBSS containing 10% heat inactivated and ultracentrifuged normal goat serum (NGS), previously absorbed with mouse Ig, at a dilution of 1:20. This dilution had been previously determined to be a saturating concentration. Fifty μl of diluted mAb were added to each tube. Cells were incubated for 30 minutes on ice and then washed ×3 in HBSS with 0.1% bovine serum albumin (BSA) and 0.01% sodium azide by cycles of centrifugation (300 g × 10 min at 4°C) and resuspension. Cell pellets were then incubated with 50 μl of goat anti-mouse IgG conjugated with FITC (FITC Gα-M IgG from Cappel, Cochranville, PA, 1:100 dilution of the ~8 mg/ml stock solution in HBSS with 10% NGS, previously determined to be a saturating concentration). Cells were again washed ×3 and resuspended in 1 ml of indicator-free HBSS with 0.1% BSA and 0.01% Na azide.

Cell Subset Enumeration and Fluorescence Intensity Determination Using FACS Analysis

Ten thousand cells exposed to a given mAb were recorded at a rate of 500 cells/second on a fluorescence-activated cell sorter (FACS: Becton Dickinson, Sunnyvale, CA) equipped with a 2-watt argon laser (Spectra-Physics, Inc., Mountain View, CA). The fluorescence intensity of each cell was assigned to one of the 128 available fluorescence channels. In preliminary experiments, fluorescence detector gain settings (amplification) were determined for each mAb so that the median fluorescence for cells from control donors fell approximately at the midpoint of the 128 channels. Monoclonal antibody-labeled cells were considered positive if their fluorescence fell to the right of the midpoint of the trough (approximately channel 17) between autofluorescent unlabeled cells and fluorescent labeled cells. Almost all (>95%) positive cells were found below channel 88.

The median fluorescence of the cells considered as positive was determined from cell-frequency histograms. For each mAb evaluated, MS patients and controls were compared with regard to the channel representing the median of fluorescence intensity. The distribution of fluorescence intensity for $T8^+$ cells could be further compared between MS patients and controls by determining the number of $T8^+$ cells found below or above the channel number (52.5) representing the median between the usual channel numbers containing cells with the lowest (channel 17) and highest (channel 88) fluorescence intensity.

Cells positive for OKT8 staining were brightest and the gain setting was set at 2.0. $OKT3^+$ cells were counted with amplification at 4.0. $OKT4^+$ cells were dim even at optimal staining conditions and it was necessary to increase electronic amplification of the fluorescence signal to 8.0. The laser output was set at 150 mW at 488 nm and the fluorescence detector at 520 V, with filters of 520 nm and 530 nm long pass and 0.45 neutral density in front of the fluorescence detector. A standard preparation of glutaraldehyde-fixed chicken red blood cells (G-CRBC) and occasionally fluorescent microspheres were used to adjust the laser output intensity to comparable levels on different days to reduce day-to-day variation. The strongly fluorescent G-CRBC exhibited a fluorescence peak at channel 42 under these conditions with the gain setting at 1.0.

Modulation Studies with OKT8

Washed and pelleted lymphocytes ($n = 4 \times 10^6$) were incubated either with 20 μl of OKT8 diluted 1:20 in HBSS plus 10% NGS (treated cells) for 30 minutes on ice or with HBSS plus 10% NGS only (untreated cells) and then resuspended in 4 ml of RPMI 1640 (GIBCO) + 10% newborn calf serum, 6 mg/ml L-glutamine, and 0.1 mg/ml gentamycin. Treated and untreated cells were incubated in 25 cm^2 tissue culture flasks (Corning, Corning, NY) for 18 hours at 37°C in a humidified 5% CO_2 atmosphere. Following incubation, 10^6 treated or 10^6 untreated cells were pelleted and then stained with OKT8 followed with FITC Gα-M IgG as described above. Treated

TABLE 1. FACS Analysis of Peripheral Blood MNCs in MS[a]

	Enumeration of Cell Subsets Percent ± SEM			Median Fluorescence Intensity Channel Number ± SEM		
mAb	Stable	Progressive	Relapse	Stable	Progressive	Relapse
T3	50.7 ± 3.7	49.1 ± 2.8	60.1 ± 3.8	46.0 ± 3.1	43.0 ± 2.9	41.9 ± 4.0
	$n = 9$	$n = 7$	$n = 7$	$n = 9$	$n = 7$	$n = 7$
	60.3 ± 2.5	*58.6 ± 1.6*[b]	*61.6 ± 2.6*	*44.4 ± 2.3*	*42.6 ± 2.8*	*42.2 ± 2.8*
T4	33.3 ± 2.9	37.6 ± 1.9	44.0 ± 1.5	55.3 ± 4.3	60.8 ± 4.6	47.5 ± 6.9
	8	8	4	8	6	6
	41.1 ± 3.4	*33.3 ± 1.9*	*39.5 ± 3.6*	*54.4 ± 2.4*	*51.5 ± 3.4*	*48.3 ± 3.8*
T8	17.3 ± 2.5	14.5 ± 7[b]	17.8 ± 3.0	58.5 ± 7.6	48.0 ± 4.4[b]	45.2 ± 3.2[c]
	8	8	6	8	8	6
	18.6 ± 1.9	*20.9 ± 2.0*	*20.7 ± 1.9*	*54.3 ± 9.4*	*54.5 ± 3.7*	*50.5 ± 3.3*

[a]Control values are shown in italics.
[b]$p < 0.05$.
[c]$p < 0.001$.

cells ($n = 10^6$) were also stained with FITC Gα-M IgG alone as a control. In some studies, treated and untreated cells were initially cultured with or without concanavalin A (Con A), 3 μg/ml for 48 hours. Cells were then treated with mitomycin and their suppressor activity assayed by culturing them with fresh responder cells plus Con A for 72 hours as previously described.[6] Suppressor effects of Con A activated OKT8-treated and nontreated cells were compared.

RESULTS

Enumeration Studies Using FACS Analysis in MS

As shown in TABLE 1, the proportion of $T8^+$ cells was significantly lower in progressive MS patients, suggestively lower in patients during relapse, and not significantly different in stable MS patients compared to paired controls. The mean percent T3$^+$ cells for both progressive and stable MS groups was lower than for the matched control group. The percent T3$^+$ cells in relapsing MS did not differ from controls. The proportion of T4$^+$ cells did not differ between any MS groups and controls.

Median Fluorescence Intensity Studies

The median fluorescence intensity (MFI), expressed as the median fluorescence channel number of OKT8$^+$ cells stained, was lower in both progressive (48.0 ± 4.4) and relapsing MS (45.2 ± 3.2) when compared to same-day controls (54.5 ± 3.7, $p < 0.05$ and 50.5 ± 3.3, $p < 0.02$, respectively). For the active MS patients overall, MFI was significantly lower than for controls (46.8 ± 2.9 *versus* 53.2 ± 2.7, $p < 0.001$). The ratio of low:high density cells, as defined on the basis of fluorescence intensity being less than or greater than 52.5, *i.e.,* the median between channels 17 and 88, was increased in the active MS patients (1.80) compared both to the control (1.25)

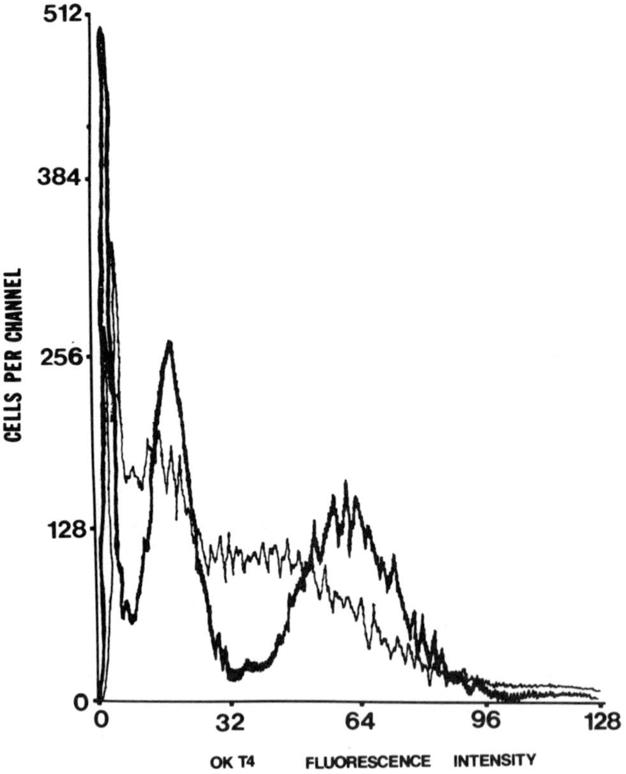

FIGURE 1. T4 antigen expression on mononuclear cells from two control donors. For donor (—), relatively bright T4$^+$ cells are clearly separated from dim autofluorescent cells. In contrast, for donor (—), the weakly staining T4$^+$ cells are difficult to distinguish from autofluorescent cells.

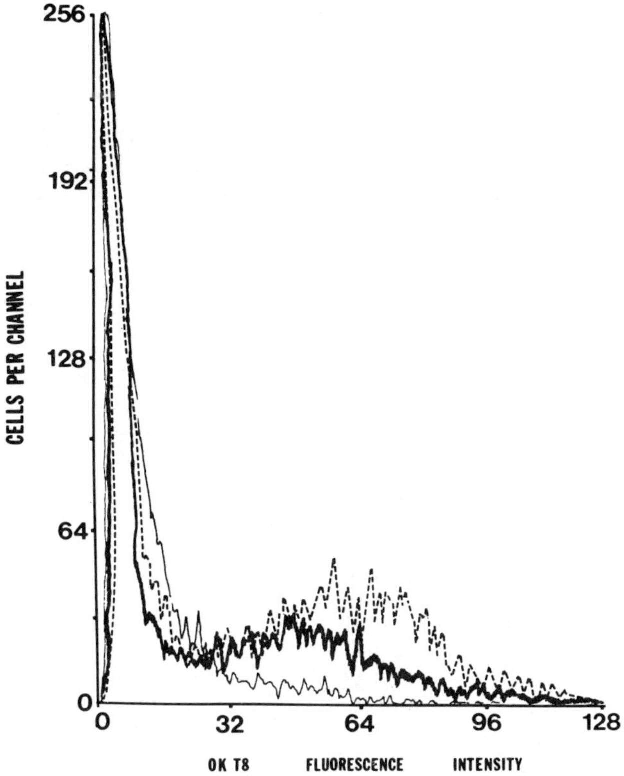

FIGURE 2. T8 antigen expression on cells of a representative patient with active MS (—) and on control OKT8-modulated (—) and nonmodulated (- - -) cells. After 18-hour OKT8 modulation, mononuclear cells were stained with OKT8 followed by FITC G α-M IgG. MS $T8^+$ cells are less numerous and have lower median fluorescence than nonmodulated controls. Modulated cells show a marked reduction in both the number of fluorescence-positive cells and in median fluorescence intensity.

and stable disease patient (0.75) groups. There was no internal correlation between the number of $T8^+$ cells and the MFI in either MS or in controls ($r = 0.08$).

OKT3-labeled cells did not differ, with respect to MFI, between any of the MS subgroups and their matched controls. OKT4-labeled cells were also not consistently different between MS subgroups and controls. With OKT4-labeled cells, however, there was considerable variation in the maximal fluorescence recorded (FIGURE 1); in addition, overlap with autofluorescent T4-negative cells sometimes obscured the more dimly fluorescent $T4^+$ cells, preventing accurate determination of MFI. This problem was a consequence of the high gain settings necessitated by the weak fluorescence of $T4^+$ cells which in turn resulted in amplification of the weak signal given off by T4-negative cells. This overlap of cell populations interfered with the accurate definition of $T4^+$ cells even if lymphocytes alone (low scatter cells) were counted after electronically gating out large cells (generally macrophages with a high scatter profile).

Modulated Cell Studies

Following 18 hours of incubation with OKT8, the mean proportion of cells in the mononuclear cell population considered as being T8$^+$ using the FACS was 7% compared to 23% for mononuclear cells cultured without antibody. The MFI of these OKT8-modulated cells was markedly reduced compared to control cells. FIGURE 2 depicts a representative FACS profile of OKT8-stained mononuclear cells from a control before and after modulation along with OKT8-stained mononuclear cells from an MS patient with progressive disease. When the same OKT8-stained modulated cells as above were enumerated using a fluorescence microscope, the mean percent positive cells was found to be 18%. For nonmodulated cells, in contrast, a close correlation existed between results of enumeration performed with the microscope compared to the FACS.

As previously reported,[6] we have found that Con A-induced suppressor activity directed toward a mitogen-induced T cell response by OKT8-modulated mononuclear cells was significantly reduced compared to the suppressor activity of nonmodulated cells (29 ± 5% *versus* 43 ± 6%, $p < 0.02$). Using a "panning" technique to prepare enriched T4$^+$ or T8$^+$ cell populations, we have shown that this suppressor activity is mediated by the T8$^+$ cell population.[7]

DISCUSSION

Our enumeration data on T cell subsets in MS do indicate that during clinically active phases of disease, there is an underrepresentation of T8$^+$ cells in the MNC population. The findings seem most apparent in patients with chronic progressive disease. Considerable overlap, however, is found in T cell subset values between stable and active MS patients, precluding the use of a given value for T8$^+$ cell number as a clear-cut indicator of active disease. Our studies did not address whether serial determinations of T_s numbers for a given individual can predict a pending exacerbation of disease. In prior studies, we have shown that the amount of *in vitro* pokeweed mitogen-induced immunoglobulin production by mononuclear cells of either MS patients or controls is not directly correlated with the absolute number of T_s (T8$^+$) cells present but rather with the functional properties of the T8$^+$ cells.[8]

The analysis of the fluorescence intensity of MS patients' mononuclear cells after staining with OKT mAbs suggests several potential mechanisms that may contribute to the functional immunoregulatory defects found in MS and provide some explanation for the apparent discrepancies in results obtained in the various studies enumerating T cell subsets. We find that in active MS, particularly with progressive disease, the proportion of cells with a high density of T8 antigen is reduced. This observation could reflect either a selective depletion of a T8$^+$ subset with high density of surface antigen, a reduction in T8 antigen expression (modulation), or masking of the T8 antigen. With regard to the first possibility, specific functional properties of T8$^+$ cells have been associated with different antigen densities. Titus *et al.*[9] reported that high antigen density T8$^+$ cells mediated high levels of cytolytic activity.

With regard to antigen modulation or masking, several lines of evidence indicate that the expression of the T8 antigen may be linked to cell function and that removal or blocking of the antigen can alter functional activity. Reinherz *et al.* found that incubation of T8-bearing cells with OKT8 blocked their cytolytic activity.[10] Interaction between the T8 antigen and the mitogen wheat germ agglutinin results in cell activation.[11] Our data indicate that modulation of the T8 antigen from the cell surface results in reduced Con A-activated suppressor activity.[6]

The data derived from enumeration of OKT8-modulated cells using both a FACS and a fluorescence microscope further indicate difficulties that arise in using immunofluorescence techniques to enumerate cells expressing low amounts of surface antigen. When the density of the T8 antigen on cells is reduced by modulating the cells, significant differences are found between the two techniques, with higher numbers being found using the microscope.[4] Dim cells are less likely to be counted as positive with a FACS than with a microscope because cells retaining even a few flecks of fluorescence are read as positive under the microscope but are not distinguished from autofluorescent cells with the FACS. Furthermore, with reduced cell fluorescence, the cutoff between positive and negative cells on the FACS becomes less sharply defined, resulting in further difficulties in segregating the cells. This difficulty is comparable to that encountered when enumerating OKT4-stained cells (see Results section). The reduced MFI which we find for T8-bearing cells from active MS patients may thus contribute to the discrepancies in results among studies, particularly if positive and negative are the only criteria used in the analysis of fluorescence.

REFERENCES

1. ANTEL, J. P., B. G. W. ARNASON & M. E. MEDOF. 1979. Suppressor cell function in multiple sclerosis—correlation with clinical disease activity. Ann. Neurol. **5:** 338–342.
2. GONZALEZ, R. L., P. C. DAU & L. E. SPITLER. 1978. Altered regulation of mitogen responsiveness by suppressor cells in multiple sclerosis. Clin. Exp. Immunol **36:** 78–84.
3. NEIGHBOUR, P. A. & B. R. STONE. 1979. Absence of virus-induced lymphocyte suppression and interferon production in multiple sclerosis. Proc. Natl. Acad. Sci. U.S.A. **76:** 476–480.
4. REDER, A. T., J. P. ANTEL, J. OGER, T. A. MCFARLAND, M. ROSENKOETTER & B. G. W. ARNASON. 1984. Low T8 antigen density on lymphocytes in active multiple sclerosis. Ann. Neurol. **16:** 242–249.
5. REDER, A. T., T. A. MCFARLAND, J. OGER & J. P. ANTEL. 1983. Cytotoxic/suppressor cell population in active multiple sclerosis: Reduction in T8 antigen density. Ann. Neurol. **14:** 116.
6. ANTEL, J. P., J. OGER, S. JACKEVICIUS, H. H. KUO & B. G. W. ARNASON. 1982. Modulation of T lymphocyte differentiation antigens: Potential relevance for multiple sclerosis. Proc. Natl. Acad. Sci. U.S.A. **79:** 3330–3334.
7. ANTEL, J. P., D. M. PEEPLES, A. T. REDER & B. G. W. ARNASON. 1984. Analysis of T regulator cell surface markers and functional properties in multiple sclerosis. J. Neuroimmunol. **6:** 93–103.
8. ANTEL, J. P., M. ROSENKOETTER, A. REDER, J. OGER & B. G. W. ARNASON. 1984. Multiple sclerosis: Relation of *in vitro* IgG secretion with T suppressor cell number and function in multiple sclerosis. Neurology **34:** 1155–1160.
9. TITUS, J. A., S. O. SHARROW & D. M. SEGAL. 1983. Analysis of Fc (IgG) receptors on human peripheral blood lymphocytes by dual fluorescence flow microfluorometry. II. Quantitation of receptors on cells that express the OKM1, OKT3, OKT4, and OKT8 antigens. J. Immunol. **130:** 1152–1158.
10. REINHERZ, E. L., R. E. HUSSEY, K. FITZGERALD, P. SNOW, C. TERHORST & S. F. SCHLOSSMAN. 1980. Antibody directed at a surface structure inhibits cytolytic but not suppressor function on human T lymphocytes. Nature **294:** 168–170.
11. BOLDT, D. H. & S. A. DORSEY. 1983. Interactions of lectins and monoclonal antibodies with human mononuclear cells. J. Immunol. **130:** 1646–1653.

Evaluation of Leukocyte Surface Antigens in Patients with Multiple Sclerosis

D. E. McFARLIN AND E. S. MINGIOLI

Neuroimmunology Branch
Intramural Research Program
National Institute of Neurological and
Communicative Disorders and Stroke
National Institutes of Health
Bethesda, Maryland 20205

Although the etiology and pathogenesis of multiple sclerosis (MS) are unknown, it has long been believed that aberrant immune function may play a role.[1] Within recent years the concept that suppressor T lymphocytes may be reduced in the disease has received considerable emphasis. During acute attacks reduced Con A-induced suppressor cell activity[2] and reduced T gamma cells[3] have been described. Impaired production of interferon has been reported.[4,5] In addition, some investigators have observed abnormalities of the natural killer cells,[4] but this area is somewhat controversial.[6] Subsequent to the development of monoclonal antibodies which recognize different subsets of T lymphocytes[7] it was reported that the subset defined by the OKT5 antiserum was reduced in patients during acute episodes of MS.[8] This was believed to be consistent with the notion of deficiency of suppressor cells in MS because the population of Con A-induced T cells which suppress the allogeneic mixed lymphocyte reaction[9] was shown to be OKT5 positive. Reduced OKT5 cells were also reported by Bach *et al.*[12]; subsequently, the OKT8 antiserum was introduced as a marker for the same set of lymphocytes defined by OKT5. With this reagent, Hauser *et al.*[11] provided evidence that variation in lymphocyte subsets correlated with disease activity. However, recently others[12] have failed to find changes in lymphocyte phenotypes during acute episodes of MS.

For the past three years lymphocyte phenotypes have been examined in patients being investigated by the Neuroimmunology Branch. In order to interpret the findings in patients, considerable effort has been devoted to the study of lymphocytes in normal individuals. The purpose of this report is to describe our findings to date in both normals and MS patients.

MATERIALS AND METHODS

Subjects. Patients satisfied the criteria for a diagnosis of clinically definite MS.[13] Three females with acute relapses were studied; these individuals had developed new neurological signs within 72 hours of the study. The remaining patients (21 female and 17 males) had chronic progressive MS with evidence of steady deterioration over the six months of study. Controls consisted of 20 normal females and 19 normal males.

Isolation of PBLs. Thirty ml venous blood was collected in a syringe containing 1000 units Panheprin (Abbott), mixed with an equal volume of Dulbecco's phosphate-buffered saline (PBS) without calcium and magnesium and divided between two 50 ml conical centrifuge tubes. Ten ml Lymphocyte Separation Medium (Bionetics) was layered beneath the cell suspension in each tube, and the discontinuous gradients were centrifuged in a horizontal rotor for 30 min at 486 ×g at 18°C. The cells at the interface were aspirated, pelleted at 250 ×g at 5°C, and washed two times with PBS under the same conditions. The cells were then suspended in a known volume of cold FACS medium (RPMI 1640 + 0.1% sodium azide, 20 mM hepes and 5% heat-inactivated fetal calf serum), counted and centrifuged as above. Finally, a suspension of 1×10^7 peripheral blood lymphocytes (PBLs) per ml FACS medium was prepared, and 0.25 ml aliquots were distributed in 15 ml conical centrifuge tubes.

Staining of PBLs. Individual PBL aliquots were treated with 12.5 μl of each of the following: a negative control (mouse anti-mouse I-A^k), anti-HLA-DR (Becton Dickinson Monoclonal Center, Inc.), anti-OKT3, OKT4 and OKT8 (Ortho Diagnostic Systems, Inc.) and antimonocyte (Bethesda Research Laboratory). The cells were incubated for 90 min in an ice bath and then suspended in 10 ml FACS medium and centrifuged as above. The pellet was then resuspended in 0.25 ml previously titrated

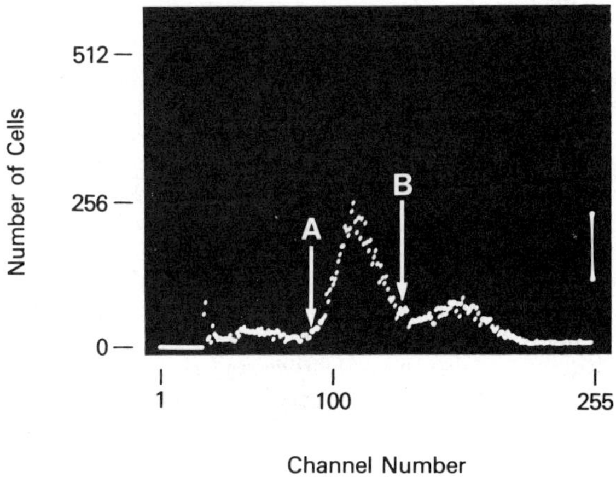

FIGURE 1. Forward light scatter histogram of human PBL preparation.

goat $F(ab')_2$ anti-mouse IgG conjugated to FITC (Boehringer-Manneheim Biochemicals). After 45–60 min in ice, the cells were washed once as above, resuspended in 1.5 ml FACS medium and filtered through 52 μ pore nylon mesh (Spectrum Medical Industries, Inc.) immediately before analysis.

Data Acquisition. A sample containing both positive and negative fluorescent cells was run through the FACS IV (Becton-Dickinson FACS Systems) to determine the suitable forward light scatter gate. For cells stained with anti-OKT3, 4 and 8, a population was chosen comparable to that between points *A* and *B* in FIGURE 1. The particles to the left of *A* were considered to be debris, platelets, dead or dying lymphocytes and/or red cells.[14] The viable lymphocytes fall largely between *A* and *B*, and the large cells to the right of *B* are mostly macrophages or monocytes. When these latter cells were being analyzed, the gate was set from *A* to channel 255. After establishment of the scatter gate, 10,000 gated cells were collected from each sample

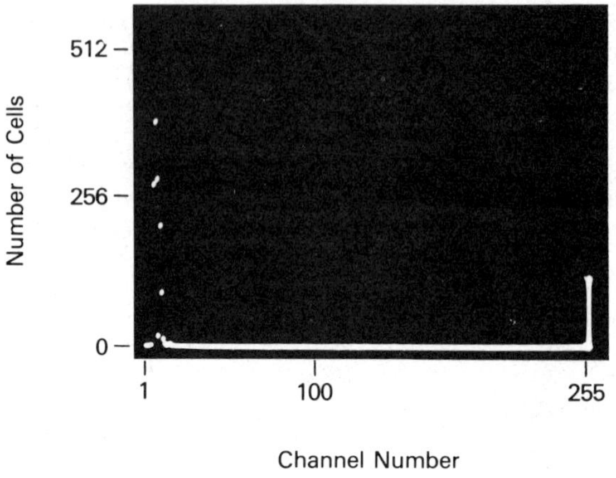

FIGURE 2. Fluorescence intensity histogram. PBLs strained with negative control serum. Linear amplification and linear display.

for fluorescence analysis, using each of two systems: a linear amplifier and a logarithmic amplifier. All data were stored on a floppy disk.

Data Analysis. The FACS IV instrument has the capacity to display two histograms simultaneously. To aid in analysis, the appropriately amplified and gated histogram generated using mouse anti-mouse I-A^k was stored and displayed in the overlap group. Histograms obtained in the same manner with each of the other antisera were displayed and compared to the negative control. The positive fluorescence window for each stained cell preparation was determined using either an overlap point or a valley point as the cutoff between positive and negative cells; these are described below. The number of cells in each window was recorded and the number of cells in the same window in the appropriate negative control histogram was subtracted from each value.

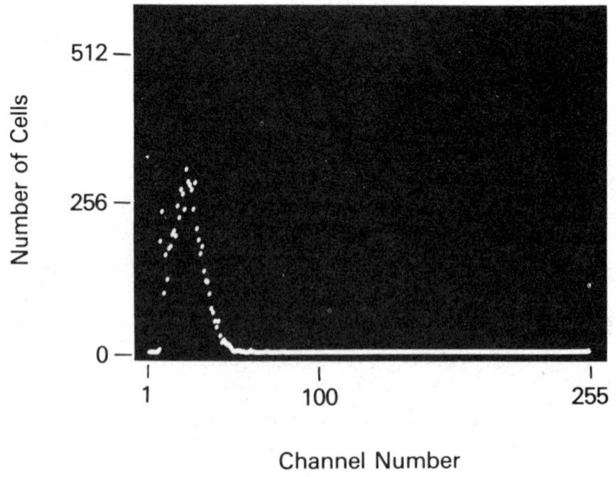

FIGURE 3. Fluorescence intensity histogram. PBLs stained with negative control serum. Log amplification and linear display.

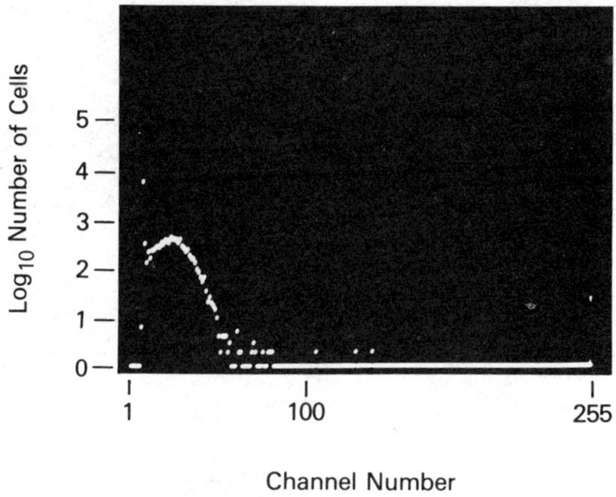

FIGURE 4. Fluorescence intensity histogram. PBLs stained with negative control serum. Log amplification and log display.

Statistical Analysis. The geometric mean, 67.5% confidence range and 95% confidence range were calculated in each group. Patient and control groups were compared by unpaired Student's t test.

RESULTS

In our early efforts to quantitate cells bearing various markers in the peripheral blood, considerable effort was devoted to determining the appropriate method for defining positive and negative cells. A number of approaches were tried. Our initial analyses were performed with a linear amplifier of fluorescence intensity which was expressed on the vertical axis. Later studies were performed using a log amplifier. With a given antiserum this resulted in slightly different values depending on the

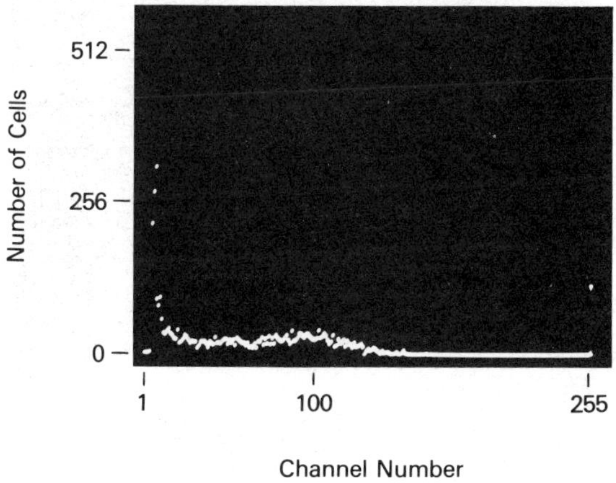

FIGURE 5. Fluorescence intensity histogram. PBLs stained with anti-OKT8. Linear amplification and linear display.

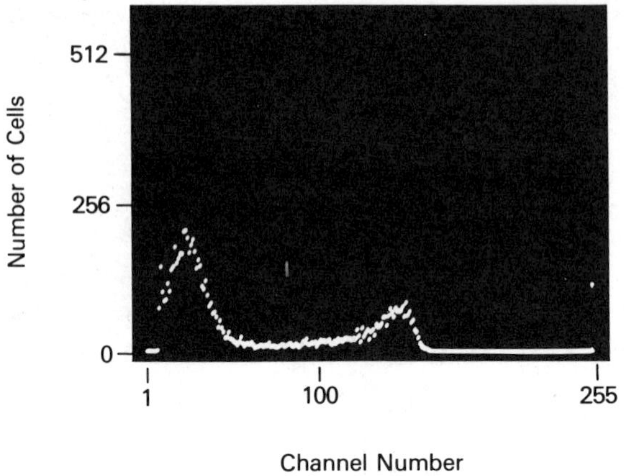

FIGURE 6. Fluorescence intensity histogram. PBL stained with anti-OKT8. Log amplification and linear display.

method of amplification. Examples of cells stained in the same manner and amplified by the various methods are shown in FIGURES 2–7.

One approach for defining positive and negative cells with a specific antiserum was to take the lowest point, *i.e.*, the channel number containing the fewest cells, between the initial negative peak and the subsequent positive peak. This channel was designated as the "valley," and all cells to the right of it were considered positive. An alternative approach was to superimpose the results obtained with the control antiserum and those obtained with specific antiserum. The point at which the two curves crossed, designated as the "overlap," was considered the endpoint and all cells falling in channels to the right of this were regarded as positive. These two approaches were used with both linear and log amplifiers. The differences between the overlap and the valley methods are illustrated in FIGURE 8.

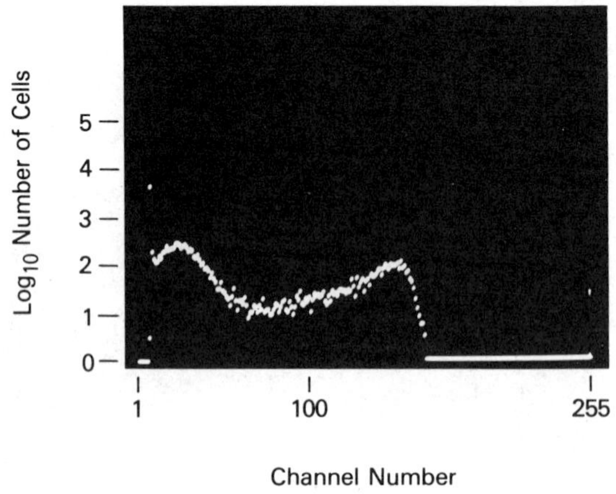

FIGURE 7. Fluorescence intensity histogram. PBL stained with anti-OKT8. Log amplification and log display.

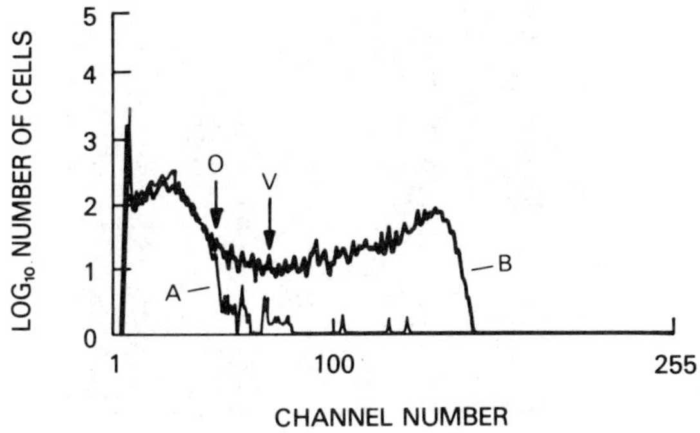

FIGURE 8. Fluorescence intensity histograms. PBLs stained with negative control serum (*A*) and anti-OKT8 (*B*). *O:* overlap channel; *V:* valley channel.

In order to determine the extent to which the analysis method affected the experimental results, PBLs from nine individuals were stained with anti-OKT3, OKT4 and OKT8; data were obtained using both linear and log amplifiers. These were analyzed by both the overlap and valley methods. The findings are shown in TABLE 1. Cells stained with anti-OKT3 and anti-OKT4 showed minimal differences; however, analyses of cells stained with anti-OKT8 consistently gave higher values by the overlap method than by the valley method. This is true regardless of whether linear or log amplifiers were used. The reason for this can be seen in FIGURES 7 and 9. In these illustrations it is apparent that there is not a sharp cutoff between cells that are not stained and those that are brightly stained with anti-OKT8. Instead, a significant portion of the cells are lightly stained with this reagent. Experiments were performed in which the forward and right angle light scattering characteristics of cells that were lightly stained with anti-OKT8 were analyzed. These experiments showed that these cells had the same size and surface characteristics as lymphocytes. In addition, consultation with other investigators at our institution[15] provided evidence that such cells were indeed T lymphocytes. Consequently, it has been concluded that there are

TABLE 1. Comparison of FACS Analysis Methods

		Overlap		Valley	
Antiserum		Linear	Log	Linear	Log
OKT3	GM	46.4	64.9	63.8	63.7
	67% CL	55.8–74.3	56.8–74.0	54.6–74.5	54.5–74.4
	95% CL	48.4–85.7	49.8–84.5	46.8–87.0	46.6–86.9
OKT4	GM	36.1	37.4	34.7	34.8
	67% CL	30.1–43.3	31.3–44.7	28.3–42.6	28.6–42.4
	95% CL	25.0–52.0	26.1–53.5	23.0–52.4	23.5–51.5
OKT8	GM	29.8	32.7	21.4	23.0
	67% CL	25.8–34.4	34.4–38.7	16.0–28.6	17.8–29.6
	95% CL	22.3–39.7	23.3–45.8	11.9–38.2	13.8–38.2

PBLs from nine normal individuals stained with a given antiserum were analyzed in a FACS using either a linear or a log amplifier. The percent positive cells were delineated using either the valley or overlap approach as described in the text. GM = geometric mean. CL = confidence limit.

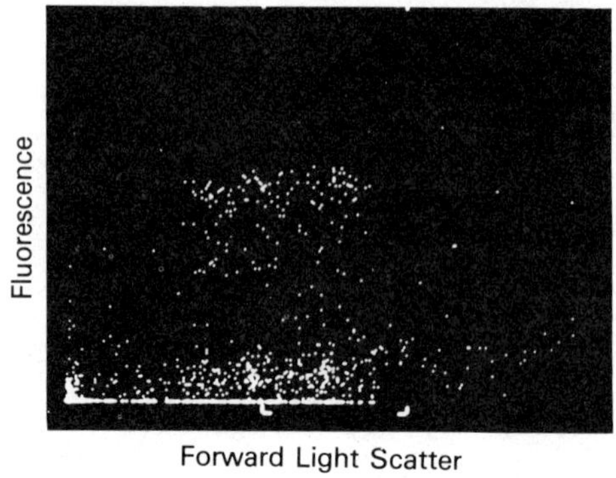

FIGURE 9. Dot display. PBLs stained with anti-OKT8. Log amplification of fluorescence intensity.

cells in the peripheral blood with varying amounts of the OKT8 antigen. It is our current practice to analyze PBLs using a log amplifier and the overlap point as the end point.

The geometric means, 67% confidence limits and 95% confidence limits of OKT3-, OKT4-, and OKT8-bearing cells in the peripheral blood of 20 normal females and 19 normal males were determined. These results are shown in TABLE 2 and illustrated in FIGURES 10, 11 and 12. These geometric means and standard deviations are in good agreement with those reported by other workers.[8,12] While these studies were in progress, PBLs from 17 males and 24 females with active MS were analyzed. The values are shown in FIGURES 10, 11 and 12. The studies with anti-OKT3 did not show a significant difference between normals and MS patients. However, significant differences were encountered between patients with MS and sex-matched controls when anti-OKT4 was used. The mean for normal males was 37.5% and for male patients was 44.0% ($p < 0.005$). This was largely due to the fact that the percentage of OKT4-bearing cells was greater than 2 SD above the mean in 5 of the male patients. The findings in females were similar; the mean of the normal females was 40.5%; for the patients it was 47.2% ($p < 0.025$). Four female patients had values greater than 2 SD above the normal mean. With anti-OKT8 no significant differences were found between normal females and female patients. However, the percentage of OKT8-positive cells was significantly less in the male patients. The mean was 31.6% for normals and 24.6% for the male patients ($p < 0.001$). The percent of anti-OKT8

TABLE 2. Normal Values for Lymphocyte Phenotypes

		OKT3	OKT4	OKT8
Males	GM	67.3	37.5	31.2
($n = 19$)	67% CL	60.8–74.4	32.9–42.8	25.7–38.0
	95% CL	55.0–82.3	28.8–48.8	21.1–46.1
Females	GM	65.2	40.5	27.7
($n = 20$)	67% CL	55.6–76.6	33.5–49.1	22.6–33.9
	95% CL	47.4–89.8	27.7–59.6	18.5–41.4

Normal values for OKT3, OKT4 and OKT8 were established using log amplification and the overlap method (see text). GM = geometric mean. CL = confidence limit.

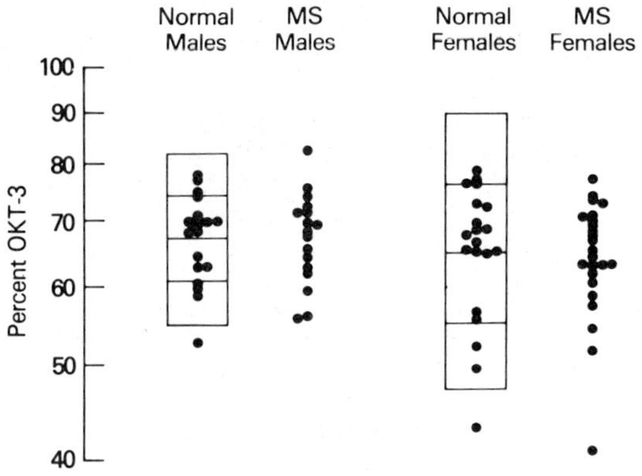

FIGURE 10. Percentage of OKT3-bearing cells in normal and MS males and females. In the normals, the geometric mean, 67% confidence limits, and 95% confidence limits are indicated.

positive cells in four of the male patients was two standard deviations below the normal mean.

The subset of T lymphocytes assessed with the anti-OKT8 reagent in this study probably can be identified with other monoclonal antisera such as anti-OKT5 (Ortho) and anti-Leu-2A (Becton Dickinson). In order to analyze this with our methods during the course of these experiments, 22 PBL preparations were also stained with anti-Leu-2A (Becton Dickinson) and the results were compared with those obtained using anti-OKT8. No significant difference was found with respect to the number of cells stained by the two reagents.

Other investigators[8,12] have expressed lymphocyte phenotype data as the ratio of OKT4/OKT8. Accordingly this was calculated in our subjects. For normal males the

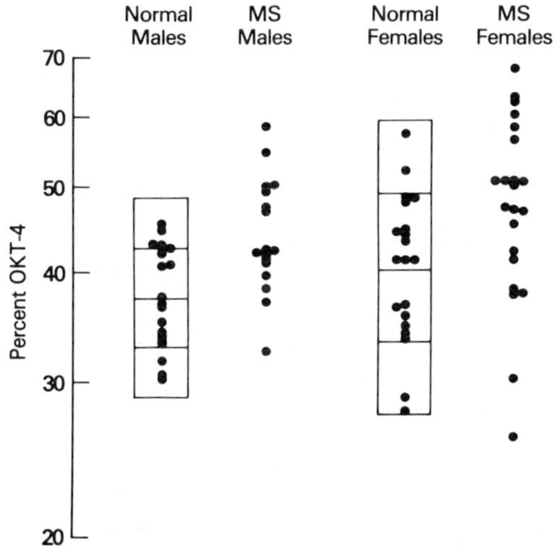

FIGURE 11. Percentage of OKT4-bearing cells in normal and MS males and females. In the normals, the geometric mean, 67% confidence limits, and 95% confidence limits are indicated.

mean was 1.2 and the 95% confidence range was 0.70 to 2.0. For normal females the mean was 1.5 and the 95% confidence range was 0.80 to 2.72. The three female patients with acute episodes had normal ratios (2.4, 1.0, 2.3). However in the chronic progressive patients, 6 of 17 males and 5 of 21 females had elevated ratios. Further, the means of both males and females were significantly higher than the normal controls.

The percentage of cells which react with the antimonocyte reagent and the anti-DR were assessed in nine normal males and in ten normal females. In these studies all cells the size of lymphocytes and larger were analyzed. For example, the scatter gate as illustrated in FIGURE 1 was set from point *A* to the final channel. With the antimonocyte reagent the means for males and females are 10.5% and 10.2%

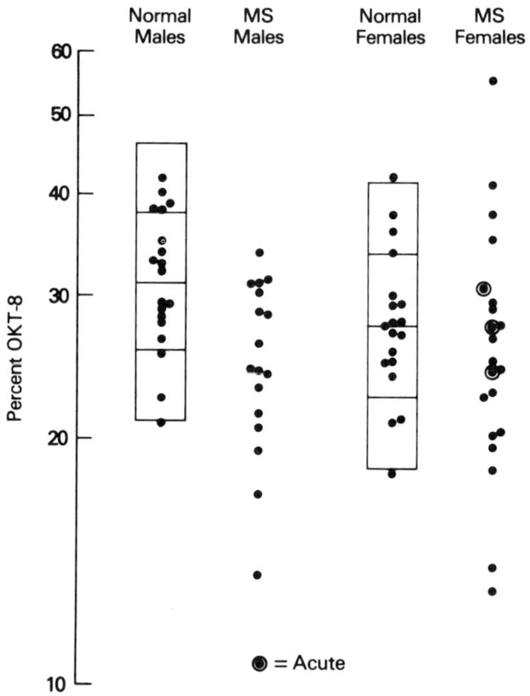

FIGURE 12. Percentage of OKT8-bearing cells in normal and MS males and females. In the normals, the geometric mean, 67% confidence limits, and 95% confidence limits are indicated.

respectively; the 95% confidence limits were 7.0–15.9% and 4.2–24.7%. Twelve male and 17 female MS patients were studied. These populations were not significantly different from the corresponding normals. The values for all patients fell within the normal 95% confidence limits except two. Both a male patient (3.0%) and a female (3.0%) were below the 95% confidence limits.

Studies on the same groups using anti-HLA-DR gave normal means for males and females of 27.4% and 23.2% respectively, with 95% confidence limits of 19.8–37.8% and 12.8–41.9%. Again the patient populations were not significantly different from normal, although three males had values below the 95% confidence limits (16.9, 18.5 and 19.0%) and one female had 43.7% DR-positive cells. The DR-positive cells probably include B cells, some T cells and macrophages. Evaluation of various populations of DR-positive cells is in progress but has not been completed. One approach currently being used is to delineate the number of DR-positive cells falling within the lymphocyte scatter gate, between points *A* and *B*, and in the light scatter gate for cells larger than lymphocytes between point *B* and the final channel (FIGURE 1). In the latter gate there was good agreement between the percentage of cells staining with the anti-DR and the antimonocyte reagent. This has led us to conclude that most, if not all, of the cells identified by the antimonocyte reagent are DR positive. In contrast only a small percentage of the cells (approximately 10–25%) in the lymphocyte scatter gate are DR positive. This includes both T and B lymphocytes. To date, no consistent differences in the percentage of DR-positive lymphocytes have been detected between MS patients and normals. A single interesting exception was the patient with 43.7% DR-positive cells. This individual had a normal number of cells that reacted with the antimonocyte reagent but an increase in the percentage of DR-positive lymphocytes. Further, the percent of B lymphocytes, as quantitated with a monoclonal anti-IgM, was elevated.

DISCUSSION

In the assessment of surface markers on PBLs in patients with multiple sclerosis a number of variables are involved. They include: (1) the status of the patient, (2) the reagents, (3) the methods for identification and quantitation of surface antigens (both fluorescence microscopy and cytofluorography have been used), (4) the gate setting when this is used to analyze selectively cells of different size, (5) the criteria for differentiating positive and negative cells. Because technical procedures undoubtedly vary among laboratories and can lead to different results, our laboratory has devoted considerable effort to standardizing our approaches and in this report the details of these have been emphasized.

Patients in general are referred to the Neuroimmunology Branch after the diagnosis of MS has been established; consequently only three patients were studied during acute attacks. It is noteworthy that the myelin basic protein in cerebrospinal fluid was elevated in these patients, which is consistent with the clinical impression. However, the lymphocyte phenotypes were normal. Although the number of acute patients was too few for meaningful independent analysis the findings in these three individuals are consistent with those described by Paty *et al.*[12] Both Reinhertz *et al.* and Bach *et al.*[10] reported reduced numbers of OKT5-bearing cells in MS patients with acute episodes of MS. Although the OKT5 and OKT8 epitopes are located on the same molecule, the former reagent detects fewer cells.[12] A recent study[16] of the T5/T8 molecule with a panel of eight monoclonal antibodies directed at different epitopes has shown that the determinant detected by OKT5 is the most susceptible to enzymatic cleavage. Because proteolytic enzymes may be increased in the serum during an acute attack of MS, the reduced number of OKT5-bearing cells could indicate loss of the OKT5 epitope rather than a reduction in a subset of cells.

Our findings that the percentage of OKT8-bearing cells is reduced in male patients with chronic progressive disease are also consistent with the findings by Paty *et al.*[12] whereas our normal values with female patients using this antiserum were at variance with their results. This discrepancy could be due to the fact that these investigators did not separate their subjects by sex. In our studies to date the means of the T4/T8 ratio are different in both male and female patients with chronic progressive MS.

Throughout this report functional designations (such as helper, inducer and suppressor) for subpopulations of lymphocytes have been avoided. It is clear that antisera directed at OKT4 and OKT8, as well as antisera directed at Leu 2A and 3A, define subsets of T cells. However, it is also clear that each subset is heterogeneous in terms of function. For example, in the subset of cells defined by anti-OKT4 or anti-Leu 3A, helper function,[7] suppressor function[17] and major histocompatibility complex (MHC)-restricted killing[18] have been demonstrated.

Currently, evidence is mounting that the OKT4 and OKT8 molecules have important functions in the interaction between lymphocytes and targets. It is established that T lymphocytes react with specific antigens present in conjugation with the major histocompatibility complex. Further, the subset of OKT4-positive T lymphocytes, regardless of function, are restricted by Class II MHC antigens[18,19,20]; similarly OKT8 lymphocytes are restricted by Class I MHC antigens. Consequently in our laboratory the practice is to refer to the two major subsets of T lymphocytes as either Class I MHC-restricted or Class II MHC-restricted rather than to assign a functional designation on the basis of phenotypic markers.

ACKNOWLEDGMENT

The authors would like to express their appreciation to Dr. John Whitaker for CSF basic protein determinations in the acute patients and Pamela Danner for her assistance in the preparation of this manuscript.

REFERENCES

1. McFarlin, D. E. & H. F. McFarland. 1982. Multiple sclerosis. N. Eng. J. Med. **307:** 1183–1252.
2. Antel, J. P., D. P. Weinrich & B. G. W. Arnason. 1978. Mitogen responses and suppressor cell function in multiple sclerosis: Influence of age and disease activity. Neurology **28:** 999–1003.
3. Huddlestone, J. R. & M. B. A. Oldstone. 1979. T suppressor (Ts) lymphocytes fluctuate in parallel with changes in the clinical course of patients with multiple sclerosis. J. Immunol. **123:** 1615–1618.
4. Neighbour, P. A., A. E. Miller & B. R. Bloom. 1981. Interferon responses of leukocytes in multiple sclerosis. Neurology **31:** 561–566.
5. Salonen, R., J. Ilonen, M. Reunanen, J. Nikoskelainen & A. Salmi. 1982. PPD PWM and PHA-induced interferon in stable multiple sclerosis: Association with HLA-DW2 antigen and clinical variables. Ann. Neurol. **11:** 219–224.
6. Neighbour, P. A. & B. R. Bloom. 1982. The interferon-natural killer cell system in multiple sclerosis. *In* Immunology and Allergy. B. Waksman, Ed: **2:** 279–295. W. B. Saunders. Philadelphia.
7. Reinhertz, E. L., P. C. Kung, G. Goldstein & S. F. Schlossman. 1979. Separation of functional subsets of human T cells by a monoclonal antibody. Proc. Natl. Acad. Sci. U.S.A. **76:** 4061–4065.
8. Reinherz, E. L., H. L. Weiner, S. L. Hauser, J. A. Cohen, J. A. Distaso & S. F. Schlossman. 1980. Loss of suppressor T cells in active multiple sclerosis analysis with monoclonal antibodies. N. Eng. J. Med. **303:** 125–129.
9. Reinherz, E. L. & S. F. Schlossman. 1979. Con A-induced suppression of MLC: Evidence for mediation by the TH_2^+ T-cell subset in man. J. Immunol. **122:** 1335–1341.
10. Bach, M. A., F. Phan-Dinh-Tuy, E. Tournier, L. Chatenoud, J. F. Back, C. Martin & J. D. Degos. 1980. Deficit suppressor T cells in active multiple sclerosis. Lancet **2:** 1221–1224.
11. Hauser, S. L., E. L. Reinherz, C. J. Hobar, S. F. Schlossman & H. L. Weiner. 1983. Immunoregulatory T-cells and lymphocytotoxic antibodies in active multiple sclerosis: Weekly analysis over a six-month period. Ann. Neurol. **13:** 418–425.

12. PATY, D. W., L. KASTRUKOFF, N. MORGAN & L. HIOB. 1983. Suppressor T-lymphocytes in multiple sclerosis: Analysis of patients with acute relapsing and chronic progressive disease. Ann. Neurol. **14:** 445–449.
13. SCHUMACHER, G. A., G. BEEBE, R. F. KIBLER, L. T. KURLAND, J. F. KURTZKE, F. McDOWELL, B. NAGLER, W. A. SIBLEY, W. W. TOURTELLOTTE & T. L. WILLMON. 1965. Problems of experimental trials of therapy in multiple sclerosis: Report by the panel on the evaluation of experimental trials of therapy of multiple sclerosis. Ann. N.Y. Acad. Sci. **122:** 552–568.
14. HERZENBERG, L. A. & L. A. HERZENBERG. 1978. Analysis and separation using the fluorescence activated cell sorter (FACS). *In* Handbook of Experimental Immunology, vol. 2. D. M. Weir, Ed.: 22.1–22.21. Backwell. Oxford.
15. TITUS, J. A., S. O. SHARROW & D. M. SEGAL. 1982. Analysis of Fc (IgG) receptors on human peripheral blood leukocytes by dual fluorescence flow microfluorometry. II. Quantitation of receptors on cells that express the OKM1, OKT3, OKT4, and OKT8 antigens. J. Immunol. **130:** 1152–1158.
16. BIDDISON, W. E., P. E. RAO, M. A. TALLE, C. M. BOSELLI & G. GOLDSTEIN. 1984. Distinct epitopes on the T8 molecules are differentially involved in cytotoxic T-cell function. Hum. Immunol. **9:** 117–130.
17. THOMAS, Y., L. ROGOZINSKI, O. H. IRIGUYEN, S. M. FRIEDMAN, P. C. KUNG, G. GOLDSTEIN & L. CHESS. 1981. Functional analysis of human T-cell subsets determined by monoclonal antibodies. IV. Induction of suppressor cells with the OKT4 population. J. Exp. Med. **154:** 459–467.
18. BIDDISON, W. E., P. E. RAO, M. A. TALLE, G. GOLDSTEIN & S. SHAW. 1982. Possible involvement of the OKT4 molecule in T cell recognition of class II HLA antigens: Evidence from studies of cytotoxic T lymphocytes specific for SB antigens. J. Exp. Med. **156:** 1065–1076.
19. MEUER, S. C., S. F. SCHLOSSMAN & E. L. REINHERTZ. 1982. Clonal analysis of human cytotoxic T lymphocytes: $T4^+$ and $T8^+$ effector T cells recognize products of different major histocompatibility complex regions. Proc. Natl. Acad. Sci. U.S.A. **79:** 4395–4399.
20. ENGLEMAN, E. G., C. J. BERIKE, E. GLICKMAN & R. L. EVANS. 1981. Antibodies to membrane structures that distinguish suppressor/cytotoxic and helper T lymphocyte subpopulations block the mixed leukocyte reaction in man. J. Exp. Med. **153:** 193–198.

Suppressor T Cells in MS: Do Changes in Numbers Vary with Clinical Activity?

D. W. PATY AND L. F. KASTRUKOFF

Department of Medicine
Division of Neurology
Health Sciences Centre Hospital
The University of British Columbia
Vancouver, British Columbia V6T 1W5, Canada

Even though most investigators agree that suppressor-cell function falls with acute relapses in multiple sclerosis (MS)[1,2] there is a controversy over what happens to suppressor T cell numbers during the various stages of clinical MS[3] (see other papers in this Part). We have studied this phenomenon in three phases using a variety of monoclonal antibodies directed toward T cell surface antigens. The initial phase[4] was a study of patients in active, stable, and chronic progressive MS compared to controls. The second portion[5] was a serial study of 12 patients with relapsing and remitting MS. Blood was tested every week for six months and correlation with disease activity determined. The third phase has been to look at the suppressor T cell phenotype using two-color techniques. Using two-color analysis, changes in the expression of two suppressor/cytotoxic-specific cell surface antigens can be monitored simultaneously.

METHODS

Patients

All MS patients satisfied the Schumacher criteria[7] for clinically definite disease. Stable MS was defined as three or more months of a stable clinical state with an overall disability rating of less than 3 on the Kurtzke DSS scale.[8] Acute relapses were defined as definite changes in the neurological examination occurring over a period of 1–5 days in a previously documented stable patient. Chronic progressive MS was defined as steady deterioration in function or neurological findings for at least three months prior to testing. Benign MS was defined as less than Kurtzke DSS 3 after 15 years of disease. Normal controls consisted of hospital and laboratory personnel.

In the initial project we now have a total of 52 normal controls, 22 spinal-injured adults as neurological controls, 72 stable MS, 33 acute relapse MS (17 studied in both stable and acute relapse phases), 36 chronic progressive MS and 5 patients in a category of benign MS. In the second phase of the study 12 patients (8 female, 4 male), selected because they suffered from relapsing and remitting MS, had enumeration of T cell subsets on a weekly basis. Each patient kept a daily diary of symptoms and this was reviewed weekly with the clinic coordinator. Relapses were evaluated by formal neurological examination and rated on the Kurtzke DSS scale. Three normal controls were also studied on a weekly basis. In the third phase of the study we did two-color analysis of the suppressor cell phenotype in selected normal subjects and in stable MS patients. We are in the process of applying this method to acute relapse patients.

Lymphocyte Preparation

Blood was collected in preservative-free heparin and separated on a ficoll-hypaque gradient. Cells were washed repeatedly in phosphate-buffered saline (PBS) and resuspended in RPM1-1640 with 2% bovine serum albumin (BSA). Cells (1×10^6) were incubated with either 0.1 μg of directly fluorescinated anti-Leu 1, 2a, or 3a (Becton Dickinson, Sunnyvale, CA) or 0.1 μg of OKT5[a] or OKT8 (Ortho Pharmaceuticals, Raritan, NJ) for 30 minutes at 4°C. Cells labeled with OKT monoclonals were washed and then incubated with 25 μg of goat anti-mouse IgG (Cappell Laboratories, Cochranville, PA) for an additional 30 minutes at 4°C.

FACS Analysis

Analysis was performed on a dual laser fluorescence-activated cell sorter (FACS IV, Becton Dickinson). Forward light scatter gating was done to eliminate dead cells, debris and the majority of large cells (monocytes). Cells (1×10^4) were counted after the cursor was set at the crossover point of the autofluorescent curve and the curve generated by specific antibody-labeled cells. The latter represented a population of lymphocytes with a 3–5% monocyte contamination. Results are reported as percent fluorescent cells minus negative control of the total cells counted. Two laser two-color studies were done in a subgroup of patients studying simultaneously the expression of two antigens such as Leu 2a and OKT5.

RESULTS

TABLE 1 displays the results in our combined experience with one-color analysis of the enumeration of T cell subsets using the Leu series of monoclonals plus a smaller group of MS patients using OKT8. The chronic progressive MS patients had an older age of onset, were older at the time of the study, had a more severe neurological deficit, and a longer duration of disease. We were unable to show any consistent changes associated with the acute relapse. In the 17 patients studied in both stable phase and acute relapse (TABLE 2) there was no consistent change. Nine relapse patients had a mean fall in percent suppressor cells of 3.88, whereas 7 had a mean rise in percent suppressor cells of 6.28.

Chronic progressive MS (TABLE 1) was associated with low Leu 2a-positive cells ($p < 0.005$), and also had a slightly low T cell level ($p < 0.02$) when compared to stable MS. The few benign patients we studied also had a slightly low number of T8-positive cells (18.75%).

In the second phase we studied 12 MS patients with an average age of 30 years, an average age of onset of 23, and an average Kurtzke DSS score of 3. Fluctuations in the percentage of suppressor cells were seen but there was no consistent association with clinical activity. In one patient there was a continuing low level of suppressor cells but no consistent association with clinical activity. In a second patient there was a reduction in suppressor cell numbers associated with an acute relapse. There were several other times when significant changes in numbers of suppressor cells were not associated with any evidence of clinical activity. One of the control subjects had the lowest level of suppressor cell numbers throughout the study.

In the third phase we looked at two colors simultaneously on the cell surface. This enabled us to demonstrate in a direct fashion that the OKT8- and Leu 2a-labeled cells were a subpopulation of the OKT3- and/or Leu 1-labeled populations. This is a direct

[a]OKT5 was kindly supplied by Mr. J. F. Egan, Ortho Pharmaceuticals, Raritan, NJ.

TABLE 1. T Cell Subsets in Normals, Neurological Controls, and MS

Category	n	% Leu 1 (SD)	% Leu 3a (SD)	% Leu 2a (SD)	% OKT8 (SD, n)
Normal controls	52	72.38 (6.65)	45.1 (8.11)	24.13 (7.75)	28.44 (7.67 $n = 16$)
Neurological controls	22	73.5 (7.5)	49.0 (7.5)	22.7 (6.1)	—
MS					
Stable	72	71.25 (8.22)	49.57 (8.49)	20.80 (7.97)	21.8 (7.48, $n = 10$)
Acute relapse	33	70.0 (9.32)	46.09 (7.32)	20.12 (7.05)	21.52 (7.68, $n = 21$)
Chronic progressive	36	67.25 (11.15)[a]	51.67 (8.72)	15.47 (6.44)[b]	19.62 (7.54, $n = 8$)
Benign	5	67.2 (11.15)	47.8 (7.29)	21.2 (5.63)	18.75 (2.75)[c]

[a]Chronic vs. stable (Leu 1), $p < 0.002$.
[b]Chronic vs. stable (Leu 2a), $p < 0.005$.
[c]Benign vs. normal (OKT8), $p < 0.01$.

demonstration that the suppressor/cytotoxic cell population is a subpopulation of T cells. Two-color studies of OKT8 and Leu 2a showed that these two monoclonals labeled the same population of cells and competitively inhibited each other's binding. This suggested that these two monoclonals were labeling the same antigen or closely linked antigenic sites on the same molecule. OKT5 and Leu 2a labeled the same population of cells but did not inhibit each other's binding. Experiments comparing OKT5 and Leu 2a showed that there were a number of Leu 2a-positive cells that were OKT5 negative. This was true in both MS and normals. Serial studies of these two antigens have shown that OKT5 routinely labels about 15–20% of peripheral blood lymphocytes (PBL) and the level fluctuates much more widely in percentage than do OKT8 and anti-Leu 2a which label about 25% of PBL.

Our overall experience with suppressor cell numbers as measured in this fashion has not confirmed previous reports that suppressor-cell numbers consistently fall during an acute relapse. We have shown that the expression of cell surface antigens is likely to be a dynamic process. The suppressor/cytotoxic population of T cells, as studied by two-color fluorescence, is not homogeneous. We have demonstrated subpopulations within this group of cells. We suspect that some of the differences in findings between the various studies noted in the literature reflect this dynamic state in the expression of cell surface antigens. Intensity of fluorescence also seems to change over time, leaving the impression that certain cells may be appearing and disappearing from the population during clinical activity.

TABLE 2. Seventeen MS Patients Studied in Both Stable Phase and Acute Relapse

Category	*n*	% Leu 2a	No. of Patients with Decrease	Mean % Change	No. with Increase	Mean % Change
Stable	17	21.23	—	—	—	—
Acute relapse	17	27.75	9	3.88	7	6.28

DISCUSSION

Multiple sclerosis is thought to be an autoimmune disease mediated by T cells that may be cytotoxic toward myelin or myelin components. Changes in the behavior and/or number of suppressor/cytotoxic T cells may have pathogenic significance. We have studied this phenomenon quite carefully and have been unable to show that suppressor-cell numbers consistently change during the acute relapse of MS. We have been able to show that cell surface antigen expression is a dynamic process, and perhaps subtle changes in the expression of these antigens occur in response to physiological stimuli.

The only consistent abnormality in the numbers of T cell subsets we have found is that patients with chronic progressive MS carry low numbers of suppressor/cytotoxic T cells. This does not appear to reflect a nonspecific change related to chronic neurological deficit because a control population of spinal-cord injured patients did not show this. These chronic progressive patients were older and perhaps an age factor had an influence because the older patients had the lowest suppressor T cell numbers. In contrast to this we did not find lower numbers in the older controls.

We now have nuclear magnetic resonance (NMR) imaging data to show that the development of new lesions on NMR does not necessarily correlate with clinical expression. This might explain some of the lack of correlation between biological markers of disease activity and clinical signs of activity. We are now in the process of using clinical and NMR studies to correlate with T cell subset enumeration. Additional detailed multicolor studies of cell-surface antigen expression in both normals and MS are also underway in this laboratory.

REFERENCES

1. ANTEL, J. P., D. P. RICHMAN, M. E. MEDOF & B. G. W. ARNASON. 1978. Suppressor cells in multiple sclerosis. Neurology **28:** 106.
2. PATY, D. W., H. K. COUSIN & B. BASS. 1980. Suppressor cell activity and mitogen responses in various phases and stages of multiple sclerosis. Can. J. Neurol. Sci. **7:** 322.
3. REINHERZ, E. L., H. L. WEINER, S. L. HAUSSER, J. A. COHEN, J. A. DISTASO & S. F. SCHLOSSMAN. 1980. Loss of suppressor T cells in active multiple sclerosis: Analysis with monoclonal antibodies. N. Engl. J. Med. **303:** 125.
4. PATY, D. W., L. F. KASTRUKOFF, N. MORGAN & L. HIOB. 1980. Suppressor T-lymphocytes in multiple sclerosis: Analysis of patients with acute relapsing and chronic progressive disease. Ann. Neurol. **14:** 445–449.
5. KASTRUKOFF, L. F. & D. W. PATY. 1984. A serial study of peripheral blood T lymphocyte subsets in relapsing-remitting multiple sclerosis (MS). Ann. Neurol. **15:** 250–256.
6. KASTRUKOFF, L. F. & D. W. PATY. 1984. A two label microfluorometric analysis of the expression of OKT5 and Leu 2 a antigens on peripheral blood lymphocytes in patients with multiple sclerosis. J. Neuroimmunol. **6:** 89–92.
7. SCHUMACHER, G. A., G. BEEBE, R. F. KIBLER, L. T. KURLAND, J. F. KURTZKE, F. MCDOWELL, B. NAGLER, W. A. SIBLEY, W. W. TOURTELLOTTE & T. L. WILLMON. 1965. Problems of experimental trials of therapy in multiple sclerosis. Report by the panel on the evaluation of experimental trials of therapy of multiple sclerosis. Ann. N.Y. Acad. Sci. **122:** 552.
8. KURTZKE, J. F. 1965. Further notes on disability evaluation in multiple sclerosis with scale modifications. Neurology **15:** 654.

The Failure of Monoclonal Antibody-defined Lymphocyte Subsets to Monitor Disease Activity in Patients with Multiple Sclerosis[a]

GEORGE P. A. RICE, JACK C. SIPE,
SHERRY L. BRAHENY, ROBERT L. KNOBLER,
DAVID A. FINNEY, AND MICHAEL B. A. OLDSTONE

Department of Immunology and Division of Neurology
Scripps Clinic and Research Foundation
La Jolla, California 92037

INTRODUCTION

Cellular immunological mechanisms have been implicated in the etiology of multiple sclerosis (MS),[1] and have been studied extensively in pursuit of an *in vitro* marker of the activity of this disease. The recent literature has focused on enumeration of T and B lymphocytes in peripheral blood and spinal fluid by means of assays reflecting the evolution and availability of new technologies. Proponents of the earliest studies examined the T cell compartment by a variety of rosetting techniques and suggested that there was in patients with MS a deficiency of T cells in the blood and an excess in the spinal fluid.[2-4] Further refinement in techniques allowed the separation of T lymphocytes into two functionally discrete groups, a population bearing a receptor for the Fc fragment of immunoglobulin G with a suppressor function (T gamma), and a population bearing a receptor for the Fc fragment of immunoglobulin M with a helper-cell function (T mu). Application of these techniques to characterization of immunoregulatory lymphocyte subsets in blood[5] and spinal fluid[6] of patients with MS indicated that during exacerbation the number of cells with the T gamma phenotype decreased. Further, during convalescence, the number of T gamma cells increased to levels above normal. Although conflicting reports of T gamma proportions have emanated from other laboratories,[7-9] all who have studied this subset have found abnormalities. However, the cumbersome nature of these assays discourages their routine usage.

The advent of monoclonal antibodies specific to human lymphocyte surface markers allowed for more exacting phenotypic characterization. Currently, human T

[a]This research was supported by USPHS grant no. NS 12428, National Multiple Sclerosis Society research grant no. 1285–A–4, NIH grant no. RR00833 to the General Clinical Research Center at Scripp's Clinic and Research Foundation and grants from the Leiper Trust and the McDonald and Hearst Foundation.

Dr. Rice is a recipient of the Centennial Fellowship from the Medical Research Council of Canada. Dr. Knobler is a recipient of a Teacher Investigator Award from the National Institute of Neurological and Communicative Disorders and Stroke (no. NS–00803).

cells can be divided into major functional classes, a helper cell compartment identified by monoclonal antibodies OKT4 and Leu 2, and a suppressor cell compartment marked by monoclonal antibodies OKT5, OKT8, and Leu 3.[10] Although the number of markers continues to increase with the burgeoning of hybridoma technology, we have focused on the markers that have been extensively studied relative to MS. With these reagents, Reinherz *et al.*[11] initially found in MS patients a rather striking diminution in the suppressor cell compartment defined by monoclonal antibody OKT5. As work in this area increased, the initial observation was questioned. We sought firsthand experience, as reported here.

MATERIALS AND METHODS

Patient Selection

Patients with MS were drawn from the Demyelinating Disease Clinic at Scripps Clinic and Research Foundation. All patients included in this study had clinically definite disease as defined by the Poser criteria[12] and these diagnoses were substantiated by at least two neurologists. Disease activity was categorized as stable, chronic progressive, or active (clinical evidence of exacerbation within three weeks). Patients receiving steroid or other immunomodulatory treatment were excluded. Age-matched control subjects were drawn from a healthy population of hospital employees. All blood sampling was performed between 0800–1000 h.

Methods

Venous blood was collected into heparinized Becton-Dickinson Vacutainer tubes and processed the same morning. Lymphocytes were isolated by density gradient centrifugation over ficoll-hypaque (Pharmacia, Piscataway, NJ), washed three times in phosphate-buffered saline, and resuspended at a concentration of 5 million cells per ml. Two hundred microliter fractions were then reacted for 30 minutes with 5 μl of the appropriate Orthoclone monoclonal antibodies (OKT3-total T cell marker; OKT4 T helper cell marker; OKT5 and OKT8 T suppressor cell markers, Ortho Diagnostics, Raritan, NJ), according to the manufacturer's instructions. The natural killer cell-specific monoclonal antibodies B73.1 and CL 45 were gifts of Drs. G. Trinchieri and R. Fox, respectively. The entire procedure was conducted at 4°C to preclude capping of cell-surface determinants. After two washes with ice-cold saline, the pellet was resuspended in an appropriate volume of an affinity purified, $F(ab)_2$ preparation of a fluoresceinated goat antibody to mouse immunoglobulin G (Boehringer-Mannheim). After 30 minutes the cells were washed twice and resuspended at a density of one million per ml in saline containing 1% formaldehyde.

The cells were counted by cytofluorographic analysis on a fluorescence-activated cell sorter (FACS IV, Becton-Dickinson, Mountain View, CA). Background fluorescence, which was determined by omitting the first antibody in the indirect immunofluorescence procedure, was consistently less than 2%. The criteria appear in the legend of FIG. 1. All analyses were performed by an operator (DF) without knowledge of the clinical status of the patient. In these experiments ten thousand cells were counted from each sample.

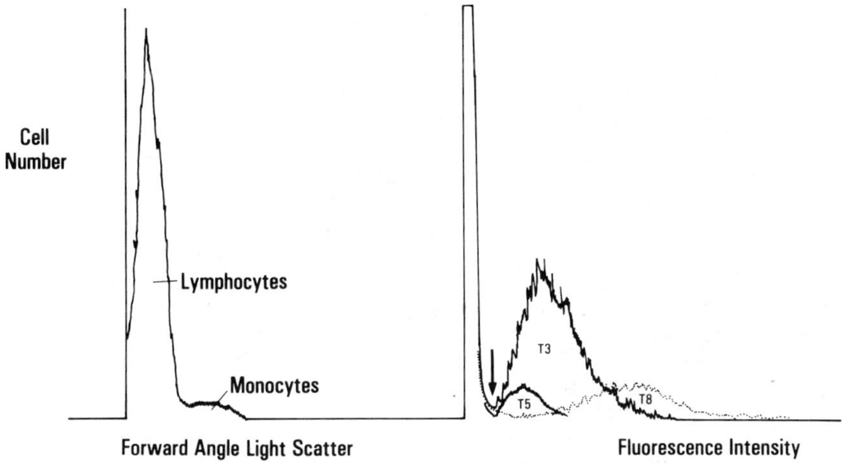

FIGURE 1. FACS analysis of cell surface phenotype. Cell number is plotted against forward angle light scatter (*left panel*) and fluorescence intensity (*right panel*). The light scatter characteristics of lymphocytes and monocytes are shown on the left. On the right are the fluorescence histograms of lymphocytes from a healthy adult (control) marked with the monoclonal antibodies OKT3, 5 and 8. For a cell to be counted as positive by automated cytofluorometry, the light scatter characteristics had to be typical of lymphocytes or monocytes, and the fluorescence intensity had to be greater than a threshold defined by the intersection of the autofluorescence curve and the OKT3 fluorescence histogram (*arrow*).

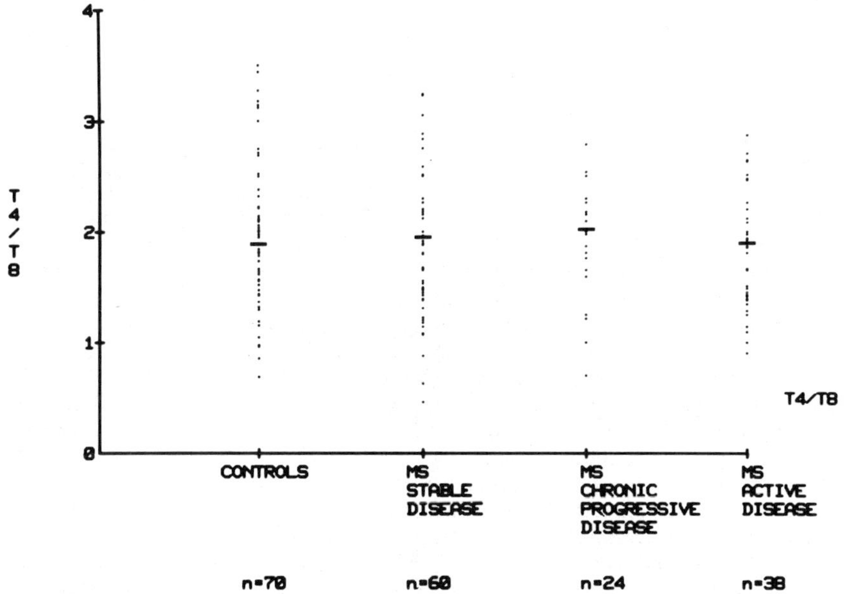

FIGURE 2. Ratios of helper cells (OKT4) to suppressor cells (OKT8) are plotted for controls (see Methods), and patients with MS, stratified according to disease activity.

RESULTS

The Ratio of Helper Cells to Suppressor Cells (OKT4:OKT8) Does Not Correlate with Disease Activity in Patients with MS

As shown in FIG. 2, we could demonstrate no differences between patients and controls in the ratio of helper cells to suppressor cells as defined by the ratio of OKT4:OKT8 positive cells. The mean ratio in 70 controls was 1.88 ± 0.08 (SE) compared to 1.96 ± 0.15 in 60 MS patients with stable disease, 2.00 ± 0.12 in 24 patients with chronic progressive disease and 1.79 ± 0.08 in 38 patients with active disease. The small differences between the patient groups were not significant when tested by Student's *t* test (all intergroup *p* values exceeded 0.3). Similar data were obtained when the OKT5-positive subset was studied in the same fashion, although fewer patients were studied with this reagent.

The OKT4:OKT8 Ratio Does Not Change in a Longitudinal Study of Patients Undergoing Exacerbation

Ten consecutive patients were followed prospectively through periods of exacerbation. All had an estimation of baseline subset ratio at some time before the exacerbation. Most were seen in the first week of the exacerbation, and all within a fortnight. Subset ratios and clinical examinations were performed subsequently on a weekly or fortnightly basis. As shown in FIG. 3, in a serial plot of these data, we could establish no consistent correlation between disease activity and subset fluctuations. Similar minor fluctuations in subset ratio occurred in a control population (data not shown).

The OKT4:OKT8 Ratio Does Not Correlate with the Development of an Antigen-specific Immune Response in Vivo

Twelve patients with relapsing and remitting disease were engaged in a two-year study designed to test the efficacy of human alpha interferon in the treatment of MS. OKT4:OKT8 T lymphocyte ratios were assessed on a monthly or bimonthly basis. Three major observations could be drawn from this study group. First, there was a poor correlation between exacerbation and change in subset ratios. In this cohort, there were 21 exacerbations over a two-year period, only five of which were associated with fluctuation in ratio greater than 1 SD from baseline (*e.g.,* FIGURE 4, panel B, exacerbation 1). Second, change in subset ratios from baseline often occurred without clinically detectable alteration in clinical status (FIG. 4B). Third, all patients in this study developed high titer of antibody to a contaminant in the partially purified interferon preparation. This antibody was shown to be directed to a 27,000 dalton protein contaminant related to the Sendai virus that was used to prepare the interferon (Rice *et al.,* 1984, manuscript in preparation). The antibody developed within three weeks of interferon administration, and continued to increase throughout the six months of daily interferon administration, after which it fell. The rise and fall of this antigen-specific immune response occurred without a correlating change in lymphocyte populations defined by monoclonal antibodies OKT4 and OKT8. This perhaps exemplifies the difficulty in using these reagents to characterize the phenotype of lymphocytes involved in the possible control of an antigenic-specific immune response.

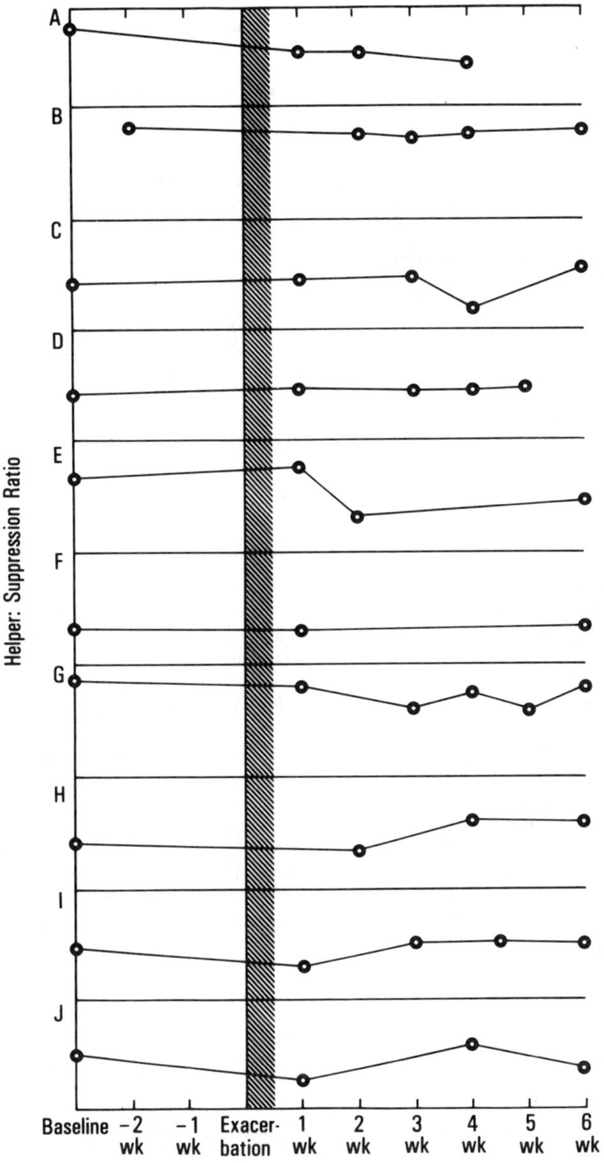

FIGURE 3. OKT4:OKT8 ratios were serially plotted against time for ten individual MS patients (*A* through *J*) who underwent exacerbation in the hatched zone and who subsequently recovered within the next several weeks. The *y*-axis (OKT4:OKT8 ratio) ranges in each panel from 0–4.

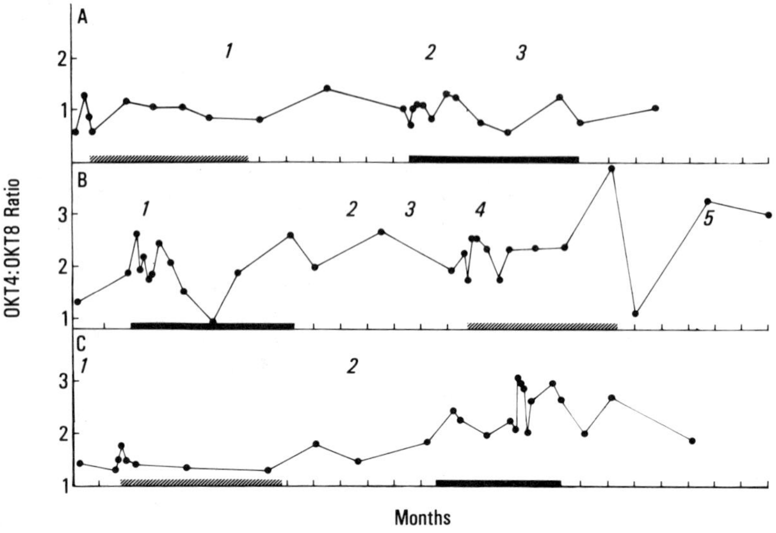

FIGURE 4. Serial determinations of OKT4:OKT8 ratios in 3 of the 12 patients engaged in a crossover trial of human alpha interferon (*solid bars*) compared to placebo (*hatched bars*). Each clinical exacerbation is indicated by number. In panel (**A**), subset ratios fluctuated within a standard deviation of the mean subset ratio for patients with stable MS (0.6), but three exacerbations occurred. The first two consisted of optic neuritis and worsening of leg weakness, and the third, deterioration in leg strength alone. Panel (**B**) illustrates that wide fluctuation in subset ratio can occur without clinically detectable deterioration in neurological performance. In this patient, there was a slight perturbation in subset ratio before exacerbation 1, manifested by loss of sensation and unilateral leg weakness. Subset data were insufficient at the time of exacerbations 2 and 3 to make further comments. Exacerbation 4, an abrupt onset of leg numbness and cerebellar ataxia, was unassociated with major change in subset ratios. Large amplitude changes in ratio occurred between the first and second and the fourth and fifth exacerbations without clinical change. We concede that subclinical exacerbations can indeed occur. At the time of the fifth exacerbation, manifested by right hemiparesis and internuclear ophthalmoplegia, the ratio increased. The patient depicted in panel (**C**) had two exacerbations unassociated with subset ratio change. The first exacerbation consisted of left arm weakness and incoordination; the second, right arm numbness and right leg weakness. All patients who received this interferon preparation developed antibody to a noninterferon 27K protein. The levels of this antibody peaked in the fourth to sixth month of treatment, often to titers exceeding 10,000, and fell to much lower levels (approximately 100–200) after treatment.

Interferon or placebo administration had no effect on the proportions of cells identified with these markers.

Monoclonal Antibodies to Other Lymphocyte Antigens Also Fail to Correlate with Disease or Disease Activity

We examined the usefulness of OKT3, which identifies about 90% of peripheral blood T cells, and OKM1, which marks a monocyte population, as predictors of disease activity in MS. No correlation could be established. Patients with chronic progressive disease tended to have fewer T cells, but this was not statistically significant.

Further, we studied monoclonal antibodies specific to natural killer cells. With the CL 45 and B73.1 reagents, we were similarly unable to identify a lymphocyte subset that correlated with disease or disease activity. These data are consistent with our previous observations that natural killer cells function normally in patients with MS.[13]

There Is No Characteristic Change in the Fluorescence Histogram during Exacerbation.

To anticipate the argument that cytofluorographic analysis might have been too sensitive in falsely considering positive dimly fluorescent cells that would have been missed by fluorescence microscopy, we studied the entire fluorescence histogram in some patients. As shown in FIG. 1, monoclonal antibodies usually stain lymphocyte surface antigens in a characteristic fashion most clearly demonstrated if cell number is plotted against fluorescence intensity. For example, the total T cell compartment marked by monoclonal antibody OKT3 is a population of homogeneously bright cells, represented graphically by a sharply defined peak in the fluorescence histogram. The OKT8-positive population has a wide spectrum of fluorescence intensity, noted in the histogram by a rather flat peak. In the data shown previously, cells were counted as positive if they were more brightly fluorescent than a threshold determined by the intersection of the autofluorescence curve and the first positive deflection in the OKT3 histogram. This point consistently represented the inflection point between the

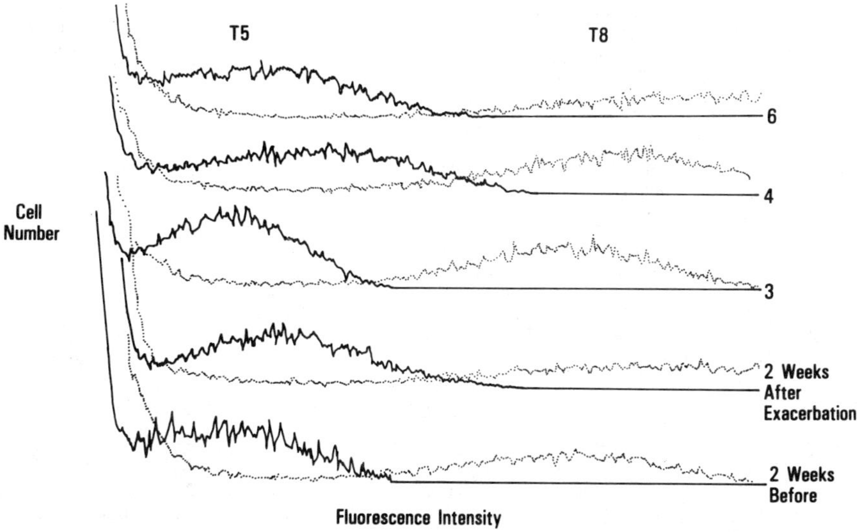

FIGURE 5. In this figure, the right panel seen in FIG. 1 is expanded to show the entire fluorescence histogram for lymphocytes stained with monoclonal reagents OKT5 (*solid lines*) and OKT8 (*stippled lines*). Superimposed on each other are the serially studied fluorescence histograms of lymphocytes from an individual studied during an exacerbation manifested by optic neuritis and worsening of myelopathy. The time intervals of these studies are indicated on the right side of the graph.

autofluorescence and fluorescence curves for the other monoclonals, but was easier to discern, as FIG. 1 shows.

When the entire fluorescence histogram was plotted in patients serially studied during exacerbation, no consistent change occurred for either OKT5- or OKT8-positive cells. The data for serial histogram monitoring of lymphocyte phenotype in a 32-year-old man undergoing a severe exacerbation manifested by optic neuritis and worsening myelopathy are plotted in FIG. 5. The evolution of the histogram in a prospectively followed age- and sex-matched control is seen in FIG. 6, and changes are minor.

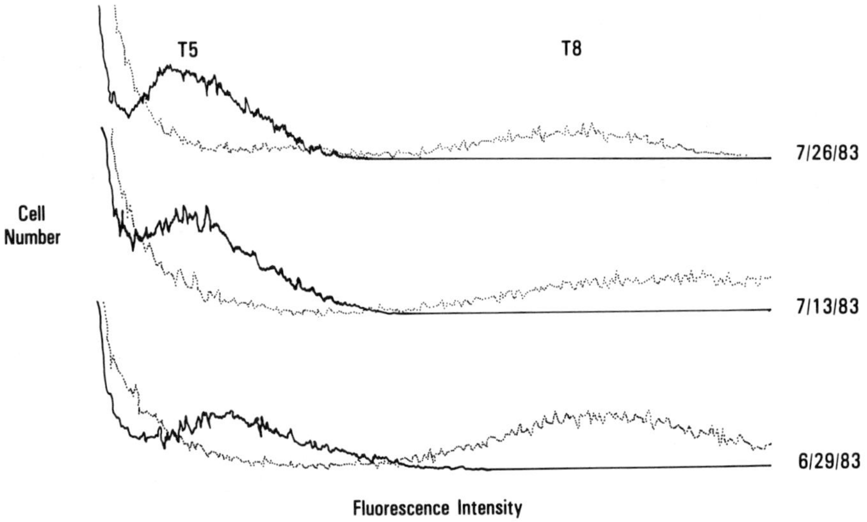

FIGURE 6. The evolution of a fluorescence histogram in an age- and sex-matched control of the patient examined in FIG. 4.

DISCUSSION

Here we report that the monoclonal antibodies OKT3, OKT4, OKT5, OKT8, OKM1, B73.1 and CL 45 fail to identify any lymphocyte subset that correlates with MS or its course. The literature concerning this issue has been controversial. Early reports, examining both populations[14–16] and individuals followed serially[17,18] appeared to support the initial observation that subset changes correlate with disease activity, especially the subset characterized by OKT5 or OKT8. More recent reports[19,20] have challenged those original observations, or have proposed other markers, such as Leu 2,[19] as more relevant to the activity of this disease. The reasons for this disparity are not immediately clear, especially because most investigators have followed the standardized methods outlined by the manufacturers of these reagents. Several possible explanations can be proposed. First, although there is generally a high correlation between enumerative analysis of the OKT8-positive subset determined by automated cytofluorometry and that by fluorescence microscopy,[21] most of the reports that have suggested a deficiency in the OKT8-positive subset have employed fluorescence microscopy. Not all have been blind studies, which is an important consideration because of the wide spectrum in fluorescence intensity of cells marked with OKT8. Further, not all studies have been careful to ensure that patient groups had only clinically definite MS, and some reports have included patients receiving therapy capable of modulating lymphocytes and their function. Another important consideration (usually not addressed in these reports) is the time of venous blood sampling, to control for the effect of circadian rhythm on these ratios.[22] There is also evidence to suggest that the surface antigen recognized by the OKT8 antibody is unstable and certainly susceptible to small variations in methodological handling. The expression of this antigen is dependent on such seemingly trivial variables as the concentration of fetal calf serum in preparatory media and monocyte activation.[23]

This controversy makes it difficult to interpret the relevance of the OKT5/8 subset to MS. At best, if subset perturbations do exist, they are not disease-specific; similar alterations have been found in other human diseases.[10] Additional caution in interpreting lymphocyte subset ratio changes as showing possible functional changes in suppressor activity is underscored by recent reports from several laboratories of functional heterogeneity within these phenotypically defined compartments.[24,25]

In conclusion, our experience with these monoclonal reagents has stayed our enthusiasm for their use in monitoring clinical course of disease and hence employing them for selection of patients for clinical trials involving immunomodulatory treatment. The shortcomings of the current reagents have refocused our attention on functional assays of suppressor-cell function, for which there is greater agreement as to their usefulness in monitoring disease activity.[1,26]

ACKNOWLEDGMENTS

We are greatly indebted to Ms. Kendis Cox and Ms. Pamela Elliott for skilled technical assistance and to the staff of the General Clinical Research Center, Kaye Smith, RN and Margaret Floyd, RN for aid in patient care. The deployment of the CLINFO system was stewarded by Mrs. Aparna Ewing. We are extremely grateful to Ms. Gay L. Wilkins for unflagging secretarial assistance.

REFERENCES

1. KNOBLER, R. L., G. P. A. RICE & M. B. A. OLDSTONE. 1983. Immunologic studies of multiple sclerosis. *In* Clinical Laboratory Assays: New Technology and Future Directions. R. Nakamura, Ed.: 377–388. Masson. New York.
2. LISAK, R. P., A. I. LEVINSON, B. ZIVELMAN & N. I ABDOU. 1975. T + B lymphocytes in multiple sclerosis. Clin. Exp. Immunol. **22:** 30–34.
3. ALLEN, J. C., M. SHEREMATA, J. B. R. COSGROVE, K. OSTERLAND & M. SHEA. 1978. Cerebrospinal fluid T + B lymphocyte kinetics related to exacerbations of MS. Neurology **26:** 579–583.
4. NAESS, A. & H. NYLAND. 1978. Multiple sclerosis T lymphocytes in cerebrospinal fluid and blood. Eur. Neurol. **17:** 61–65.
5. HUDDLESTONE, J. R. & M. B. A. OLDSTONE. 1979. T suppressor (Tg) lymphocytes are fluctuate in parallel with changes in the clinical course of patients with multiple sclerosis. J. Immunol. **123:** 1615–1619.
6. COYLE, P. K., B. R. BROOKS, R. HIRSCH, S. R. COHEN, P. O'DONNELL, R. T. JOHNSON & J. S. WOLINSKY. 1980. Cerebrospinal fluid lymphocyte populations and immune complexes in active multiple sclerosis. Lancet **2:** 229–231.

7. SANTOLI, D., L. MORETTA, R. LISAK, D. GILDEN & H. KOPROWSKI. 1978. Imbalances in T-cell subpopulations in multiple sclerosis patients. J. Immunol. **120:** 1369–1371.
8. GOUST, J. M., P. M. HOFFMAN, J. PRYJMA, E. L. HOGAN & H. H. FUNDENBERG. 1980. Defective immunoregulation in multiple sclerosis. Ann. Neurol. **8:** 526–533.
9. MERRILL, J., G. BIBERFELD, A. LANDIN, A. SIDEN & E. NORRBY. 1980. Identification of three FcR positive T cell subsets (T, T and T) in the cerebrospinal fluid of multiple sclerosis patients. Clin. Exp. Immunol. **42:** 345–354.
10. REINHERZ, E. L. & S. F. SCHLOSSMAN. 1980. Regulation of the immune response: Inducer and suppressor T lymphocyte subsets in human beings. N. Engl. J. Med. **303:** 370–373.
11. REINHERZ, E. L., H. L. WEINER, S. L. HAUSER, J. A. COHEN, J. A. DISTASO & S. SCHLOSSMAN. 1980. Loss of suppressor T cells in active multiple sclerosis. N. Engl. J. Med. **303:** 125–129.
12. POSER, C. M., D. W. PATY, L. SCHEINBERG, W. I. MCDONALD, E. A. DAVIS, G. C. EBERS, K. P. JOHNSON, W. A. SIBLEY, D. H. SILBERBERG & W. W. TOURTELLOTTE. 1983. New diagnostic criteria for multiple sclerosis: Guidelines for research protocols. Ann. Neurol. **13:** 227–231.
13. RICE, G. P. A., P. CASALI, T. C. MERIGAN & M. B. A. OLDSTONE. 1983. Natural killer cell activity in patients with multiple sclerosis given alpha interferon. Ann. Neurol. **14:** 333–338.
14. BACH, A., T. PHAN-DIN-TUY, E. TOURNIER, L. CHATENAUD & J. BACH. 1980. Deficit of suppressor T cells in active multiple sclerosis. Lancet **ii:** 1221–1223.
15. SANDBERG-WOLLHEIM, M. 1983. Lymphocyte populations in the cerebrospinal fluid and peripheral blood of patients with multiple sclerosis and optic neuritis. Scand. J. Immunol. **17:** 575–583.
16. BOCCI, L., R. GOREN, R. VALENZUELA, R. TURINIC & S. DEADHAR. 1983. Multiple sclerosis: Evaluation of T cell subsets in peripheral blood by flow cytometry. Neurology **33:** 122.
17. HAUSER, S. L., E. L. REINHERZ, C. J. HOBAN, S. F. SCHLOSSMAN & H. L. WEINER. 1983. Immunoregulatory T cells and lymphocytotoxic antibodies in active multiple sclerosis: Weekly analysis over a six month period. Ann. Neurol. **13:** 418–425.
18. COMPSTON, A. 1983. Lymphocyte subpopulations in patients with multiple sclerosis. J. Neurol. Neurosurg. Psychiatry **46:** 106–114.
19. PATY, D. W., L. KASTRUKOFF, N. MORGAN & L. HIOB. 1983. Suppressor T-lymphocytes in multiple sclerosis: Analysis of patients with acute relapsing and chronic progressive disease. Ann. Neurol. **14:** 445–449.
20. CASHMAN, N., C. MARTIN, J. F. EISENBAUM, J. D. DEGOS & A. BACH. 1982. Monoclonal antibody defined immunoregulatory cells in multiple sclerosis cerebrospinal fluid. J. Clin. Invest. **70:** 387–392.
21. LINDSAY, A., G. L. GARTLAND, T. ABO & M. D. COOPER. 1983. Enumeration of human lymphocyte subpopulations by immunofluorescence: A comparative study using automated flow macrofluorometry and fluorescence microscopy. J. Immunol. Meth. **58:** 337–347.
22. LEVI, F., C. CANON, J. P. BLUM, A. REINBERG & G. MATHE. 1983. Large amplitude circadian rhythm in helper:suppressor ratio of peripheral blood lymphocytes. Lancet **ii:** 462–463.
23. DORE-DUFFY, P., H. H. KUO & M. M. DOWLING. 1983. Role of prostaglandin E in modulation of T cell differentiation antigens. Implication for multiple sclerosis. Neurology **33**(Suppl. 2): 142.
24. THOMAS, Y., L. ROGOZINSKI, O. H. IRIGOYEN, H. H. SHEN, M. A. TALLE, G. GOLDSTEIN & L. CHESS. 1982. Functional analysis of human T-cell subsets defined by monoclonal antibodies. J. Immunol. **128:** 1386–1390.
25. JACOBY, D. R. & M. B. A. OLDSTONE. 1983. Delineation of suppressor and helper activity within the OKT4 defined T-lymphocyte subset in human newborns. J. Immunol. **131:** 1765–1770.
26. HUDDLESTONE, J. R. & M. B. A. OLDSTONE. 1982. Suppressor T cells are activated *in vivo* in patients with multiple sclerosis coinciding with remission from acute attack. J. Immunol. **129:** 915–917.

T Cell Subsets in Patients with Multiple Sclerosis

An Overview[a]

HOWARD L. WEINER, DAVID A. HAFLER, ROBERT J. FALLIS, DAVID JOHNSON, KENNETH A. AULT, AND STEPHEN L. HAUSER

Multiple Sclerosis Clinical and Research Unit
Division of Neurology
Department of Medicine
Brigham and Women's Hospital
Harvard Medical School
Boston, Massachusetts 02115

INTRODUCTION

Over the past four years we have been involved in the study of immunoregulatory T cell abnormalities in patients with multiple sclerosis (MS).[1-6] These studies have focused on the quantitation of T cell phenotypes in the peripheral blood, cerebrospinal fluid (CSF), and more recently in brain sections using monoclonal antibodies (mAbs). The mechanism(s) by which these T cell phenotypes change in the peripheral blood of MS patients and the pathophysiologic significance of these changes to the disease process itself have not yet been defined. Nonetheless, it is now possible to draw some conclusions concerning the mechanism(s) by which they may occur and to address the usefulness and role of these changes, both in the diagnosis and clinical management of patients with multiple sclerosis and in basic immunologic investigations into disease pathogenesis. The present overview consists of a summary of our published data to date as reported in the *Journal of Neuroimmunology,*[6] plus preliminary data from ongoing experiments in our laboratory.

T Cell Changes in the Peripheral Blood of Patients with MS, Other Neurologic Diseases, and Controls

We have analyzed T cell subsets over the past four years in 197 patients with multiple sclerosis. These results are summarized in TABLE 1. T cell subpopulations were determined with monoclonal antibodies and indirect immunofluorescence using an automated cell sorter, as previously described.[1,5] For each blood specimen analyzed, the percentage of inducer (T4-positive) and suppressor/cytotoxic (T8-positive) cells was determined, and the ratio of T4- to T8-positive cells (T4:T8) was calculated. Abnormalities are expressed as changes in the T4:T8 ratio, with a ratio greater than 4

[a]This work was supported by NIH grant no. NS–17182. Dr. Hafler is the recipient of NIH National Research Service Award no. NS07170; Dr. Fallis is a Fellow of the National Multiple Sclerosis Society. We would like to thank Ms. Pat Lamy-Gilbreath for her excellent support in the preparation of the manuscript.

TABLE 1. Analysis of T Cell Subsets in Neurological Disease

Group	Elevated T4:T8 Ratio[a]	
	Number	Percent
Normal subjects ($n = 90$)	3/90	3%
Inactive multiple sclerosis ($n = 60$)	5/60	8%
Acute relapse, multiple sclerosis ($n = 22$)	15/22	68%
Chronic progressive multiple sclerosis ($n = 115$)	47/115	41%
Acute Guillain-Barré syndrome ($n = 12$)	0/12	0%
Active myasthenia gravis ($n = 12$)	1/12	8%
Other neurological diseases[b] ($n = 35$)	1/35	3%

[a]The T4:T8 ratio reflects the relative numbers of helper to suppressor T cells in peripheral blood and represents cumulative data obtained over the past four years. When standardized against normal controls, ratios of greater than 4 were considered elevated in previously published work.[1,3-5] In the past year, some T cell subsets have been measured in the clinical laboratory of the hospital (Dr. Ault) in which a ratio of greater than 3 is considered abnormal.

[b]Includes vascular, inflammatory, infectious, degenerative, and malignant diseases.

considered abnormal. (In the past year, some T cell subsets have been measured in the clinical laboratory of the hospital in which a ratio greater than 3 is considered abnormal.) In patients with inactive multiple sclerosis 5/60 had abnormal ratios; in patients with acute relapse, 15/22; in chronic progressive MS, 47/115. These changes occurred in 0/12 patients with acute Guillain-Barré, in 1/11 patients with myasthenia gravis and in 1/35 patients with other neurologic diseases. In normal subjects 3/90 had abnormal T4:T8 ratios. Of note is that identical changes were found in three children during active phases of acute multiple sclerosis, suggesting that the same pathophysiologic process that occurs in MS in adults occurs in young children as well.[3]

Longitudinal Study of T Cell Subsets in Multiple Sclerosis Patients

Immunoregulatory T cell subsets were measured at weekly intervals over a four- to six-month period in six patients with MS and four age- and sex-matched controls.[5] These studies were performed to determine whether fluctuations of T cells in the peripheral blood occur in normal individuals, the degree to which they occur in multiple sclerosis patients who are in an inactive *versus* active stage of disease, and the relationship of these changes, if any, to attacks of multiple sclerosis. Our studies demonstrated that there were no changes in T cell subsets in the normal controls studied or in two patients who were neurologically stable during the study period. Two patients with intermediate disease activity of the relapsing-remitting type had elevated ratios on three to four occasions (FIG. 1) and the patient with the most clinically active multiple sclerosis had an abnormal ratio 12 of 27 times tested (FIG. 2). Of particular note from these studies was the demonstration of the dynamic nature of T cell subset changes in active relapsing-remitting multiple sclerosis, *viz.*, the rapid depletion and repopulation of T8 cells in the peripheral blood over a week's period. Even during acutely evolving MS attacks, subset ratios fluctuated between normal and abnormal when measured at weekly intervals. In our studies, on three occasions abnormal ratios appeared to precede an acute relapse by 1.5 to 7 days. In addition, one patient with chronic progressive MS specifically chosen for the study had an abnormal ratio on each occasion tested (FIG. 3) and one patient had what appeared to be an exacerbation of neurologic symptoms not associated with peripheral blood T cell changes.

Phenotype of T Lymphocytes in the Central Nervous System in MS

T lymphocyte phenotypes were studied, both in the cerebrospinal fluid and in the brains of MS patients, using monoclonal antibodies. Mononuclear cells were analyzed in the CSF and blood of 102 patients with multiple sclerosis and it was found that the majority (78%) of cells in the CSF were T lymphocytes and the ratio of T4 to T8 cells was approximately 2:1. No characteristic alterations in CSF phenotypes could be related to changes in circulating T8 cells or to disease activity. However, in a group of 75 patients studied, the CSF cell count was higher in patients with low numbers of circulating T8 cells than in those with normal T8 cells. These data demonstrate that decreases of T8 cells in the blood of multiple sclerosis patients are associated with CSF pleocytosis but we did not demonstrate fluctuations in the ratio of different subsets in the CSF,[4] although others have reported a decrease of T8 cells in the spinal fluid.[7]

We have recently completed the analysis of over 30 MS brains containing plaques of various ages via immunohistochemical staining using monoclonal antibodies (see ref. 8 for methodology). Immunohistochemical staining was performed using monoclonal antibodies, T8 (suppressor/cytotoxic cell), T4 and Leu 3a (inducer cell), M1 (macrophage), anti-HLA-DR (Ia^+ cell), and B1 (B cell). Lymphocyte perivascular cuffs were most prominent at the edge of active plaques and were occasionally seen in histologically normal areas. Perivascular cuffs consisted of $T8^+$ cells, Ia^+ cells, variable

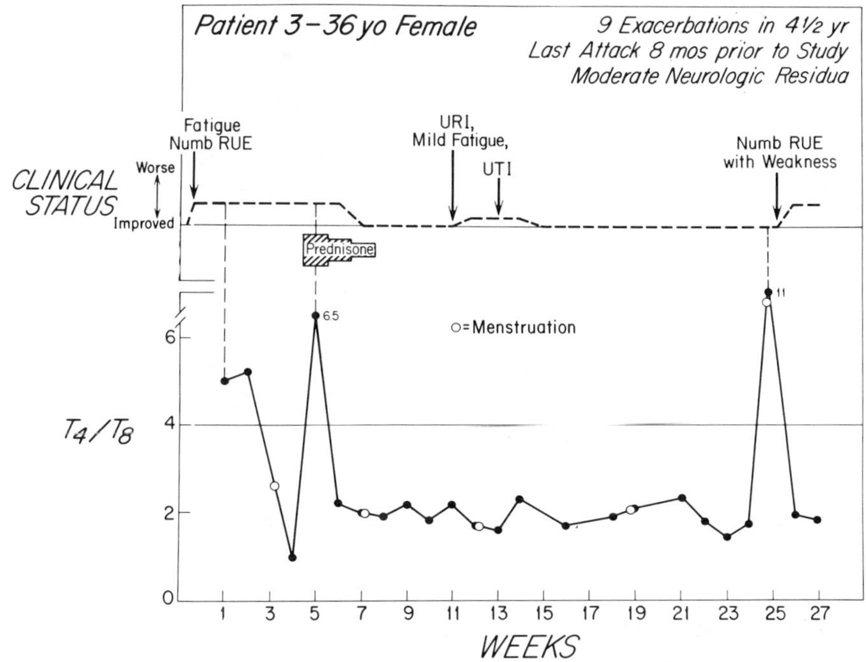

FIGURE 1. Serial analysis of T cell subsets and clinical course of Patient 3. *RUE* = right upper extremity; *URI* = upper respiratory infection; *UTI* = urinary tract infection. Prednisone was administered for a three-week period beginning three days prior to subset analysis on week 5. Prednisone dosage is indicated on the figure by the thickness of the hatched bar; wide width = 60 mg per day; medium width = 40 mg per day; narrow width = 20 mg per day.

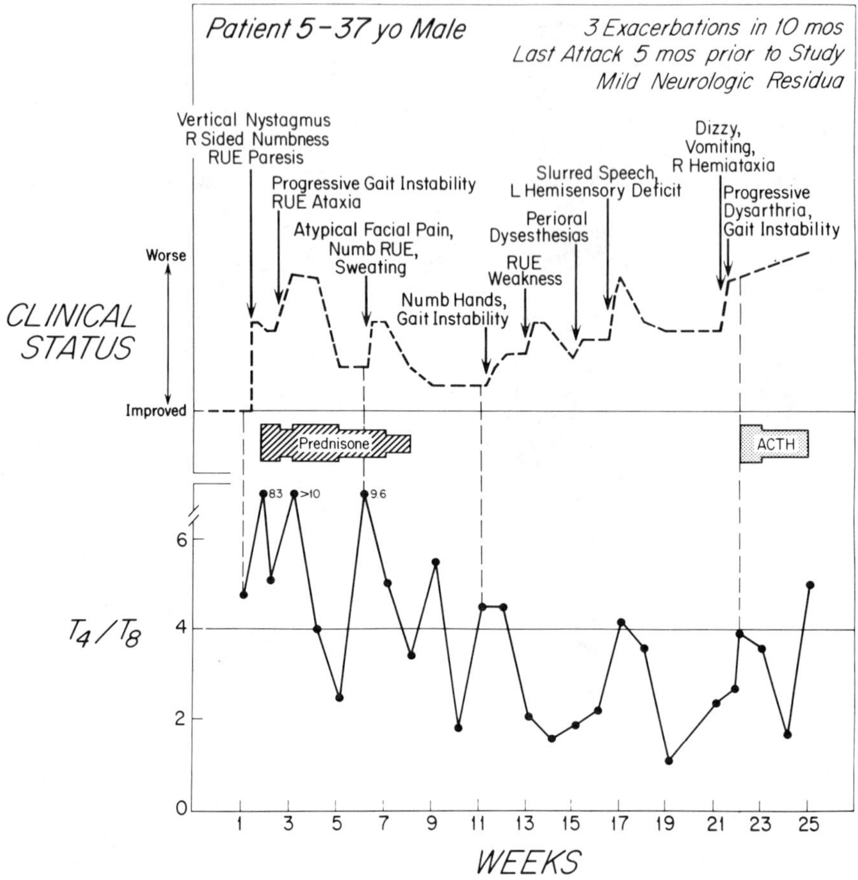

FIGURE 2. Serial analysis of T cell subsets and clinical course of Patient 5. *RUE* = right upper extremity; *L* = left; *R* = right. In this patient, prednisone was begun immediately following the second T cell subset determination at week 1.5; dosages are as described in FIGURE 1. At week 22, treatment with adrenocorticotropic hormone (ACTH) was begun (following blood drawing for subsets) and continued for three weeks; dosages administered: 40 units intravenously, daily for seven days (*thick hatch*), followed by a tapering intramuscular schedule.

numbers of $M1^+$ cells, and variable numbers of $T4^+$ cells. T8:T4 ratios in cuffs varied between 1:1 to 50:1. In normal-appearing white matter, cuffs were sparse and were predominantly T8-positive. The distribution of T cells in the parenchyma resembled that seen in perivascular cuffs, namely, predominantly $T8^+$ cells and variable numbers of $T4^+$ cells. Many Ia^+ cells were present in active lesions and the majority of these cells were macrophages. Some macrophages were also stained lightly by T4. No brain had more $T4^+$ than $T8^+$ cells using both T4 and Leu 3a mAbs to measure inducer cells. $B1^+$ cells were rare. An example of T8 staining of an MS brain is contained in FIG. 4. These results suggest that the cellular infiltrate in multiple sclerosis consists predominantly of T cells and macrophages and that there is an overrepresentation of T8 cells compared to T4 cells.[9]

Mechanism of Changes of Immunoregulatory T Cells in Multiple Sclerosis

Possible mechanisms to explain the decrease of T8 cells in the peripheral blood of MS patients include: (1) destruction by antibody, (2) modulation and (3) sequestration. We have been unable to demonstrate antibodies directed against isolated T8 cells in patients with active MS in whom there were rapid changes in T cell subsets,[5] even though we have previously found lymphocytotoxic antibodies in multiple sclerosis patients.[10] Thus, there is no evidence for antibody-mediated destruction of T cells in MS patients. Of note is that changes in the numbers of immunoregulatory T cell subsets in the peripheral blood could be caused by other humoral factors besides antibody, and we have demonstrated changes in T4 cells in healthy individuals following injection of epinephrine.[11]

A second possible mechanism relates to modulation of surface markers *in vivo.*[12] We have carried out a number of investigations looking for re-expression of the T8 marker following culture of T cells *in vitro* from patients with decreased T8 cells in the peripheral blood and have been unable to demonstrate consistently re-expression of the T8 marker following *in vitro* culture, although further work is needed in this area.

Our current hypothesis is that changes of T4:T8 ratios in peripheral blood may represent the migration of T8 cells from the peripheral blood into the central nervous system and perhaps into lymphoid tissue as well. This conclusion is based on the finding

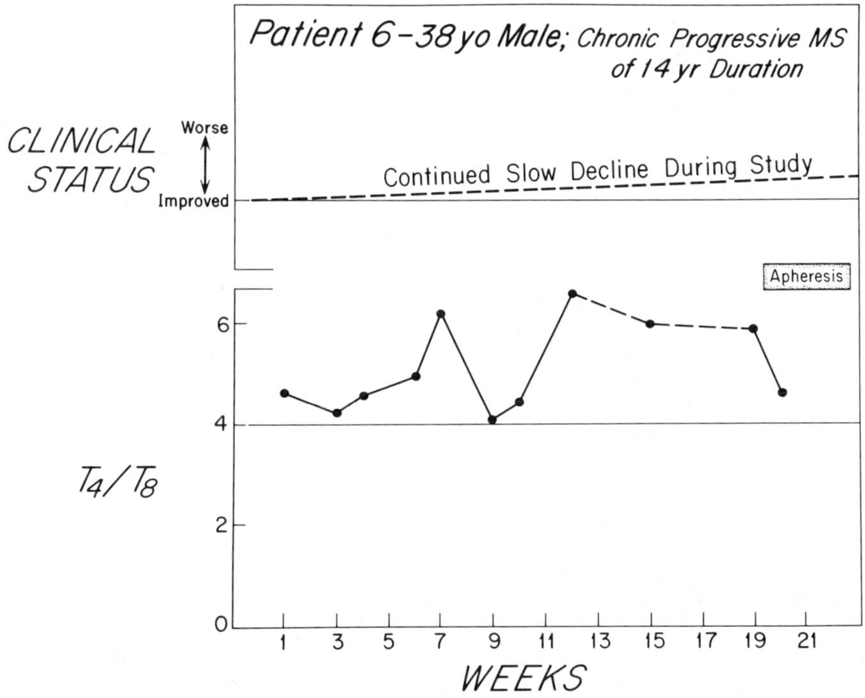

FIGURE 3. Serial analysis of T cell subsets and clinical course of Patient 6. No subset analysis was performed between weeks 12 and 15 and 15 and 19 (*dashed lines*). Ten lymphocytapheresis (apheresis) treatments were administered between weeks 19 and 21.

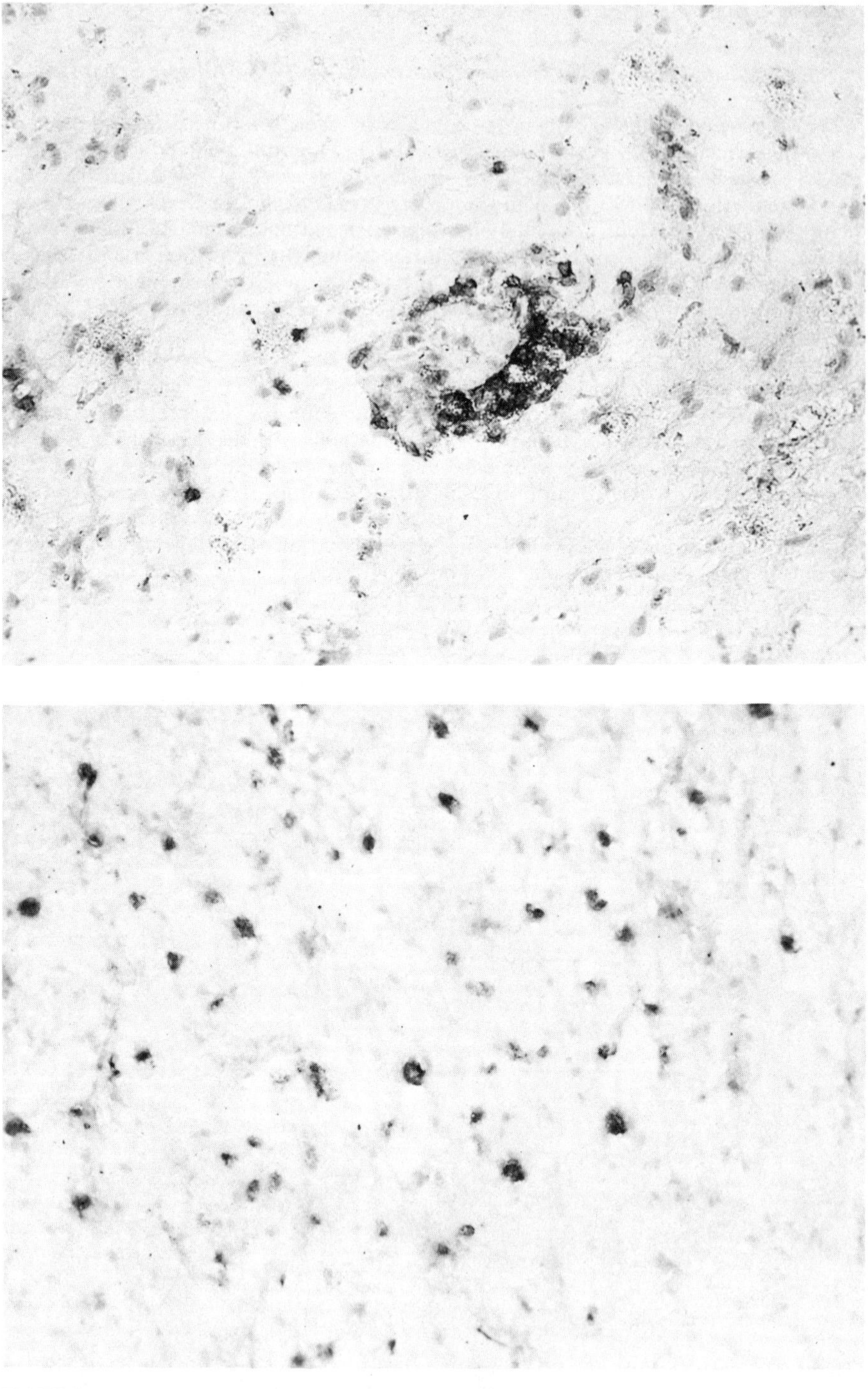

FIGURE 4. Immunoperoxidase staining of MS brain tissue with anti-T8 monoclonal antibody. *Top:* Perivascular infiltrate from acute MS plaque demonstrating T8-positive cells in the perivascular cuff. *Bottom:* T8-positive cells in the parenchyma.

of increased or equal numbers of T8 cells compared to T4 cells in the brains of MS patients in the face of episodic decreases of T8 cells in the peripheral blood.[9,13,14] Furthermore, the clinical pattern of T4:T8 ratio changes, *viz.*, the relatively rapid appearance and disappearance of cells from the peripheral blood of patients with relapsing disease, presents a temporal picture consistent with such an explanation. Of note is that one patient with progressive MS had persistent abnormalities of T4:T8 ratios in the peripheral blood (FIG. 3). If these changes are secondary to migration of cells, this theoretically would imply continued movement of cells from the peripheral blood to the CNS or other compartments in some cases of progressive MS. We have not, however, found major fluctuations of specific subsets in the spinal fluid of MS patients, which may represent an inconsistent correlation between cells infiltrating brain parenchyma and those that make their way to the spinal fluid. A recent study did not show a correlation between the cells infiltrating the brain and those in the spinal fluid in Sindbis viral encephalitis.[15] Nonetheless, in MS patients there is a correlation between the decrease of T8 cells in the peripheral blood and the degree of inflammation in the central nervous system as measured by CSF pleocytosis.[4]

Of note is that in the murine model of experimental allergic encephalomyelitis (EAE), we have found a decrease of the Lyt 1 T cell subset in the blood of animals prior to their appearance in the brain.[15a] It is known that Lyt 1 cells are required for adoptive transfer of murine EAE[16] and that Lyt 1 cells preferentially accumulate in the brain.[17] In the rat model of EAE, the Lyt 1 analogue also preferentially accumulates in the spinal cord.[18] In the guinea pig model of EAE, a decrease in the peripheral blood of "early T cells" occurs in association with the appearance of these cells in the central nervous system.[19] In sarcoidosis, T4 cells are decreased in the blood and appear to be sequestered in the lung.[20]

Several questions remain to be answered concerning T cell changes in the peripheral blood of MS patients. If T8 cells migrate to the CNS, this does not imply that these cells mediate CNS damage or that enough cells migrate to the brain to account for the decrease in the blood. Clearly there may be more than one mechanism for T cell changes in the blood of MS patients. Furthermore, the T8 cell is a "suppressor/cytotoxic" cell and recent evidence suggests that the majority of cells measured by the T8 monoclonal antibody in normals are of the cytotoxic rather than suppressor phenotype.[21] This also appears to be true in patients with multiple sclerosis.[22] Of note is that accompanying the decrease of T8 cells in the peripheral blood of MS patients is an associated decrease of a small number of T4 cells as well.[1]

Clinical Studies

The measurement of T cell subsets requires sophisticated laboratory techniques in which tests are performed routinely with appropriate controls and monitoring of immunologic reagents. Although some investigators have found T cell subset changes primarily in patients with chronic progressive MS,[23,24] other investigators have found changes in both acute and progressive cases.[25–28] Of note is that a decrease of T cells in the peripheral blood of MS patients was reported as early as 1975 using sheep red blood cell rosetting techniques as a marker.[29] In our experience, changes in T4:T8 ratios in the peripheral blood are not of benefit in the diagnosis of multiple sclerosis, something that is best done using neurologic examination in conjunction with laboratory tests such as spinal fluid evaluation, neuroimaging techniques, and electrophysiologic studies. T4:T8 ratios may be of benefit in monitoring patients with active disease who are being treated with immunotherapy or in determining the stage of disease when a patient receives treatment.[30,31] At present, however, decisions concerning who receives experimental treatment and the determination of response to therapy are made primarily on clinical grounds, with T cell changes in the peripheral blood and spinal fluid used in an investigational manner. Nonetheless, patients who have repeatedly abnormal blood T4:T8 ratios tend to be more active clinically. Thus, blood T cell subsets might be important in an individual patient being treated if that patient has had repeated abnormalities. If T4:T8 ratio changes represent movement of cells from the blood to the central nervous system and these changes in the blood do not persist in the face of ongoing clinical deterioration, it is possible that disease activity is related to ongoing cellular events in the central nervous system that are not accessible to the study of peripheral blood.

A more important role of blood T cell subsets relates to studies of basic immunologic abnormalities in MS. It is our general practice to measure T cell subsets at the time functional studies, other phenotypic analyses, and T cell cloning procedures are being performed. We have found results that may be quite different if blood is studied from a patient who has normal T cell subsets as opposed to one with abnormal subsets (TABLE 2). For example, in a recent study of spontaneous immunoglobulin production in patients with MS, increased production of immunoglobulin was observed in patients with abnormal subsets as compared to those whose subsets were normal.[32] In addition, we have found a decreased autologous mixed lymphocyte reaction in

TABLE 2. Correlation of T Cell Subset Changes with Parameters of Immune Function

	Elevated T4:T8 Ratios	Normal T4:T8 Ratios
Pleocytosis in spinal fluid	increased	minimal
Spontaneous immunoglobulin production *in vitro*	increased	normal
Autologous mixed lymphocyte reaction	decreased	normal

patients with MS who have abnormal T4:T8 ratios (Hafler and Weiner, unpublished).

In summary, repeated monitoring of T cell subset changes may be helpful in categorizing disease activity of individual patients and as a marker when other phenotypic and functional studies are performed. At the present time, they are not useful as a routine diagnostic test for multiple sclerosis. Their ultimate place in the treatment and management of MS awaits larger scale clinical experience and reliable and available phenotypic analysis that can be carried out in a hospital laboratory.

REFERENCES

1. REINHERZ, E. L., H. L. WEINER, S. L. HAUSER, J. A. COHEN, J. A. DISTASO & S. F. SCHLOSSMAN. 1980. Loss of suppressor T cells in active multiple sclerosis: Analysis with monoclonal antibodies. N. Engl. J. Med. **303:** 125–129.
2. WEINER, H. L. & S. L. HAUSER. 1982. Neuroimmunology I: Immunoregulation in neurological disease. Ann. Neurol. **11:** 437–449.
3. HAUSER, S. L., M. J. BRESNAN, E. L. REINHERZ & H. L. WEINER. 1982. Childhood multiple sclerosis: Clinical features and demonstration of changes in T cell subsets with disease activity. Ann. Neurol. **11:** 463–468.

4. HAUSER, S. L., E. L. REINHERZ, C. J. HOBAN, S. F. SCHLOSSMAN & H. L. WEINER. 1983. CSF cells in multiple sclerosis: Monoclonal antibody analysis and relationship to peripheral blood T-cell subsets. Neurology **33:** 575–579.
5. HAUSER, S. L., E. L. REINHERZ, C. J. HOBAN, S. F. SCHLOSSMAN & H. L. WEINER. 1983. Immunoregulatory T-cells and lymphocytotoxic antibodies in active multiple sclerosis: Weekly analysis over a six-month period. Ann. Neurol. **13:** 418–425.
6. WEINER, H. L., D. A. HAFLER. R. J. FALLIS, D. JOHNSON, K. A. AULT & S. L. HAUSER. 1984. Altered blood T-cell subsets in patients with multiple sclerosis. J. Neuroimmunol. **6:** 115–121.
7. CASHMAN, N., C. MARTIN, J.-F. EIZENBAUM, J.-D. DEGOS & M.-A. BACH. 1982. Monoclonal antibody- defined immunoregulatory cells in multiple sclerosis cerebrospinal fluid. J. Clin. Invest. **70:** 387–392.
8. HAUSER, S. L., A. K. BHAN, F. H. GILLES. C. J. HOBAN, E. L. REINHERZ, S. F. SCHLOSSMAN & H. L. WEINER. 1983. Immunohistochemical staining of human brain with monoclonal antibodies that identify lymphocytes, monocytes, and the Ia antigen. J. Neuroimmunol. **5:** 197–205.
9. WEINER, H. L., A. K. BHAN, J. BURKS, F. GILLES, C. KERR, E. REINHERZ & S. L. HAUSER. 1984. Immunohistochemical analysis of the cellular infiltrate in multiple sclerosis lesions. Neurology. **34**(1): 112.
10. SCHOCKET, A. L., H. L. WEINER, J. WALKER *et al.* 1977. Lymphocytotoxic antibodies in multiple sclerosis. Clin. Immunol. Immunopathol. **7:** 15–23.
11. CRARY, B., S. L. HAUSER, M. BORYSENKO, I. KUTZ, C. J. HOBAN, K. A. AULT, H. L. WEINER & H. BENSON. 1983. Epinephrine-induced changes in the distribution of lymphocyte subsets in peripheral blood of humans. J. Immunol. **131:** 1178–1181.
12. OGER, J., S. JACKEVICIUS, J. P. ANTEL *et al.* 1982. MS: Regeneration of T suppressor cell markers in culture. Ann. Neurol. **12:** 81.
13. TRAUGOTT, U., E. L. REINHERZ & C. S. RAINE. 1983. Multiple sclerosis. Distribution of T cells, T cell subsets and Ia-positive macrophages in lesions of different ages. J. Neuroimmunol. **4:** 201–221.
14. BOOSS, J., M. M. ESIRI, W. W. TOURTELLOTTE & D. Y. MASON. 1983. Immunohistochemical analysis of T-lymphocyte subsets in the central nervous system in chronic progressive multiple sclerosis. J. Neurol. Sci. **62:** 219–232.
15. MOENCH, T. R. & D. E. GRIFFIN. 1984. Immunohistochemical identification and quantitation of the mononuclear cells in the cerebrospinal fluid, meninges, and brain during acute viral meningoencephalitis. J. Exp. Med. **159:** 77–87.
15a. HAUSER, S. L., A. K. BAHN, M. CHE, F. GILLES & H. L. WEINER. 1984. Redistribution of Lyt-bearing T cells in acute murine allergic encephalomyelitis: Selective migration of Lyt-1 cells to the central nervous system is associated with a transient depletion of Lyt-1 cells in peripheral blood. J. Immunol. **133:** 3037–3042.
16. PETINELLI, C. B. & D. E. MCFARLIN. 1981. Adoptive transfer of experimental allergic encephalomyelitis in SJL/J mice after in vitro activation of lymph node cells by myelin basic protein: Requirement for Lyt 1^+2^- T lymphocytes. J. Immunol. **127:** 1420–1423.
17. SRIRAM, S., D. SOLOMON, R. V. ROUSE & L. STEINMAN. 1982. Identification of T cell subsets and B lymphocytes in mouse brain experimental allergic encephalomyelitis lesions. J. Immunol. **129:** 1649–1651.
18. HICKEY, W. F., N. K. GONATAS, H. KIMURA & D. B. WILSON. 1983. Identification and quantitation of T lymphocyte subsets found in the spinal cord of the Lewis rat during acute experimental allergic encephalomyelitis. J. Immunol. **131:** 2805–2809.
19. TRAUGOTT, U., S. H. STONE & C. S. RAINE. Experimental allergic encephalomyelitis—T cell migration to the central nervous system. J. Neurol. Sci. **36:** 55–61.
20. HUNNINGHAKE, G. W. & R. G. K. CRYSTAL. 1981. Pulmonary sarcoidosis. A disorder mediated by excess helper T lymphocyte activity at sites of disease activity. N. Engl. J. Med. **305:** 429–439.
21. MORETTA, A., G. PANTALEO, L. MORETTA, J.-C. CEROTTINI & M. C. MINGARI. 1983. Direct demonstration of the clonogenic potential of every human peripheral blood T cell. Clonal analysis of HLA-DR expression and cytolytic activity. J. Exp. Med. **157:** 743–754.

22. HAFLER, D. A., M. BUCHSBAUM, A. BENSUSSAN & H. L. WEINER. 1984. Phenotype distribution of cytotoxic T lymphocytes in multiple sclerosis peripheral blood and spinal fluid using T cell lines. Neurology **34**(1): 113.
23. PATY, D. W., L. KASTRUKOFF, N. MORGAN & L. HIOB. 1983. Suppressor T-lymphocytes in multiple sclerosis: Analysis of patients with acute relapsing and chronic progressive disease. Ann. Neurol. **14:** 445–449.
24. OGER, J., R. ROOS & J. P. ANTEL. 1983. Immunology of multiple sclerosis. *In* Neurologic Clinics. J. P. Antel, Ed.: 655–679. W. B. Saunders. Philadelphia.
25. HUDDLESTONE, J. R. & M. B. A. OLDSTONE. 1978. T suppressor (Ts) lymphocytes fluctuate in parallel with changes in the clinical course of patients with multiple sclerosis. J. Immunol. **123:** 1615–1618.
26. HUDDLESTONE, J. R. & M. B. A. OLDSTONE. 1982. Suppressor T cells are activated in vivo in patients with multiple sclerosis coinciding with remission from acute attack. J. Immunol. **129:** 915–917.
27. BACH, M. A., F. PHAN-DINH-TUY, E. TOURNIER, L. CHATENOUD & J.-F. BACH. 1980. Deficit of suppressor T cells in active multiple sclerosis. Lancet **2:** 1221–1224.
28. COMPSTON, A. 1983. Lymphocyte subpopulations in patients with multiple sclerosis. J. Neurol. Neurosurg. Psychiat. **46:** 105–114.
29. LISAK, R. P., A. I. LEVINSON, B. ZWEIMAN & N. ABDOU. 1975. T and B lymphocytes in multiple sclerosis. Clin. Exp. Immunol. **22:** 30–34.
30. HAUSER, S. L., D. M. DAWSON, J. R. LEHRICH, M. F. BEAL, S. V. KEVY, R. D. PROPPER, J. A. MILLS & H. L. WEINER. 1983. Intensive immunosuppression in progressive multiple sclerosis. A randomized, three-arm study of high-dose intravenous cyclophosphamide, plasma exchange, and ACTH. N. Engl. J. Med. **308:** 173–180.
31. HAUSER, S. L., M. FOSBURG, S. KEVY & H. L. WEINER. 1982. Plasmapheresis, lymphocytapheresis, and immunosuppressive drug therapy in multiple sclerosis. *In* Therapeutic Apheresis and Plasma Perfusion. Alan R. Liss. New York. pp. 239–254.
32. HAUSER, S. L., C. J. HOBAN, E. L. REINHERZ & H. L. WEINER. 1983. Increased spontaneous IgG production by cultured mononuclear cells in multiple sclerosis. Neurology **33**(Suppl. 2): 180.

GENERAL DISCUSSION

UNIDENTIFIED SPEAKER: I think we can state it, in a way, that there is no clear relationship between the abnormalities of T cell subsets in the blood and the sum of the clinical parameters of multiple sclerosis. We know it has something to do with the severity of the process but further than that we cannot go. This morning, Dr. Arnason showed that there is no relationship between the percentage of T_H cells in the blood and IgG production, but as he said, the blood is one step farther away from the brain than the CSF. My suggestion would be that if we are looking for significance of these changes and subsets of T cells, we should look more closely at CSF and especially at relations of these subsets to the parameters of the CSF. Now we had a series of patients where we did the typing in the CSF and in the blood simultaneously. The first slide shows that in the CSF, the percentage of T_H cells is inversely correlated with the number of cells. It was already demonstrated by Dr. Weiner's group that as you have more cells in the CSF in MS, the percentage of T_H is lower. The next slide shows a population of 15 untreated MS patients which demonstrated an inverse relationship between the intrathecal IgG synthesis and the percentage of T_H cells. This is something we should expect. At least what we find in the cerebrospinal fluids has some correlation with what is happening in the brain. The correlation is lost in immunosuppressed MS where the relative number of T_H cells is increased and there seems to be some indication that the IgG is lower. I think that if we are talking about significance of T cell subsets in MS, we should look very carefully into the relationship of these subsets with analysis of the spinal fluid.

D. M. MARCUS (*Baylor College of Medicine, Houston, TX*): I think that there are clearly some areas of disagreement that ought to be addressed in a constructive way and I would like to suggest a mechanism that was used at a workshop held about a year ago at the International Leukocyte Differentiation Conference, a monoclonal antibody workshop modeled on the histocompatibility workshops. I think the mechanism that could be used would be to distribute to a half-dozen or so laboratories doing these studies a panel of cells and a panel of reagents, and have them submit the results for computer analysis. I think the role model for this is now in place; the second monoclonal antibody workshop is going to occur next year and look at it from that point of view. In addition to whatever reagents are distributed, individual laboratories could use their reagents in parallel. The interesting thing that came out of the Paris meeting, which unfortunately is not published yet, is that although the laboratories participating in this study were really hard-core professional monoclonal laboratories whose major interest has been in the generation and characterization of antibodies, there was an absolutely hair-raising variation in the values that were obtained with the same reagents and the same antibodies. One is never going to resolve this kind of difference without some kind of collaborative study of these same cells with the same reagents and it would be useful if either the NIH, the MS Society or some national organization might consider undertaking such a study.

D. MCFARLIN (*NINCDS, Bethesda, MD*): I had the impression that we all agree that T cell subsets are of no diagnositic value in the disease. Does anyone disagree with that?

H. L. WEINER (*Harvard Medical School, Boston, MA*): I would agree with that.

MCFARLIN: Well the point is that although I think it's a very nice suggestion, I'm just not sure we could convince the MS society to sink a lot of money into carrying out a study like this if it's of no practical value to the patients.

I. MCDONALD (*National Hospital, London, England*): Dr. Waksman, would you like to comment on the question of variability in the standard of antibodies? Are we absolutely confident that the things labeled in a particular way remain constant?

B. H. WAKSMAN (*National Multiple Sclerosis Society, New York*): There certainly is a suggestion that the OKT8 antiserum that's being used today is not the same agent that was being used a couple of years ago. The company changed cell clones without telling anybody, sort of in midstream so people who laid in a good supply of OKT8 two or three years back are using a different reagent from those who are using a newer supply. When you have good labs who get different results with the same technique, after you've matched up the technique, you have to worry about whether the reagent is really the same. Unfortunately for this kind of reagent, we don't really have very satisfactory quality control methods at the disposal of the investigators and they're somewhat at the mercy of the providers.

A. COMPSTON (*University of Cardiff, Wales*): One of the problems that's arising is that some people are basing their interpretations on single observations made on groups of patients and others are using serial observations—given the inherent, enormous potential for technical problems and the fact that is there such a thing as an abnormal T8 result. About 80% of observations on normal controls come well under 20% and if you study the people who are in very close contact with MS patients, this proportion is even higher. Is it really possible to say anything about single observations, and shouldn't we only be concentrating on serial measurements?

J. ANTEL (*Pritzker School of Medicine, Chicago, IL*): I think your comment about serial observations was particularly needed if this test is going to move towards being a clinically usable test and it seems by agreement that we're not at this point. Dr. Hommes mentioned it, and our own data suggested that there was no correlation between functional secretion of immunoglobulins and T8 cell numbers. Now that was a population study and in fact what we can show in our system is that if we take T8 cells from a given individual and add them in increasing numbers, we get a dose response curve. So that for any individual I think that the number of T8 cells does play a role in regulating the immune response. In that sense we've really concocted an *in vitro* method of showing that serial variations do contribute to immune reactivity. From a research study, each of us is somewhat going our own way depending upon the problem we've defined, from a clinical role at this point with this given reagent, I don't think any of us are using it as a diagnostic test and therefore don't need serial studies.

R. P. LISAK (*University of Pennsylvania School of Medicine, Philadelphia, PA*): Two points related to the spinal fluid study. One is that counts on expanded cells are being done on 20 to 50 per aliquot which is fine if you have an all or none phenomenon, but it's pretty dicey if you're trying to detect a little change. The second point is that, based on Dr. Antel's work, if you have a correlation between the machine and the microscope, that's fine when one compares normals but if one has abnormals and is measuring blood T8 levels or other antigens on the cell sorter and looking down a microscope at 20 to 50 cells per aliquot in the spinal fluid looking for minor changes, I think you have to be very cautious.

WEINER: I wanted to make a couple of points. One relates to what's going on in the brain and what's going on in the spinal fluid. We don't know that they are necessarily the same. The one case in point would be the large number of macrophages that we see in the brains of MS patients and we don't really see that many of them in the spinal fluid. The second point that I would make is that all the investigators who looked at the T cell changes in MS are not represented here and we have to really look at all the data that all different laboratories have done and see there is a general agreement among most laboratories. People in general have been able to find these changes and Dr. Lisak had data on this without using these monoclonal reagents when he initially studied T cells and found in active MS that the total numbers of T cells were down. This suggested decreases in T cells in the blood during activity. One question I'd like to ask in terms of the work presented by Dr. Rice is that the Scripps group published initially on T gamma cell fluctuations in the peripheral blood, and also published a paper in September 1982, in the *Journal of Immunology,* using the T4 and T8 ratios (Huddlestone and Oldstone) which showed that in seven out of eight patients with an acute attack, there were changes in these T cells. There are two publications from the Scripps group showing it, and yet your statements here are different from that. I wonder if you could comment on that?

G. RICE (*Scripps Clinic and Research Foundation, La Jolla, CA):* The first observation, which was published in the *Journal of Immunology,* was basically Dr. Huddlestone's experience with the first ten patients. As we looked at 122 patients, the experience changed. This is a common phenomenon. One other point I'd like to address: I challenge the manufacturers of these orthoclonal reagents that there may have been some product change midstream in their distribution of Orthoclone product T8. They confirmed the fact that initially there were several clones, subclones, all which radio-immunoprecipitated the same epitope on lymphocyte surfaces; but all the material that's been marketed called Orthoclone T8 has originated from the same clone. Now some of the original investigators who produced this material have access to some products of the other clones but all material ever marketed by the Ortho Company represented material derived from a single clone. They do quality control checks on this material and their antibody continues to immunoprecipitate the same protein and stain in the same fashion.

G. HASHIM (*St. Luke's Hospital, New York*): In all these studies presented by the five speakers, we are essentially looking at an antibody-identified subset or subpopulation. We are really looking for a needle in a haystack if we are going to expect a change in the subset; 21 *versus* 21.8 means nothing to me, and the only way you're going to see it is when it's 21 *versus* 51, or the absence of such a subset. With regard to Dr. Weiner's statement about sequestration, when these subsets can be identified in terms of antigenic specificity, we then begin to make some sense out of it. Your suggestion of sequestration is about five years old. We've done a similar experiment. We didn't look at the level *per se,* we also looked at the MBP-sensitive cell and in fact so long as you provide antigen to this animal, be it in saline or whatever, we find that these cells disappear from the circulation; you don't find them. In an animal that does not have any of these responses, which I call antigen-responsive cells, if you introduce a little antigen, you recall them and as such, I do not see that they got to the brain. I think your later statement that they got sequestered in some lymphoid tissue is perhaps much more to the point.

WEINER: I'm very happy that you brought up this particular issue because I think the focus of our discussion should be what do these changes represent and how it relates to multiple sclerosis as opposed to what the diagnostic value is, or why some laboratories can find them and some laboratories can't. I raised the issue of sequestration but I didn't say it was a new issue. It's something that's been mentioned before, Drs. Raine and Traugott have very nice data in the guinea pig using E-rosetting cells showing decrease of cells in the blood and appearing in the brain in the guinea pig, so that isn't new. But if it is true that one of the mechanisms relates to the movement of cells out of the blood into the brain then that's a very important conception in terms of thinking about MS; it raises a lot more questions. All of those cells are probably not antigen specific, so why are they moving to the brain? Are those cells causing any damage? If they are not going to the brain, are they going somewhere else and if they're going somewhere else, why? So I think the importance in my own mind of that relates to new questions that can be asked in terms of trying to understand what's going on with these particular changes. We haven't been able to find other explanations, for example, lymphocytotoxic antibodies or modulation of surface antigens.

Magnetic Resonance Imaging and CT Scanning in Multiple Sclerosis

BURTON P. DRAYER AND LYNN BARRETT

Departments of Radiology and Medicine (Neurology)
Duke University Medical Center
Durham, North Carolina 27710

INTRODUCTION

Prior to the development of cranial computed tomography (CT), the major role for neuroimaging was the exclusion of other pathologic processes that might mimic multiple sclerosis (MS). Cerebral angiography was generally normal or showed nonspecific mass effect with no evidence for arteriopathy or venopathy. Pneumoencephalography was either normal or defined dilated sulci and ventricles with longstanding disease. Myelography was normal even in the face of significant myelopathic clinical findings and only revealed cord (intramedullary) swelling or complete block on rare occasions with acute, severe disease. All of these techniques had the additional disadvantage of being traumatic and thus potentially leading to iatrogenic exacerbation of the disease process.

With the advent of high resolution, cross-sectional imaging over the past decade, a powerful approach was made available for the diagnosis of demyelinating disease. These imaging methods are safe, relatively noninvasive, and able to provide exquisitely detailed anatomic information of even submillimeter structures routinely. Information obtained by CT or magnetic resonance (MR) imaging is thus an *in vivo* representation of gross pathology. Precise pathoanatomic studies in living patients have the additional advantage of permitting repeated examinations during the various stages of lesion development and of providing a better understanding of the dynamics (*e.g.*, blood-brain barrier integrity) of this remitting and exacerbating disease process.

As both the specificity and sensitivity of CT and MR imaging improve, the results of these tests will need to be integrated into the diagnostic criteria schemas used to detect, prognose, and evaluate therapeutic response in demyelinating disease.[1] It is, however, important to recognize that the positive information derived from CT or MR imaging, if not used in careful conjunction with clinical acumen, may further complicate rather than facilitate patient care. The additional psychosocial dilemma exists of the patient with a minimal neurologic deficit or complete remission with an unequivocally abnormal imaging study.

NEUROIMAGING AND NEUROPATHOLOGIC CORRELATION

Pathoanatomy

Pathologic Findings[2]

Multiple sclerosis is a disease of the oligodendroglia-myelin system in which the lesions are often closely associated with a venule. Initial presentation is generally in the second to fifth decade and is characterized by a clinical remission and exacerbations with pathologic central nervous system lesions of various ages and in multiple locales.

There is often a lack of correspondence between the location of a lesion and the expressed clinical symptomatology.

On gross pathologic inspection, a chronic case of multiple sclerosis may show significant loss of brain substance, particularly involving the cerebral white matter. There is mild to moderate enlargement of the cortical sulci and lateral ventricles secondary to the atrophic changes in the central white matter. In addition, severe shrinkage may occur over large segments of the spinal cord. The MS plaques have an irregular, sharply outlined edge and are scattered in a fairly symmetric fashion throughout the white matter and in a small percentage of cases within the gray matter. Many plaques are extremely difficult to detect on gross inspection as they may only be a few millimeters in size, whereas others are larger and may spread as finger-like extensions ("Dawson's fingers") through the white matter. "Shadow plaques" are extremely difficult to detect grossly and are commonly found in the brainstem. In addition, acute plaques are more difficult to detect on gross pathologic inspection than chronic sclerotic ones.

The distribution of lesions in MS includes all portions of the central nervous system but can be arbitrarily divided into four anatomic locales: (a) the optic nerves, chiasm, and tracts, (b) the cerebrum, (c) the brainstem and cerebellum, and (d) the spinal cord. The prototype lesions are best delineated in the myelinated brain substance in close relationship to the ependymal lining of the ventricular system (especially the lateral angles of the lateral ventricles, the aqueduct, and the floor of the fourth ventricle), the cerebral and cerebellar white matter with sparing of the immediately subcortical white matter, and the cortical and basal ganglia gray matter with many of the cortical lesions adjacent to the pial surface. The distribution of lesions is roughly symmetrical, particularly within the supratenorial brain substance.[3]

Histopathologic findings are often difficult to detect in the early days following an insult to the oligomyelin system. The paradoxical situation exists in which microscopic alterations in relatively well-defined MS lesions are often best delineated on a delayed (few weeks later) basis during clinical remission. Lesions of the oligomyelin system generally occur in a perivenular distribution involving ependymal venules (periventricular white matter), medullary venules (cerebral white matter) and pial venules (cortical gray matter). Phagocytic macrophages and perivenular lymphocytes and plasma cells are prominent in the acute and subacute MS lesion. These lesions contain myelin debris as well as globules of sudanophilic lipid (*i.e.*, triglycerides and cholesterol esters) material. The presence of intracellular and extracellular neutral fat at the border of the lesion coincides with lesion activity. There is mounting evidence that the macrophages, rather than merely acting as secondary scavengers, may actually cause receptor-mediated myelin destruction. Proliferation of protoplasmic astrocytes is maximal at the periphery of the MS plaque with chronic fibrillary gliosis most common in the center of the plaque.

The correlation of MS lesions with disease symptomatology is often imprecise. This lesion-symptom dichotomy is highlighted by the fact that the gross and histopathologic delineation of the MS plaque is optimal in the subacute phase when remission of symptoms has often begun. The chronic disability associated with MS may often be more related to associated axonal degeneration than acute oligomyelin disruption. The difficulties in correlating lesions with symptomatology is highlighted by the fact that the common site of MS lesions adjacent to the angles of the lateral ventricles has no known classical clinical manifestations. The multiple diffuse lesions in the cerebral white matter may account for the neurobehavioral aberrations and declining memory. These lesion-symptom disassociations highlight one of the major difficulties encountered when performing therapeutic trials based on clinical or nonspecific CSF responses.

CT Scanning

Multiple studies have reported the use of CT scanning in the diagnosis of MS. CT safely provides unique information concerning brain morphology and even function that has never previously been available prior to autopsy. This has opened a window to expand our understanding of the course and development of MS lesions rather than merely to provide a view of the final devastation. There have been three basic abnormalities described in CT reports: (a) enlargement of cerebrospinal fluid spaces (ventricles and/or sulci); (b) white matter hypodensities; and (c) abnormal contrast enhancement (described below in the "Blood-Brain Barrier" section).

In a retrospective analysis of 85 patients studied at Duke University with definite, probable, or possible MS (Poser classification), enlargement of the ventricles and/or sulci occurred in 33 (definite MS 20/34, probable MS 5/18, and possible MS 8/33).[4] There was a significant ($p < 0.005$) correlation between duration of disease and CSF space enlargement (TABLE 1). Of the 53 patients with an abnormal CT scan, 28% exhibited only enlargement of ventricles or sulci without associated white matter lucencies or abnormal enhancement.

TABLE 1. CT and MS: Duke Experience

	Definite	Probable	Possible	Total
Mean age at CT	40	43	38	40
Mean age at onset	31	34	32	32
Mean duration of MS (yrs)	9	9	6	8
CSF protein (>45)	6/26	0/14	2/28	8/68
CSF WBC (>5)	10/22	2/10	7/21	19/53
CSF IgG/Alb (>12%)	5/16	3/12	3/21	11/49
+ Evoked response	25/26	15/17	21/32	61/74
CT hypodensity	16/34	4/18	6/33	26/85
CT enhancement[a]	15/34	3/18	7/33	25/85
CT CSF spaces	20/34	5/18	8/33	33/85
CT abnormal	29/34	7/18	17/33	53/85

[a]In a subgroup of 18 patients with definite MS and recent (>8 weeks) exacerbation, abnormal enhancement was significantly correlated ($p < 0.025$) whereas CSF parameters did not correlate with exacerbation.

Hypodensity of the brain white matter was noted in 26/85 patients in the Duke study[4] (TABLE 1, FIG. 1). The mean number of discrete areas of white matter hypodensity was approximately 4 per patient. The lesions seen by CT were predominantly in the periventricular (~50%) and central cerebral (~35%) white matter with a small percentage at the gray-white junction, brainstem, and cerebellar peduncles. There were no distinctive characteristics of any given brain hypodensity that was pathognomonic of MS or that could definitively distinguish MS from other disorders involving the white matter.

Anatomic maps of the distribution of low-density regions presumably representing demyelination and gliosis tabulated from our CT studies correlate closely with autopsy series, with a few exceptions. Our results correlated with the neuropathologic reports that suggest a relative symmetry of plaque distribution. The incidence of hypodensities on brain CT is particularly underrepresented in four anatomic locations:

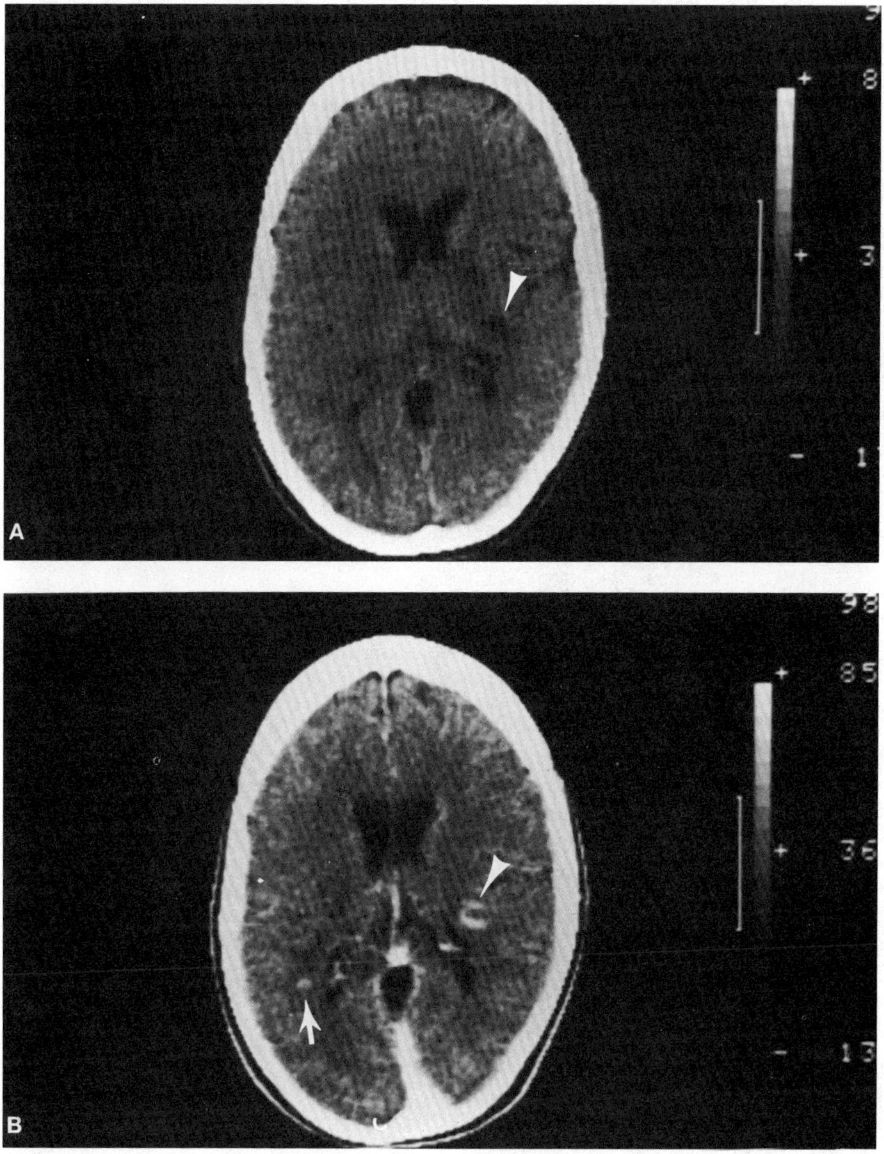

FIGURE 1. Multiple sclerosis enhanced vs. nonenhanced CT. (**A**) Nonenhanced: abnormal hypodensity typical of foci of demyelination in the posterior limb of the internal capsule (*arrowhead*). No other CT abnormality is noted. (**B**) Enhanced: in addition to abnormal enhancement in the posterior limb of the internal capsule (*arrowhead*), a foci of enhancement is noted in the parietal white matter adjacent to the atrium of the lateral ventricle (*arrow*).

1. *Brainstem/cerebellum.* In autopsy series, approximately 20% of lesions are in the posterior fossa while in the Duke and other CT studies only approximately 5% of abnormalities were in this location. Anatomic definition in the posterior fossa is degraded by artifacts related to the petrous bones and CT algorithms. In addition, "shadow plaques" (incomplete demyelination) are far more common in the brainstem than in the cerebrum and therefore may be more difficult to detect on CT than a completely demyelinated plaque.
2. *Optic nerves.* Although involvement of the optic nerves and chiasm is common in multiple sclerosis, CT abnormalities have rarely been reported. Even with thin section (1.5 mm) CT scanning with special attention to the optic nerves, it is difficult to detect the subtle abnormalities that might occur in optic nerve size, contour, and texture with atrophy or swelling.
3. *Spinal cord.* The spinal cord is another common pathologic focus of MS. CT studies have not been productive in defining abnormalities in the spinal cord, as differentiation of the spinal cord from its surrounding subarachnoid spaces is particularly difficult in the lower cervical and thoracic regions. With the limited degree of anatomic specificity for spinal cord structures using CT without intrathecal contrast enhancement, the difficulty in defining the subtle regions of hypodensity with the spinal cord is apparent.
4. *Peripheral gyral.* Autopsy studies[2] suggest that peripheral gyral regions (pure cortical, gray-white junction, superficial white matter) are considerably smaller (often only a few millimeters) than periventricular lesions. This factor, in addition to the potential artifacts near the inner table of the skull, accounts for decreased detection by CT.

When analyzing CT studies in patients with MS, additional pitfalls particularly related to the overly zealous diagnosis of white matter lesions which merely represent normal white matter with high resolution scanners must be assiduously avoided. Two central areas of decreased density in the midbrain are commonly seen with high resolution CT and represent the normal termination of the superior cerebellar peduncles. Following intravenous contrast enhancement, the distinction between gray and white matter becomes extremely prominent because of the four times greater capillary density in the gray matter. The centrum semiovale, internal capsule, and cerebellar white matter are then particularly well visualized and this should not be mistaken for demyelination.

The use of more sophisticated CT scanning equipment has improved diagnostic sensitivity and specificity. Hershey *et al.*[5] reviewed a group of 66 patients with suspect or definite multiple sclerosis that had been scanned on an early generation CT unit. They found hypodensity in 21% of patients with definite multiple sclerosis and 7% of patients with probable or possible multiple sclerosis. Using high resolution (GE 8800) CT scanning in a group of patients selected for acute exacerbations, Vinuela *et al.*[6] found focal hypodensities in 51% of patients studied with definite MS.

Magnetic Resonance Imaging

Due to certain limitations of CT scanning, particularly in the analysis of central nervous system structures adjacent to bone (*e.g.*, spinal cord, brainstem, inferior temporal lobe) and the improved contrast sensitivity of MR as compared to CT, MS has been one of the initial disease processes studied using MR imaging.[7] When analyzing an MR image, it is important to recognize that the image is dependent upon three general factors: (1) the field strength and homogeneity of the magnet, (2) basic tissue parameter interrelationships (proton density, T1 relaxation time, T2 relaxation time, flow); (3) the operator-selected radiofrequency (RF) pulse sequence (repetition time, TR; echo delay, TE). Parameters 1 and 2 cannot be altered by the operator, however, the selection of the optimal RF pulse sequence is the critical element that must be established prior to evaluating an individual with MS in an MR experiment.

Young *et al.*[7] studied 10 patients with definite MS comparing CT (Siemens Somatom II) to MR (0.17 Tesla, inversion recovery pulse sequences) imaging. They reported three lesions in the supraventricular white matter by CT and nine lesions by MR, 16 periventricular white matter lesions by CT and 84 by MR, and no brainstem lesions by CT and 38 by MR. Even though double-dose delayed CT scanning was not used and the number of lesions per patient in each location was lower than in other CT studies,[4,6] the advantages in contrast sensitivity of MR for the detection of MS lesions is apparent.

Lukes *et al.*[8] also reported on 10 patients studied using CT and MR with multiple sclerosis. CT scanning was positive in 7/10 whereas MR was positive in all 10 patients. A total of 13 lesions was seen by intravenously enhanced CT and 158 lesions were seen by MR. Although only a limited number of patients were studied and only a limited number of pulse sequences were tested, this article suggested that a spin echo pulse sequence with a TR of 1.5 sec and TE of 56 ms is superior to any inversion recovery pulse sequence for the detection of MS plaques (FIG. 2). Further study is certainly needed to better delineate the optimal scanning parameters for the evaluation of demyelinating disease. The sensitivity for the detection of posterior fossa lesions seems a particularly useful feature of MR imaging. It is hoped that MR will also assist in improving the visualization of abnormalities in the spinal cord and optic nerves. The major limitations of MR imaging at present are the cumbersome aspects of providing a site for a high field strength magnet, the longer scanning times with MR as compared to CT, and the difficulties encountered when imaging a sicker or less cooperative patient.

The abnormalities noted to date in MS are nonspecific and consist of a prolongation of the T1 and T2 relaxation times. In terms of image analysis, prolongation of the T1 relaxation time results in decreased signal intensity (darker than normal brain) on a T1 weighted image (*e.g.*, inversion recovery, partial saturation, saturation recovery or short TE spin echo) and prolongation of the T2 relaxation time results in increased signal intensity (whiter than normal brain) on a T2 weighted image (*e.g.*, spin echo sequence with a long TE). The T2 relaxation time can be calculated with a reasonable degree of accuracy from a multiple echo, spin echo sequence.

The mechanisms of T1 and T2 relaxation time abnormalities have not yet been definitively resolved. Young *et al.*[7] suggested that the destruction of lipids in the myelin altered the chemical environment of the protons in the region causing a subsequent increase in their T1 and T2 relaxation times. Normal myelin is approximately 78% lipid by dry weight and is composed of cholesterol, phospholipid and galactolipid in an approximately 4:3:2 molar ratio. The acute or subacute MS plaque consists of neutral lipids, principally cholesterol esters and triglycerides, which represent myelin breakdown products. The formation of esterified cholesterol from free (unesterified) cholesterol is a hallmark of demyelination. In contrast, a chronic plaque contains no myelin breakdown products, but rather consists of replacement of myelin by a dense gliotic network. In acute and subacute MS, there is also an associated membrane instability of the blood-brain barrier causing an increase in free brain water either related to a release of bound water or an increase in passage of water into the extracellular brain space. The prolongation of the T1 and T2 relaxation times in acute and subacute MS as noted by MR proton imaging is thus potentially due to an increase in free water, an increase in neutral lipids, or a decrease in myelin lipids (*e.g.*,

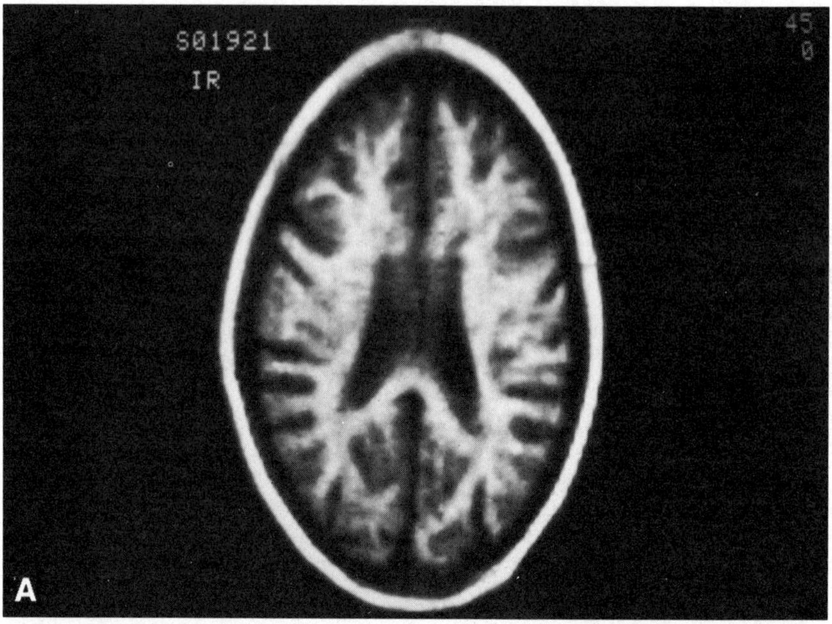

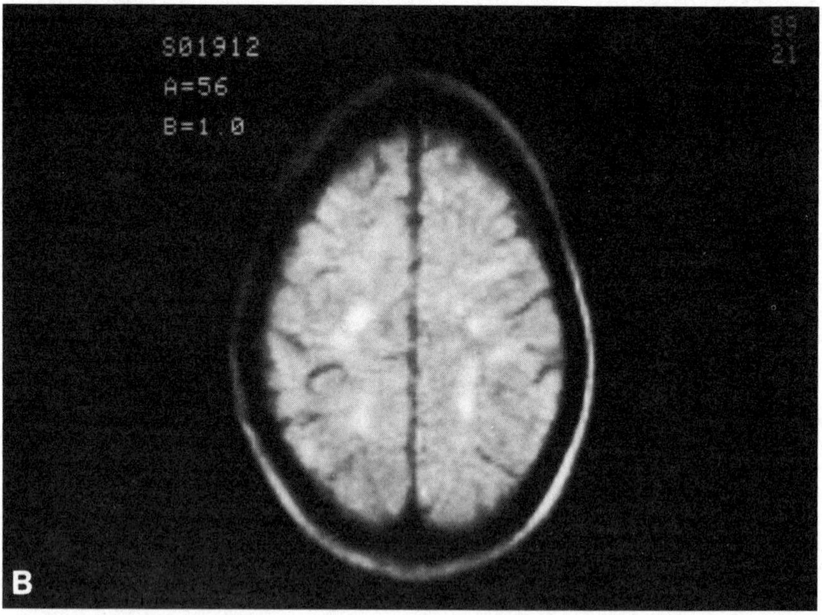

FIGURE 2. Multiple sclerosis, magnetic resonance imaging. Comparison of an inversion recovery image at the level of the lateral ventricle to a spin echo image (TR 1.0 s, TE 56 ms) at the level of the centrum semiovale. Subtle, small regions of decreased signal intensity are noted within the white matter on the inversion recovery image consistent with demyelinating plaque (**A**). The plaques are better seen on the spin echo sequence as high-signal intensity foci (**B**). A CT scan performed in this patient was normal. (Courtesy of Michael Brant-Zawadzki, University of California San Francisco Medical Center.)

phospholipids). Recent studies by our group at Duke using a high field strength (1.5 Tesla) General Electric unit have shown that there is not a homogeneous increase in the T1 and T2 relaxation times within a given MS plaque. In some plaques there existed a central core that had an even greater prolongation of the T1 relaxation time, suggesting chronic fibrillary gliosis (FIG. 3). The MR findings were fully consistent with pathologic data which show that a chronic dense central glial network may be surrounded by subacute or acute changes of edema, myelin breakdown products, and inflammatory macrophage response.

Blood-Brain Barrier

Pathophysiology

Experimental models reveal a close interrelationship between alterations of the blood-brain barrier and demyelination. Following the intracarotid injection of hyperosmotic materials to disrupt the blood-brain barrier experimentally, sequential pathologic changes are noted which consist of initial vasodilatation followed by capillary endothelial cell alterations and white matter edema. Venous stasis is then seen associated with the vasodilatation followed by a macrophage response and finally perivascular demyelination.[9,10] The possibility exists that intermittent episodes of blood-brain barrier disruption and concomitant vasogenic edema may play a similar role in the pathogenesis of demyelination in MS. Broman[11] has reported barrier disruption in MS using a nondiffusible indicator. Experimental allergic encephalomyelitis is also known to cause blood-brain barrier disruption and associated brain edema.[12,13] Brain[14] suggested that there is an increased incidence of cervical spondylosis in association with MS and that this might be due to repeated trauma to the cervical spinal cord from bony spurs leading to blood-brain barrier breakdown. Some individuals may have a myelinolytic factor in the bloodstream which enters the brain when there is abnormal permeability of the blood-brain barrier. Intermittent barrier opening may occur with sympathetic stimulation related to stressful episodes such as fatigue, sickness and fever, emotional upset, excessive heat, or trauma. These factors are known to precipitate exacerbations in MS patients. The central adrenergic system regulates the cerebral microcirculation and adrenergic agonists (*e.g.*, amitriptyline) have been noted to increase the permeability of the blood-brain barrier.[15] The remissions and exacerbations as well as the relative symmetry of brain lesions in MS might thus be explained by a theory invoking intermittent episodes of increased permeability of the blood-brain barrier.

CT Scanning

Following the intravenous infusion of a single (42 g I) or double (84 g I) dose of iodinated contrast material, there is no accumulation of contrast medium in a normal brain. As the capillary density of the gray matter is approximately 4 times that of the white matter, gray matter areas will initially show greater CT enhancement than adjacent white matter. This enhancement is due to iodinated contrast material within the capillary bed and not within the brain substance. With an abnormally increased permeability of the cerebral capillary endothelial cells which represent the blood-brain barrier, iodinated contrast medium will accumulate in abnormal areas of the brain[16] (FIG. 4). By delaying the performance of the CT scan for 30–60 minutes, delineation of even subtle abnormalities in the blood-brain barrier is improved due to the combined effect of an exponentially increasing passage of contrast medium into the lesion with a

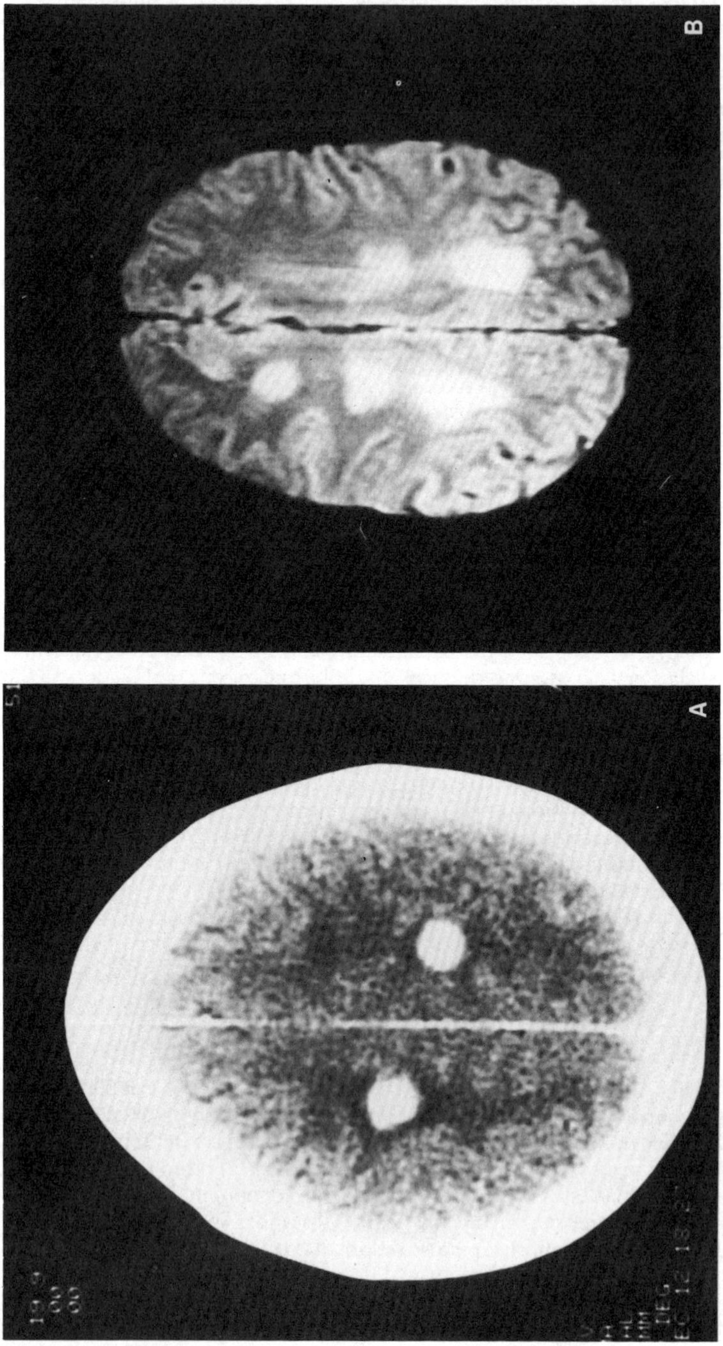
B
A

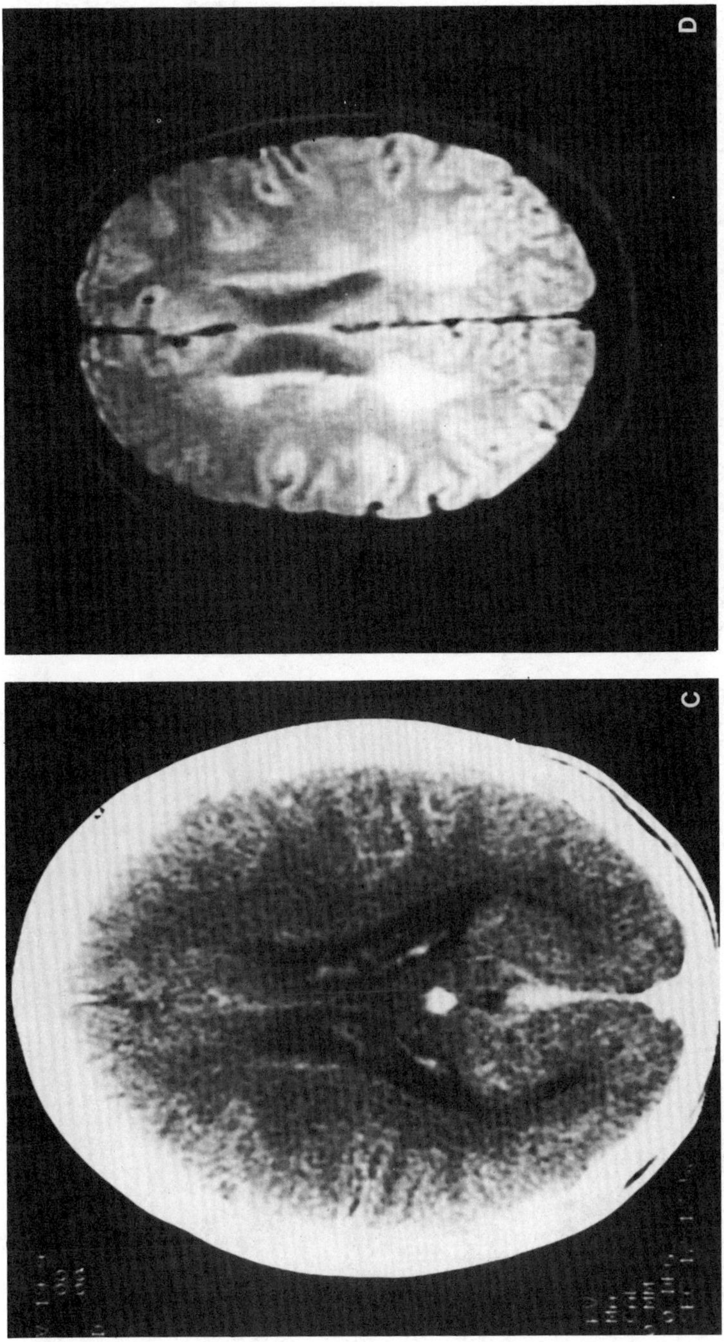

FIGURE 3. Multiple sclerosis, proton MR vs. intravenously enhanced CT. **(A)** Enhanced CT: two large enhancing abnormalities in the cerebral white matter. In addition, there are some low densities in the adjacent white matter. **(B)** MR spin echo (TR 1500 s, TE 75 ms). MR scan at approximately the same level as the CT scan shows three additional large areas of high-signal intensity consistent with MS plaques. **(C)** Intravenously enhanced CT scan: high resolution (GE 9800) CT scan showing no abnormalities at this body of lateral ventricle level. **(D)** MR spin echo (TR 1500 s, TE 75 ms). Approximately the same level as in **(C)** showing multiple areas of high-signal intensity consistent with MS plaques in the cerebral white matter.

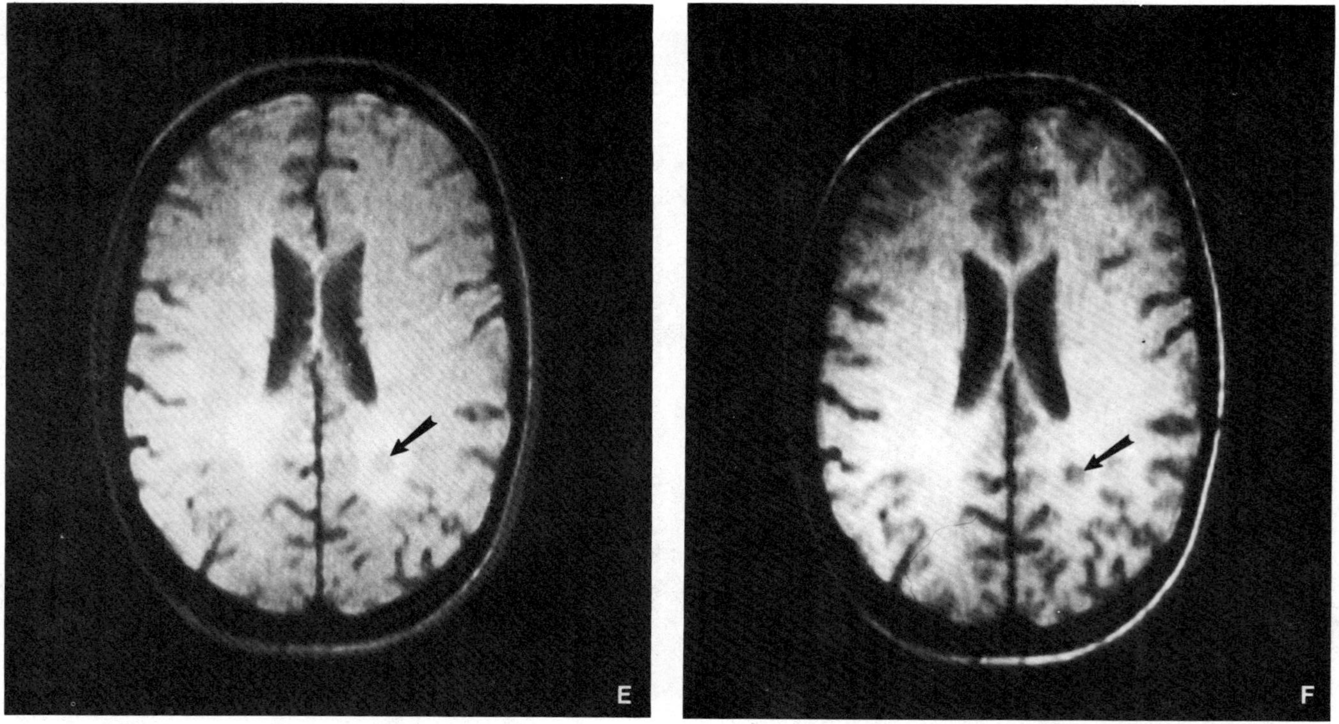

FIGURE 3 (*con't.*). (**E**) MR spin echo (TR 1000 s, TE 25 ms). MR at the same level as (**D**). The lesions are not as well visualized because of the shorter TR and TE pulse sequence. However, a central area is noted in the left occipital MS plaque in which the signal intensity is less than that in the surrounding lesion. This is an area of higher T1 relaxation time and consistent with the central fibrillary gliosis seen in the chronic portion of an MS lesion. (**F**) MR spin echo (TR 500 s, TE 25 ms). The same level as (**D**) and (**E**) exhibiting even poorer delineation of the MS lesions. Many lesions would be overlooked if only this pulse sequence were used. However, the central area of even greater decreased T1 relaxation time is better visualized (*arrow*).

far more rapid clearance of the contrast material from the bloodstream than the diseased brain (FIG. 5). This strategy of obtaining delayed CT scans after infusing a double dose of contrast medium to improve lesion contrast has been widely utilized to detect the disruption of the blood-brain barrier that is associated with MS.[4,6,17]

Abnormal contrast enhancement was delineated in 44% of definite MS patients, 17% of probable MS patients, and 21% of possible MS patients in the Duke series (TABLE 1). The distribution of enhancing lesions was similar to that of cerebral hypodensities with 36% in a periventricular location, 30% in a central white matter or internal capsule location, 20% in the white matter at the gray-white junction, 7% in the deep or cortical gray matter, and 7% in the brainstem or cerebellum. In patients with abnormal enhancement, a mean of 6.4 enhancing abnormalities were noted per patient. The distribution of enhancing abnormalities was relatively symmetric with an approximately equal number involving each cerebral hemisphere. Although a higher percentage of patients who received a double dose of contrast material as compared to a single dose exhibited contrast enhancement, there was no statistically significant difference between the single vs. the double-dose strategy if delayed scanning was used. In a selected group of patients with double-dose delayed CT scanning and CSF studies (protein, WBC, IgG), a statistical correlation ($p < 0.025$) was noted between recent exacerbation and abnormal contrast enhancement. There was no significant correlation between exacerbation and CSF findings. The determination of acute or subacute disease activity based on abnormal contrast enhancement is one of the most important reasons for obtaining a CT scan in a patient with MS. Corticosteroid therapy, possibly related to membrane stabilization, may result in a dramatic reduction in contrast enhancement[17,18] (FIG. 6).

The use of high resolution CT scanning has improved the yield of positive studies in MS. Hershey *et al.*,[5] using an early generation CT scanner, standard, single-dose contrast enhancement, and immediate scanning found a 9% incidence of abnormal contrast enhancement. Vinuela *et al.*,[6] using high resolution CT scanning, double-dose contrast enhancement, and delayed imaging, described abnormal contrast enhancement in 82% of definite MS patients selected for relatively recent onset of clinical symptomatology and acute exacerbation at the time of scanning. In a selected group of patients within the Duke series studied using high resolution, double-dose delayed CT scanning, 89% showed abnormal contrast enhancement if a clinical exacerbation had occurred within the prior 8 weeks.[4] Only 12% of patients in this series with abnormal contrast enhancement had an elevated CSF protein level. This finding is consistent with that of Tourtellotte[19] who found only 23% of patients had an elevated CSF protein and supports the concept that the measurement of CSF protein is an extremely poor marker for the detection of disruption of the blood-brain barrier.

MR Imaging

One of the shortcomings of MR has been the inability to evaluate the integrity of the blood-brain barrier. As stated above, analysis of blood-brain barrier integrity appears to be an important criterion for disease activity. There have been two strategies evaluated to date for evaluating the blood-brain barrier. The first involves the use of a paramagnetic compound which does not cross an intact blood-brain barrier. A paramagnetic compound should decrease the T1 relaxation time with proton MR imaging. The brain abnormality with a damaged blood-brain barrier will therefore have an increased signal intensity (appear white) on a T1-weighted image sequence.

Various nitroxide stable free radicals (NSFR) have been tested as paramagnetic

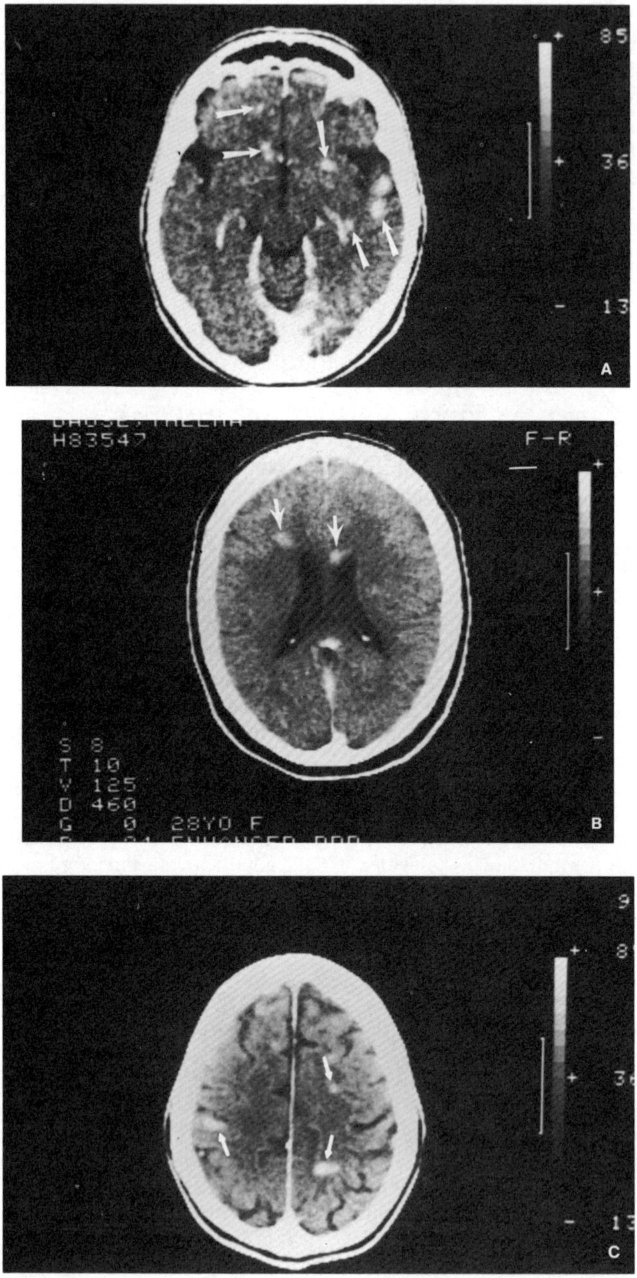
85
36
13
A
H83547
F-R
S 8
T 10
V 125
D 460
G 0 28YO F
B
C

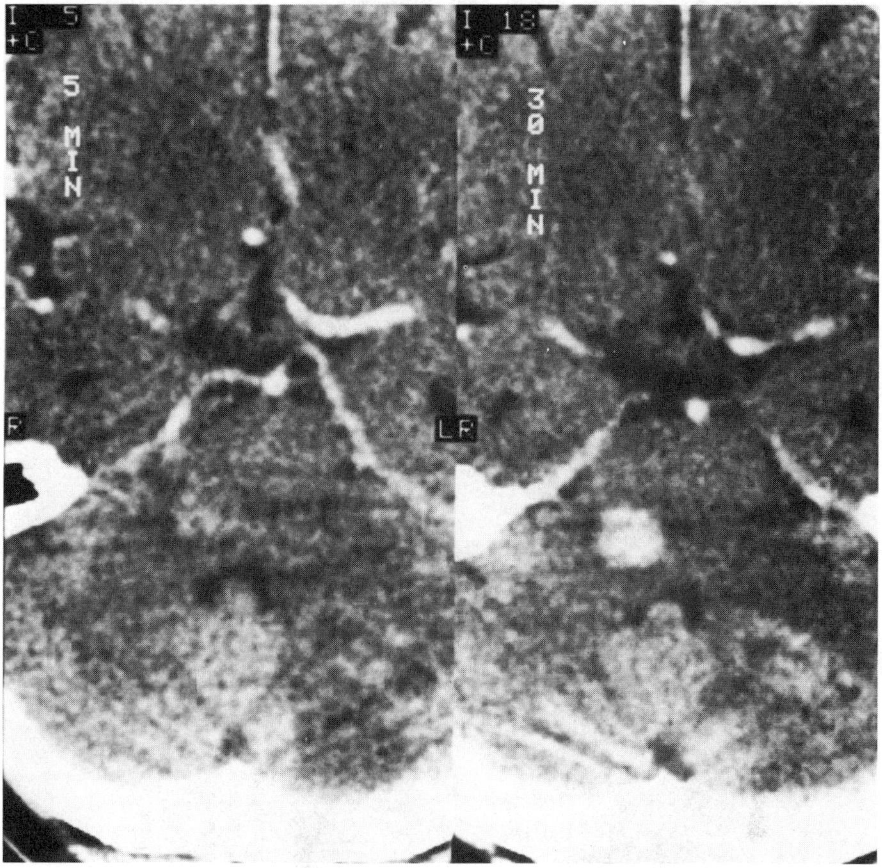

FIGURE 5. Intravenous enhancement, delayed CT in multiple sclerosis. A comparison of a CT scan performed 5 minutes and 30 minutes following the intravenous infusion of iodinated contrast material. The delayed (30 minute) scan shows marked improved delineation of the circular enhancing abnormality in the cerebellar peduncle. Even using a single dose (42 g I) of iodinated contrast material as in this patient, the performance of a delayed CT scan greatly improves the detection of blood-brain barrier abnormalities.

FIGURE 4. Multiple enhancing abnormalities (*arrows*) are present throughout the white matter at the (**A**) midbrain, (**B**) body of lateral ventricle, and (**C**) stock supraventricular level. The enhancing abnormalities adjacent to the sylvian fissure may be in either gray or white matter. The ventricles and cortical sulci are prominent for a 34-year-old woman. The multiple areas of enhancement are consistent with disruption of the blood-brain barrier. This patient was studied during an acute exacerbation.

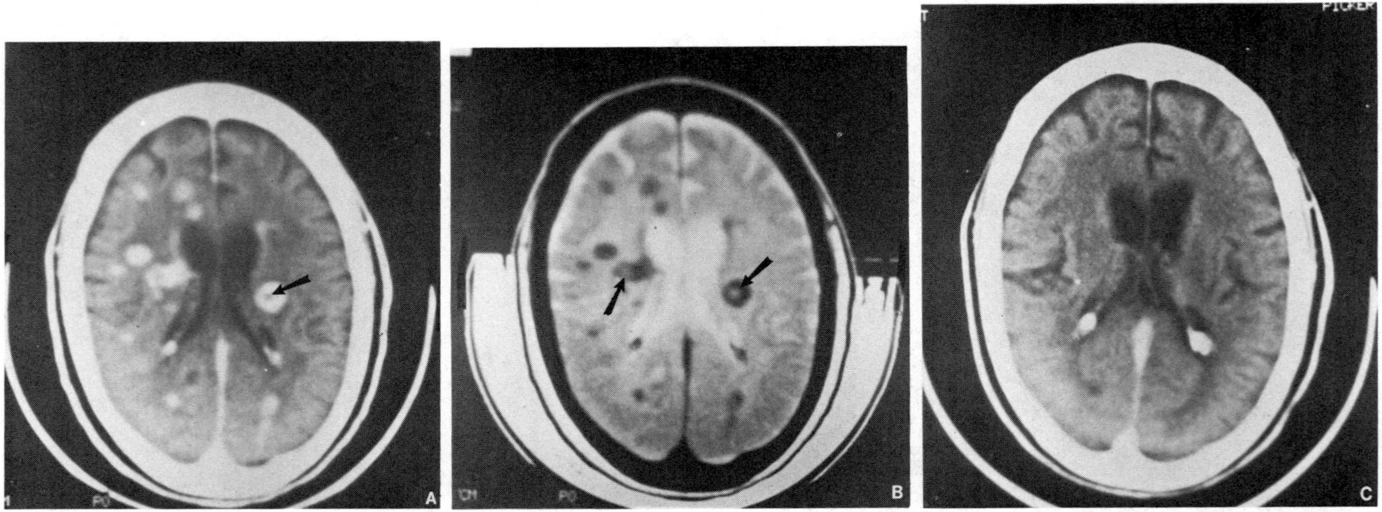

FIGURE 6. Multiple sclerosis: enhancement and steroid therapy. (**A**) Intravenously enhanced CT. Multiple enhancing abnormalities are noted, particularly in the periventricular cerebral white matter during an acute exacerbation of multiple sclerosis. This enhancement is consistent with multiple areas of disruption of the blood-brain barrier. (**B**) Intravenously enhanced CT scan, reversal mode. The same enhancing abnormalities are now noted in a reversal mode. The reversal mode may highlight the central area of nonenhancement (*arrow*) that is most likely related to fibrillary gliosis in a chronic portion of the MS plaque. (**C**) Intravenously enhanced CT scan; a CT scan performed nine days later. During this period the patient was receiving corticosteroid therapy. There are no longer any areas of abnormal enhancement suggesting there has been membrane stabilization because of the corticosteroid effect. This case illustrates the importance of utilizing contrast enhancement whether for CT or MR to better understand therapeutic efficacy. (Courtesy of Richard Fernandez, Medical College of Virginia.)

agents. When used in extremely high concentrations that are potentially toxic to living systems, they have been shown to decrease the T1 relaxation time in a manner sufficient to increase the signal intensity on a proton MR image.[20] The major problem with most of these NSFR agents has been the rapid reduction in the bloodstream to a nonparamagnetic compound and thus the dosage required is extremely high. New compounds are now being developed with a goal of decreasing reduction yet retaining the strong paramagnetic qualities.[21]

Certain metallic ions may also be used as paramagnetic contrast agents as they decrease the T1 relaxation time. Initially transition metals such as manganese (Mn^{++}) were tested in animal models. Lanthanide series metallic ions such as gadolinium (Gd^{+++}) are more paramagnetic when used in equal concentrations. The major problem with the metallic ions has been their potential toxicity. However, recently a gadolinium DTPA compound has been tested in both animal models and man with excellent results. In 12 patients studied by the Hammersmith group in London, gadolinium DTPA was equivalent or superior to iodinated contrast material in causing lesion "enhancement."[22] This enhancement by MR is an increase in signal intensity on

TABLE 2. Comparison of MR and CT Imaging

	MR	CT
Ionizing radiation	no	yes
Patient convenience	poor	good
Hospital convenience	poor	good
Outpatient convenience	good	good
Imaging parameters[a]	T1, T2, H	U
Spatial resolution (FWHM)	0.5	0.5
Contrast sensitivity	+++	++
Imaging time	slow	fast
Direct sagittal/coronal	simple	difficult
Contrast media[b]	+	++

[a]The signal intensity in an MR image is dependent upon the T1 and T2 relaxation times, proton density, and flow, whereas the CT image is related to the attenuation coefficient (U).

[b]Paramagnetic compounds (*e.g.*, Gd^{+++} DTPA) are presently being tested for MR while iodinated contrast media are routinely used for CT to analyze blood-brain barrier integrity.

the T1-weighted image. They reported no adverse reactions to the gadolinium DTPA contrast material.

The second strategy for analyzing blood-brain barrier integrity involves the use of proton chemical shift MR. The brain contains predominantly a water peak with only a negligible lipid peak on a proton spectra. This differs from many other organs in the body that have both a water and lipid peak. It has been proposed that with membrane instability, as might be seen with disruption of the blood-brain barrier, an abnormal area of brain might contain both a proton and lipid peak.[23] If this hypothesis is verified, the potential might exist to analyze membrane instability without the infusion of a paramagnetic contrast material.

CONCLUSION

Initial studies using MR imaging suggest that this methodology may prove even more sensitive than CT scanning for the anatomic detection of lesions in multiple

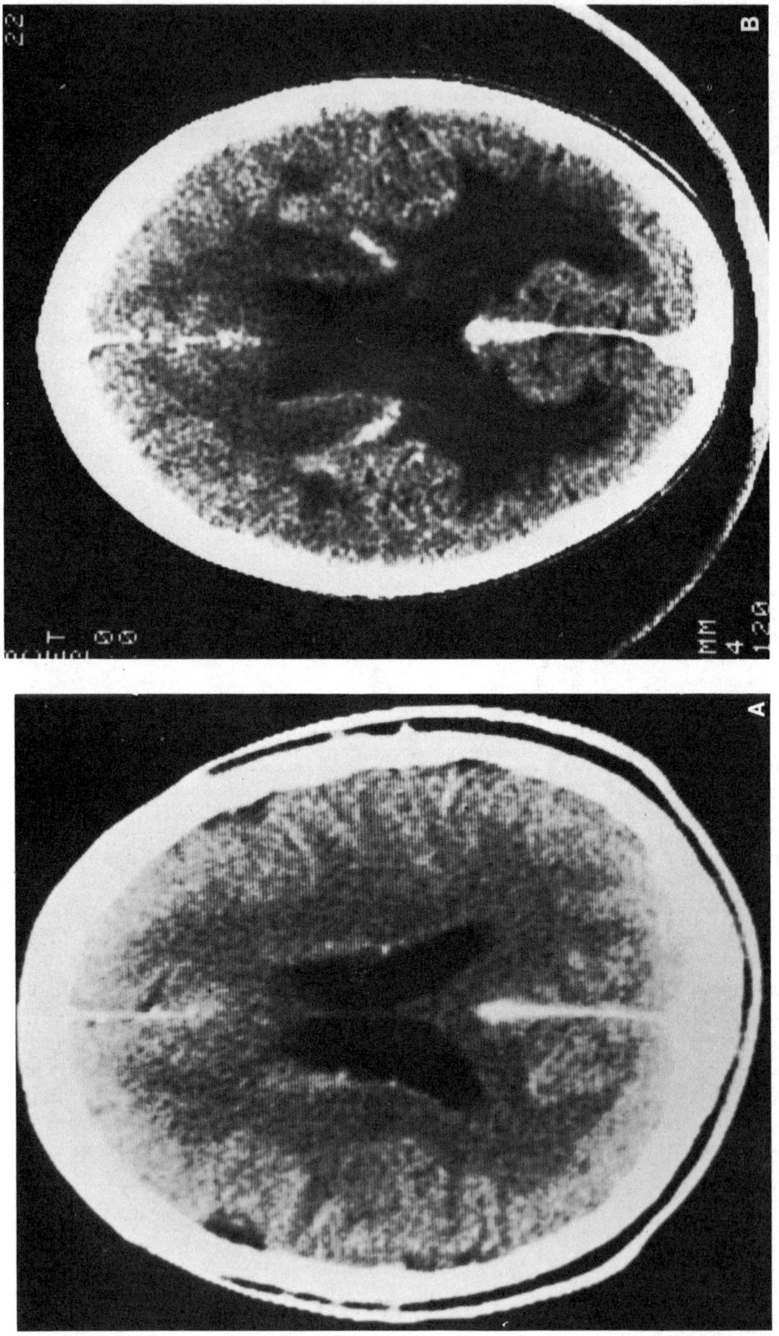

FIGURE 7. Non-MS white matter disease. **(A)** Normal intravenously enhanced CT scan showing the prominent distinction between the gray matter capillary bed and white matter that may normally be highlighted following the infusion of iodinated contrast material. This should not be mistaken for white matter disease on a high resolution CT scan. **(B)** Adrenoleukodystrophy. Ten-year-old boy with hypodensity involving most significantly the parietal periventricular white matter but also involving the frontal periventricular white matter. Two linear strands of enhancement are noted just prior to their crossing the corpus callosum as it is typical of the CT intravenously enhanced appearance of adrenoleukodystrophy.

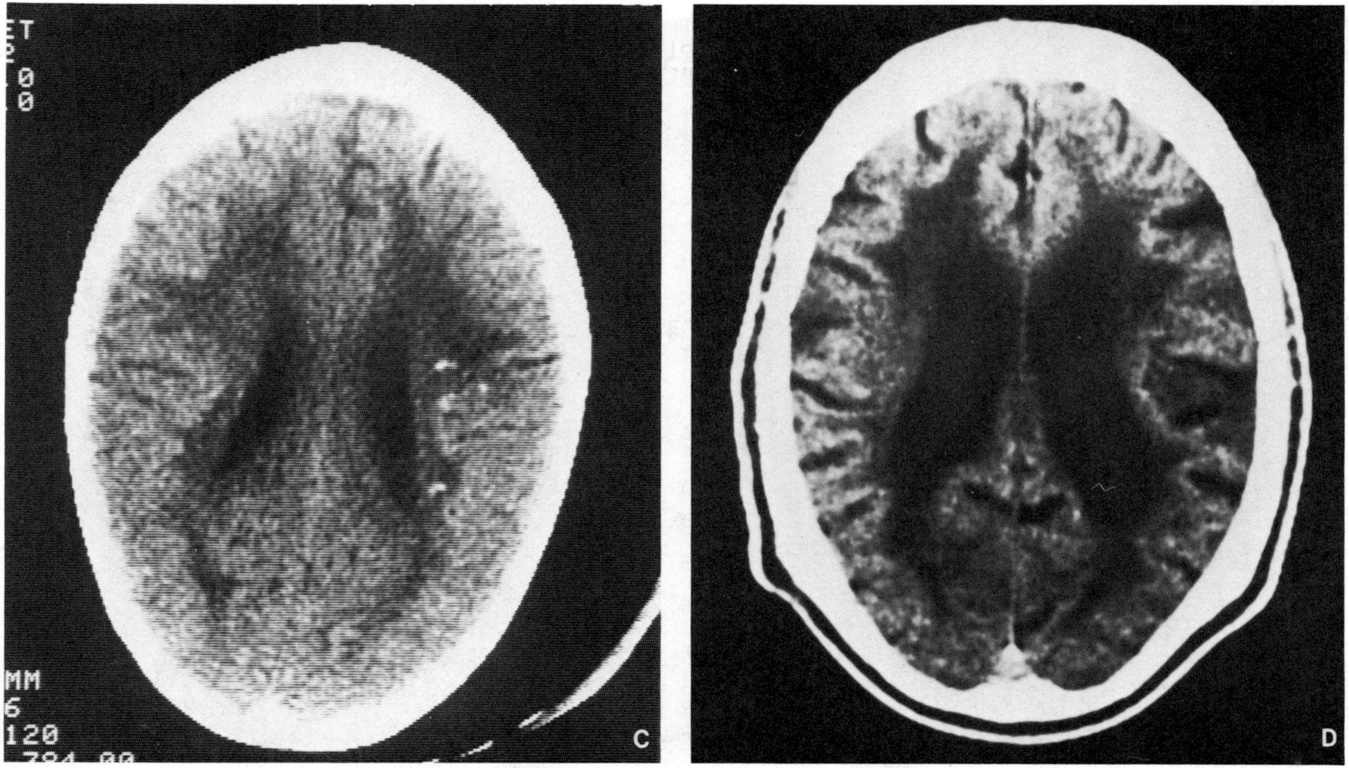

FIGURE 7 ***(con't.).*** (**C**) Disseminated necrotizing leukoencephalopathy (DNL). Hypodensity in the frontal and parietal white matter. Increased density on this nonenhanced scan represents calcification in this patient with leukemia who has been treated with methotrexate and radiation. (**D**) Subcortical arteriosclerotic encephalopathy (Binswanger). Multifocal, confluent hypodensity throughout the cerebral white matter with associated enlargement of the lateral ventricles and cortical sulci. On sections at the basal ganglia level lacunar infarcts are seen. These CT findings are typical for SAE in a 67-year-old with hypertension, dementia, and a pseudobulbar affect.

sclerosis by improving the visualization of plaques not only in the cerebral white matter, but also in the brainstem and spinal cord. A comparison of MR *versus* CT imaging characteristics is presented in TABLE 2. At present, there is no indication that any given white matter abnormality seen by either CT or proton MR imaging will prove specific for multiple sclerosis as compared to other disorders involving the white matter. In all situations there will be a nonspecific prolongation of the T1 and T2 relaxation times. However, it is important to realize that by improving sensitivity and detecting lesions in previously silent locales, the potential of making a diagnosis of MS is greatly improved, particularly if multiplicity is established. In addition, the distribution or other characteristics of a white matter abnormality when evaluated in conjunction with the clinical history may prove quite specific (FIG. 7).

When evaluating putative therapeutic agents for the treatment of MS, knowledge of the integrity of the blood-brain barrier may contribute to our understanding of pathophysiology and prove a useful marker of therapeutic efficacy. The use of iodinated contrast material and CT scanning has proved extremely valuable in this regard over the past years. Although extremely promising, the use of paramagnetic nondiffusible indicators to delineate disruption in the blood-brain barrier is at an early experimental stage. Recent studies using gadolinium DTPA in man suggests that contrast enhancement strategies will prove useful for MR.

With the improving sensitivity of noninvasive imaging techniques for the detection of MS plaques, the need to incorporate findings from imaging studies in any new classification of MS seems apparent. The frequently striking dichotomy between clinical symptomatology and the locations of MS lesions highlights the important role of imaging techniques when evaluating the utility of therapeutic protocols. Noninvasive imaging not only provides unique information concerning the natural history of MS when long-term follow-up studies are obtained but also provides important information concerning disease activity by analyzing the integrity of the blood-brain barrier.

REFERENCES

1. POSER, C. M., D. W. PATY, L. SCHEINBERG, W. I. MCDONALD, F. A. DAVIS, G. C. EBERS, K. P. JOHNSON, W. A. SIBLEY, D. H. SLIBERBERG & W. W. TOURTELLOTTE. 1983. New diagnostic criteria for multiple sclerosis: Guidelines for research protocols. Ann. Neurol. **13:** 227–231.
2. LUMSDEN, C. E. 1970. The neuropathology of multiple sclerosis. *In* Handbook of Clinical Neurology, vol. 9. P. J. Vinken & G. W. Bruyn, Eds.: 217–309. North-Holland. Amsterdam.
3. BARRETT, L. & B. P. DRAYER. 1984. High resolution computed tomography in multiple sclerosis. Ann. Neurol. In press.
4. FOG, T. 1965. The topography of plaques in multiple sclerosis. Acta Neurol. Scand. (Suppl. 41) **15:** 1–162.
5. HERSHEY, L. A., M. H. GADO & J. L. TROTTER. 1979. Computerized tomography in the diagnostic evaluation of multiple sclerosis. Ann. Neurol. **5:** 32–39.
6. VINUELA, F. V., A. J. FOX, G. M. DEBRUN, T. E. FEASBY & G. C. EBERS. 1982. New perspectives in computed tomography of multiple sclerosis. Am. J. Neuroradiol. **3:** 227–281.
7. YOUNG, I. R., A. S. HALL, C. A. PALLIS, N. J. LEGG, G. M. BYDDER & R. E. STERNER. 1981. Nuclear magnetic resonance imaging of the brain in multiple sclerosis. Lancet **2:** 1063–1066.
8. LUKES, S. A., L. E. CROOKS, M. J. AMINOFF, L. KAUFMAN, H. S. PANITCH, C. MILLS & D. NORMAN. 1983. Nuclear magnetic resonance imaging in multiple sclerosis. Ann. Neurol. **13:** 592–601.

9. KLATZO, I., A. PIRAUX & E. J. LASKOWSKI. 1958. The relationship between edema, blood-brain barrier and tissue elements in local brain injury. J. Neuropathol. Exp. Neurol. **17:** 548–564.
10. POSER, C. M. 1969. Disseminated vasculomyelinopathy. Acta Neurol. Scand. (Suppl. 7) **45:** 1–44.
11. BROMAN, T. 1964. Blood-brain barrier damage in MS: Supravital test observation. Acta Neurol. Scand. **40:** 21–24.
12. CUTLER, R. W. P., A. V. LORENZO & C. F. BARLOW. 1967. Brain vascular permeability to I-125 gamma globulin and leukocytes in allergic encephalomyelitis. J. Neuropath. Exp. Neurol. **26:** 558–571.
13. FIELD, E. J. & C. S. RAINE. 1966. Experimental allergic encephalomyelitis. Am. J. Pathol. **49:** 537–553.
14. BRAIN, R. & M. WILKINSON. 1957. The association of cervical spondylosis and disseminated sclerosis. Brain **80:** 456–478.
15. PRESKORN, S. H., B. K. HARTMAN, G. H. IRWIN & C. W. HUGHES. 1982. Role of the central adrenergic system in mediating amitriptyline-induced alteration in the mammalian blood-brain barrier in vivo. J. Pharm. Exp. Therap. **223:** 388–395.
16. DRAYER, B. P. 1981. Functional applications of CT of the central nervous system. Am. J. Neuroradiol. **2:** 495–510.
17. SEARS, E. S., R. S. TINDALL & H. ZARNOW. 1978. Active multiple sclerosis: Enhanced computerized tomographic imaging of lesions and the effect of corticosteroids. Arch. Neurol. **35:** 426–434.
18. TROIANO, R., M. HAFSTEIN, M. RUDERMAN, P. DOWLING & S. COOK. 1984. Effect of high dose intravenous steroid administration on contrast enhancing computed tomographic scan lesions in multiple sclerosis. Ann. Neurol. **15:** 257–263.
19. TOURTELLOTTE, W. W. 1970. Cerebrospinal fluid in multiple sclerosis. *In* Handbook of Clinical Neurology, vol. 9. P. J. Vinken & G. W. Bruyn, Eds.: 324–382. North-Holland. Amsterdam.
20. BRASCH, R. C. 1983. Methods of contrast enhancement for NMR imaging and potential applications. A subject review. Radiology **147:** 781–788.
21. GRIFFETH, L. K., G. M. ROSEN, E. J. RAUCKMAN & B. P. DRAYER. 1984. Pharmacokinetics of nitroxide NMR contrast agents. Invest. Radiol. In press.
22. CARR, D. H., J. BROWN, G. M. BYDDER, H. J. WEINMANN, U. SPECK, D. J. THOMAS & I. R. YOUNG. 1984. Intravenous chelated gadolinium as a contrast agent in NMR imaging of cerebral tumours. Lancet **1:** 484–486.
23. PYKETT, I. L. & B. R. ROSEN. 1983. Nuclear magnetic resonance: In vivo proton chemical shift imaging. Radiology **149:** 197–201.

DISCUSSION OF THE PAPER

D. PATY (*University of British Columbia, Vancouver, BC*): With nuclear magnetic resonance we have begun to do serial studies on a group of MS patients which I think is going to give us the most information on this and I'd like to point this out because it's perhaps relevant to some of our other discussions for trying to detect abnormalities in immune parameters and other parameters that may or may not parallel clinical activity.

There was a young man who had an exacerbation, a severe exacerbation involving one leg and we began doing serial NMR studies. One was done in July. Another was done in September, at which time he was asymptomatic but there was this very large new lesion back in the occipital lobe that obviously was silent. We've heard already the frequency with which subclinical lesions develop and I think biologically that is important; clinically it doesn't represent itself in any way and I can't see why the T cells should behave differently under this circumstance from one that develops clinical activity because the lymphocytes don't know whether or not they're producing a hemiparesis or no symptoms at all. Thanks.

B. DRAYER (*Duke University Medical Center, Durham, NC*): Just one comment on that. That's really been the experience with CT as well and we're seeing multiple lesions, often multiple enhancing lesions of which we have no clinical correlate. This is a problem and in fact, when the patients are getting better, the lesions are often still showing up and we're seeing new areas of abnormal enhancement.

Secondly, it's probably worth it for you to see Dr. Paty's exhibit. I think they've done 29 cases now at the University of British Columbia, and are confirming a lot of the data that is coming out of other centers. It's very difficult to accumulate large numbers of patients and as any of you know who have NMR scanners right now, it's difficult to get time on the scanner.

C. POSER (*Boston University School of Medicine, Boston, MA*): Dr. Drayer, what's the NMR equivalent of contrast enhancing?

DRAYER: That's important. One of the advantages right now of CT certainly is the ability to do contrast enhancement and whatever you feel the mechanism is we happen to believe it is a breakdown in the blood-brain barrier that we are seeing; that's been very useful with CT. How can we do this with NMR? Right now there's no way but there are really two potential things coming up and I think within the next year or two we'll hear much more about these.

First is doing chemical shift proton NMR. If you look at chemical shift spectra the brain mainly has a water peak. If you start to see a lipid peak you may surmise membrane instability.

Number two, every major pharmaceutical company and university is working on new contrast materials. These are so-called paramagnetic substances that will decrease the T_1 and T_2 relaxation time of an area of the brain with abnormal barrier. There are really two groups, one of the transition metals and the first of these will be gadolinium DTPA. Gadolinium DTPA will be tested in the next six months in clinical trials. The second group is the nitroxite stable free radicals. There are multiple stable free radicals that have been tried. The ones tried to date have not been very useful because they have been reduced in the bloodstream.

Our group is working on an agent which we think is excellent; they will be very interesting because not only will they be nondiffusable indicators to look at blood-brain barrier but we might be able to alter them as well and look at other brain functions using these.

The third technique which will probably be three or four years in the future will be to use one of the other nuclei that's normally not diffusable across the blood-brain barrier and then look at spectra or an image. So I think the possibility of evaluating the blood-brain barrier, to answer your question, is definitely there; with magnetic resonance it's just going to take a little time until we establish the best way to do it.

Pattern-Shift Visual, Brainstem Auditory and Short-Latency Somatosensory Evoked Potentials in Multiple Sclerosis

KEITH H. CHIAPPA

Harvard Medical School
Boston, Massachusetts 02115
and
Clinical Neurophysiology Laboratory
Massachusetts General Hospital
Boston, Massachusetts 02114

INTRODUCTION

An evoked potential (EP) is the brain's electrical response to stimulation of a sensory system, recorded via scalp electrodes, biologic amplifiers and signal averaging computers. Pattern-shift visual, brainstem auditory, and short-latency somatosensory evoked potentials have developed into reliable diagnostic tests that yield reproducible results in routine clinical practice. Since they provide an objective measure of function in their related sensory systems and tracts, they have been studied in large groups of normal subjects and in patients with a wide variety of neurologic diseases. The clinical utility of EPs in multiple sclerosis (MS) is based on their ability (1) to demonstrate abnormal sensory system function when the history and/or neurological examination are equivocal, (2) to reveal the presence of clinically unsuspected malfunction in a sensory system when demyelinating disease is suspected because of symptoms and/or signs in another area of the central nervous system (CNS), (3) to help define the anatomic distribution of a disease process, and (4) to monitor objective changes in a patient's status. Latencies and amplitudes of the various waves provide numerical data; sometimes the absence of a wave or an abnormal configuration of its potential field also provides useful information.

PATTERN-SHIFT VISUAL EVOKED POTENTIALS

The pattern-shift visual EP (PSVEP) is obtained with a reversing checkerboard pattern and recorded from the scalp overlying visual cortex where a prominent positive peak appearing at about 100 ms in normal subjects (see FIGURE 1) is used for clinical interpretation. PSVEPs provide a sensitive extension of the clinical examination and commonly used clinical tests (visual acuity, clinical and formal visual fields, pupillary responses, fundoscopic examination, and red color desaturation). To demonstrate the relative sensitivity of the PSVEP, 198 patients with multiple sclerosis who had had PSVEP testing were studied retrospectively by extracting pertinent aspects of the neuro-ophthalmologic examination from their medical records.[1] When the PSVEP was normal, there was never an abnormality found on the clinical examination. Even when the PSVEP was abnormal, various clinical examinations were often normal. For example, in those patients with abnormal PSVEPs, the visual fields by usual clinical examination (confrontation) were normal in 96%, formal fields were normal in 55%, pupillary responses were normal in 74%, fundus appearance was normal in 39% and there was no red color desaturation in 27% (only 22 patients had this test reported). These figures convey the degree of sensitivity that the test can add to the routine clinical ophthalmological examination. However, if the formal visual field examination is done carefully a greater incidence of clinical abnormalities can be found even in asymptomatic patients,[2-4] although it never matches that of the PSVEP.

However, PSVEP abnormalities produced by the demyelinating plaques of optic neuritis and MS are indistinguishable from abnormalities produced by many other retinal, compressive and degenerative diseases. Thus, abnormal findings demonstrated by the PSVEP must be carefully integrated into the clinical situation by a physician familiar with the clinical use of this test. He or she must decide if other procedures (*e.g.*, electroretinography, formal visual fields, radiologic studies, subspecialty consultation) are indicated to differentiate the possible causes of the conduction delay.

A large number of clinical studies attest to the sensitivity of the PSVEP in revealing demyelinating lesions in the optic nerve, and in our experience about 90% of

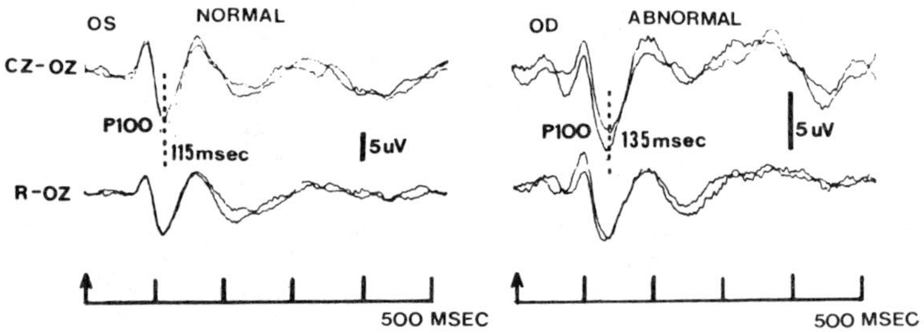

FIGURE 1. PSVEPs recorded from a patient with MS showing a monocular latency abnormality. Left eye response (OS) was normal at 115 ms, right response (OD) was abnormal with P100 peak delayed in latency at 135 ms (normal mean plus 3 standard deviations with this pattern-shift stimulator was 117 ms). Each trace is the average of 128 stimuli, with a repetition superimposed. Cz and Oz refer to International 10–20 System positions (vertex and occiput, respectively); reference was linked ears; relative positivity at G2 caused a downward trace deflection. (Reprinted, with permission, from ref. 1.)

patients who have a clear history of optic neuritis (ON) have abnormal PSVEPs. Of the more than 400 patients with optic neuritis presented in the literature, 89% had PSVEP abnormalities. In some studies, the percentage is closer to 100%. When there was no clinical evidence for optic nerve involvement, the incidence of PSVEP abnormalities was 51% (of 715 patients). In addition, these abnormalities are present whatever the time interval since the clinical episode of optic neuritis; Shahrohki *et al.*[5] reported PSVEP abnormalities five years after the clinical episode and Halliday *et al.*[6] reported patients who had abnormal PSVEPs 15 years later. For a comprehensive index to the literature on ON and MS, see ref. 7.

Less than 5% of patients with abnormal PSVEPs have the P100 absolute latency (stimulus to EP waveform peak) return to normal even 10 or 15 years after visual acuity has returned to normal following an episode of optic neuritis. When the latency difference between the two eyes can be used for interpretation (sometimes patients will have binocular PSVEP abnormalities when first studied) then the percentage of patients in whom the PSVEP returns to normal drops to below 1%. Thus, if optic neuritis is suspected and the patient complains of moderate to severe visual difficulty but the PSVEP is normal, that diagnosis is highly unlikely.

Tackmann *et al.*[8] tested 32 patients with isolated optic neuritis using brainstem auditory evoked potentials (BAEPs), somatosensory evoked potentials (SEPs) and blink reflexes. Eleven patients were shown to have additional lesions in the CNS outside the optic nerve. Halliday and McDonald[9] have followed patients with serial recordings over several years, noting step-like increases in latency associated with relapses characterized by visual impairment; if there was no visual system involvement, PSVEPs tended to remain unchanged.

When the diagnosis of MS is suspected because of typical symptoms and/or signs referrable to other central nervous system locations, then the demonstration by an abnormal PSVEP of a clinically silent conduction defect in the optic nerve can further delineate the anatomic distribution of the disease process and thus narrow the range of diagnostic possibilities. Optic nerve demyelination is a common finding in autopsy material of MS patients,[10,11] and this is paralleled by the incidence of PSVEP abnormalities, which ranges from a high of 96%[6] to a low of 47%.[12] In a large number of clinical studies encompassing almost 2000 patients with all MS classifications, the average abnormality rate found was 63%. Of 464, 322 and 799 patients classified as possible, probable and definite MS the average abnormality rates were 37%, 58% and 85%, respectively. These figures reflect the greater likelihood of optic nerve lesions with more definite clinical diagnoses. Of 744 patients reported as having no history or clinical findings of optic neuritis, 51% had PSVEP abnormalities (ranging from a high of 93%[6] to a low of 34%.[13] The differences between studies are best explained by the different definitions of MS used, some studies being composed of a preponderance of one class of patients. Note also that screen and check sizes differed greatly between the studies mentioned above. Contrasts, when reported, were all above 74%. Luminance levels varied so much that the reliability of the measurements has to be doubted.

The major change associated with ON is prolongation of P100 latency. The mean latency in MS patients in a representative study exceeded the normal mean by about 10 (possible MS) to 30 (definite MS) ms,[14] and delays exceeding 100 ms have also been reported.[5]

Interocular latency difference is probably the most sensitive indicator of optic nerve dysfunction in the PSVEP and has been used to provide evidence of optic nerve pathology.[5,12] Failure to utilize this parameter in a comparative study of flight of colors testing *versus* PSVEPs[15] resulted in erroneously low sensitivity of the PSVEP. Shahrohki *et al.*[5] found that 8 of 100 ON and MS patients had abnormal PSVEPs based on this parameter alone. Amplitude has not proved to be a reliable measure.

There have been various attempts to increase the sensitivity of the test in this clinical area, including the use of smaller stimulus fields, partial-field stimulation, changes in body temperature and light-emitting diode array stimulation, all without consistent or convincing improvement.

Cant *et al.*[14] and Camisa *et al.*[16] found that lower luminance levels revealed more abnormalities and suggested routine use of more than one intensity level. However, this effect was not observed by others[17,18] except for restricted foveal stimulation.[18] For discussions of the (inconsistent) relationship between visual acuity and PSVEP findings, the use of PSVEP to follow the course of MS, and the findings with this test in spinal cord disease, see ref. 7.

Patients with acute transverse myelitis show PSVEP abnormalities in only a small proportion of cases. Blumhardt *et al.*[19] studied 31 patients in whom the spinal cord symptoms developed over hours to days (nine of these were classified as transverse myelitis) and found PSVEP abnormalities in 10%. Ropper *et al.*[20] found no PSVEP or BAEP abnormalities in 12 patients with acute transverse myelitis.

The chronic, progressive myelopathies have a greater incidence of abnormal PSVEPs. The abnormality rates ranged from 76% in the series of Bynke *et al.*[21] to 35% in the 100 patients with disease of more than six months duration studied by Blumhardt *et al.*[19] (see also ref. 7).

It has been suggested that PSVEP data can be used clinically in the setting of undiagnosed spinal cord disease to help decide whether or not myelography is necessary.[22] Bynke *et al.*[21] suggested that if the clinical neuro-ophthalmological examination and the PSVEP are abnormal, and the CSF shows oligoclonal IgG banding, then radiological investigations can be limited or avoided. However, the possibility of concurrent diseases dictates very careful assessment of the clinical situation before an abnormal PSVEP (with or without other tests) should be used as presumptive evidence of MS to delay myelography. In fact, Blumhardt *et al.*[19] found five patients with abnormal PSVEPs and abnormal myelograms. Three had only borderline narrowing of the cervical canals and spondylotic changes (two of these have subsequently developed further signs of MS) but two had cord compression caused by prolapsed intervertebral disks. After laminectomy one of these patients had little clinical change but the other had a marked improvement.

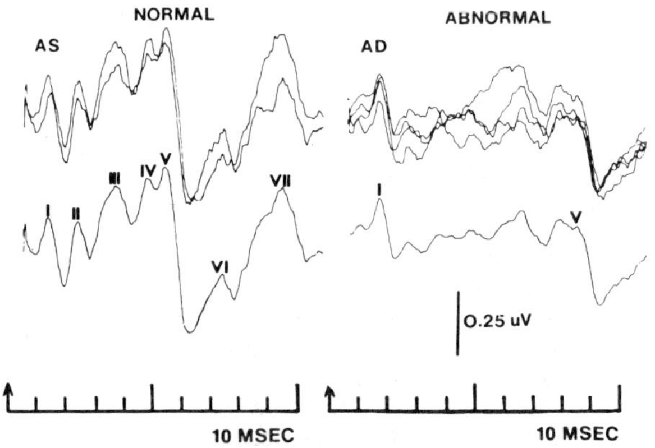

FIGURE 2. BAEPs from an MS patient showing the marked asymmetry that can be present with monaural stimulation. The left ear response (AS) is normal; the right ear response (AD) illustrates one of the several types of abnormality seen in BAEPs in MS: wave III absent and the I–V interval markedly abnormal (6.7 ms; upper limit of normal was 4.7 ms for the stimulus parameters used here). AS superimposed trials have $n = 1024$ clicks each; in AD, $n = 2048$ clicks each. The single trace below each is the sum of the superimposed trials. Recorded with the usual bipolar derivation, ipsilateral earlobe to vertex; vertex positivity yielding an upward deflection. (Reprinted, with permission, from ref. 23.)

BRAINSTEM AUDITORY EVOKED POTENTIALS

The brainstem auditory evoked potential was recorded in response to a 10/s click stimulus, most often using a vertex-to-earlobe derivation, and shows five peaks in the first 10 ms after the stimulus (see FIG. 2), arising in brainstem auditory structures from nerve VIII to inferior colliculus. Its clinical utility stems from the close relationship between the EP waveforms and specific anatomic structures. This specificity allows localization of conduction defects in the brainstem to within a centimeter or so. In addition, BAEPs are very resistant to alteration by anything other than structural pathology in the brainstem auditory tracts. For example, barbituate doses sufficient to render the EEG "flat" (isoelectric) and general anesthesia do not significantly affect BAEPs. These factors of anatomic specificity and physiologic and metabolic immutability are the basis of the clinical utility of BAEPs.

Brainstem auditory evoked potentials offer a look at "physiologic anatomy." They provide a sensitive tool for assessment of brainstem auditory tracts and nearby structures. As with PSVEPs and SEPs, abnormalities demonstrated by BAEPs are etiologically nonspecific and must be carefully integrated into the clinical situation by a physician familiar with the clinical use of this test. He or she must decide if other procedures (*e.g.*, conventional audiometric studies, electrocochleography, electronystagmography, radiologic studies, subspecialty consultation) are indicated to differentiate the possible causes of the conduction delay.

In demyelinating disease, BAEPs are potentially useful in three ways: (1) in patients with a nonbrainstem locus of CNS involvement, an abnormal BAEP signals the presence of another clinically unsuspected lesion, thus helping to define the disease process, (2) when the clinical findings are equivocal or otherwise uncertain, an abnormal BAEP provides objective evidence of disturbed function, and (3) various treatments can be monitored objectively by following abnormal BAEPs.

There have been a large number of studies of BAEPs in patients with MS (see ref. 7). Of 1000 patients in the literature with varying classifications of MS, 46% had abnormal BAEPs. For patients classified as definite, probable and possible MS the average abnormality rates were 67%, 41% and 30%, respectively. Of patients reported as having no history of brainstem findings, 38% had BAEP abnormalities; abnormality rates varied from 21% to 55%. Thus, in one-fifth to one-half of MS patients without brainstem symptoms or signs, BAEP testing will reveal evidence of clinically unsuspected lesions. Differences in definitions of MS, patient populations and techniques account for the variations among studies.

In a large group of MS patients, the reliability of BAEP techniques was demonstrated by the fact that all parameters in the MS patients with BAEPs interpreted as normal (the BAEP-normal MS group) showed no statistical differences from the normal values.[23] Those MS patients who had BAEPs with abnormal interwave separations had latency values which were a mean of 4.9 SDs above the normal mean and those MS patients who were determined to have abnormal BAEPs on the basis of an abnormal I/V amplitude ratio (17% of the BAEP-abnormal MS group) had ratios which were a mean of 5.5 SDs above the normal mean. These facts, and the higher incidence of abnormalities in the definite MS group suggest that the BAEP is a reliable test for clinical usage.

Although the normal mean plus 3 SDs was used in the above study[23] as the upper limit of normal, the BAEP-normal MS patients (including those in the definite MS group) had values for both interwave latency and amplitude parameters which were essentially identical to the normal values. The fact that the values for the MS patients had a bimodal distribution (also noted for absolute wave V latency by Robinson and Rudge[24]) either completely normal or markedly abnormal, suggests that the smallest MS plaques in this part of the auditory system are sufficient to produce a marked conduction abnormality.

A majority of the BAEP abnormalities in MS patients are wave V amplitude abnormalities (absence or abnormally low amplitude of wave V was seen in 87% of the BAEP-abnormal MS patients[23]). The next most frequent abnormality, increased III–V IPL, was seen in 28% of the BAEP-abnormal MS patients. The presumed generators of waves III and V are the superior olivary complex and inferior colliculus, respectively, and thus the majority of the conduction abnormalities were found to occur between them, as would be expected since this is the longest segment of white matter in the tracts being tested. However, in those patients who had recognizable waves V, there was no significant correlation between the III–V separation and the wave I/V amplitude ratio, contrary to our expectations. In fact, in 17% of the BAEP-abnormal MS patients the III–V separation was normal and the I/V amplitude ratio was abnormal. In addition, three patients had the unusual combination of no wave III, a recognizable wave V of normal amplitude, and an abnormal I–V separation. The disparity between these different kinds of abnormalities is not easily resolved merely by consideration of the known conduction deficits in demyelinated axons such as slow conduction across the demyelinated segment and increased refractory period. Multiplicity of lesions, possible contributions to the BAEP waveforms from conduction in separate but parallel tracts, and possible synchronous activation of different auditory tract structures need to be considered.

The importance of monaural stimulation is evident since 45% of the BAEP abnormalities were seen with stimulation of one ear only.[23] The prevalence of monaural abnormalities suggests that, with respect to the BAEP waveform generators, there is relatively little bilateral conduction, although the anatomy had suggested otherwise.

Faster rates of stimulation alter all BAEP parameters, including interwave separations. It has been noted previously[25,26] that increased click repetition rate revealed a higher incidence of abnormalities in the BAEPs of MS patients. However, in our group of MS patients, more BAEP abnormalities were not seen with 70 clicks per second, although abnormalities seen at 10/s were sometimes worse at 70/s.[23] Elidan *et al.*[27] recently reported similar findings. The relative difficulty of waveform recognition at 70/s, with increased waveform duration and indistinct peaks, restricted the clinical utility of that stimulus rate. In a few patients with diseases other than MS we have noted the reverse situation, *i.e.*, the I–V separation was abnormal at 10/s and normal at 70/s. This "normalization" may be due to complete failure of conduction in the abnormal fibers at the faster rate, possibly due to an increased refractory period. With their abnormal contribution removed from the resultant waveforms the activity manifest is only that from the normally conducting fibers, hence the normal appearance. Although this effect was sought in the MS patients, it was not found.

Emerson *et al.*[28] noted that some patients with MS show BAEP abnormalities with only one click polarity, usually rarefaction clicks. Some of these patients have normal hearing on conventional audiometric tests and this effect is presumably due to central conduction abnormalities.

In spite of obvious abnormalities in the BAEP, none of the MS patients studied here had clinical complaints of hearing difficulties, and click thresholds were essentially normal (formal audiograms were rarely obtained but those which were obtained were normal). This is consistent with the findings of routine audiological testing in MS patients[29] but detailed auditory and vestibular testing[30] and interaural time discrimination and auditory localization testing[31] may reveal functional abnormalities in MS patients. In the latter study almost all MS patients with abnormal BAEPs also had abnormal interaural time discrimination. Occasionally MS patients do have symptomatic hearing difficulties and abnormal BAEPs apparently related to the disease[32] but none were seen in our group. The occurrence of grossly abnormal BAEPs in conjunction with subjectively normal hearing may reflect the production of BAEP abnormalities by temporal dispersion of the click-induced volley as it ascends the affected tracts. It may be that, although these asynchronous potentials do not sum to generate a discrete peak of activity discernible at the scalp, the integrity of conduction, albeit deranged, is sufficient to sustain functionally normal hearing.

However, this does not explain those cases where the amplitude and waveform shape are essentially normal and there is an abnormally large interwave separation. Perhaps in these cases the demyelination involves a majority of the fibers equally. Also, of course, BAEP waveform generation might have little to do with functional hearing.

Matthews *et al.*[33] followed for 38 months after BAEP testing 84 patients in whom the diagnosis of MS was under consideration. In nine of these patients an abnormal BAEP at initial presentation subsequently proved to be of diagnostic value in that it revealed a separate, clinically silent lesion, indicating a multifocal disease (and the patient on follow-up proved to have MS).

It should be reiterated here that a large part of the clinical utility of the BAEP lies in its ability not only to reveal unsuspected, and thereby multiple, lesions, but also to document clinically equivocal findings. For example, some of our patients with MS initially presented with symptoms and/or signs which could have been produced by disease in the labyrinths. Other than absence of wave I in three of the patients with Ménière's disease, no abnormalities of interwave separations or amplitude ratios in the BAER were seen in those 21 patients with labyrinthine diseases.[23] Thirty-seven percent of the MS patients who presented with nystagmus at the time of testing had BAEP abnormalities. Similarly, van Buggenhout *et al.*[4] found BAEP abnormalities in half of their patients who had vestibular lesions. Thus the BAEP can be helpful in this setting: if abnormal, then the lesion is clearly centrally rather than peripherally located. Conversely, 56% of the patients with an INO at the time of testing had abnormal BAEPs[23] so that the BAEP does not help to distinguish MS from the other causes of an INO (infarction and tumor[34]) which might also affect both medial longitudinal fasciculus and auditory tracts.

The BAEP is abnormal in some patients with system disorders affecting cerebellar function, particularly those who have spasticity, and thus is not helpful in differentiating possible MS in that setting.

Amyotrophic lateral sclerosis (ALS) sometimes presents initially with symptoms and/or signs that might be suggestive of MS; in our nine patients with ALS there was none with abnormal BAEPs.[23] Optic neuritis and cervical transverse myelitis may have etiologies closely related or identical to that of MS; all of the patients in those groups had normal BAEPs, and the ON patients tested also had normal SEPs (the cervical transverse myelitis patients all had abnormal SEPs). Also, in a different study 12 consecutive patients with inflammatory acute transverse myelitis (virtually or completely transverse lesions) had normal BAEPs.[20] Trigeminal neuralgia has also been associated with MS; in our 15 patients with trigeminal neuralgia there was none with abnormal BAEPs. Thus, as is also the case clinically, at the time of onset of ON, cervical transverse myelitis and trigeminal neuralgia, there may be no EP evidence of lesions elsewhere in the CNS.

The consistency of the BAER when followed over time in normals suggests that it could be used to follow the activity of lesions affecting these tracts and might possibly provide assistance in evaluating the effectiveness of therapeutic measures, although one study has suggested that the main value of BAEPs in patients with MS was to indicate clinically silent lesions and that its value in monitoring the clinical condition of the individual patient was less.[35]

SHORT-LATENCY SOMATOSENSORY EVOKED POTENTIALS

Short-latency somatosensory EPs are usually evoked with a 2/s to 5/s brief electrical pulse delivered transcutaneously to median, tibial or other nerves, and recorded at several points along the sensory pathway (*e.g.*, for upper limb testing, over the brachial plexus, dorsal columns and somatosensory cortex). See FIGURE 3 for the waveforms obtained with these derivations. The peak labeled EP is generated in the brachial plexus, P/N13 in the lower medulla, and N19–P22 in the thalamus cortex. The clinical utility of SEPs is related to the same factors of anatomic specificity and physiologic and metabolic immutability as were discussed above for BAEPs. SEPs offer a look at "physiologic anatomy" and thus provide a sensitive tool for assessment of spinal cord and brainstem posterior columns and medial lemniscal tracts and nearby structures. Again, abnormalities demonstrated by SEPs are etiologically nonspecific and must be carefully integrated into the clinical situation by a physician familiar with the clinical use of this test, who can decide whether or not other procedures (*e.g.*, electromyography, radiologic studies, subspecialty consultation) are indicated to

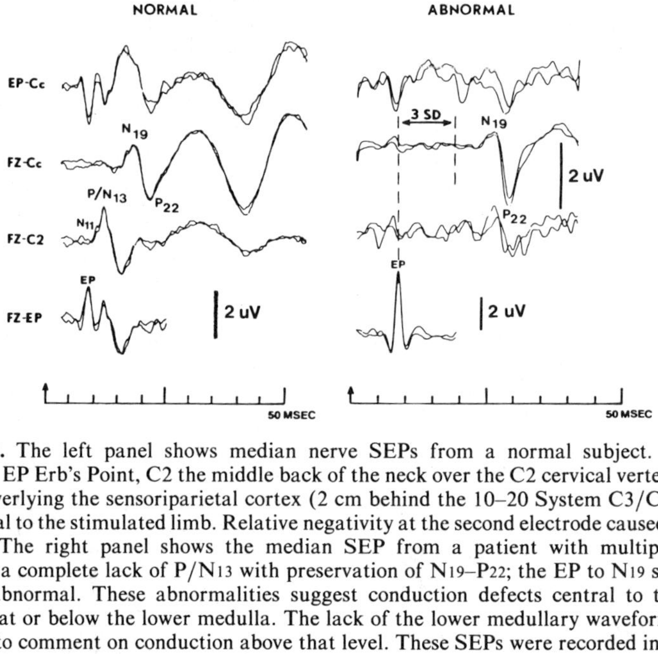

FIGURE 3. The left panel shows median nerve SEPs from a normal subject. Fz denotes midfrontal, EP Erb's Point, C2 the middle back of the neck over the C2 cervical vertebra, and Cc the scalp overlying the sensoriparietal cortex (2 cm behind the 10–20 System C3/C4 positions) contralateral to the stimulated limb. Relative negativity at the second electrode caused an upward deflection. The right panel shows the median SEP from a patient with multiple sclerosis, illustrating a complete lack of P/N13 with preservation of N19–P22; the EP to N19 separation is markedly abnormal. These abnormalities suggest conduction defects central to the brachial plexus and at or below the lower medulla. The lack of the lower medullary waveforms makes it impossible to comment on conduction above that level. These SEPs were recorded in response to unilateral stimulation at the wrist at 5/s. (Reprinted, with permission, from ref. 44.)

differentiate the possible causes of the conduction delay. In demyelinating disease, SEPs are potentially useful in the same three ways as noted above for BAEPs.

There have been a large number of studies of SEPs in patients with MS (see ref. 7). Of 1000 patients with varying classifications of MS reported in the literature, 58% had abnormal median/digital SEPs and 76% had abnormal peroneal/tibial SEPs. In patients classified as definite, probable or possible MS the average abnormality rates were 77%, 67% and 49%, respectively.

Although the effect of stimulus rate has been studied in normals, there has been no study of rate effects in patients with MS. In published studies on the relationship between clinical sensory findings and SEPs in patients with MS, 42% (249/598) of patients reported to have no symptoms or signs referrable to the sensory system had abnormal SEPs whereas 75% (250/335) of patients with sensory system symptoms and/or signs had abnormal SEPs (both upper and lower limbs included). Note that there is a higher incidence of clinically silent SEP abnormalities found on testing the lower limbs (as compared with the upper limbs).

Data from a group of 114 MS patients seen in our laboratory exemplify the findings that can be expected when using SEPs to test patients with (or suspected of having) MS. Twenty-nine percent of the patients had completely normal tests (both upper and lower limb). Upper limb SEPs were abnormal in 54% of patients, lower limb SEPs in 64%. In 18% of the patients, upper limb SEPs were normal when lower limb SEPs were abnormal, whereas the converse was true in 7%. Only 2% of patients had bilaterally abnormal upper limb and bilaterally normal lower limb SEPs, but the reverse was found in 11% of the patients. Thirty-seven percent of normal upper limb SEPs were associated with abnormal lower limb SEPs on the same side, whereas only 12% of normal lower limb SEPs were associated with abnormal upper limb SEPs ipsilaterally. Some of the conclusions that may be drawn from these results are: (1) when lower limb testing is normal, upper limb testing will reveal abnormalities in an additional, although small, group of patients, (2) SEP abnormalities in one limb (upper or lower) are not necessarily associated with SEP abnormalities in the other limb on the same side, although lower limb abnormalities will be more commonly associated with upper limb abnormalities than *vice versa*. Others have had similar results, the yield of abnormalities being greater with lower limb stimulation.[36–38]

Patients with suspected MS have been tested and the finding that all EPs were normal, except for SEPs pointing to an upper cervical cord conduction defect, has prompted a myelogram that revealed significant cervical cord compression from spondylotic bars; some of these patients have improved with surgical decompression. Conversely, of course, multiple EP abnormalities do not necessarily indicate MS (see Fig. 7-20 in ref. 7 for a patient who had multiple EP abnormalities caused by multiple meningiomas).

Although every conceivable abnormality is seen in the SEPs of the MS patients, the most interesting is the absence of P/N13 (lower medullary component) with preservation of N19–P23 (thalamus cortex) and a normal brachial plexus to N19 separation. The pathophysiology of such a finding and how it relates to the generation of the SEP waveforms are matters of pure speculation. In our group of patients,[7] 30% of the abnormalities were unilateral and 70% were bilateral, an incidence quite similar to the average in the literature. Of the bilateral abnormalities, 79% were identical and 21% were different on the two sides.

Matthews *et al.*[33] followed for 38 months after SEP testing 84 patients in whom the diagnosis of MS was under consideration. In only three of these patients did an abnormal SEP at initial presentation subsequently prove to be of diagnostic value, in that it revealed a separate, clinically silent lesion, indicating multifocal disease (and the patient on follow-up proved to have MS).

Ropper *et al.*[20] studied EP abnormalities in 12 consecutive patients with inflammatory acute transverse myelopathy (ATM) as their first neurological illness. All nine patients tested with median SEPs had normal findings, the lesions being below cervical levels mediating that response. Five of six patients tested with peroneal SEPs had abnormal findings (the sixth was tested eight months after onset when there was no residual neurological deficit). All of these patients had normal PSVEPs and BAEPs and none developed new neurological signs during 18 months mean follow-up. The authors felt that the lack of other lesions by EP testing and the failure to develop new clinical lesions indicates that ATM, when defined as a virtually or totally complete transverse inflammatory lesion of the cord, is a different process from MS.

Attempts have been made to use SEPs—and other EPs—to gauge the effectiveness of plasmapheresis therapy in MS but only a few patients have been studied so far and it is not yet possible to draw conclusions.[39,40]

Effects on SEPs of raising body temperature in patients with MS have been studied by Matthews *et al.*[41] and Kazis *et al.*[42] The former authors used intercurrent extra-CNS infection (viral or bacterial) as the hyperthermic agents and the effect of toxins cannot be discounted as the cause of the observed SEP changes. Matthews *et al.*[41] used external heat to raise the body temperature of their subjects and found that P/N13 amplitude was markedly diminished by the temperature increase.

COMBINED EVOKED POTENTIAL STUDIES

The comparative utility of PSVEPs, BAEPs and SEPs has been studied in groups of patients.[8,13,22,23,33,37,38,43] As might be postulated on the basis of length of white matter tracts involved, the order of relative utility of the tests in revealing evidence of clinically unsuspected lesions was SEP, PSVEP and BAEP. These data suggest that there is not a specific differential susceptibility to demyelination in the systems involved in the tests. Rather it is the length and amount of white matter tracts being tested that determine the likelihood of detection of a lesion in a given system.

REFERENCES

1. Brooks, E. B. & K. H. Chiappa. 1982. A comparison of clinical neuro-ophthalmological findings and pattern shift visual evoked potentials in multiple sclerosis. *In* Clinical Applications of Evoked Potentials in Neurology. J. J. Courjon, F. Mauguiere & M. Revol, Eds.: 435–437. Raven Press. New York.
2. Patterson, V. H. & J. R. Heron. 1980. Visual field abnormalities in multiple sclerosis. J. Neurol. Neurosurg. Psychiatr. **43:** 205–208.
3. Meienberg, O., J. Flammer & H. P. Ludin. 1982. Subclinical visual field defects in multiple sclerosis. J. Neurol. **227:** 125–133.
4. van Buggenhout, E., P. Ketelaer & H. Carton. Success and failure of evoked potentials in detecting clinical and subclinical lesions in multiple sclerosis patients. Clin. Neurol. Neurosurg. **84:** 3–14.
5. Shahrokhi, F., K. H. Chiappa & R. R. Young. 1978. Pattern shift visual evoked responses: Two hundred patients with optic neuritis and/or multiple sclerosis. Arch. Neurol. **35:** 65–71.
6. Halliday, A. M., W. I. McDonald & J. Mushin. 1973. Visual evoked responses in the diagnosis of multiple sclerosis. Br. Med. J. **4:** 661–664.
7. Chiappa, K. H. 1983. Evoked Potentials in Clinical Medicine. Raven Press. New York.
8. Tackmann, W., Th. Ettlin & H. Strenge. Multimodality evoked potentials and electrically elicited blink reflex in optic neuritis. J. Neurol. **227:** 157–163.
9. Halliday, A. M. & W. I. McDonald. 1981. Visual evoked potentials. *In* Neurology I: Clinical Neurophysiology. E. Stalberg & R. R. Young, Eds.: 228–258. Butterworths. London.
10. Lumsden, C. E. 1970. The neuropathology of multiple sclerosis. *In* Handbook of Clinical Neurophysiology, vol. 9. North-Holland. Amsterdam. pp. 175–234.
11. McAlpine, D., C. E. Lumsden & E. D. Acheson, Eds. 1972. Multiple Sclerosis: A Reappraisal. Churchill Livingstone. Edinburgh.
12. Hoeppner, T. & F. Lolas. 1978. Visual evoked responses and visual symptoms in multiple sclerosis. J. Neurol. Neurosurg. Psychiatr. **41:** 493–498.
13. Purves, S. J., M. D. Low, J. Galloway & B. Reeves. 1981. A comparison of visual,

brainstem auditory, and somatosensory evoked potentials in multiple sclerosis. Can. J. Neurol. Sci. **8:** 15–19.

14. CANT, B. R., A. L. HUME & N. A. SHAW. 1978. Effects of luminance on the pattern visual evoked potential in multiple sclerosis. Electroencephalogr. Clin. Neurophysiol. **45:** 496–504.
15. SWART, S. & P. MILLAC. 1980. A comparison of flight of colours with visually evoked responses in patients with multiple sclerosis. J. Neurol. Neurosurg. Psychiatr. **43:** 550–551.
16. CAMISA, J., I. BODIS-WOLLNER & L. MYLIN. 1980. Luminance-dependent pattern VEP delay in human demyelinating disease. Soc. Neurosci. Abstr. **6:** 596.
17. DIENER, H. CH., W. KOCH & J. DICHGONS. 1982. The significance of luminance on visual evoked potentials in diagnosis of MS. Arch. Psychiatr. Nervenkr. **231:** 149–154.
18. HENNERICI, M. & E. R. WIST. 1982. A modification of the visual evoked response method involving small luminance decrements for the diagnosis of demyelinating disease. *In* Clinical Applications of Evoked Potentials in Neurology. J. Courjon, F. Mauguiere & M. Revol, Eds.: 433–441. Raven Press. New York.
19. BLUMHARDT, L. D., G. BARRETT & A. M. HALLIDAY. 1982. The pattern visual evoked potential in the clinical assessment of undiagnosed spinal cord disease. *In* Clinical Applications of Evoked Potentials in Neurology. J. Courjon, F. Mauguiere & M. Revol, Eds.: 463–471. Raven Press. New York.
20. ROPPER, A. M., T. MIETT & K. H. CHIAPPA. 1982. Absence of evoked potential abnormalities in acute transverse myelopathy. Neurology **32:** 80–82.
21. BYNKE, H., J. E. OLSSON & I. ROSEN. 1977. Diagnostic value of visual evoked response, clinical eye examination and CSF analysis in chronic myelopathy. Acta Neurol. Scand. **56:** 55–69.
22. MASTAGLIA, F. L., J. L. BLACK & D. W. K. COLLINS. 1976. Visual and spinal evoked potentials in the diagnosis of multiple sclerosis. Br. Med. J. **2:** 732.
23. CHIAPPA, K. H., J. L. HARRISON, E. B. BROOKS & R. R. YOUNG. 1980. Brainstem auditory evoked responses in 200 patients with multiple sclerosis. Ann. Neurol. **7:** 135–143.
24. ROBINSON, K. & P. RUDGE. 1980. The use of the auditory evoked potential in the diagnosis of multiple sclerosis. J. Neurol. Sci. **45:** 235–244.
25. STOCKARD, J. J. & V. S. ROSSITER. 1977. Clinical and pathologic correlates of brain stem auditory response abnormalities. Neurology **27:** 316–325.
26. ROBINSON, K. & P. RUDGE. 1977. Abnormalities of the auditory evoked potentials in patients with multiple sclerosis. Brain **100:** 19–40.
27. ELIDAN, J., H. SOHMER, M. GAFNI & E. KAHANA. 1982. Contribution of changes in click rate and intensity on diagnosis of multiple sclerosis by brainstem auditory evoked potentials. Acta Neurol. Scand. **65:** 570–585.
28. EMERSON, R. G., E. B. BROOKS, S. W. PARKER & K. H. CHIAPPA. 1982. Effects of click polarity on brainstem auditory evoked potentials in normal subjects and patients: Unexpected sensitivity of wave V. Ann. N.Y. Acad. Sci. **388:** 710–721.
29. LEZAK, R. J. & B. SELHUB. 1966. On hearing in multiple sclerosis. Ann. Otol. Rhinol. Laryngol. 1102–1110.
30. NOFFSINGER, D., W. OLSEN, R. CARHART, C. W. HART & V. SAHGAL. 1972. Auditory and vestibular aberrations in multiple sclerosis. Acta Otolaryngol. Suppl. (Stockholm) **303:** 4–63.
31. HAUSLER, R. & R. A. LEVINE. 1980. Brain stem auditory evoked potentials are related to interaural time discrimination in patients with multiple sclerosis. Brain Res. **191:** 589–594.
32. LEDERMAN, R. J., R. H. NODAR, J. P. CONOMY & W. T. DAUGHERTY. 1978. Hearing loss in multiple sclerosis. Neurology **28:** 406.
33. MATTHEWS, W. B., J. R. B. WATTAM-BELL & E. POUNTNEY. 1982. Evoked potentials in the diagnosis of multiple sclerosis. J. Neurol. Neurosurg. Psychiatr. **45:** 303–307.
34. COGAN, D. G. & S. H. WRAY. 1970. Internuclear ophthalmoplegia as an early sign of brainstem tumors. Neurology **20:** 629–633.
35. KJAER, M. 1980. Variations of brain stem auditory evoked potentials correlated to duration and severity of multiple sclerosis. Acta Neurol. Scand. **61:** 157–166.

36. EISEN, A. & K. ODUSOTE. 1980. Central and peripheral conduction times in multiple sclerosis. Electroencephalogr. Clin. Neurophysiol. **48:** 253–265.
37. KHOSHBIN, S. & M. HALLETT. 1981. Multimodality evoked potentials and blink reflex in multiple sclerosis. Neurology **31:** 138–144.
38. TROJABORG, W. & E. PETERSEN. 1979. Visual and somatosensory evoked cortical potentials in multiple sclerosis. J. Neurol. Neurosurg. Psychiatr. **42:** 323–330.
39. DAU, P. C., J. H. PETAJAN, K. P. JOHNSON, H. S. PANITCH & M. B. BORNSTEIN. 1980. Plasmapheresis in multiple sclerosis: Preliminary findings. Neurology **30:** 1023–1028.
40. WEINER, H. L. & D. M. DAWSON. 1980. Plasmapheresis in multiple sclerosis: A preliminary study. Neurology **30:** 1029–1033.
41. MATTHEWS, W. B., D. J. READ & E. POUNTNEY. 1979. Effect of raising body temperature on visual and somatosensory evoked potentials in patients with multiple sclerosis. J. Neurol. Neurosurg. Psychiatr. **42:** 250–255.
42. KAZIS, A., N. VLAIKIDIS, D. XAFENIOS, J. PAPANASTASIOU & P. PAPPA. 1982. Fever and evoked potentials in multiple sclerosis. J. Neurol. **227:** 1–10.
43. GREEN, J. B., R. PRICE & S. G. WOODBURY. 1980. Short-latency somatosensory evoked potentials in multiple sclerosis. Comparison with auditory and visual evoked potentials. Arch. Neurol. **37:** 630–633.
44. CHIAPPA, K. H. & A. H. ROPPER. 1982. Evoked potentials in clinical medicine. N. Eng. J. Med. **306:** 1140–1150, 1205–1211.

DISCUSSION OF THE PAPER

I. MCDONALD (*National Hospital, London, England*): Well thank you very much, that was a very good note to end on. Now, questions, comments?

J. FOLEY (*University Hospital, Cleveland, OH*): I don't want to be difficult but I'd like to ask Dr. Drayer and Dr. Chiappa both, what is the cost of such a procedure, and how do you prevent the utilization of these expensive resources by house staff and indeed by physicians when they're not necessary?

Finally if you used it only when you absolutely needed it for diagnosis, treatment or prognosis could you keep your laboratory going?

K. CHIAPPA (*Harvard Medical School, Boston, MA*): I'd like to take the last point first. There have been in some publications (*e.g.*, recently the *New England Journal of Medicine* and *Neurology*) similar statements based on no data, erroneous data or irrelevant data. As far as I know I have the only data on this topic.

I took all of the patients who were tested in our laboratory in the month of March, and went back over their medical records and assessed whether or not the test was indicated and what the disease was. And if you disagree with my data I'd be happy to have you come and do the same thing. What I found was that 40% of patients in our laboratory were tested because of a question of demyelinating disease. So to take care of your third question, the lab wouldn't shut down if we never saw a patient because of a question of demyelinating disease. As far as utilization is concerned, I think that study also answered that question. In the total group of patients, the test was clinically not indicated for about 10%, which is about the same as most laboratory tests. As far as cost is concerned, that varies a great deal in different areas of the country. In our region that runs about $100 per test.

MCDONALD: Dr. Drayer.

B. DRAYER (*Duke University Medical Center, Durham, NC*): I guess I should answer cost first because our techniques are certainly more expensive, we're talking the 500 to 700 dollar range. I think cost has two aspects and I think in both aspects neuroimaging and CT, and I think NMR, are going to do very, very well. The first aspect is dollars and cents, how much does it cost? And I think there's no question that if you can increase the number of outpatients that will be done on these types of tools and decrease hospital admissions you're going to save money. Nuclear magnetic resonance is the perfect example of the ideal outpatient procedure. It uses no contrast materials. In the NMR particularly, there's no radiation, there's not the risk of contrast material and it's a very useful diagnostic tool. We all forget so fast about doing pneumoencephalograms, and angiograms. What's the cost to the patient of not having to do a pneumoencephalogram. So it's my feeling that number one, in dollars and cents it's cost effective, and number two, to the patient themselves it's extremely cost effective.

McDONALD: Yes.

P. TSAIRIS (*Cornell University*): I'd like to ask Dr. Chiappa whether or not he feels the evoked potential studies are useful in following patients who are treated for multiple sclerosis, specifically those who have received plasma pharesis or lymphocyte pharesis because I think you've discussed this in the literature and said that they do improve sometimes, and whether or not you think it's worthwhile doing it and secondly, what do you think the mechanism of that is? Speculatively.

CHIAPPA: I don't think I can really give you the answer. You can certainly see changes and obviously they are not going to follow the clinical symptomatology perfectly; that data is just being gathered and I don't have the answer.

McDONALD: Yes, one more question.

A. BLITZKEY: My question is related to your last comment on the specificity of the etiology. I know in the context of brainstem auditory responses you had reasonably specific levels of generators. With regard to the visual evoked response I'd like to know how you can eliminate the contributions of the retinal component, particularly with NMS and along the same lines, where specifically in the visual pathway do you see this pattern response coming from? Is it possible to emphasize that it's strictly the optic nerve?

CHIAPPA: I think with the monocular abnormalities the lesion is somewhere anterior to the chiasm. When one is faced with that pattern of abnormalities, although you know that the conduction defect is anterior to the chiasm, it can be any lesion anterior to the chiasm and it's then necessary to utilize one's clinical skills in deciding how much further one has to go to rule out the other possible diseases that could involve the retina, or be a compressive lesion on the optic nerve. So that one might simply take the history and look at the retina through an ophthalmoscope and if all that looked perfectly normal that might be enough. If there are still some suspicious elements then one might want to go on to an electroretinogram or ophthalmological consultation or whatever.

Multiple Sclerosis Bladder

Studies and Care

JERRY G. BLAIVAS,[a] NANCY J. HOLLAND,[b]
BARBARA GIESSER,[b] NICHOLAS LAROCCA,[b]
MICHELE MADONNA,[b] AND LABE SCHEINBERG[b]

[a]*Department of Urology*
Columbia Presbyterian Medical Center
New York, New York 10032

[b]*Department of Neurology*
Albert Einstein College of Medicine
Bronx, New York 10461

INTRODUCTION

Symptomatic bladder dysfunction occurs at some time during the course of multiple sclerosis (MS) in 50–80% of patients.[1–10] Approximately 10% of patients have bladder dysfunction as part of the initial presentation with 2% having it as the sole first complaint.[9] In addition to the high incidence of urinary symptoms, attention is warranted because of the severe handicap from incontinence, and the increased morbidity and shortened life expectency resulting from urinary complications.[11]

The diagnosis of "clinically definite multiple sclerosis" is based on the history of two attacks and clinical evidence of two distinct lesions involving central myelin. In the absence of signs of two distinct lesions, laboratory tests, *e.g.*, pattern-shift evoked response or neuroimaging may substitute for one lesion and the diagnosis is then "laboratory supported definite multiple sclerosis." If there is history of only one episode or evidence of only one lesion, the diagnosis is "probable multiple sclerosis."[12] The high prevalence of bladder symptoms from a variety of causes in the general population necessitates a firm diagnosis of MS before attributing any findings to this disease. Since urinary tract infection (UTI) is the commonest cause of urinary bladder symptoms, it must be excluded by urinalysis and appropriate cultures before subjecting any patient, including one with MS, to more sophisticated urologic procedures.

SYMPTOM ANALYSIS

Urinary bladder symptoms are usually described as being either irritative or obstructive in nature. However, we find it more practical to consider symptoms as being related to either problems with the storage of urine or problems related to bladder emptying.[4,10] Irritative symptoms, *e.g.*, frequency, urgency, urge-incontinence, and dysuria are generally associated with storage problems, and obstructive symptoms, *e.g.*, hesitancy, diminished size and force of stream, "double voiding," postvoid dribbling, and postvoid feeling of fullness with emptying problems. Storage symptoms are often associated with detrusor hyperactivity or sphincter insufficency whereas emptying symptoms are usually associated with either a poor detrusor contraction or bladder outlet obstruction.

In many cases the function of the detrusor and external sphincter are dyssynergic so that as the detrusor contracts, the sphincter also contracts. This is called detrusor-external sphincter dyssynergia (DESD) and the symptomatology may mimic both failure-to-store and failure-to-empty dysfunctions.

The relationship between MS urinary symptoms and the underlying pathophysiology is inexact.[4,5,13] In these series, treatment based on history and physical examination alone was ineffective in over 50% of patients. Because of this disparity we believe that persistent symptoms (in an uninfected patient) should serve to alert the physician to the need for further studies.

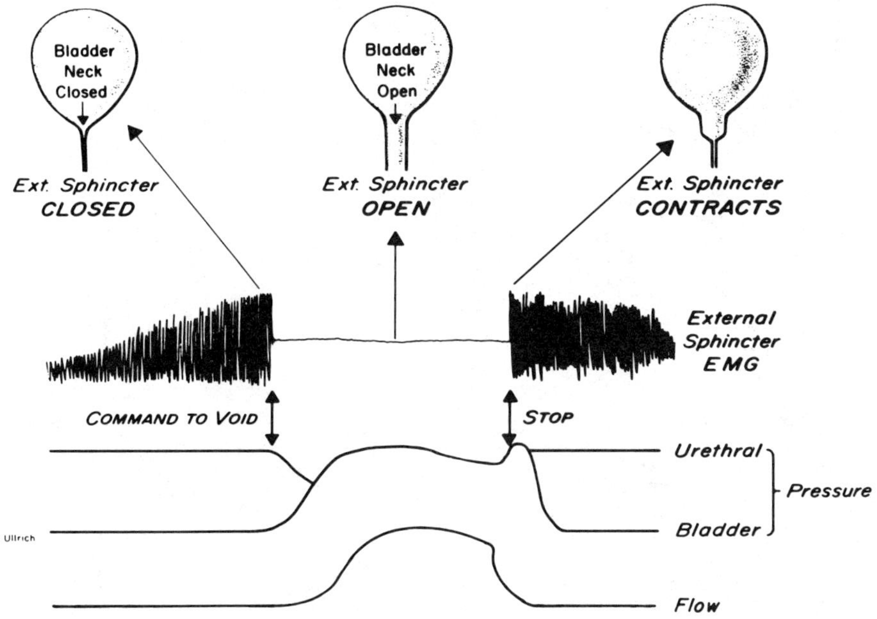

FIGURE 1. Basic bladder evaluation and management.

VESICOURETHRAL PHYSIOLOGY

The bladder and its sphincter function is a single physiologic unit whose main purpose is the storage and timely expulsion of urine (FIG. 1). It is generally agreed that the primary continence mechanism in both sexes is the smooth muscle of the vesicle neck and proximal urethra. The urinary stream can be voluntarily interrupted by contracting the striated periurethral musculature or "external sphincter," but this muscle plays only an ancillary role in serving preserving continence and, when the proximal smooth muscle is deficient, the external sphincter is incapable of maintaining continence.

During the last decade there has been a major change in our understanding of vesicourethral innervation. It had been previously taught that the "micturition center" was located in the sacral spinal cord and that suprasacral pathways were necessary only to provide voluntary control of the micturition reflex. It is now well documented both in the cat and in humans that the micturition reflex is integrated not in the sacral cord, but in the rostral brain stem. What follows is a summary of the available data about vesicourethral innervation (FIG. 2).

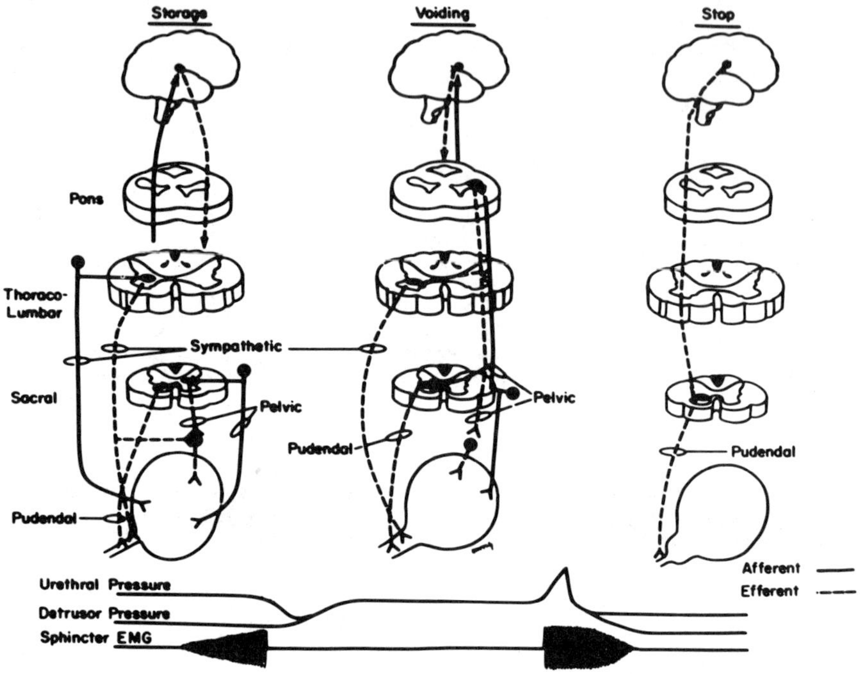

FIGURE 2. Summary of major neurologic pathways involved in voiding. *Storage:* bladder distension results in afferent pelvic nerve discharge. After synapse in pudendal nucleus efferent pudendal nerve impulses result in contraction of external urethral sphincter. At same time afferent sympathetic discharges traverse hypogastric nerve. After synapse in sympathetic nuclei efferent firing causes (1) inhibition of transmission at postganglionic parasympathetic neuron, which inhibits detrusor contraction, and (2) increased tone at bladder neck. Net effect is that urethral pressure remains greater than detrusor pressure, facilitating urine storage. *Voiding:* afferent pelvic nerve discharges ascend in spinal cord and synapse in pontine micturition center. Descending efferent pathways cause (1) inhibition of pudendal firing, which relaxes external sphincter, (2) inhibition of sympathetic firing, which opens bladder neck and permits postganglionic parasympathetic transmission, and (3) pelvic parasympathetic firing, which causes detrusor contraction. Net result is that relaxation of external sphincter causes decrease in urethral pressure followed almost immediately by detrusor contraction and voiding ensues. *Stop:* voluntary interruption of urinary stream. Descending corticospinal pathways emanating from motor cortex synapse in pudendal nucleus, resulting in contraction of external urethral sphincter. Urethral pressure increases above detrusor pressure, interrupting stream.

Voiding Pathways

As mentioned above, the micturition reflex is not a simple sacral cord reflex, but rather, it is integrated in the rostral brain stem, probably in the pontine mesencephalic reticular formation in an area designated as the pontine micturition center (PMC).[14–18] During bladder filling afferent pelvic parasympathetic impulses ascend in the lateral white matter of the spinal cord and synapse in the PMC.[19] Descending pathways from the PMC synapse with neurons of the hypogastric (sympathetic), pelvic (parasympathetic) and pudendal (somatic) nuclei.[17,22] These integrated neurologic events result in a micturition reflex—relaxation of the external urethral sphincter, a fall in urethral pressure, a rise in detrusor pressure, opening of the vesical neck and coordinated micturition (see FIG. 1).[14] This reflex may be initiated or abolished at will. Neurologic lesions that interrupt the neural connections between the PMC and the "sacral micturition center" result in detrusor-external sphincter dyssynergia, a condition in which there is involuntary contraction of the external urethral sphincter during the detrusor contraction. These patients are obstructed because of the sphincter contraction, yet incontinent because of the involuntary detrusor contraction.[14,23]

The "sacral micturition center" is located in the second through fourth segments of the sacral spinal cord and consists of the pelvic and pudendal reflex arcs.[18,24] The pelvic nerve is the major motor nerve to the bladder. Stimulation of the efferent pelvic nerve results in detrusor contraction. The pudendal nerve is the major motor and sensory nerve to the striated external urethral sphincter. Stimulation of these efferent fibers results in contraction of the external urethral sphincter. Neurologic lesions of the sacral spinal cord or its roots result in detrusor areflexia and urinary retention.

Storage Pathways

There are four major storage pathways—suprapontine, fronto-pudendal, sympathetic and pelvic-pudendal (FIG. 2).[14,16–18]

Suprapontine pathways emanate from many poorly described regions of the brain—frontal cortex, thalamus, hypothalamus, basal ganglia, limbic system, cerebellum and other parts of the central nervous system. The net result of all of these pathways is modulation and voluntary control of the micturition reflex. Corticospinal connections between the motor cortex and the pudendal nucleus permit voluntary control of the external urethral sphincter.[14,16–18] Interruption of these neural pathways releases the micturition reflex from voluntary control.

The role of the sympathetic nervous system continues to be a controversial subject.[16,20,21,25–29] What follows is what we believe to be the most reasonable interpretation of the available data. During bladder filling sympathetic receptors in the bladder wall send afferent discharges via the hypogastric nerve to the sympathetic neurons in the thoracolumbar portion of spinal cord. Efferent sympathetic firing has two important effects. Firstly, via an alpha-mediated receptor, tonic contraction of the smooth muscle of the proximal urethra is maintained. Secondly, via another alpha receptor, there is inhibition of transmission of excitatory impulses from the preganglionic to the postganglionic parasympathetic neuron. The net result of the sympathetic stimulation is promotion of continence by helping to keep the vesical neck closed and by inhibiting parasympathetic stimulation of the detrusor. However, from a clinical standpoint, neurologic lesions that interfere with sympathetic pathways generally result in sphincteric incontinence.

The major storage pathway centered in the sacral cord is a pelvic-pudendal reflex. During bladder filling afferent pelvic nerve stimuli (probably via an interneuron) cause increased efferent activity in the pudendal nerve which causes the external sphincter to increase its tone.

INITIAL BLADDER MANAGEMENT

The goals of initial treatment are: (1) the control of micturition by means of medication or techniques, such as intermittent catheterization (IC); (2) the relief of bladder symptoms; (3) the prevention of urinary tract infection; (4) the elimination of risk factors for subsequent urinary complications.

After routine neurological evaluation, the diagnosis of the underlying bladder dysfunction is accomplished in most cases by a combination of bladder, bowel, and sexual history, voided and residual urine determinations and cystometric/uroflow estimation. Bladder history includes previous symptoms, frequency of UTI, urodiagnostic and surgical procedures, and previous medical management. Current symptoms are also identified, as well as medical and self-management measures such as restricted fluid intake. Bladder capacity and residual urine volumes are obtained by postvoid urethral catheterization in well-hydrated patients, who void when the urge to urinate is experienced. The voided amount, plus the postvoid volume, provide an estimation of bladder capacity. Following residual measurement, normal saline is instilled in the bladder through a 50 ml catheter-tipped syringe (barrel removed) until the desire to urinate occurs. An involuntary rise of fluid in the syringe suggests uninhibited detrusor contractions. The catheter is then removed and the patient voids into a commode or urinal, while flow is directly observed and timed. When visualization is inhibiting for the patient, timing without observing will suffice. The Einstein MS Center utilizes the following values in defining parameters which guide management decisions:

1. Normal capacity range: 350 to 500 ml.[30]
2. Low residual: under 100 ml.
3. High residual: over 100 ml.[31]
4. Capacity needed for adequate uroflow determination: 200 ml.

Intravenous urogram (IVP) and other evaluations of upper tract status are reserved for those patients with long-standing bladder dysfunction, persistent symptoms despite adequate therapy, recurrent UTIs, or risk factors. These studies are not routinely performed since significant urinary tract deterioration is uncommon in MS.[1]

A minimally invasive screening method for assessing bladder capacity, postvoiding residual, renal size and perfusion is the radioisotope renal function/residual urine scan.[32] This procedure gives very accurate total bladder capacity and residual urine volume and useful information about kidney size and perfusion. It may be performed in any nuclear medicine facility and requires no preparation except adequate hydration. Its major shortcoming is the failure to detect bladder stones, but otherwise is a rapid, minimally invasive and useful procedure for renal tract evaluation.

Prior to classifying the patient as having a storage or emptying problem, there are several considerations. Urinary tract infection must be tested for and treated, if present. There should be screening for non-neurogenic factors such as stress incontinence, iatrogenic features such as the use of diuretics and functional components such as difficulty in reaching the toilet or transferring to the commode.[33] Once these problems have been ruled out or treated, diagnosis and management of neurogenic dysfunction can proceed.

MS CENTER MANAGEMENT

In a simplified format, the MS Center's treatment protocol is as follows:

1. Storage (failure-to-store) problem: anticholinergic medication.
2. Emptying (failure-to-empty) problem: intermittent catheterization (IC).
3. Combined problem (detrusor-external sphincter dyssynergia): IC and anticholinergic medication.

Failure to store urine usually results from involuntary bladder contractions that signify detrusor hyperreflexia.[4,34] Therefore, management utilizing anticholinergic therapy is aimed at reducing this phenomenon which causes varying degrees of urgency, frequency and incontinence. Once satisfactory symptom relief is attained, periodic check of capacity/residual volumes is necessary to assure that iatrogenic urinary retention does not occur.

Emptying problems most commonly result from impaired detrusor contractions, detrusor-external sphincter dyssynergia, or, less commonly, from bladder outlet obstruction. Diminished detrusor activity sometimes may result from prolonged bladder distention, rather than being a primary neurologic deficit.[35] It is also recognized that absent detrusor contractions in the testing situation may represent psychic inhibition. Approximately fifty percent of normal women and five percent of normal men do not demonstrate detrusor contractions under these circumstances.[36] Regardless of speculated neuropathological components, management interventions are aimed at eliminating urinary retention. Aseptic or "clean" IC has been widely proposed and employed for this purpose[31,34,37] and is the primary treatment utilized at the MS Center for emptying problems. The procedure is clean rather than sterile, and no. 14 French clear plastic catheters are recommended for both males and females.[37] Females are instructed to locate the urinary meatus using a mirror prior to initial attempts at self-catheterization, but are discouraged from continued use of the mirror. The procedure is more easily accomplished by the woman seated on toilet or commode, with a technique similar to tampon insertion. Males generally have little technical difficulty, but may need to overcome initial psychological resistance. When the patient is unable to catheterize him/herself because of incoordination, weakness or other MS impairment, a family member or other caretaker may assume this task. It is surprising that patients are able to catheterize themselves despite severe upper extremity incoordination by stabilizing the forearm or hand on the thigh during self-catheriza-tion. The protocol followed at the Einstein MS Center for urinary antisepsis during IC includes ascorbic acid, four grams per day and methenamine hippurate, two grams per day, both in divided doses. Methenamine mandelate may be substituted for methena-mine hippurate, but twice as much is required.[31,38] This regimen is based upon the impression that results of IC are better when urinary antiseptics are used.[31] Urinary acidification is also prophylactic against calcium calculi.[39] Stone formation secondary to hypercalcuria is a particular problem for less mobile patients who tend to develop demineralization of bone.[40] Additionally, a marked decrease in stone formation has been reported when IC rather than indwelling catheterization is employed.[39] When IC alone fails to relieve symptoms of urgency, frequency and incontinence between catheterizations (in the absence of UTI), combined dysfunction is suspected, with uninhibited detrusor contractions superimposed upon DESD or inadequate detrusor force. Addition of anticholinergic agents usually relieves persistent symptoms by reducing uninhibited detrusor contractions. Since bilateral plantar reflexes were predictive of DESD in 70% of patients studied urodynamically, this finding suggests the possibility of neurogenic obstruction and resultant failure-to-empty or combined dysfunction.[5]

Although some clinicians believe that urinary dysfunction in MS is progressive,[41] experience at thc Einstein MS Center militates against this. In failure-to-empty or combined dysfunction treated with IC, gradual reduction of residual volumes may lead to return of nearly normal urologic function.[35] Follow-up of patients with storage problems has demonstrated, for some, a resumption of normal volume parameters and absence of urinary symptoms. A progressive deterioration of urinary status should not, therefore, be a foregone conclusion. The fluctuation in MS bladder function, as with other MS impairments, necessitates periodic review of bladder status by assessment of

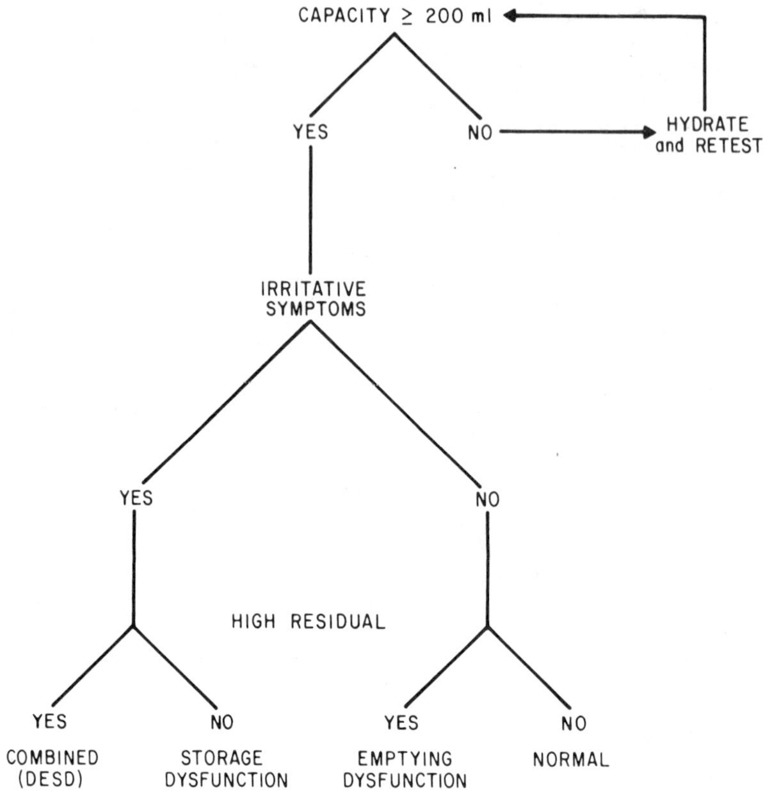

FIGURE 3. Algorithm for determination of types of bladder dysfunction in multiple sclerosis.

capacity/residual volumes and patient-reported clinical manifestations.[35] FIGURE 3 illustrates the formula for determination of the specific type of MS bladder dysfunction.

Specific Treatment Measures

For storage or combined dysfunction due to detrusor hyperreflexia, several anticholinergic or similar acting medications are employed, until the most effective drug or combination of drugs is identified. Individual response varies, and for the same patient, a successful regimen may diminish in effectiveness, requiring modification after several weeks or months. The drug of choice for detrusor hyperreflexia is propantheline, with dosages ranging from 7.5 mg to 105 mg four times per day needed to achieve symptom relief (J. Blaivas, personal communication). Dry mouth at the higher dosage is intolerable for some patients, necessitating a lower than optimal dosage. Constipation is generally a less bothersome side effect because of enhanced ability to tolerate adequate fluid intake, and pre-existing bowel programs practiced by many chronically constipated MS patients. However, for some patients, severe constipation may also necessitate reduced dosage. Combined anticholinergic and smooth muscle relaxants such as oxybutynin or dicyclomine are also useful.[42,43] The tricyclic antidepressant, imipramine, is another agent widely utilized at the MS Center for its anticholinergic effect on detrusor hyperreflexia.[43] Twenty-four-hour symptom relief has been achieved with single dose bedtime administration of 50 to 200 mg, and the primary antidepressant action is beneficial for appropriate patients. When mild anxiety is an additional patient complaint, Librax®, a combination of chlordiazepoxide and clidinium (anticholinergic/spasmolytic) has provided relief of both symptoms associated with detrusor hyperreflexia and manifestations of anxiety.

Mild emptying problems that are due to detrusor-external sphincter dyssynergia (residual lower than 100 ml) occasionally may respond to low dosage baclofen (15 mg per day). Most failure-to-empty situations require intermittent catheterization, with frequency dependent upon patient reports of capacity/residual, rate of infection,[40] and relief of urinary symptoms.

FIGURE 4 details the diagnostic methodology and management interventions.

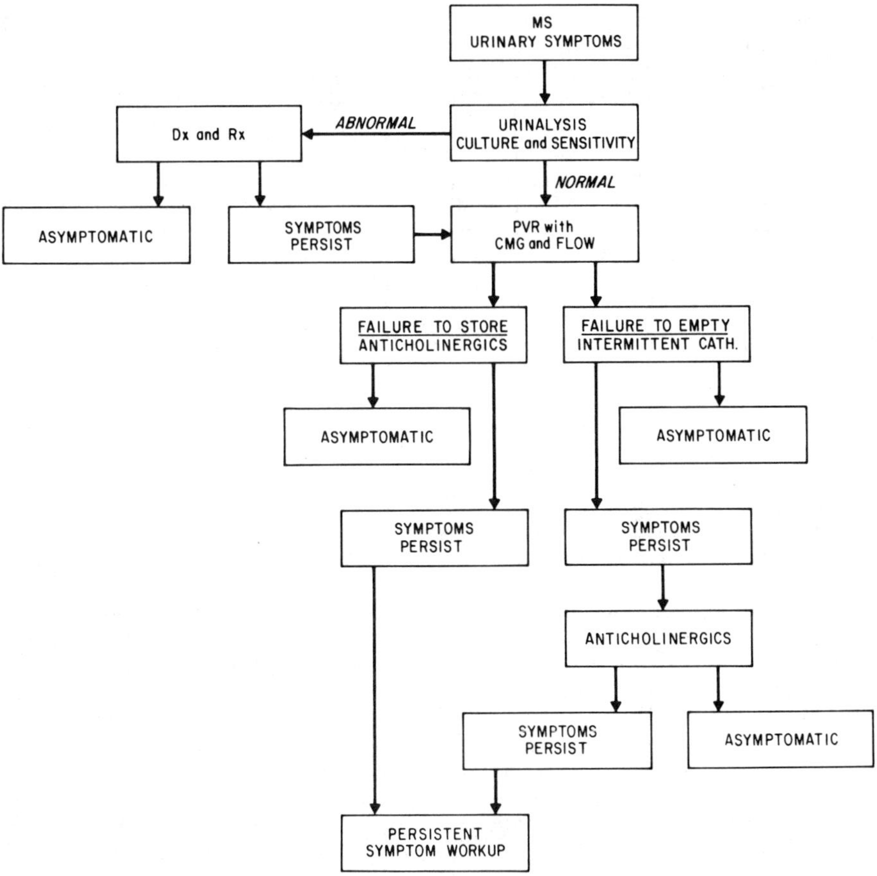

FIGURE 4. Algorithm for analysis of bladder symptoms.

For persistent urinary symptoms, or situations where upper tract involvement or other complications are suspected because of a history of pyelonephritis or urolithiasis, a more comprehensive workup is indicated. The following section elaborates on the specific methodology for such an evaluation.

Persistent Symptom Workup

Because of the relatively poor correlation between urinary bladder symptoms and underlying pathophysiology, it is necessary to perform physiologic tests of bladder and sphincteric function in order to define the etiology of the patient's symptoms.

Cystometry

Cystometry is the graphic representation of bladder pressure as a function of volume.[44] If one considers that the main goal of urodynamic investigation is to reproduce the patient's symptoms while physiologic observations and measurements are being obtained, the cystometric examination is the prototype. The technique of cystometry is straightforward. The patient voids, a catheter is placed in the bladder and postvoid residual urine is measured. Infusion of fluid is begun and during bladder filling the patient is instructed neither to try to void nor inhibit micturition, but to report his sensations to the examiner. Normally detrusor pressure remains almost constant during filling unless the fluid is infused very rapidly. The volume at the first sensation of bladder filling, first urge and severe urge to void are variable and serve as only a subjective guideline. If the patient experiences his usual symptoms, such as urgency, pain or incontinence, the physiologic measurements of pressure and volume serve as objective data to explain the etiology of the symptoms. Bladder capacity and the presence or absence of involuntary detrusor contractions are important objective parameters that enable a firm diagnosis to be made.

Sphincter Electromyography

When precise neurologic information is desired, sphincter electromyography should be performed with needle electrodes by an experienced electromyographer using oscilloscopic or audiographic control.

Electromyography of the external urethral sphincter should always be performed with simultaneous cystometry.[44–47] It has two main applications in urodynamic testing. Firstly, it can be used to detect whether the perineal floor muscles are contracting or relaxing at any given instant. Secondly, the integrity of these muscles and their nerve supply can be assessed. On the basis of standard electromyographic criteria, combined with clinical findings, the innervation of the external urethral sphincter (and by implication the bladder) may be classified as normal, upper motor neuron lesion, lower motor neuron lesion or mixed lesion.[45] It should be remembered, however, that the pelvic floor consists not only of the external urethral sphincter, but also of the bulbocavernosus muscle, the ischiocavernosus muscle, the external anal sphincter and the levator ani. In multiple sclerosis there may be a disparity between the EMG findings in these muscles.[3,48] For that reason multiple sampling sites may be necessary when diagnostic neurologic information is desired.

Voiding Cystourethrography

The radiographic visualization of the lower urinary tract during both storage and voiding is an extremely useful diagnostic procedure, especially when performed with fluoroscopic monitoring. Once bladder outlet obstruction has been diagnosed by urodynamic studies, the site and nature of the obstruction is usually apparent radiographically. The presence or absence of vesicoureteral reflux may be detected and the diagnosis of sympathetic decentralization may be suggested by the finding of an open vesical neck during bladder filling. There is usually a characteristic radiographic appearance to detrusor-external sphincter dyssynergia, prostatic obstruction and urethral strictures.

Combined Studies

For those patients who are unresponsive to conventional therapy, the simultaneous measurement of multiple urodynamic parameters offers the most reliable methodology for diagnosing their lower urinary tract condition. Synchronous video/pressure/flow/EMG studies are currently employed at only a handful of diagnostic centers throughout the world.[44,49] It is our opinion that the initial expense and extra personnel necessary to run such a diagnostic unit is well worth the investment of time, personnel and money, but this has not yet been widely accepted, especially in the United States.

Persistent Symptom Management

Although urologic symptoms respond to pharmacologic manipulation and/or intermittent catheterization in the majority of patients, there are complicating conditions that can cause management problems. In these cases, a more extensive workup as described above must be pursued.

Patients may continue to have frequency, urgency, nocturia and incontinence despite treatment, or these symptoms may appear acutely in patients who were previously urologically well controlled. The most common cause of this problem is an acute urinary tract infection (UTI). The most common organism is *E. coli*. Chronic or recurrent infections tend to be caused by *Klebsiella, Proteus* and *Pseudomonas* species.[39] In patients with recurrent symptoms of UTI with pyuria, or in whom a routine urine culture and sensitivity does not grow out an organism, urine should also be sent for special cultures for tuberculosis and occasionally for chlamydia or mycoplasma. Other sources of UTI may be vaginitis or prostatitis.

In patients who are symptomatic and infection-free, investigation must be undertaken to look for a structural lesion. Intravenous pyelography may reveal lesions such as calculi, abscess or tumor. Cystoscopy should be done to investigate intravesicular pathology, *e.g.*, tumor, calculi or diverticula. Sometimes, low-grade chronic bladder inflammation of indeterminate etiology is responsible for the patients' symptoms, and can be treated with a few weeks of high-dose steroids, (*e.g.*, Prednisone—60 mg/day) and then tapered to a low dose for several months. An alternate-day regimen helps avoid systemic complications. In those patients who continue to be symptomatic despite treatment, without obvious infectious or structural pathology, sophisticated urodynamics are indicated to determine further management.

Patients who continue to have recurrent UTI in the absence of demonstrable structural pathology should be placed on chronic urinary suppression. Any one of several antibiotics in low doses may be used; among those recommended is trimethoprim/sulfa methoxazole (one tablet/day).[50]

Women with persistent frequency or incontinence may be symptomatic because of uterine prolapse, or other pelvic/perineal pathology, and hesitancy, urgency and frequency in men may be caused by an enlarged prostate.

The MS Center has had experience with several patients whose primary urologic

TABLE 1. Treatment Guidelines for Patients with Persistent Symptoms (Surgical Procedures)

Treatment of Storage Disorders	Comment
Functional electrical stimulation[a]	experimental
Neural ablation[b]	sexual and sensory function lost
Destruction of nerve roots[c,d,e]	results inconsistent; danger of chemical arachnoiditis
Peripheral denervation of bladder	clinically unproved
Transvaginal denervation[f,g]	rarely used; 60% success reported
Detrusor transection[h,i]	60% success reported
Cystolysis[j]	favorable results reported; one-third of patients require IC
Urinary diversion	last option; long-term complications (30%)
Treatment of Emptying Disorders	
External sphincterotomy	gravitational incontinence; males require condom catheters
Transurethral resection of the bladder neck	further clinical studies needed
Treatment of Emptying and Storage Disorders	
External sphincterotomy	used only when conservative measures have failed

[a]Fall, M., B.E. Erlanson, A.E. Nilson & T. Sundin. 1978. Long term intravaginal electrical stimulation in urge and stress incontinence. Scand. J. Urol. Nephrol. Suppl. **44:** 55.

[b]McGuire, E.J., J.R. Woodside, T.A. Borden & R.M. Weiss. 1981. Prognostic value of urodynamic testing in myelodysplastic patients. J. Urol. **124:** 205.

[c]Manfredi, R.A. & J.F. Leal. 1968. Selective sacral rhizotomy for the spastic bladder syndrome in patients with spinal cord injuries. J. Urol. **100:** 17.

[d]Rockswold, G.L., C.N. Shelly & W.E. Bradley. 1978. Re-evaluation of differential sacral rhizotomy for neurological bladder disease. J. Neurosurg. **48:** 773–778.

[e]Torrens, N.J. 1974. The effect of selective sacral nerve blocks on vesical and urethral function. J. Urol. **112:** 204.

[f]Hodgkinson, C.P. & B.H. Drukker. 1977. Intravesical nerve resection for detrusor dyssynergia. Acta Obst. Gynecol. Scand. **56:** 401–408.

[g]Ingleman-Sundberg, A. 1959. Partial denervation of the bladder. A new operation for the treatment of urge incontinence and similar conditions in women. Acta Obst. Gynecol. Scand. **38:** 487.

[h]Hindmarsh, J.R., D.M. Essenhigh & W.K. Yates. 1977. Bladder transection for adult enuresis. Br. J. Urol. **49:** 515–521.

[i]Parsons, K.F., P.J. O'Boyle & N.O.K. Gibbon. 1977. A further assessment of bladder transection in the management of adult enuresis and allied conditions. Br. J. Urol. **49:** 509–514.

[j]Freiha, F.S. & T.A. Stamey. 1980. Cystolysis: A procedure for the selective denervation of the bladder. J. Urol. **123:** 360.

symptom is persistent nocturia resistant to all previously mentioned forms of treatment. These patients have responded well to a low dose of antidiuretic hormone (lypressin) taken intranasally at bedtime.

TABLE 1 outlines the surgical procedures that may need to be considered for those cases in which all conservative measures have failed.

Bladder Management for the Severely Disabled

MS patients with severe motor deficits tend to have severe bladder dysfunction as well. Unfortunately, these patients are generally unable to perform intermittent self-catheterization, and if there is no aide or family member available to do this, then continuous urinary drainage must be employed. Even when IC is feasible, it is sometimes insufficient to control severe incontinence, and alternative methods are used.

Indwelling Catheter. An indwelling urethral catheter is the simplest method of achieving continence and proper urinary drainage in the severely disabled patient. However, it carries with it the risk of several serious complications, including chronic infection, urethral stricture, calculus formation or urethrocutaneous fistula.[31] It has also been reported that patients on long-term indwelling catheterization have a 5–10% risk of developing squamous cell carcinoma.[40] A short-term indwelling catheter is useful in promoting healing of sacral or buttock decubiti in incontinent individuals.

Guidelines for indwelling catheter care include use of a moderate size catheter, which is connected to a closed system drainage bag. The catheter tubing and urinary meatus should be cleansed daily with antiseptic solution.[31] The catheter should be irrigated periodically to prevent clot or stone formation; use of continuous bladder irrigation is not recommended. Some authors advocate changing the catheter on a weekly basis but usually 2–4 week intervals are adequate.[38] Acidification of the urine with ascorbic acid and antisepsis with methenamine hippurate may help to prevent urine infection.

Condom Catheter. In male patients without obstruction, an external drainage device, the condom catheter, is often an acceptable solution. The main disadvantages are leakage and the potential for penile ulceration. In men who cannot retain a condom catheter because of small penis size, silastic penile implants usually correct the problem.[51]

Surgical Intervention. When conservative measures of bladder management have been ineffective, surgical procedures may be necessary. The oldest type of urinary diversion is the intubated suprapubic cystostomy. Although some authors claim a similar incidence of complications with cystostomy as with indwelling urethral catheterization,[40] the experience with cystostomy at the MS Center has been that it is easier to manage than an indwelling catheter and has a lower rate of infection.

Methods of supravesical diversion, including nephrostomy, ureterostomy, ureterosigmoidostomy and ileal conduit diversion carry multiple complications, including ascending infection, calculus, reflux and progressive renal deterioration, and are not recommended.[40]

DATA ANALYSIS

Specific parameters of MS bladder function were examined in the Einstein MS Center patient population. Areas explored included the types of urinary symptoms experienced and their rate of occurrence, the temporal stability of symptoms, and the outcomes of management. The charts of 50 patients who were seen at the MS Center between 1 July 1982 and 1 July 1983 were reviewed. Selection was random, and

TABLE 2. Fluctuations in Urinary Symptoms[a]

Symptom	Symptom Present at Time 1, but Absent at Time 2	Symptom Absent at Time 1, but Present at Time 2
Urgency	16%	8%
Frequency	18%	11%
Hesitancy	33%	7%
Incontinence	15%	22%
Nocturia	23%	14%
Bowel	25%	8%

[a]Figures represent the percent of the total sample ($n = 50$).

included patients both with and without urinary complaints. It is possible that this sample is not representative of the general MS population, since it is likely that relatively asymptomatic or stable MS patients seek specialized medical help less often.

In addition to outpatient charts, hospital records were also reviewed, when hospitalization occurred between the initial visit (Time 1) and follow-up visit (Time 2). The average age of these patients was 45 years, and average duration of MS 11 years. The average Kurtzke, or Disability Status Score was 5, indicating that the typical patient was ambulatory without assistive devices. Seventy-four percent reported some bladder problems, with duration of symptoms from several months to 14 years, the median duration being 2 years.

As part of the initial assessment, a history of urinary tract infection was elicited. Nearly one-third of the sample reported previous UTIs and about the same number had had exposure to prior medical efforts at bladder management. Only four patients reported bladder or kidney surgery, and previous urodiagnostic evaluation was limited to a few cystoscopies, urodynamics and radiologic or radioisotope studies.

The symptoms most commonly reported were irritative, and included urgency (52%), frequency (50%), and incontinence (44%). Nocturia was present in 34% of cases, hesitancy in 22%, and dysuria was not reported by any patient. Bowel dysfunction, primarily constipation, was identified in 20% of the sample.

The temporal variation of symptoms between Time 1 and Time 2 is illustrated in TABLE 2. These figures suggest that in both untreated patients and patients receiving symptomatic treatment, old symptoms may disappear and/or new ones appear over a relatively short interval. At Time 2, many patients were beginning efforts at bladder management and some were noncompliant with recommendations. Others had presented with priority problems in another area at Time 1, *e.g.*, severe spasticity, so that Time 2 for these patients reflects no efforts at bladder management. Time 2 incidence is therefore a mixture of conventional intervention and nonintervention outcomes. The presence of irritative symptoms at two points in time is depicted in TABLE 3. This table shows that the disappearance of one irritative symptom does not

TABLE 3. Presence of Urinary Sumptoms at Two Points in Time

	Follow-up	
	Present	Absent
Initially present	48%	16%
Initially absent	14%	22%

TABLE 4. Presence of Bladder Problems at Two Points in Time

	Follow-up	
	Present	Absent
Initially present	58%	16%
Initially absent	14%	12%

necessarily herald the appearance of a different type of irritative symptom. Instead, patients may become symptom-free or develop symptoms of retention. The overall incidence of reported bladder dysfunction at Times 1 and 2 is represented in TABLE 4. A sizeable proportion of patients may become completely symptom-free after a short interval whereas others, previously symptom-free, develop symptoms. The 58% of patients who reported bladder problems at Times 1 and 2, and the 14% who were asymptomatic at Time 1, but symptomatic at Time 2, reflect a 72% incidence rate for urinary complaints at Time 2 for our sample, which is comparable with reports of other studies. TABLE 5 examines in somewhat more precise terms the change in bladder symptoms over time. In a random sample of clinic patients the majority will have bladder problems and of these, the majority will improve or stay the same, even if their symptoms do not completely disappear. Of particular interest is the 35% improvement group, which argues against considering all MS bladder dysfunction progressive over the short term. The findings further suggest that therapeutic trials which report improvement of bladder function as a significant outcome should take into account improvement or stability that may be achieved with no more than simple symptomatic treatment.

To summarize, two types of change were noted. One was the shift between presence (absence)/absence (presence) of symptoms. The other shift was in the type of urinary complaint reported.

At Time 2, 23% of the patients in the sample were receiving prophylactic urinary antiseptics, and 44%, urinary acidifiers, chiefly ascorbic acid. These measures were generally employed by patients with a history of UTI or those requiring intermittent or indwelling catheterization. Out of 50 patients 15 were utilizing IC, whereas 4 had an indwelling catheter, either Foley type or cystostomy. The latter group are considered management failures, since indwelling catheterization is the last option employed at the MS Center. Chronic suppression with a low dose antibiotic was reported in 13% of cases, reflecting patients with recurrent UTI, or chronic, resistant UTI. Sixty-one percent of the sample was receiving antispastic medication, almost exclusively baclofen. It is likely that only a small subgroup was utilizing antispastic agents for bladder management, while the remaining patients were being treated for lower extremity spasticity. Anticholinergic medications were taken by 46% of the sample, indicating intervention for uninhibited detrusor contraction.

TABLE 5. Change in Bladder Problems over Time

	Follow-up		
	Improved	No Change	Worse
Initially no problems	0	8%	12%
Initially had problems	35%	37%	8%

Age correlated with duration of the bladder symptoms of urgency, frequency and incontinence. No relationship was found between the duration of MS and the duration of bladder symptoms, suggesting that clinicians should look for urinary dysfunction in all MS patients, regardless of the length of time MS has been manifest. History of UTI was likewise unrelated to duration of MS, whereas it was positively correlated with duration of bladder symptoms. Review of symptoms revealed that incontinence rarely appeared as the sole urinary complaint, and was associated with urgency, frequency and hesitancy. The findings suggest that MS bladder function is both complex and variable. A patient who initially reports a single urinary complaint is likely to develop one or more symptoms or to experience other bladder problems at a later time. Spasticity in the lower extremities was correlated with irritative bladder symptoms, suggesting that patients with lower limb spasticity should be carefully interviewed for manifestations of urgency, frequency and incontinence.

Analysis of the Kurtzke Functional Systems revealed a positive correlation between the presence of bladder and bowel symptomatology and Kurtzke score, as well as pyramidal, visual, mental and sensory scores. Bladder and bowel problems were unrelated to cerebellar and brainstem scores. These findings agree with clinical impressions of MS Center staff that patients demonstrating predominantly spinal cord

TABLE 6

	Grade of MS		
Complication	I	II	III
None	3	8	6
Sepsis	0	1	6
Reflux	1	1	0
Stones	0	0	1
Hydronephrosis	0	0	1
Total	4	10	14

disease are more likely to experience bladder/bowel dysfunction than those patients who exhibit cerebellar/brainstem disease.

In a previous series, MS Center staff analyzed the records of 50 patients who had undergone radioisotope renal function/residual urine scans (RRF/RU).[52] Patients with a higher Kurtzke score tended to have a higher residual urine, suggesting that the failure-to-empty problem is associated with greater disability. A subgroup of 11 patients had catheterized residuals measured within a three-month interval of the radioisotope study. Whereas the radioisotope and catheterization methods of measuring urine residuals yielded slightly different numerical values, they corresponded in their identification of storage and emptying dysfunction. The residual urine determined by radioisotope studies was therefore found to be interchangeable with catheterized samples for separating storage from emptying dysfunction. It should be noted that the hospital of the Albert Einstein College of Medicine utilizes a precise formula for determining residual amount.[32] This method may be easily replicated by other nuclear medicine departments, many of whom provide only an estimate of residual urine volume.

The renal scan component of the RRF/RU of 140 patients with urinary complaints was reviewed, with only five found to be suggestive of upper tract abnormalities. Follow-up intravenous urograms were performed on these five patients, with one abnormality verified. With this low yield of positive findings in the upper urinary tract, routine screening by radioisotope procedures does not seem justified, since lower tract dysfunction can be satisfactorily classified by urethral catheterization for residual urine volume.

In another previous series, Blaivas and Barbalias studied 27 men as part of a prospective study of voiding dysfunction in MS.[53] Patients were categorized according to disability level. Those patients in Grade I had minimal neurologic disease, Grade II patients had moderate neurologic findings that interfered with lifestyle, but they remained ambulatory and self-sufficient, and Grade III patients were wheelchair or bed confined. Complications were found to increase significantly with the severity of MS as scored by the above system (TABLE 6).

DISCUSSION

Several important findings emerged from data analysis that have particular relevance for the clinician. The tendency of bladder symptoms to improve or totally remit with appropriate management supports the value of active intervention in MS urinary dysfunction. Since symptoms may also remit spontaneously, therapeutic claims which base efficacy on reduction of urinary complaints should take into account improvement that can occur spontaneously or with only symptomatic treatment.

The high incidence of bladder dysfunction in our sample (74%), and the lack of association between duration of MS and occurrence of symptoms, suggest that all MS patients are at risk for development of urinary problems. Experience at the MS Center has shown that direct questioning regarding presence of urinary complaints is not always successful in eliciting accurate information. Patients frequently deny symptoms initially or attribute them to other causes. In order to select those patients for whom additional probing may be fruitful, a profile of the MS patient most likely to develop urinary symptoms is postulated: predominantly spinal cord disease, spasticity in the lower extremities, positive plantar response, higher Kurtzke score and history of UTI.

It is hoped that these efforts will ultimately improve the quality of life for MS patients by relieving urinary symptoms and reducing associated morbidity and mortality.

REFERENCES

1. ANDERSON, J. T. & W. E. BRADLEY. 1976. Abnormalities of detrusor and sphincter function in multiple sclerosis. Br. J. Urol. **48:** 193–8.
2. BECK, P. R., K. G. WARREN & P. WHITMAN. 1981. Urodynamic studies in female patients with multiple sclerosis. Am. J. Obstet. Gynecol. **139:** 273–276.
3. BLAIVAS, J. G. & G. BHIMANI. 1979. Vesicourethral dysfunction in multiple sclerosis. J. Urol. **122:** 342–347.
4. BLAIVAS, J. G. 1979. Management of bladder dysfunction in multiple sclerosis. Neurology **30**(2): 12–18.
5. GOLDSTEIN, I., M. B. SIROKY, D. S. SAX & R. J. KRANE. 1982. The urodynamic characteristics of multiple sclerosis. J. Urol. **128:** 541.
6. PHILP, T., D. J. READ & R. H. HIGSON. 1981. The urodynamic characteristics of multiple sclerosis. Brit. J. Urol. **53:** 672–675.
7. PIAZZA, D. H. & A. C. DIOKNO. 1979. Review of neurogenic bladder in multiple sclerosis. Urology **14:** 33.
8. SUMMERS, J. L. 1978. Neurogenic bladder in the woman with multiple sclerosis. J. Urol. **120:** 555.
9. MILLER, H., C. A. SIMPSON & W. K. YEATES. 1965. Bladder dysfunction in multiple sclerosis. Brit. Med. J. **1:** 1265.

10. BRADLEY, W. E., J. L. LOGOTHETIS & G. W. TIMM. 1973. Cystometric and sphincter abnormalities in multiple sclerosis. Neurology **23:** 1131–1139.
11. SCHEINBERG, L. & C. ABISSI. 1981. Multiple sclerosis: Diagnosable and treatable. Resident and Staff Physician **27:** 75–81.
12. POSER, C., D. PATY, L. SCHEINBERG *et al.* 1983. New diagnostic criteria for multiple sclerosis: Guidelines for research protocols. Ann. Neurol. **13:** 227–231.
13. KATZ, G. P. & J. G. BLAIVAS. 1984. A diagnostic dilemma: When urodynamic findings differ from the clinical impression. J. Urol. In press.
14. BLAIVAS, J. G. 1982. The neurophysiology of micturition: A clinical study of 550 patients. J. Urol. **127:** 948.
15. BRADLEY, W. E. & C. J. CONWAY. 1966. Bladder representation in the pontine-mesencephalic reticular formation. Exp. Neurol. **16:** 237.
16. BRADLEY, W. E., G. W. TIMM & F. B. SCOTT. 1974. Innervation of the detrusor muscle and urethra. Urol. Clin. N.A. **1:** 3.
17. DEGROAT, W. C., A. M. BOOTH, J. KRIER, R. J. MILNER, C. MORGAN & I. NADELHAFT. 1979. Neural control of the urinary bladder and large intestine. *In* Integrative Functions of the Autonomic Nervous Systems. C. McBrooks, K. Koizumi & A. Sato, Eds. Elsevier/North-Holland, Amsterdam. Chap. 4.
18. FLETCHER, T. F. & W. E. BRADLEY. 1978. Neuroanatomy of the bladder-urethra. J. Urol. **119:** 153.
19. BARRINGTON, F. J. F. 1983. The localization of the paths serving micturition in the spinal cord of the cat. Brain **56:** 126.
20. DEGROAT, W. C. & R. J. THEOBALD. 1976. Reflex activation of sympathetic pathways to vesical smooth muscle and parasympathetic ganglia by electrical stimulation of vesical afferents. J. Physiol. (London) **259:** 223.
21. DEGROAT, W. C. & P. M. LALLEY. 1972. Reflex firing in the lumbar sympathetic outflow to activation of vesical afferent fibers. J. Physiol. (London) **226:** 289.
22. MORGAN, C., W. C. DEGROAT & I. NEDELHAFT. 1978. Identification of visceral afferents to the sacral cord of the cat using horseradish peroxidase. Soc. Neuroscience **4:** 23.
23. BLAIVAS, J. G., H. P. SINHA, A. A. H. ZAYED & K. B. LABIB. 1981. Detrusor-external sphincter dyssynergia. J. Urol. **125:** 542.
24. KURU, M. 1965. Nervous control of micturition. Physiol. Rev. **45:** 425.
25. DEGROAT, W. C. & W. R. SAUM. 1971. Adrenergic inhibition of mammalian parasympathetic ganglia. Nature **231:** 188.
26. DEGROAT, W. C. & W. R. SAUM. 1972. Sympathetic inhibition of the urinary bladder and of pelvic ganglionic transmission in the cat. J. Physiol. (London) **214:** 297.
27. DEGROAT, W. C. & A. M. BOOTH. 1980. Inhibition and facilitation in parasympathetic ganglia of the urinary bladder. Fed. Proc. **39:** 2990.
28. EDVARDSEN, P. 1968. The nervous control of the urinary bladder. I. The collecting phase. Acta Physiol. Scand. **72:** 157.
29. NORLEN, L. 1982. Influence of the sympathetic nervous system on the lower urinary tract and clinical implications. Neurourol. Urodynamic. **1:** 125.
30. KENDALL, A. R. & L. KARAFIN. 1974. Classification of neurogenic bladder disease. *In* The Urologic Clinics of North America. J. Lapides, Ed. W. B. Saunders Co. Philadelphia.
31. KHANNA, O. 1979. Nonsurgical therapeutic modalities. *In* Clinical Neurology. R. J. Krane & M. B. Siroky, Eds. Little, Brown and Co. Boston.
32. STRAUSS, B. S. & M. D. BLAUFOX. 1970. Estimation of residual urine and urine flow rates without urethral catheterization. J. Nucl. Med. **11:** 81.
33. WILLIAMS, M. E. & F. C. PANNILL. 1982. Urinary incontinence in the elderly. Ann. Int. Med. **97:** 895–907.
34. PARSONS, C. L. 1983. The bladder in multiple sclerosis. *In* Multiple Sclerosis. J. F. Hallpike, C. W. M. Adams & W. W. Tourtellotte, Eds. Williams and Wilkins. Baltimore.
35. ABRAMSON, A. S. 1983. Neurogenic bladder: A guide to evaluation and management. Arch. Phys. Med. Rehabil. **64:** 6–10.
36. MERRILL, D. C., W. E. BRADLEY & C. MARKLAND. 1972. Air cystometry II. A clinical evaluation of normal adults. J. Urol. **108:** 85.

37. LAPIDES, J. 1974. Neurogenic bladder: Principles of treatment. *In* The Urologic Clinics of North America. J. Lapides, Ed. W. B. Saunders Co. Philadelphia.
38. BORS, E. & A. E. COMARR. 1971. Neurological Urology. University Park Press. Baltimore.
39. BOYARSKY, S., L. PEREGRINA, P. HANICK, A. ABRAMSON & R. BOYARSKY. 1979. Care of the patient with neurogenic bladder. *In* Clinical Neuro-Urology. R. Krane & M. Siroky, Eds. Little, Brown and Co. Boston.
40. HALD, T. & W. BRADLEY. 1982. The Urinary Bladder: Neurology and Dynamics. Williams and Wilkins. Baltimore.
41. BRADLEY, W. E. 1979. Neurologic disorders affecting the urinary bladder. *In* Clinical Neuro-Urology. R. J. Krane & M. B. Siroky, Eds. Little, Brown and Co. Boston.
42. SIROKY, M. B. & R. J. KRANE. 1983. Rehabilitation of the patient with neurogenic bladder dysfunction. Seminars in Neurology, vol. 3, no. 2.
43. DEVER, D., W. HULBERT, M. J. STUBBINGS, J. VOLVO & A. COCKETT. 1983. Urinary incontinence. Am. Fam. Physician. August. pp. 123–132.
44. BLAIVAS, J. G. 1979. A critical appraisal of specific diagnostic techniques. *In* Clinical Neuro-Urology. R. Krane & M. Siroky, Eds. Little, Brown and Co. Boston. Chap. 5.
45. BLAIVAS, J. G., K. B. LABIB, S. B. BAUER & A. B. RETIK. 1977. A new approach to electromyography of the external urethral spincter. J. Urol. **117:** 773.
46. DIOKNO, A. C., S. A. KOFF & L. F. BENDER. 1977. Periurethral striated muscle activity in neurogenic bladder dysfunction. J. Urol. **122:** 361.
47. BRADLEY, W. E., F. B. SCOTT & G. W. TIMM. 1974. Spincter electromyography. Urol. Clin. N.A. **1:** 69.
48. NORDLING, J. & H. H. MEYHOFF. 1979. Dissociation of urethral and anal sphincter activity in neurogenic bladder dysfunction. J. Urol. **122:** 52.
49. BLAIVAS, J. G. & D. M. FISHER. 1981. Combined radiographic and urodynamic monitoring. Advances in technique. J. Urol. **125:** 693.
50. KEYS, T. F. & R. S. EDSON. 1983. Antimicrobial agents in urinary tract infections. Mayo Clinic Proc. **58:** 165.
51. HACKLER, R. 1979. Surgical treatment of the adult neurogenic bladder dysfunction. *In* Clinical Neuro-Urology. R. Krane & M. Siroky, Eds. Little, Brown and Co. Boston.
52. HOLLAND, N. J., P. WIESEL-LEVISON, G. MILLER & B. GIESSER. Radioisotope studies of neurogenic bladder in multiple sclerosis. Neuroscience Nursing Journal. In press.
53. BARBALIAS, G. A. & BLAIVAS, J. G. Neurologic implications of the pathologically open bladder neck. J. Urol. **129:** 780.

DISCUSSION OF THE PAPER

J. BLAIVAS (*Columbia University, New York, NY*): To answer Dr. Foley's question before he asks, the urodynamic studies we do are indicated in about 100% of the patients that I refer to the study and about 40% of the patients that other people refer. They're very time consuming and very expensive to perform and the more that we do the more money we lose, so the lab is something that has become an economic burden to us. The mainstay of treatment is not a Foley catheter but intermittent cathertization which is really very satisfactory to the overwhelming majority of patients that use it. And I think that's revolutionized how we do things.

If you look at men and women differently, men we can just about always find a socially acceptable way of managing. The detrusor-sphincter dyssynergia can be managed either by paralyzing the bladder and intermittent cathertization, or by external sphincterotomy and condom catheter. There are really numbers of ways of handling men. We can say with a certain degree of pride that not in a single man in our practice (which consists of a lot of spinal cord injury patients and a lot of multiple sclerosis) have we used an indwelling catheter other than on a temporary basis, *e.g.*, postoperatively.

As for women, again in my very select group of difficult patients, we only have about 20% on indwelling catheters and there are a number of different operations that we're doing but again, unfortunately I don't know what the long-term results are.

The common one is something called cystolysis where you simply do what you do in a cystectomy, you remove the whole bladder except you leave it in, just hanging by the urethra and the uterus. You cut all the nerves to the bladder; that generally stops the bladder from contracting in those patients who had hopeless problems with urinary frequency and urgency due to involuntary bladder contractions. So there really are lots of things that can be done.

The electrical stimulation has worked very well in stopping involuntary bladder contractions. Extraordinarily well, but not in our experience in multiple sclerosis though it's worked in just about every other group of patients. So I think at least to date the electrical stimulation has not been very promising. In the hopeless kind of MS patients, we can expect about an 80% rate of changing the life of the person and having them not dependent upon the bathroom.

L. SCHEINBERG (*Albert Einstein College of Medicine, Bronx, NY*): I'd just like to respond for a moment to Dr. Davis's comment about "not really doing anything." It's one of the more gratifying things that when a chronic MS patient comes to you with a Kurtzke of 6–8, bladder management is the only thing that we can do to help the patient.

Disability Rating Scales in Multiple Sclerosis

JOHN F. KURTZKE

Neurology Service
Veterans Administration Medical Center
Washington, D.C. 20422
and
Departments of Neurology and Community and Family Medicine
Georgetown University School of Medicine
Washington, D.C. 20007

Measuring the degree of involvement in our patients does not come naturally to neurologists. We are much more concerned with establishing the presence of particular neurologic deficits, from which we derive diagnosis. As to the course of illness, in clinical practice we are often satisfied with a statement that the patient has improved or not, sometimes qualifying the change by adding "much" or "slight." But outside of formal therapeutic trials, there is usually little effort to quantitate the degree of involvement or of changes therein.

Impairments to health have many facets, in their nature, their cause, their effects on the affected person, and their effects on his family and on society. The World Health Organization (WHO) has divided the consequences of an individual's disease, like all Gaul, into three parts: impairments, disabilities, and handicaps.[1] The rationale for this division is that a disease directly causes certain impairments, such as abnormalities on neurologic examination. These impairments result in disability or altered performance, such as in locomotion, which in turn provides a disadvantage or handicap to the patient in terms of his role in society.

The International Federation of Multiple Sclerosis Societies (IFMSS) has been attempting to establish a Uniform Minimum Record of Disability that would be acceptable as a method of characterizing all patients with MS. There is no attempt to supplant any schema in use in any center, but rather to incorporate an additional data set that would be uniform but simple, and express it in a common vocabulary.[2] For this purpose three separate systems have been proposed, one for each of the tripartite divisions of the WHO. The first is a rating scheme that summarizes the neurologic abnormalities (impairments), the next is a scale that codifies the physical dysfunction (disabilities) and the last measures the societal impact of the disease (handicaps).

As to the first, the system recommended by the IFMSS panel[3,4] is the Disability Status Scale (DSS) plus Functional Systems (FS).[5–8] For the second an Incapacity Status Scale (ISS) was devised,[9] and for the third a Socio-Economic Scale,[10] now called the Environmental Status Scale (ESS).

Within each system there are a number of items. Each item is subdivided in an ordinal or rank scale with 0 representing the normal state. Increasing deviations from normal are specified by consecutive numbers up to the maximum grade for that item.

The ordinal nature of these systems should be stressed. In fact, it would have been preferable to have designated the steps by letters instead of numbers, in order to avoid the temptation to treat them as if they were true numerical scales that could be added, and for which means and standard deviations would be appropriate.

TABLE 1. Environmental Status Scale (1983 Revision)

1. Actual work status
2. Financial/economic status[a]
3. Personal residence/home[a]
4. Personal assistance required[a]
5. Transportation[a]
6. Community services[a]
7. Social activity

[a]MS-related.

ENVIRONMENTAL STATUS SCALE

The original specifications for what was then called a Socio-Economic Scale were laid out in 1980.[10] Since then there have been several revisions, and the 1983 version of the Environmental Status Scale consists of seven items: work, finances, residence, assistance, transportation, community, and socialization (TABLE 1). Each of these has a six-step, 0–5 rank scale. Grade 0 is defined as no needs or normal performance. Grade 5 is maximal support needs or lack of performance, and the intervening grades are also specified.

This scale does provide a measure of how the patient's MS affects his role in society, and on the needs of society to respond. The separate items are clearly not additive, but together they provide a profile of the MS patient *vis-à-vis* his environment. They are also obviously far too remote from the illness and can be influenced by too many extraneous factors to be of any practical value as measures of treatment effects. And they are redundant. Similar neurologic impairment will be reflected in most of the separate items. For these reasons this scale would be of little use in assessing the effects of treatment in MS.

INCAPACITY STATUS SCALE

The Incapacity Status Scale as published consisted of 16 items, each rated on a 0–4 basis.[9] Here too the content has been amended (TABLE 2). Transfer functions, formerly

TABLE 2. Incapacity Status Scale (1983 Revision)

1. Stair climbing
2. Ambulation
3. Toilet/chair/bed transfer
4. Bowel function
5. Bladder function
6. Bathing
7. Dressing
8. Grooming
9. Feeding
10. Vision
11. Speech and hearing
12. Medical problems
13. Mood and thought disturbances
14. Mentation
15. Fatigability
16. Sexual function

two in number, are now one. The new item 12 is now called "medical problems" in place of the old item 13, "physical problems." The old item 14, "societal role," was deleted, having been much better defined by the Environmental Status Scale.

Items 1 through 11 cover ambulation and other activities of daily living, as well as communication. Mood and thought disturbances (item 13) and mentation (item 14) were separated into two from one item (old item 16) of the published version. Fatigability remains as item 15, and the new sexual function is 16.

General criteria for rating the first nine items of the ISS are that for grade 1, performance is impaired but accomplished without aid. For grade 2 mechanical aids are required, and for grade 3 human assistance is required, whereas for grade 4 performance is lost. For items 10–15, and somewhat modified for item 16 (sexual), the criteria are as follows: grade 1 is minimal impairment; grade 2 is moderate impairment or need for some personal care or special aids; grade 3 is marked impairment or need for extensive personal care; grade 4 is inability to perform.

The ISS, and in particular its first nine items, was derived from several scales in use in rehabilitative medicine.[9] The next six items cover aspects that, *inter alia,* might well influence rehabilitation. Sexual function was included as an important phase of WHO disabilities.

The items on the scale refer to the present level of function regardless of cause. Mental retardation calls for grades in item 14, mentation, as does schizophrenia in item 13. Amputees are scored in several items.

The nonspecificity of the content is one reason why the ISS would be a poor index of treatment effects in MS. Another is that change in grade can well occur for reasons other than change in the severity of the disease. Most important, though, is the redundancy of the items. The first nine reflect primarily involvement of motor and coordination functions.

The scoring, too, is problematical. Most orthodox is to handle this scale as a 16-item profile of the patient, just as with the 7-item Environmental Status Scale. However, we are attempting to assess the utility of adding the item scores, with each score weighted by its grade. A maximal score then would be 16×4 or 64. With much experience, it might be possible in the future to validate either this scoring or an alternative item-weighted scoring system.

It is probable that major changes in neurologic function will be reflected by similar changes in ISS item grades, and thus in their sum as well. But the converse is not true; as stated above, changes in grades clearly can occur without changes in neurologic function. Below we shall consider further the validity of rating scales as indicators of the state of the disease.

DISABILITY STATUS SCALE AND FUNCTIONAL SYSTEMS

In 1955 a Disability Status Scale was proposed for use in MS.[5] The scale had steps or grades from 0 (normal) to 10 (death due to MS), and it was completely based upon neurologic deficits as elicited at examination. It was, in fact, devised only after efforts proved unrewarding to handle the neurologic examination directly, or as it was encoded into Functional Systems. The Functional Systems were a means of collapsing the neurologic examination into categories that were mutually exclusive and yet together comprised all deficits found in MS; they were, however, not additive.[11] The Functional Systems are eight in number.[6–8]

The DSS has now been elaborated into a 20-step Expanded Disability Status Scale by subdividing each of the original steps 1–9 into two parts.[8] The EDSS is obligatorily defined in its lower ranges by FS scores, a procedure that had also been a recommendation for the DSS.[6] If one uses the EDSS, the addition of any two half-steps, such as 2.0 and 2.5, gives the same step (2) as the original Disability Status Scale.

The method that should be used to establish the appropriate step on the EDSS—or the DSS—is to repeat its ontogeny: (1) perform the neurologic examination, (2) code the exam into Functional Systems, and only then (3) assign the EDSS score on the basis of FS scores and ambulation.

Functional Systems

The eight Functional Systems are: pyramidal (P), cerebellar (Cℓℓ), brain stem (BS), sensory (S), bowel and bladder (BB), visual (V), cerebral (Cb), and other (O). The last system, other, is dichotomous, with a grade of 0 assigned when no neurologic deficits are found that cannot be assigned to another system. Grade 1 represents the presence of any such deficits, which are then specified but not coded. All the other FS have either six grades (Cℓℓ, BS, Cb) or seven grades (P, S, BB, V), and thus range from 0–5 or 6. The revised criteria for all FS are in Appendix A of the paper on the EDSS.[8] The frequency of involvement by FS, regardless of degree, is given in TABLE 3 for an early bout in one series of male MS patients. In terms of frequency, the four major systems are P, Cℓℓ, BS, and S, the other four being notably less commonly involved. This pattern holds throughout the course of illness.

The Functional Systems, then, are merely a method of encoding abnormalities found at neurologic examination into discrete, exclusive packets that cover all deficits to be found in MS. The delineation of the specific Functional Systems followed the assessment of the neurologic findings in a series of over 300 hospitalized MS patients, and the findings were then condensed into categories that were separate according to functional neuroanatomy, such as pyramidal and sensory systems. The number of FS required was defined by the need to cover the entire CNS as it is clinically affected in MS within a minimum of categories, but so that there would be only a few instances in which a specific finding could not be incorporated therein and would have to be relegated to a residual or "other" class.

After the categories were chosen, a means of indicating increasing involvement had to be specified that also followed the patterns of impairment seen in multiple sclerosis. The first series of MS cases on which this was based and then published numbered over 400,[6] and later experience has led to some further revisions.[7,8] The impairments observed are the reason why, for example, the "long tract" systems emphasize the lower extremities as their first and their most severely involved parts. From these considerations came the specific grades for each FS.

Therefore, the Functional Systems were designed to measure the frequency and intensity of clinical involvement in MS based upon findings at neurologic examination, with the intent that these scales would then reflect both the location and the extent of CNS dysfunction. The inference is that the greater the qualitative and quantitative FS involvement, the greater is the amount of tissue damage caused by the lesions of MS.

Now we know that there are MS plaques in clinically silent areas, as well as new ones being laid down in already nonfunctioning regions. However, it is still reasonable to hold that the greater the neurologic deficit, the greater are the quanta of plaques. I believe, therefore, that the Functional Systems do give a valid estimate of how much disease is present, and changes for the worse or for the better should then reflect more or less disease. If this is so, then the Functional Systems do provide a measurement tool of use in therapeutic trials.

But how should they be handled? We can, as with the prior systems, provide a profile of involvement within each system. However, this does not give one index of overall impairment. Can the scores be added? My answer is no for several reasons.

First, when this was attempted with several series, the sums did not increase with obviously increasing clinical deficits. Rather, they reached a plateau long before the theoretical maximum score, which is now 48. Second, as we shall see, the individual scales behave differently and have differing frequency configurations over their ranges. Third, some patients improve in one area while worsening in another. Fourth, and perhaps most important, as stated earlier these are all ordinal scales and therefore not subject to addition.

These points were the basic reasons why a scale for overall involvement had to be constructed, but one that was still based on the observed patterns of the neurologic deficits in this disease. The FS should remain as the profile of specific defects, and as such each system should be treated individually.

TABLE 3. Percentage Frequency of Involvement according to FS from Neurologic Examinations at Admission to Hospital for an Early Bout of MS[a]

Functional Systems (FS)	Percent Involved	Total n Known
Pyramidal (P)	84.9	511
Cerebellar (Cℓℓ)	76.9	481
Brain stem (BS)	73.0	514
Sensory (S)	55.2	478
Bowel and bladder (BB)	22.6	517
Visual[b] (V)	33.9	425
Cerebral-total[c] (Cb)	20.7	487
Cerebral-mentation[d]	2.9	487
Other (O)	14.9	523

[a] Army WW II series.[12]
[b] Neuropathic signs either/both eyes (from Army WW II series[12]).
[c] Includes mood changes only (step 1).
[d] Steps 2+ on the scale.

Disability Status Scale

The Disability Status Scale (DSS), then, was the scale devised in order to provide the overall assessment of neurologic impairment in MS. A summary statement of FS equivalents underlying the scale is in TABLE 4. The specific equivalents for the EDSS, and hence the DSS, are detailed in ref. 8.

The frequency distribution of the DSS in two series of MS patients is presented in TABLE 5. Each DSS step is well represented, and there is a tendency toward a normal or Gaussian configuration. It is for this latter reason that one could perhaps justify treating the DSS as a true numerical scale, and mean values would not be the absurdity they are for the FS grades. However, the structure of this scale is still ordinal, and it should be handled as such, as further discussed below.

FS and DSS Interrelationships

Some 2,000 neurologic examinations of more than 500 males with MS during a 20-year course of illness have been coded to the FS and DSS (TABLE 6). This series is

TABLE 4. Approximate FS Grades and Ambulation Equivalents for DSS Scores[a]

DSS	FS Grades/Ambulation
0	grade 0 in all FS[b]
1	grade 1 in any/all FS
2	grade 2 in 1 or 2 FS; others 0/1
3	grade 3 in 2 FS; grade 3 in 1 FS c/s 1/2 FS grade 2; grade 2 in 3–5 FS
4	ambulation 300m + without aid; FS exceed DSS 3
5	limited ambulation without aid; FS usually exceed DSS 4
6	ambulatory with aid; FS combinations with 3+ grade 3+
7	wheelchair; FS combinations with 2+ grade 4+
8	bed patient; FS combinations with several grade 4+
9	helpless bed patient; FS combinations with most FS grade 4+
10	death due to MS

[a]Specific EDSS (hence DSS) criteria in Kurtzke (1983).[8]
[b]May be cerebral grade 1.

independent of the ones on which the scales were based. For the FS the frequency of involvement overall, the DSS 0–9 column, is quite similar to that recorded for an early bout in this same series (TABLE 3), with the same preponderance of involvement in the four major systems (P, Cℓℓ, BS, S). When subdivided by DSS scores, this pattern generally persists, although the smallest differences among the FS are for DSS 1–2. In general, the frequency of involvement, regardless of severity, clearly increases with increasing DSS scores for every Functional System (FIGURE 1).

In the succeeding four figures are the distributions by grade for each FS according to DSS group. For DSS 1–2 the most common score is grade 0, then 1, and then 2, with grade 3 only rarely attained (FIGURE 2). For DSS 3–4, grade 0 still predominates for the four minor systems (BB, V, Cb, O), but the major ones, and especially P, Cℓℓ and S, are shifting to the right (FIGURE 3). With DSS 5–6 there is clearly a movement toward increasing severity as well as increasing frequency of involvement, and this is particularly manifest for the four major systems (FIGURE 4). Even further rightward shifts are seen for DSS 7–9 (FIGURE 5).

TABLE 5. DSS: Percentage Frequency Distribution in Two Series of MS Patients at Examination

DSS	Series 1[a]	Series 2[b]
0	0.3	5.4
1	0.6	3.7
2	6.9	8.3
3	12.6	19.8
4	16.0	19.8
5	16.0	15.7
6	13.1	9.1
7	18.3	7.7
8	12.3	4.8
9	4.0	5.6
10	na	na
Total	100.1	99.9
n	(350)	(1665)

[a]VA Hospital series, admission status.
[b]Army WW II series, overview for some 20 years.

TABLE 6. FS Involvement according to DSS Scores at Neurologic Examination, Army World War II Series[a]

FS	DSS 0–9	1–2	3–4	5–6	7–9	Total n
			(percentage involved)			
Pyramidal	80.2	48.3	81.5	97.9	99.3	1695
Cerebellar	70.0	34.2	73.5	94.4	99.0	1373
Brain stem	68.6	51.5	70.2	80.8	82.1	1637
Sensory	51.6	20.4	50.6	70.2	71.9	1455
Bowel and bladder	33.8	9.3	22.6	40.7	79.7	1623
Visual[b]	30.6	15.9	33.7	33.8	54.6	1374
(Visual[c])	38.3	31.8	39.4	39.6	45.9	(392)
Cerebral[d]	21.0	8.1	19.7	27.4	32.5	1440
Cerebral[e]	4.8	0.5	2.9	6.7	15.1	1440
Other	21.4	13.4	15.2	27.9	42.1	2015

[a]Overview of some 2,000 examinations of 527 males over a 20-year period; data from ref. 13.
[b]"Neuropathic signs" and not FS (see ref. 13).
[c]VA Hospital series.
[d]Cerebral total including grade 1 (mood).
[e]Cerebral excluding grade 1.

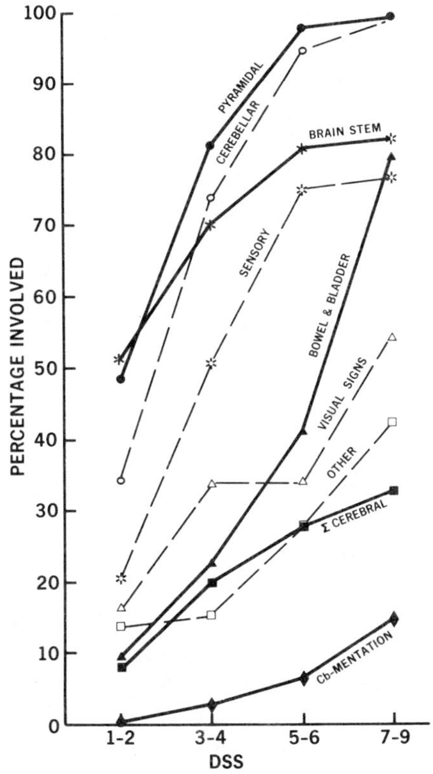

FIGURE 1. Percentage frequency involvement of each Functional System according to Disability Status Scale scores of the patients, based on some 2,000 neurologic examinations among 527 males during a 20-year course of illness. Data from ref. 13.

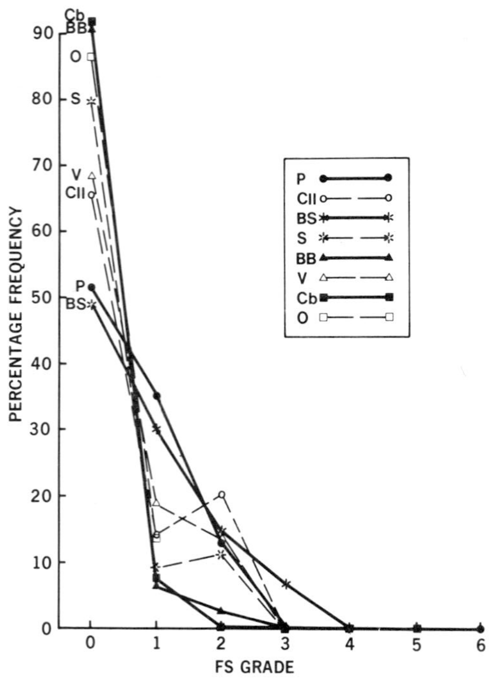

FIGURE 2. Percentage frequency distribution by grade for each FS (pyramidal, cerebellar, brain stem, sensory, bowel and bladder, visual, cerebral, other) among patients with DSS 1–2. Data as in FIG. 1.

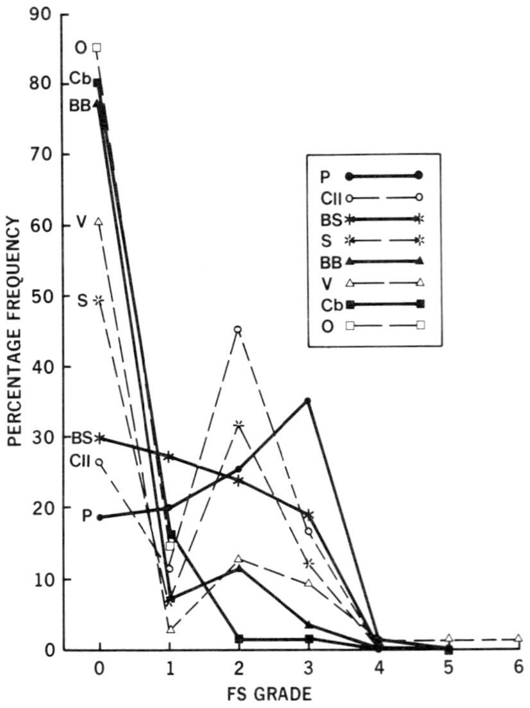

FIGURE 3. Percentage frequency distribution by grade for each FS among patients with DSS 3–4, as in FIG. 2.

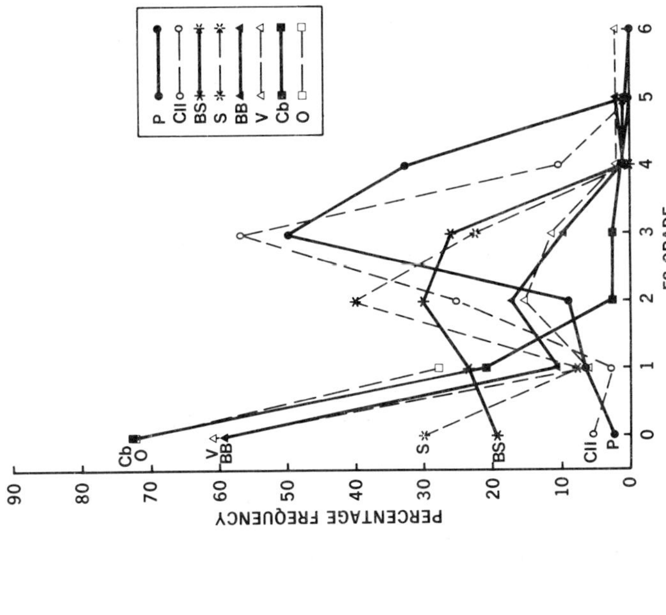

FIGURE 4. Percentage frequency distribution by grade for each FS among patients with DSS 5–6, as in FIG. 2.

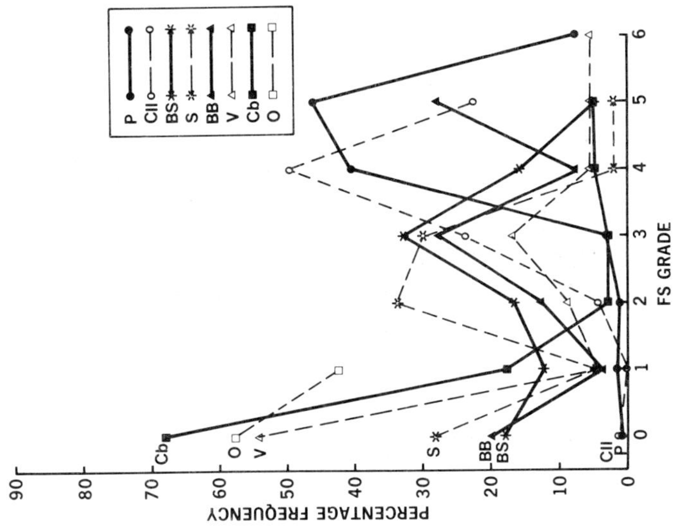

FIGURE 5. Percentage frequency distribution by grade for each FS among patients with DSS 7–9, as in FIG. 2.

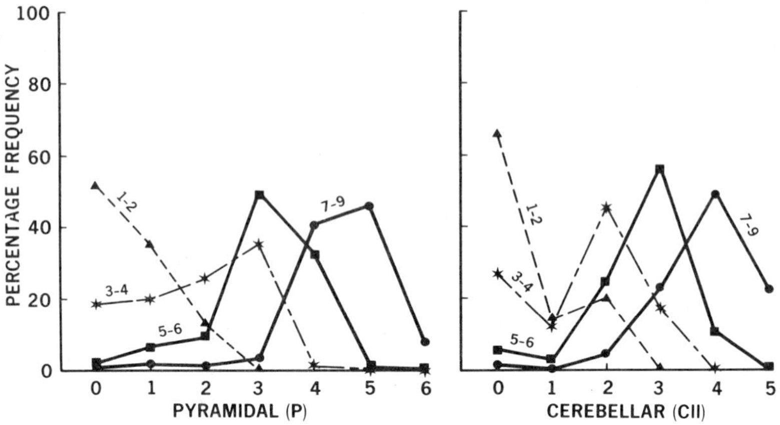

FIGURE 6. Percentage frequency distribution of pyramidal (*left*) and cerebellar (*right*) function grades according to DSS scores (1–2, 3–4, 5–6, 7–9) among all patients. Data as in FIG. 1.

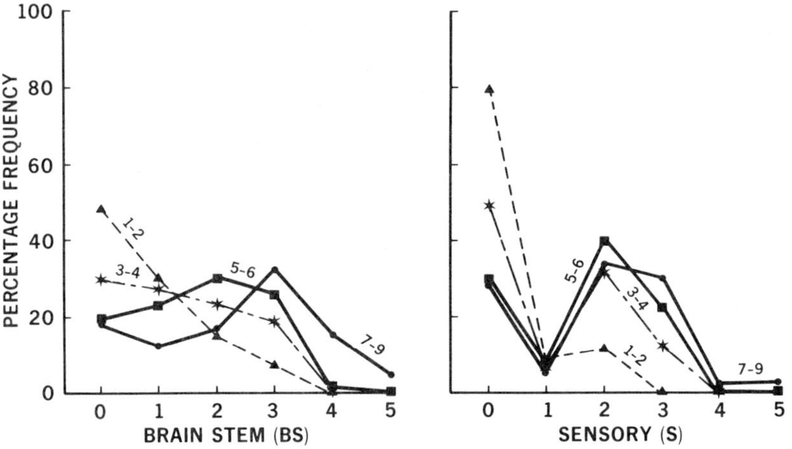

FIGURE 7. Percentage frequency distribution of brain stem (*left*) and sensory (*right*) function grades according to DSS scores, as in FIG. 6.

On these bases, one can conclude that the DSS does reflect quite well the overall severity of involvement in MS insofar as it can be defined clinically.

These data also suggest that the emphasis on ambulation in the DSS is not misplaced. Further evidence to this point arises when we consider each FS pattern according to the DSS range. For pyramidal and cerebellar functions there is a regular and marked increase in both the frequency and severity of involvement with increasing DSS scores (FIGURE 6). This is also the case for brain stem and sensory, although the proportions affected are lower for all grades, even with the highest DSS steps (FIGURE 7). Bowel and bladder and visual functions follow similar patterns, though with still lower proportions involved throughout the DSS range and for most grades of impairment (FIGURE 8). Even cerebral and other functions tend in the same direction despite the low frequency of severe involvement in the former (FIGURE 9).

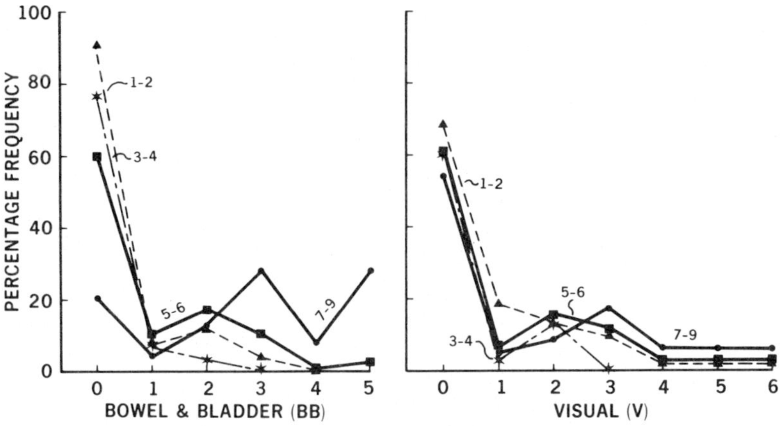

FIGURE 8. Percentage frequency distribution of bowel and bladder (*left*) and visual (*right*) function grades according to DSS scores. Data for the former as in FIG. 1; the latter is based on 392 VA Hospital patients.

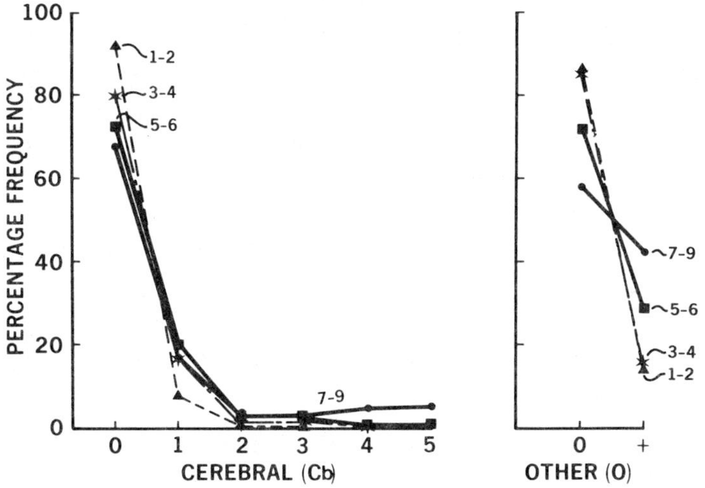

FIGURE 9. Percentage frequency distribution of cerebral (*left*) and other (*right*) function grades according to DSS scores, as in FIG. 6.

Here are the reasons why the Incapacity Status Scale, or an ambulation scale, or indeed any of the many other rating systems proposed for MS, will appear to be valid indicators of change. As groups of patients worsen, they tend to worsen in all measurable aspects. Any scheme, then, that reflects even a part of the neurologic involvement in at least an ordinal manner will demonstrate in groups some changes compatible with improvement or worsening. That a system can show change, then, is far from sufficient to conclude that it is measuring that which we are really after, the amount of dysfunctional and hence lesioned tissue.

For any rating scheme proposed one should have the following questions answered: What is its rationale or basis in MS-related neurologic function? Do changes in grade reflect changes in such neurologic function? Does it cover all that should be covered in MS or are major areas of impairment omitted? Is there a valid single figure to characterize overall impairment for each patient? Is this scheme "better" than others? And, if this should be one of several measures used in a treatment trial, will this be the principal one on which the conclusions of the study will be based, and what will be done if results from all the measurement systems used are not in agreement?

THE (E)DSS AND FS IN TREATMENT TRIALS

As mentioned, the DSS and FS should be treated as the ordinal scales they are. Improvement or worsening in each is defined as a gain or loss of at least one step on the scale. For overall patient assessment, this gain/loss is in the DSS; however, such DSS changes should not occur without similar change in at least one FS. For the EDSS, the least change is measured by the 0.5 step the scale permits. I have no data yet as to whether one can insist on FS changes for such a small increment within the higher steps of the scale. For lower steps, the FS grades define the EDSS.

Plotting of cases at two intervals is done most easily with a grid correlate of each patient's score at time 1 vs. time 2 (FIGURE 10). Cases lying off the major diagonal of

DISCHARGE	ADMISSION DSS										
DSS	1	2	3	4	5	6	7	8	9	V	T
0		1	4	2		1					8
1	6	7	16	2	1	1		2			35
2	1	23	19	15	1	2		1			62
3		6	105	13	10	1	2				137
4		3	15	118	8	5		1			150
5			9	16	57	3		1			86
6				3	8	6	1		1		19
7					4	2	2	2			10
8			1	1	1	1	1	4			9
9				1							1
V		2	3	3	1					1	10
T	7	42	172	174	91	22	6	11	1	1	527

FIGURE 10. Grid correlate to DSS at admission to and discharge from hospital for an early bout of MS; Army World War II series.[12] Numbers along the main diagonal (0,0. . .9,9) indicate no change in DSS between admission and discharge; those above the diagonal improved and those below worsened, by the number of steps off diagonal for each locus. From ref. 8.

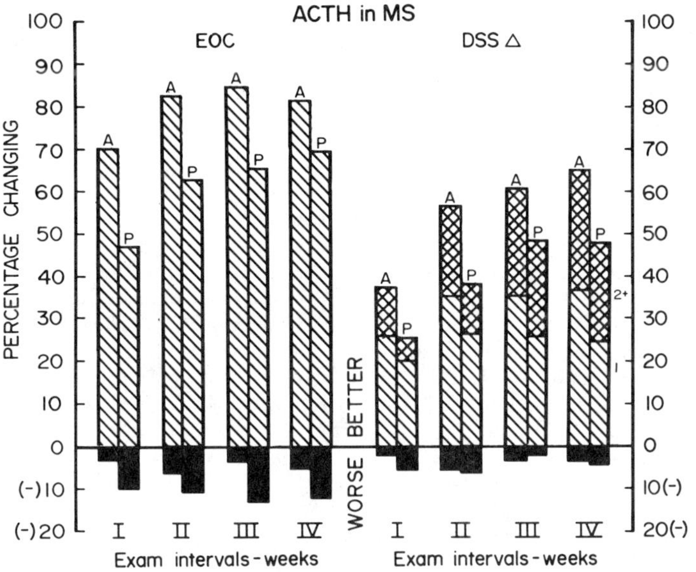

FIGURE 11. Percentage frequency of patients improved and worsened *versus* baseline status after one (I) to four (IV) weeks of study. Therapy (ACTH = *A* or placebo = *P*) given one week (I) and tapered the next (II), with none thereafter (III, IV). Measurement systems are Estimate of Overall Condition (EOC) on left and Disability Status Scale (DSS) scores on right. Data of the nationwide Cooperative ACTH Study.[14]

"no change" provide the numbers that have improved or worsened by one or more increments on whichever scale is used. This also permits identification of the locus at which such changes are most common, whether at one end of the scale or throughout its range. The improved, unchanged and worse proportions are then calculated, and for comparisons between groups it is these proportions that are the most easily assessed.

An example of such an application comes from the data of the nation-wide cooperative ACTH study of acute bouts of MS.[14] In that randomized, double-blind, placebo-controlled investigation the active drug regimen was ACTH at 80 units a day for week 1, tapering doses during week 2, and no drugs in weeks 3 and 4. Results with two of the methods of comparison used in the study are drawn in FIGURE 11. The Estimate of Overall Condition (EOC) was a summary judgement as to whether the patient was better, the same, or worse at the point of inquiry than he was at entry into the study, without the need to document the decision. The other method shown is the DSS change, with gains of one and of two or more steps.

The EOC shows higher frequency of change in both directions than does the DSS. However, the drug-placebo difference narrows with time according to EOC. This is not the case with the DSS, where the treatment difference is maintained throughout the study. Based on the EOC, the conclusion of the study was that ACTH "hastens improvement," the corollary being that the same improvement would have occurred, although later, without the drug. Taking the DSS comparison, though, would lead to the conclusion that ACTH really had a beneficial effect in terms of the frequency of improvement.

The EDSS and each FS should be handled in the same manner as exemplified for the DSS: laid out as correlations of grades "in" vs. "out," and the proportions changing compared. For the FS, this was also done in the ACTH study, and results similarly favoring the drug were found in each comparison, although not all of the differences were of statistical significance.

SUMMARY

The International Federation of Multiple Sclerosis Societies has been attempting to define a Minimal Data Set for multiple sclerosis following the tripartite scheme of the World Health Organization, with one rating scheme for neurologic signs, one for physical disabilities, and one for the societal impact of the disease. Current recommendations are the Disability Status Scale or the Expanded DSS plus Functional Systems for the first, Incapacity Status Scale of 16 items for the second, and Environmental Status Scale of 7 items for the third. All are graded in an ordinal (rank) scale from 0 (normal) with larger numbers for greater involvement. ISS scores range from 0–4 and ESS from 0–5 for each item. The only part of this scheme useful for measurement in clinical trials is the (E)DSS + FS. The DSS ranges from 0–10; EDSS subdivides each DSS grade 1–9 into two. FS are pyramidal, cerebellar, brain stem, sensory, bowel and bladder, visual, cerebral, or other; all save the last are graded 0–5 or 0–6. The DSS correlates well with both frequency and severity of involvement in all FS, which in turn represent a coded standard neurologic examination.

REFERENCES

1. Wood, P. H. N. 1980. Appreciating the consequences of disease: The international classification of impairments, disabilities, and handicaps. WHO Chronicle **34:** 376–380.
2. Slater, R. J. 1981. Functional disability ratings: Medical, social, and economic implications. Acta Neurol. Scand. **64** (Suppl. 87): 3–4.
3. Slater, R. J., T. Fog & L. Bergmann, Eds. 1981. Functional disability ratings: Medical, social and economic implications. A festschrift for Professor Tore Broman. International Federation of Multiple Sclerosis Societies. Acta Neurol. Scand. **64:** (Suppl. 87): 1–138.
4. Slater, R. J. 1983. Scoring techniques and problems in the evaluation of change in patients. Arch. Neurol. **40:** 675–677.
5. Kurtzke, J. F. 1955. A new scale for evaluating disability in multiple sclerosis. Neurology **5:** 580–583.
6. Kurtzke, J. F. 1961. On the evaluation of disability in multiple sclerosis. Neurology **11:** 686–694.
7. Kurtzke, J. F. 1965. Further notes on disability evaluation in multiple sclerosis, with scale modifications. Neurology **15:** 654–661.
8. Kurtzke, J. F. 1983. Rating neurologic impairment in multiple sclerosis: An expanded disability status scale (EDSS). Neurology (Cleveland) **33:** 1444–1452.
9. Kurtzke, J. F. 1981. A proposal for a uniform minimal record of disability in multiple sclerosis. Acta Neurol. Scand. **64:** (Suppl. 87): 110–129.
10. Mellerup, E., T. Fog, N. Raun, P. Colville, B. De Rham, B. Hannah & J. Kurtzke. 1981. The socio-economic scale. Acta Neurol. Scand. **64:** (Suppl. 87): 130–138.
11. Kurtzke, J. F. 1956. Course of exacerbations of multiple sclerosis in hospitalized patients. Arch. Neurol. Psychiat. **76:** 175–184.
12. Kurtzke, J. F., G. W. Beebe, B. Nagler, T. L. Auth, L. T. Kurland & M. D. Nefzger. 1972. Studies on the natural history of multiple sclerosis. 6. Clinical and laboratory findings at first diagnosis. Acta Neurol. Scand. **48:** 19–46.
13. Kurtzke, J. F. 1970. Neurologic impairment in multiple sclerosis and the Disability Status Scale. Acta Neurol. Scand. **46:** 493–512.
14. Rose, A. S., J. W. Kuzma, J. F. Kurtzke, N. S. Namerow, W. A. Sibley & W. W. Tourtellotte. 1970. Cooperative study in the evaluation of therapy in multiple sclerosis: ACTH vs. placebo. Final report. Neurology **20** (Part 2): 1–59.

Therapeutic Trials in Multiple Sclerosis: Azathioprine[a]

GEORGE W. ELLISON,[b] LAWRENCE W. MYERS,[b]
M. RAY MICKEY,[c] MARGARET V. FRANE,[b]
WALLACE W. TOURTELLOTTE,[b] CELSA A. SPINA,[d]
AND JOHN L. FAHEY[d]

[b]*Department of Neurology*
[c]*Department of Biomathematics*
[d]*Department of Microbiology and Immunology*
UCLA School of Medicine
Los Angeles, California 90024

Since the reviews by Ellison and Myers[1,2] several controlled studies of azathioprine have been reported. In January 1982, Patzold *et al.*[4] gave the results of an open, randomized, controlled follow-up study with a fixed dose of azathioprine (2 mg/kg/day) for up to 600 days. Treatment was effective in slowing the rate of progression in people with relapsing-progressive type multiple sclerosis. The authors could demonstrate no benefit in patients with intermittent (relapsing-remitting) or chronically progressive disease without exacerbations.

Mertin *et al.*[5] reported the results of anti-lymphocyte globulin, prednisolone, and azathioprine *versus* placebo. In 43 patients there were no significant changes in exacerbation rate after 15 months of azathioprine (3 mg/kg/day). There were changes in lymphocyte function and in visual evoked potentials. Although statistical significance was not achieved, there was a trend and the authors have decided to proceed with a larger double-blind placebo-controlled randomized trial with azathioprine alone.

Zeeberg *et al.*[6] have treated 22 patients in a double-blind placebo-controlled experiment. After 18 months of azathioprine for chronic progressive type multiple sclerosis a statistically significant reduction in the rate of progression was found in both groups but not between groups.

In our reviews in 1978 and 1980 we interpreted the reports to indicate that azathioprine did appear to slow the rate of progression.[1,2] Consultation with rheumatologists at UCLA resulted in the opinion that the addition of high-dose "pulse" methylprednisolone along with relatively high alternate-day doses of steroids might give a more rapid induction of benefit that could be maintained by azathioprine. The azathioprine would be given to reduce the white count below 4000 per cubic millimeter.[7] We embarked upon a phase I (preliminary) trial to test the drug regimen and to gain some impression of the toxicity of these agents. The results after two years treatment are to be published.[3] Here we report the results after three years of treatment.

[a]This work was supported by grants from the Kroc Foundation and the National Institute of Neurological and Communicative Disorders and Stroke (no. NS 08711).

METHODS

Patients who appeared to be having "active" multiple sclerosis were selected for participation in this study. Both those with relapses and remissions and those with steady progression were selected. The study was open. A control group was selected from the remaining clinic population of nearly 200 people by matching according to gender, activity (deterioration in preceding six months), age ±5 years, type of clinical course, and general degree of disability. The matching for the controls took place shortly after the patients had been started on azathioprine and methylprednisolone and the controls were followed concurrently. Relapse rates cover two years before entry and the duration of treatment after entry. Progression measures are equal before and after entry.

After informed consent, patients received 1 g of methylprednisolone intravenously within 30 minutes for the first three days of each of the first three months. They also were started on either 48 mg (initial three patients) or 96 mg of methylprednisolone every other day. This was decreased to 72, then 48 mg each month if the higher regimen was started. By the beginning of the fourth month, methylprednisolone was tapered 4 mg every two weeks so that a total of nine months of treatment with adrenal steroids was accomplished. Azathioprine at 2 mg per kilogram was started simultaneously with the first intravenous medication. Each month the dose was increased 25 mg a day until the target white cell count was achieved or toxicity became manifest. Clinical measurements were the Standard Neurological Examination, Kurtzke's Functional Systems Scales, and Disability Status Scales scores and the Illness Severity Score.[3,9] Slopes of the scores measure progression. Cerebrospinal fluid IgG synthesis and oligoclonal band patterns were measured at three-month intervals. Tests for lymphocyte proliferation, natural killer and killer cell activity and serum IgG were also done.[8]

RESULTS

Twelve patients were treated but three were withdrawn within six weeks of the start—two for allergic reactions, one for chemical hepatitis. In the nine pairs continued, the groups were comparable for gender, age in years, Standard Neurological Examination, Disability Status Scale and Illness Severity Score at entry, and for

TABLE 1. Grouped Patient Data

	Control	Azathioprine	p Value[a]
Females	5	5	
Males	4	4	
Frequently exacerbating group	4	4	
Progression phase group	5	5	
Age in years at entry	41.0 ± 7.6[b]	40.6 ± 9.3	0.81
Duration of illness at entry	10.4 ± 4.6	15.6 ± 11.8	0.22
Disability Status Scale score at entry	6.8 ± 0.7	6.8 ± 0.7	1.00
Standard Neurological Examination score at entry	47.2 ± 11.5	58.3 ± 14.7	0.07
Illness Severity Score at entry	55.2 ± 4.7	57.9 ± 6.7	0.11

[a]Paired Student's t test (two-tailed).
[b]Mean ± standard deviation.

TABLE 2. Trial Results

	Control	Azathioprine	*p* Value
Follow-up period			
(in years)	2.3 ± 0.9[a]	3.3 ± 0.7	0.03[b]
Exacerbation rate (all patients)			
before entry	0.94	1.17	0.52[c]
after entry	0.52	0.63	0.62
p value	0.27[d]	0.18	
Exacerbation rate (frequently exacerbating group of 4 pairs)			
before entry	1.25	2.12	0.18[c]
after entry	1.09	1.11	0.52
p value	0.92[d]	0.10	
Progression rate (all patients, avg. slope of Disability Status Scale scores)			
before entry	0.75 ± 0.63	1.11 ± 2.10	0.65[b] (0.28)[e]
after entry	0.25 ± 0.53	0.11 ± 0.43	0.47 (0.68)
p value	0.16[b] (0.21)[e]	0.15 (0.09)	0.54 (0.97)[f]
Progression rate (progression phase group of 5 pairs)			
before entry	0.81 ± 0.82	1.70 ± 2.78	0.57 (0.67)[e]
after entry	0.29 ± 0.40	0.20 ± 0.53	0.29 (0.08)
p value	0.32[b] (0.59)[e]	0.25 (0.07)	0.52 (0.84)[f]
Progression rate (all patients, avg. slope of Standard Neurological Exam scores)			
before entry	1.88 ± 3.71	5.15 ± 13.00	0.47[b] (0.92)[e]
after entry	5.10 ± 7.38	5.79 ± 3.76	0.81 (0.76)
p value	0.90[b] (0.15)[e]	0.87 (0.02)	0.57 (0.63)[f]
Progression rate (progression phase group of 5 pairs)			
before entry	1.84 ± 3.60	8.36 ± 17.14	0.44[b] (0.67)[e]
after entry	2.38 ± 5.45	5.66 ± 4.26	0.31 (0.46)
p value	0.90[b] (0.15)[e]	0.70 (0.09)	0.69 (0.39)[f]
Progression rate (all patients, avg. slope of Illness Severity Scores)			
before entry	3.07 ± 2.20	4.56 ± 7.23	0.59[b] (0.51)[e]
after entry	2.19 ± 3.93	0.98 ± 1.80	0.41 (0.67)
p value	0.64[b] (0.34)[e]	0.12 (0.03)	0.40 (0.58)[f]
Progression rate (progression phase group of 5 pairs)			
before entry	3.53 ± 2.70	6.66 ± 9.56	0.56[b] (0.60)
after entry	1.70 ± 2.52	1.46 ± 2.24	0.37 (0.62)
p value	0.39[b] (0.63)	0.23 (0.06)	0.53 (0.77)[f]

[a]Mean ± standard deviation.
[b]Paired Student's *t* test (two-tailed).
[c]Mantel-Haenszel tests.
[d]Chi-square based on Poisson distribution assumptions.
[e]Trimmed paired Student's *t* test (two-tailed).
[f]Test of the difference of the differences by trimmed paired Student's *t* test.

type of clinical course (TABLE 1). The azathioprine group was ill longer than the control group.

In TABLE 2 the trial results are given. The nine patients receiving azathioprine have been followed somewhat longer than the control group on the average. This is because of a death within the control group, and the later assignment. No censoring has been applied.

The exacerbation rate for all patients has declined to approximately the same extent. The azathioprine-treated group of frequently exacerbating patients approached statistical significance when their relapse rate before entry is compared to that after entry and if a one-tailed test is used. However, the comparison between the azathioprine-treated and the control group after entry reveals almost identical clinical exacerbation rates.

When Kurtzke's Disability Status Scale is used as the measurement there is a trend toward stabilization (less rapid deterioration) if the treated patients are compared to themselves before and after. With the Standard Neurologic Examination there was the same trend. With the Illness Severity Score the progression rate for all people also appears changed if the azathioprine-treated patients are compared to themselves before entry. If those exhibiting progression phase are compared the azathioprine-treated group again approached a statistically significant difference before as opposed to after treatment. But when matched against the control group no difference is demonstrated.

A sensitive indicator of difference (a test of the difference of the differences) does not show any effect of the azathioprine treatment with any of the scales.

We were unable to reach the target of less than 4000 WBC/mm^3 because of hepatic toxicity in four patients and arthralagia in one patient. In four people we did achieve the leukopenia.

Treated patients who had elevated CSF IgG synthesis before entry into the protocol had a dramatic drop in their synthesis rate that persisted. There was a gradual increase in the IgG synthesis rate but it never returned to its pre-entry levels. Patients who had low IgG synthesis initially had received steroids and no significant drop or elevation was detected. Oligoclonal bands did not appear to change if constant amounts of IgG were applied to the gels.

At a dose of around 2.5 mg of azathioprine per kilogram a drastic fall in natural killer cell and killer cell functions was observed.[8]

Adverse effects were quite common during the treatment with the methylprednisolone. These included: acne, moon facies, buffalo hump, hirsutism, pedal edema, increased bruising, insomnia, and headache. More moderate problems included organic brain syndrome in two patients, euphoria in one patient, diminution in night vision, severe headache, cataracts, and indigestion. Usually these adversities were dealt with by reduction in dose or addition of other medication.

With azathioprine, however, there were moderate increases in alkaline phosphatase, LDH, SGOT, and SGPT in two of the nine patients. Leukopenia below 3000/mm^3 was seen in four patients and a moderate anemia in three. One patient had thrombocytopenia.

One man receiving azathioprine died, probably secondary to respiratory failure after using a "hot tub." There was no laboratory or autopsy evidence that the azathioprine had contributed to his death. One of the control patients also died.

DISCUSSION

If one compares the azathioprine-treated patients before and after treatment there is an apparent slowing in the rate of progression. However, with this small number of patients no claims are made that azathioprine is effective treatment for MS. There were numerous side effects as well.

However, had several of these studies, perhaps with 7–14 matched pairs, been started in 1966 we might today have a clear answer on the purported efficacy of azathioprine in multiple sclerosis. Now we must wait for larger double-blind placebo-controlled trials.

CONCLUSION

We have concluded that there is some indication of clinical benefit but that a larger study will be necessary to demonstrate a significant medical effect. This trial began in June 1980 and will be completed in 1986. The risk is tolerable over the short term but unknown over 5–10 years.

ACKNOWLEDGMENTS

Marie Holevoet, R.N. and Beate Stubbings, R.N. helped with data acquisition, cleaning, processing, and analysis. Pat Jeffryes and Richard Burger typed the manuscript.

REFERENCES

1. Ellison, G. W. & L. W. Myers. 1978. A review of systemic non-specific immunosuppressive treatment of multiple sclerosis. Neurology (New York) **28**(2): 132–139.
2. Ellison, G. W. & L. W. Myers. 1980. Immunosuppressive drugs in multiple sclerosis: Pro and con. Neurology (New York). **30**(2): 28–32.
3. Myers, L. W., M. R. Mickey & G. W. Ellison. A preliminary trial of azathioprine and steroids in multiple sclerosis using a matched pairs experimental design. *In* Immunosuppressive Treatment of Multiple Sclerosis. O. R. Hommes, Ed. In press.
4. Patzold, U., H. Hecker & P. Pocklington. 1982. Azathiophrine in treatment of multiple sclerosis. J. Neurol. Sci. **54:** 377–394.
5. Mertin, J., P. Rudge, N. Karmer, N. J. R. Healey, S. P. C. Knight, A. Compston, J. R. Batchelor, B. J. Thompson, A. M. Halliday, M. Denman & P. B. Medawar. 1982. Double-blind controlled trial of immunosuppression in the treatment of multiple sclerosis: Final report. Lancet **3:** 351–353.
6. Zeeberg, I., A. Heltberg, J. H. Kristensen, N. E. Raun & T. Fog. *In* Immunosuppressive Treatment of Multiple Sclerosis. O. R. Hommes, Ed. In press
7. Rosen, J. A. 1979. Prolonged azathioprine treatment of nonremitting multiple sclerosis. J. Neurol. Neurosurg. Psychiatry **42:** 338–344.
8. Shih, W. W. H., G. W. Ellison, L. W. Myers, D. Durkos-Smith & J. L. Fahey. 1982. Locus of selective depression of human natural killer cells by azathioprine. Clin. Immunol. Immunopath. **23:** 672–681.
9. Mickey, M. R., G. W. Ellison & L. W. Myers. 1984. An illness severity score for multiple sclerosis. Neurology (Cleveland) **34**(10): 1343–1347.

Clinical Trials of Copolymer I in Multiple Sclerosis

M. B. BORNSTEIN,[a] A. I. MILLER,[a] S. SLAGLE,[a]
R. ARNON,[b] M. SELA,[b] AND D. TEITELBAUM[b]

[a]*The Albert Einstein College of Medicine*
Bronx, New York 10461

[b]*The Weizmann Institute*
Rehovot, Israel

INTRODUCTION

The understanding of the pathogenetic mechanisms involved in multiple sclerosis (MS) and the search for an effective treatment have been intimately associated with the laboratory model, experimental allergic encephalomyelitis (EAE). The validity of EAE as such a model system has been clearly and convincingly presented by Paterson in a series of scholarly publications.[1–4] Our own work in tissue culture[5] also served to relate MS, as a naturally occurring disorder, to its laboratory counterpart, EAE. Organotypic cultures of mammalian CNS tissue respond with identical patterns of demyelination,[6] swollen myelin sheaths,[7] and eventual "sclerosis"[8] when exposed to serum from EAE (whole white matter)-affected animals and MS patients. The demyelinating effect is not produced by these EAE sera on cultured peripheral nerve which, nevertheless, are responsive to serum from animals with experimental allergic neuritis.[9,10] The cultures also demonstrated the capacity of mammalian CNS to remyelinate after being demyelinated by antisera.[5,8] These laboratory demonstrations provided further support for the extension to MS patients of therapeutic possibilities arising from animal studies.

The synthetic polypeptide, copolymer I (COP I), was prepared from alanine, glutamic acid, lysine, and tyrosine (TABLE 1) as one of a series of compounds which, alone or in combination with various lipids, might simulate the ability of myelin basic protein (MBP) to induce EAE (Sela, personal communication). None of the preparations proved to be encephalitogenic, *i.e.,* capable of inducing EAE, but some, particularly COP I, did suppress EAE in animals challenged with either whole white matter or MBP in complete Freund's adjuvant. The numerous laboratory investigations of the effectiveness of COP I in EAE, involving mice, rats, guinea pigs, rabbits, monkeys, chimpanzees and baboons are of particular interest to the clinical trials and have recently been reviewed by Arnon and Teitelbaum.[11] In addition, extensive laboratory studies failed to demonstrate any toxicological or other undesirable side reactions in experimental animals exposed to COP I under a variety of testing situations (A. Meshorer, personal communication). Finally, Abramsky *et al.*[12] first examined COP I for its effect on three patients with acute disseminated encephalomyelitis (ADE) and four with terminal MS. The three ADE patients recovered rapidly and completely. The MS patients may have demonstrated slight improvements. What is more important in these first clinical studies was the absence of any significant undesirable side reactions.

This report presents the data derived from a preliminary trial of the effectiveness of copolymer I in patients with the exacerbating-remitting (ER) and chronic progressive

(CP) types of MS. It will also describe the extensions of that study to pilot trials in each group of patients, their organizational aspects and present position.

A preliminary trial is

> . . . conducted for the purpose of establishing dosages, studying toxicity, and obtaining a lead as to the possible efficacy of a new treatment which may be a new investigative drug . . . Different dosages with different schedules . . . are tried on a few patients who are very closely monitored for toxic reactions. For the assessment of therapeutic dosages, the patient with MS will serve as his own control. Therefore, the physician-investigator should be well acquainted with the medical history and past clinical course of MS in each patient . . . in most instances, it will not be necessary to involve more than perhaps 10 patients in a given preliminary trial. If the preliminary trial brings forth evidence of therapeutic efficacy and little or no evidence of serious toxicity, it would be reasonable to move onto the next stage of investigation, the pilot trial.[13]

CONDUCT OF THE PRELIMINARY TRIAL

Sixteen MS patients participated in the preliminary trial. They represented a broad spectrum of neurological involvement ranging from those of the chronic

TABLE 1. Composition of Copolymer I[a]

Amino Acid	*N*-Carboxyanhydride Used for Reaction	Amount Used in the Reaction (mM)		Molar Ratio of Amino Acid in Copolymer
alanine	alanine	8.6	75	6.0
glutamic acid	benzyl glutamate	6.0	23	1.9
lysine	*N*-trifluoroacetyl-lysine	14.0	52	4.7
tyrosine	tyrosine	3.0	14	1.0

[a]Molecular weight: 23,000.

progressive type, some of whom were essentially bed or wheelchair bound, to those of the exacerbating-remitting type who were fully active and employed between attacks. There were four of the ER type and twelve of the CP type. All patients had been well known to the principal investigator (MBB) for years prior to their entry into the study. Some had participated as volunteers in earlier clinical and laboratory studies whereas others had been unsuccessfully tried on immunosuppressant therapy.

The preliminary trial was conducted as an open study.[14] All patients were given the COP I and all knew they were receiving it. The evaluating neurologist (AM) was also aware that this was an open study and that all patients were being treated. The initial dosage schedule was suggested by the group at the Weizmann Institute on the basis of their previous studies with laboratory animals,[11] such as nonhuman primates, as well as the brief trial that was performed by Dr. Oded Abramsky.[12] Thus, it was planned to prepare the COP I at a concentration of 5 mg per ml of sterile saline solution. This was to be given to each patient intramuscularly five times a week for the first three weeks, three times a week for the next three weeks, twice a week for the next three weeks, and, finally, once a week for the balance of a six-month period, at which time we originally planned to terminate the trial.

At the time of introduction into the study, the first five patients were hospitalized at the General Clinical Research Center of the Albert Einstein College of Medicine.

They were examined and evaluated by Dr. Miller, samples of peripheral blood and cerebrospinal fluid were taken, and the copolymer injections were started. In the beginning, the patients were hospitalized during the first three weeks of treatment, because we had no knowledge as to whether or not there would be any significant local or systemic effects in patients who had multiple sclerosis. We did not, however, note any undesirable side reactions of any significance and soon found it unnecessary to keep the participants in the hospital for any period longer than was prudent following the lumbar puncture, usually 24 to 48 hours. The patients were seen, however, on an outpatient basis at the Clinical Research Center and their neurological status reevaluated at various times during the course of the following months.

The specific aims of the preliminary trial were to determine the following: (1) Did COP I produce any apparent significant or undesirable side reactions? (2) Did COP I produce any apparent desirable effects? (3) Could a dosage schedule be established for further (pilot) trials should they appear to be warranted?

RESULTS OF THE PRELIMINARY TRIAL

During the institution of the copolymer treatment, many patients reported and, in fact, demonstrated early improvements in various neurological functions. As time went on, however, and the dosage of COP I was reduced as originally planned, these early improvements disappeared and most patients returned to their previous neurological status and continued their chronic progressive course. Over the period of the next months, the dosage was gradually increased in an effort to determine whether or not the previously observed effect was dose related. By the end of the first eighteen-month period, those patients who were still on the copolymer were receiving 20 mg a day in 1 ml of saline, 7 days a week. Three patients are still on this schedule, some 3–4 years later. This is the dosage currently being used in the pilot study.

As for undesirable side reactions, patients occasionally reported transient slight pain, discomfort, itching, swelling or redness at the injection site. No systemic or general reactions of any kind were noted or reported during the preliminary trial. Examinations of urine were unremarkable. Of the sixteen patients, two of the ER type withdrew from the study at the time of an acute attack. One later returned. Of the balance, all remained in the study for at least six months as originally planned. Finally, three patients have been maintained to this date on 20 mg daily. In general, 11 of the 16 patients demonstrated no apparent favorable effects in that they either had an exacerbation during the course of the study or continued their chronic progressive course. On the other hand, 5 of the 16 patients have demonstrated a definite change for the better. (See TABLE 2.)

Nine patients received COP I for over two years, a few for over four years. No patient in this group has had any significant or undesirable local or systemic side reaction.

LABORATORY DATA

Laboratory examinations have included CBC, routine urinalysis and culture and blood chemistry analyses (SMA 6 and 12) VDRL, CSF protein and glucose and cells. Except for an occasional and transient eosinophilia (reaching 16% in one instance) no significant changes have been noted in any of these clinical tests. There has been no evidence of albuminuria or other evidence of altered kidney function. No pertinent alteration of the patient's serum demyelinating potency on CNS cultured tissues has been observed. Several sera have been examined for antibody titers against COP I. In general, they have not been elevated. Lymphoblast transformation in response to phytohemagglutinin, MBP and COP I has not occurred.

EXTENSION TO PILOT TRIALS

The question now is whether or not the demonstrated improvements were, in fact, due to the polypeptide. As stated by Brown *et al.*,[13] the aim of a pilot trial is "to

TABLE 2. Results of Preliminary Trial of Copolymer I Therapy in 16 Patients with Multiple Sclerosis

Patient	Type	Age	Sex	Date of Entry	Date of Termination	Results
IY	CP[a]	46	F	4/25/78	5/27/81	no effect
RH	CP	25	M	5/15/78	5/29/79	no effect
GT	CP	35	F	5/30/78	9/20/79	no effect
PP	ER[b]	30	F	5/30/78	2/5/79 (6/83)	no effect
AT	CP	23	M	6/27/78	2/8/79	no effect
PM	CP	39	F	7/18/78	—	arrested (not terminated) marked improvement
JP	ER	39	F	7/18/78	10/27/78	withdrew at time of exacerbation
JW	CP	32	M	6/27/78	6/5/78	no effect
KJ	CP	33	F	7/31/78	12/30/80	no effect
CN	ER	32	M	8/7/78	5/1/82	cessation of characteristic attacks
WR	CP	49	M	10/3/78	5/16/82	arrest (slight improvement)
SM	CP	42	F	10/16/78	9/20/82	no effect
HW	CP	36	M	10/24/78	11/13/78	no effect
SR	CP	38	F	10/24/78	1/28/80	no effect
FH	ER	27	F	11/7/78	—	cessation of characteristic attacks (not terminated)
JM	CP	34	F	11/20/78	—	arrest and improvement (not terminated)

[a]Chronic progressive.
[b]Exacerbating-remitting.

determine whether a treatment that 'looked good' in a preliminary trial still 'looks good' when tested under more rigorously controlled conditions." For this purpose a double-blind, placebo-controlled, randomized pilot trial was started about three years ago. Since another purpose of a pilot trial is to determine whether or not a full clinical trial is justified and, in addition, how it may be structured, the following brief description presents the current organization of the pilot trial.

The clearly defined objectives of the pilot trial of the ER patient are (1) whether or not the frequency of attacks is different between the COP I and the saline-injected groups, and (2) whether there is a difference in the degree of disability developed after two years of participation in the trial.

The patient population of 50 ER MS patients was selected from 935 volunteers to have at least one and preferably two attacks a year in each of the two years prior to entry into the trial, to be between the ages of 20 and 35, to be ambulatory, to be emotionally stable, and to have had no prior treatment with immunosuppressive drugs. The selected patients were matched for age, sex, frequency of attacks and degree of disability and randomly distributed by the statistician (SS) into the placebo or COP I groups. All information collected is sent to the Coordinating Center where it is edited, coded and stored in a data base specifically designed and constructed for this study.

The organizational structure for the pilot study includes an External Advisory Board, Steering Committee, Coordinating Center and Clinical Center. The External Advisory Board, an outside independent group which serves the trial in an advisory and consultative capacity, includes Dr. John Kurtzke, Professor of Neurology and Community Medicine, Georgetown University School of Medicine and chief of Neurology Service, Veterans Administration Medical Center; Dr. William Weiss, chief of Biometry and Field Studies at the National Institute of Neurological and Communicative Disorders and Stroke, NIH; and Dr. I. Herbert Scheinberg, chairman of the Clinical Investigation Committee at Albert Einstein College of Medicine. This group receives periodic reports from the Coordinating Center that describe the results of the trial to date and keep the members informed as to the conduct of the trial.

The Steering Committee is composed of Murray Bornstein, M.D., principal investigator (who is blinded); Dr. Sylvia Wassertheil-Smoller, Ph.D., head of the Division of Epidemiology and Biostatistics; and Ms. Susan Slagle, M.P.H., biostatistion. It is their function to monitor the progress of the trial on an ongoing basis as well as to make decisions as to the design and conduct of the trial. At the Clinical Center, patients are examined routinely every three months and more frequently at the time of exacerbations. The investigating neurologists and the principal investigator, as well as the patients themselves, are unaware of the treatment assignments to placebo or COP I. This blinding of patients and examiners is maintained through the use of a Coordinating Center, which is a separate unit responsible for matching, randomization, procedures, assignment to treatment and data management.

The pilot trial of the ER patients will end in December 1984. The code will be broken, the data analyzed and the results published.

A report summarizing the status of the ER trial as of 1 January 1983 was submitted to the External Advisory Committee. An excerpt from this report that shows current enrollment status of the pilot trial is presented in TABLE 3. Based on the recommendations from the External Advisory Committee after reviewing the report of January 1 and the fact that there have been few significant undesirable side effects or reactions observed or reported to date, the ER pilot trial is now being extended to chronic progressive (CP) patients. For this purpose, 80 participants will be entered into the trial, varying from 25 to 55 years of age. The conduct of the multicenter CP pilot trial differs in some respects from the ER pilot trial.

During a pretrial observation period, each CP patient must demonstrate a predetermined and sustained degree of worsening, specifically, at least two units in any one of Kurtzke's eight functional groups or one unit in any two unrelated functional groups. Once this is demonstrated and maintained, the patient becomes eligible to enter the trial and will then be randomly distributed into placebo or COP I groups. The dosage of COP I will be 15 mg in 0.75 of bacteriostatic saline subcutaneously, twice a day. The placebo consists of 0.75 ml of bacteriostatic saline. Patients will be evaluated at 1, 4, 8, 12, 16, 20 and 24 months after admission to the trial. The evaluation will be the same as those listed for the current ER pilot trial. The trial will of course be conducted in a double-blind manner.

The central statistic for the CP patients will be arrest of progression, which currently is defined as a change of not more than one unit in the eight functional groups over the two-year period. Any degree of improvement will also be recorded and reported, but is not being used to determine the overall effectiveness of COP I. The essential reasons for this limitation are both theoretical and practical. Theoretically, COP I is thought to interfere with the immunological attack on the nervous system by promoting the development of antigen-specific suppressor T cells. Whether or not these cells can eventually be demonstrated in human subjects, the point is that an arrest of clinical progression can be interpreted as an arrest of the immunological attack. A number of factors of structural, biochemical or bioelectrical nature, many of which are unknown, may contribute to the degree of clinically manifest neuronal dysfunctions. Moreover, they are not only unknown, but also uncontrolled in this trial. Thus, although improvements in function will be noted and reported, only arrest of progression (as stated) will be used as the central statistic to evaluate the effectiveness of COP I in the CP patient.

TABLE 3. Pilot Trial of COP I in ER Patients[a]

	Placebo	COP I	Total
Number entered	25	25	50
Average age	30.96	29.96	30.44
Sex[b]			
males	10	11	21
females	15	14	29
Race			
white			48
black/hispanic			2
Kurtzke DSS[b]			
0–2	13	13	26
3–4	5	5	10
5–6	7	7	14
mean DSS	3.2	3.2	3.2
Previous attack rate[b]			
attacks/year	2.02	1.96	1.99
Time in study			
total patient mos.	412	460	872
total patient years	34.33	38.33	72.66
average no. mos. in the study	18.40	16.48	17.44

[a]Baseline characteristics of the study population and the accumulated time in the study as of 1 January 1983.
[b]Matching variables.

Meanwhile, on the basis of current data, the Steering Committee with the advice of the External Advisory Committee is beginning to plan a full, multicenter—probably international—clinical trial of COP I in the ER type of MS patient.

If COP I should prove to be effective in arresting the progression of MS in a significant number of MS patients without evidence of unacceptable side reactions, two further possibilities may be considered.

COP I may represent a protein component of CNS tissue acting as an encephalitogen. Evidence of the possible involvement of a lipid factor, galactocerebroside, as an antigen has been demonstrated.[15] Proteolipid lipoprotein (PLP) may also be considered a candidate in this regard. A carbohydrate moiety, *e.g.*, myelin-associated glycoprotein (MAG), may have similar properties. Consequently, if COP I proves to be effective in a given proportion of patients, the addition of other antigens such as lipid (GC and

PLP) and carbohydrate (MAG) substances may prove even more effective in altering the course of MS.

Finally, if the synthetic polypeptide, COP I, proves valuable in MS as a disease involving an autoallergic mechanism, one can suggest that other synthetic polypeptides should be examined for their potential therapeutic effects in other diseases known or suspected to result from similar immunological factors.

REFERENCES

1. PATERSON, P. Y. 1977. Autoimmune neurologic disease: Experimental animal systems and implications for multiple sclerosis. *In* Autoimmunity. Genetic, Immunologic, Virologic and Clinical Aspects. N. Talmage, Ed.: 643–692. Academic Press. New York.
2. PATERSON, P. Y. 1978. The demyelinating diseases: Clinical and experimental studies in animals and man. *In* Immunologic Diseases. 3d ed. M. Samter, N. Alexander, B. Rose, W. B. Sherman, D. W. Talmage & J. H. Vaughn, Eds.: 1400–1435. Little, Brown and Company. Boston.
3. PATERSON, P. Y. 1979. Neurological disorders. *In* Medical Immunology. W. J. Irvine, Ed.: 361–381. Teviot Scientific Publications. Edinburgh.
4. PATERSON, P. Y. 1980. The immunopathology of experimental allergic encephalomyelitis. *In* The Suppression of Experimental Allergic Encephalomyelitis and Multiple Sclerosis. A. N. Davison & M. C. Cuzner, Eds.: 11–30. Academic Press. New York.
5. BORNSTEIN, M. B. 1963. A tissue culture approach to demyelinative disorders. Nat. Cancer Inst. Monogr. **11:** 197–214.
6. BORNSTEIN, M. B. 1973. The immunopathology of demyelinative disorders examined in organotypic cultures of mammalian central nerve tissues. *In* Progress in Neuropathology, vol. 2. H. M. Zimmerman, Ed.: 69–90. Grune & Stratton. New York.
7. BORNSTEIN, M. B. & C. S. RAINE. 1976. The initial structural lesion in serum: Induced demyelination *in vitro*. Lab. Invest. **35:** 391–401.
8. RAINE, C. S. & M. B. BORNSTEIN. 1970. Experimental allergic encephalomyelitis. A light and electron microscope study of remyelination and "sclerosis" *in vitro*. J. Neuropath. Exp. Neurol. **29:** 552–574.
9. BORNSTEIN, M. B. & C. S. RAINE. 1977. Multiple sclerosis and experimental allergic encephalomyelitis. Specific demyelination of CNS in culture. Neuropathology and Applied Neurobiology **3:** 359–367.
10. RAINE, C. S. & M. B. BORNSTEIN. 1979. Experimental allergic neuritis ultrastructure of serum-induced myelin aberrations in PNS cultures. Lab. Invest. **40:** 423–432.
11. ARNON, R. & D. TEITELBAUM. 1980. Desensitization of experimental allergic encephalomyelitis with synthetic peptide analogues. *In* The Suppression of Experimental Allergic Encephalomyelitis and Multiple Sclerosis. A. N. Davison & M. L. Cuzner, Eds.: 105–177. Academic Press. London, New York.
12. ABRAMSKY, O., D. TEITELBAUM & R. ARNON. 1977. Effect of a synthetic polypeptide (COP I) on patients with multiple sclerosis and with acute disseminated encephalomyelitis. Preliminary report. J. Neurol. Sci. **31:** 433–438.
13. BROWN, J. R., G. W. BEEBE, J. F. KURTZKE, R. B. LOEWENSON, D. H. SILBERBERG & W. W. TOURTELLOTTE. 1979. The design of clinical studies to assess therapeutic efficacy in multiple sclerosis. Neurology **29**(Part 2): 3–23.
14. BORNSTEIN, M. B., A. I. MILLER, D. TEITELBAUM, R. ARNON & M. SELA. 1982. Treatment of multiple sclerosis with a synthetic polypeptide. Preliminary results. Ann. Neurol. **11:** 317–319.
15. FRY, J. M., S. WEISSBARTH, G. M. LEHRER & M. B. BORNSTEIN. 1974. Cerebroside antibody inhibits sulfatide synthesis and myelination and demyelinates in cord tissue cultures. Science **183:** 540–542.

The Use of Cyclophosphamide in the Treatment of Multiple Sclerosis[a]

HOWARD L. WEINER,[b,d] STEPHEN L. HAUSER,[b,d]
DAVID A. HAFLER,[b,d] ROBERT J. FALLIS,[b,d]
JAMES R. LEHRICH,[c,d] AND DAVID M. DAWSON[b,d]

[b]*Multiple Sclerosis Clinical and Research Unit*
Division of Neurology
Department of Medicine
Brigham and Women's Hospital
Boston, Massachussetts 02115

[c]*Department of Neurology*
Massachusetts General Hospital
Boston, Massachussetts 02114

[d]*Harvard Medical School*
Boston, Massachussetts 02115

Over the past four years we have been involved in a number of clinical trials of immunosuppression in the treatment of multiple sclerosis (MS).[1-4] Our work has focused on patients with chronic progressive disease and we have found in a randomized study that a short course of high-dose intravenous cyclophosphamide can stabilize the majority of patients treated when followed for a one-year period.[3] Our work is an outgrowth of uncontrolled studies carried out by European investigators[5-6] and by other investigators who have attempted various forms of immunosuppression in MS on the assumption that disease pathogenesis is related to autoimmunity and that appropriate immunosuppressive therapy might control the disease.[7] Since the publication of our work a much larger number of patients has been treated, new protocols adopted, and longer follow-up on patients achieved. Furthermore, other physicians in the United States have begun to use high-dose cyclophosphamide for the treatment of multiple sclerosis, both in controlled and uncontrolled fashions. In the present report we will summarize our experience to date, discuss the practical and theoretical considerations raised by our studies, summarize the experience of others, and discuss the implications for the future.

Predictability of the Clinical Course of Multiple Sclerosis and Factors Associated with Poor Prognosis and Disease Progression

The two major clinical categories of MS consist of the relapsing-remitting form and the chronic progressive or progressive form of the disease.[8-9] In general, the more predictable and disabling form of the disease appears to be the progressive form, which may evolve after a series of attacks or may be the clinical pattern from the onset of the disease. Progressive MS leads to permanent disability, generally within five years after

[a]This work was supported by NIH grant no. NS-17182.

the onset of progression and often earlier, depending on the rapidity of progression.[8–11] In the vast majority of patients who have entered the progressive stage, there are no spontaneous remissions and this form of MS is generally not responsive to corticosteroid treatment. For these reasons, we have focused our clinical studies on patients with the progressive form of MS. Other, less common, subcategories of MS include patients whose course includes both progression and superimposed attacks, or multiple attacks within a relatively short period of time with accumulating deficits. The clinical course of MS in these groups appears to be as malignant as the progressive form, if not more so, and we have included such patients in our treatment protocols.

Treatment of Acute Attacks and Relapsing-Exacerbating Disease

It would seem reasonable to assume that an acute attack, when the disease is most active, may be the most appropriate time for therapeutic intervention. Nonetheless, the majority of patients recover from such attacks, and even though many are left with some degree of permanent disability, it is difficult to ascertain the benefit of a particular treatment unless large numbers of patients are studied, usually in a double-blind fashion. In this regard, we are currently involved in a double-blind study of plasma exchange plus oral cyclophosphamide and ACTH in acute attacks of MS.[12] A pilot study of high-dose cyclophosphamide did not show a benefit during the acute phase of disease, although follow-up was not carried out in this study.[13] To demonstrate an effect of treatment on patients with relapsing-exacerbating disease, one must distinguish number of relapses and severity of relapses. Thus, a patient may have many small attacks in a two-year period leaving no disability, while another patient may have two attacks leading to a major disability. In addition, it is known that a significant number of patients (approximately 50%) will enter a progressive phase following a number of defined attacks, making it difficult to monitor response to therapy in terms of numbers of attacks. Long-term follow-up of patients after treatment is generally required to resolve these issues.[14] There are uncontrolled reports of high-dose cyclophosphamide being of benefit in patients with relapsing-exacerbating disease.[5]

Current Protocols

In our initial study, approximately 75% of patients treated with high-dose cyclophosphamide/ACTH and followed for one year received benefit. Fifty percent of

TABLE 1. Composite Data (No. of Patients) of Clinical Response and Treatment Failure in Each Treatment Group

	Clinical Response[a]				Treatment Failure[b]	
	6 Months		12 Months			
Group	Stabilized	Worse	Stabilized	Worse	6 mo.	12 mo.
ACTH	8	12	4	16	8	14
Cyclophosphamide/ACTH	18	2	16	4	0	2
Plasma exchange regimen	11	7	9	9	4	7

[a]Defined as improved or unchanged according to clinical response.
[b]Defined as worsening on the Disability Status Scale to Grade 6 or greater. Number of patients with treatment failure at 12 months includes those with failure at 6 months.
Note: for details of study see ref. 3.

TABLE 2. Outline of Current Protocols for the Treatment of Multiple Sclerosis with Cyclophosphamide

Design of Protocols	Induction	Maintenance and/or Retreatment
Group 1	yes	no
Group 2	yes	yes

A. Induction of Remission
1. "Published" IV cyclophosphamide/ACTH in-hospital[3]; 500 mg cyclophosphamide/day in 4 divided doses for 10–14 days
2. "Modified" IV cyclophosphamide/ACTH in-hospital; 500–600 mg cyclophosphamide/m^2 (~1g) once/day ×5 given over 5–8 days
3. Outpatient IV cyclophosphamide/oral prednisone; 700 mg cyclophosphamide/m^2 once/week for 6 weeks

B. Maintenance and/or Retreatment
1. Full retreatment in-hospital at defined intervals or when patient begins reprogressing
2. Outpatient maintenance; 700 mg IV cyclophosphamide/m^2 once every two months for two years
3. Outpatient re-induction

patients treated did not progress further, 25% of patients improved, and 25% of patients received no benefit. These results are summarized in TABLE 1. Continued follow-up of the patients who were stabilized or improved at one year demonstrated that the majority of patients began progressive worsening again between one and three years following treatment. In addition, there appeared to be some benefit in the group treated with plasma exchange, ACTH, and low-dose cyclophosphamide, although not as dramatic as that in the high-dose cyclophosphamide/ACTH group. Based on these results, the next study we initiated was a three-armed protocol designed to ask two questions: (1) Does retreatment at one year prevent reprogression and maintain stabilization of disease? (2) Can a more prolonged remission be obtained with plasma exchange given concomitantly with high-dose cyclophosphamide/ACTH? To answer these questions a three-armed, randomized trial has been initiated, with group 1 receiving high-dose cyclophosphamide/ACTH therapy, group 2 receiving high-dose cyclophosphamide/ACTH plus five plasma exchanges given concomitantly, and group 3 receiving high-dose cyclophosphamide/ACTH therapy plus retreatment at one year irrespective of clinical status, or retreatment earlier should reprogression or deterioration occur. To date, approximately 70 patients have been entered into this study. Although there has not been sufficient follow-up for final conclusions to be drawn, it appears that the response rate in chronic progressive patients to high-dose cyclophosphamide/ACTH is similar in this group of patients as in the initial 20 patients treated. In addition, patients have undergone a second course of therapy without any untoward side effects. Preliminary data suggest that the inclusion of plasma exchange at the time of administering high-dose cyclophosphamide does not offer a significant advantage over high-dose cyclophosphamide and ACTH alone. In those patients followed long enough after receiving only one treatment, resumption of progression between one and two years following therapy continues to be observed.

The use of cyclophosphamide in chemotherapeutic doses does not necessarily require hospitalization. To this end, we have initiated pilot studies of outpatient cyclophosphamide treatment. In one protocol, cyclophosphamide is administered on an outpatient basis in a single IV bolus given at a dose of 700 mg/m^2. This procedure is identical to methods of administration used in some patients undergoing chemotherapy for cancer. In another protocol (of Dr. Lehrich), cyclophosphamide is given orally on a limited outpatient basis for a 12-week period in conjunction with prednisone using a program similar to one used for the treatment of rheumatological diseases. Should an out-patient regimen be shown to be efficacious, it would allow patients to be treated in a manner that would not interrupt daily activities in the way prolonged hospitalization does. It must be emphasized however, that the efficacy of these programs has not been demonstrated.

Design of Protocols

The design of our current protocols is contained in TABLE 2. Following induction of a remission, strategies to maintain stability and prevent progression involve either retreatment or maintenance therapy. Groups receiving maintenance or retreatment are compared to groups receiving only induction. A variety of induction regimens and retreatment and/or maintenance regimens is being tested, involving both inpatient and outpatient therapy. For example, a "modified" high-dose cyclophosphamide/ACTH in-hospital regimen is being compared to "published" high-dose cyclophosphamide/ACTH in-hospital.[3] If efficacious, the "modified" regimen has the advantages that it requires a shorter period of hospitalization and could be given on an outpatient basis in future protocols.

Characterization of Patients Treated

Thus far, we have treated 143 patients at the Brigham and Women's Hospital with short courses of high-dose cyclophosphamide designed to induce leukopenia of less than 2,000; 121 patients were treated as part of ongoing protocols, the remainder were not treated on protocol (TABLE 3). Twenty-four patients have been treated twice; two have been treated three times. Patients not treated on protocol were generally those with Disability Status Scales of 7 or greater (wheelchair-confined) who were beginning to lose function of upper extremities. Fifty-six percent of those treated were female.

TABLE 3. Patients Treated with High-Dose Cyclophosphamide/ACTH

Brigham and Women's Hospital		143
On protocol	121	
Off protocol	22	
Retreatment	(24)	
Patients Treated in Other Centers		171
Boston, MA	35	
Rochester, NY	26	
Philadelphia, PA	23	
Washington, DC	19	
Allentown, PA	18	
Burlington, VT	17	
Fargo, ND	12	
Waterbury, CT	11	
Atlanta, GA	10	
Total Patients Treated		314

TABLE 4. Characterization of Patients Treated with Cyclophosphamide/ACTH

DSS at Time of Treatment	
3	3%
4	7%
5	16%
6a	27% (unilateral support)
6b	34% (bilateral support)
7	13%
Years of Progression prior to Treatment	
less than 1 year	36%
1–2 years	18%
2–3 years	15%
3–6 years	20%
6–10 years	11%
Age of Patients Treated	
under 20	1%
20–25	7%
26–30	8%
31–35	26%
36–40	17%
41–45	18%
46–50	12%
51–60	9%
over 60	2%

Since the publication of our work a number of physicians has begun to treat selected patients with severe progressive disease with the cyclophosphamide/ACTH regimen. TABLE 3 also lists the number of patients treated by nine physicians who have been in contact with us and who have treated 10 or more patients. We have records of 171 patients treated by other physicians. Although it must be emphasized that all of these patients were treated in an uncontrolled fashion, the response to therapy in terms of stabilization or improvement of patients with progressive disease has, for the most part, been consistent with our published results. In addition, complications and side effects of treatment have been similar to our experience (discussed below).

Characterization of the 143 patients we have treated thus far in terms of age, disability status at the time of treatment, and years of progression prior to treatment is contained in TABLE 4. TABLE 5 records the white blood cell count nadir following both first and second treatments. As follow-up is obtained, it may be possible to determine the extent to which these parameters affect clinical response.

Risks Associated with Therapy

The toxicity of cyclophosphamide is well known in terms of its bone marrow suppressive effects, its potential bladder toxicity, and the potential risks for later malignancies.[15–21] In the 314 patients we have on record as having been treated with this regimen there have been no fatalities. There have been five incidents of minor infections controlled with antibiotics, and one report of osteomyelitis that developed in a patient 12 days after discharge from the hospital. Virtually all patients have had temporary alopecia. There has been no reported lung, cardiac, or liver toxicity. In terms of bladder toxicity, microscopic hematuria has been observed on urinalysis in approximately 3% of patients, and three patients developed frank bleed which responded to discontinuation of medication. Approximately one-third of patients experienced nausea and 5% have had vomiting. Disturbances in menstruation, decreased sperm counts, and early cessation of menses have also been observed. It is too early at this time to assess long-term toxic effects in terms of later-developing malignancies.

TABLE 5. Nadir of White Blood Count Following Treatment

	First Treatment	Second Treatment
Greater than 3,000	2%	—
2,500–3,000	7%	6%
2,000–2,500	12%	19%
1,500–2,000	25%	26%
1,000–1,500	23%	15%
500–1,000	15%	19%
Below 500	16%	15%

It should be noted that there are not much data in the literature on the effects of short-course high-dose cyclophosphamide given in patients who are not being treated for malignant disease. European studies do not report an increased incidence of malignancy in MS patients treated and followed for 5 to 10 years.[5,6] Most investigators feel that prolonged oral administration of cyclophosphamide is of greater risk than intermittent intravenous therapy. This has led us to refrain from using prolonged oral cyclophosphamide in MS patients. A recent editorial in the *New England Journal of Medicine* has addressed the issue of administering cyclophosphamide in a manner that will increase its efficacy and reduce its potential toxicity.[22] As stated in the editorial:

> Daily cyclophosphamide treatment puts the patient at risk every day with regard to bladder complications, infections, and chromosomal abnormalities that may lead to lymphoma or leukemia. In contrast, treatment with intermittent boluses of cyclophosphamide (*e.g.*, 0.75 to 1.0 g per square meter of body-surface area every three to four weeks) limits the risk of those complications to only a dozen or so days a year. Moreover, the risk of bladder irritation may be guarded against by intravenous administration of large volumes of fluids in the 24 hours after treatment (given with saline, since cyclophosphamide has an antidiuretic hormone-like effect). Prophylactic administration of antiemetics can reduce the nausea that follows large intravenous boluses of cyclophosphamide. Careful monitoring of the white cell count and appropriate alteration of the next drug dose may minimize the chance of infection. It is not yet clear whether the risk of malignant disease is also decreased by intermittent bolus treatment; however, preliminary studies in animals and human subjects suggest that the risk is not increased and may well be decreased.[22]

In summary, it appears that acute complications associated with therapy, apart from alopecia, occur in between 1–3% of patients and long-term effects remain unknown at the present time. One factor that we have noticed, and that other physicians have reported as well, is the tendency to unrealistic hopes in patients undergoing therapy. It must be repeatedly explained to any patient and to any physician who elects to treat with this form of therapy, whether on or off protocol, that the purpose of treatment is to stabilize disease progression and that the treatment does not represent a cure.

Requirements for Administration of ACTH Concomitantly with Cyclophosphamide

It is impossible to tell from our studies whether ACTH is needed for the effect seen with high-dose cyclophosphamide, although some physicians who have treated patients without ACTH have reported similar effects using cyclophosphamide alone.

Placebo Effect and Measurement of Clinical Response

Because it was impossible for us to carry out these studies in a double-blind fashion, the issue of placebo effects in this treatment must be considered. We feel that placebo effects are unlikely to be responsible for the positive effects we have observed for the following reasons: (1) patients have been randomized to different treatment groups; (2) chronic progressive multiple sclerosis rarely remits spontaneously, and the patients treated in whom a positive response has occurred have been patients whose disease has inexorably progressed, despite previous treatments with prednisone, ACTH, and other agents; (3) we have treated chronic progressive patients on other protocols which we have not found to be effective, including ACTH alone, lymphocytapheresis, and ACTH in association with plasmapheresis. These patients had identical hopes for a positive response and were hospitalized and given identical care and physician attention. Nonetheless, further controlled studies with cyclophosphamide in chronic progressive MS are required.

We have used a variety of scales to measure the clinical response and have found that the most valuable of these are the Ambulation Index and the Kurtzke Disability Status Scale. Quantitative neurological examination and functional status scales have not been as helpful in assessing response to therapy.

What is the Role of Cyclophosphamide in the Treatment of Multiple Sclerosis and How Should It Be Used?

We feel that the use of cyclophosphamide should be restricted to experimental treatment programs or to carefully selected patients with severely progressive disease who have not responded to conventional treatment programs. The issue of acute toxicity from administration of the medicine has been reasonably well addressed in over 300 patients treated thus far and remains minimal, although clear risks are present. Long-term risks and risks from multiple retreatments have not yet been defined. The major therapeutic question that must be addressed relates to retreatment and maintenance programs. It is clear that one 10–14 day treatment is not sufficient to halt progression of disease indefinitely. To this end, current treatment programs involve retreatment at defined intervals and programs involving maintenance therapy in the form of intravenous boosters given every two months following induction. Whether these maintenance or retreatment programs will be of benefit, and the long-term toxic effects of treatment, remain to be determined. In addition, a variety of physicians is beginning to treat selected patients with high-dose cyclophosphamide. We feel it is imperative that records be kept of such patients in order to assess long-term toxicity and, furthermore, it is most appropriate that patients be treated as part of specific randomized protocols. To this end, a Northeastern Cooperative Multiple Sclerosis Treatment Group has been created for the purpose of treating patients uniformly and gathering data according to specific randomized protocols.

The issues confronting us in the use of cyclophosphamide are illustrated by the case of a 16-year-old girl who was admitted to the hospital with a malignantly progressive case of multiple sclerosis that did not respond to high doses of prednisone. The patient was confined to her hospital bed. Following treatment with a course of ACTH, high-dose cyclophosphamide and plasma exchange, there was cessation of progression and recovery to preillness clinical status. The patient was able to return to school. Four months following treatment, disease progression recommenced and again was unresponsive to a course of prednisone. The patient was retreated with ACTH/high-dose cyclophosphamide, with a clear response to therapy and a return to virtually normal neurologic status. The patient was then followed without treatment and six months thereafter began progressing again, with new neurologic findings. At this time, the patient was treated over a six-week period as an outpatient with six weekly injections of cyclophosphamide (700 mg/m^2 per injection). This regimen induced a remission. The patient was then placed on maintenance IV boosters every two months. However, after three boosters the patient's symptoms began again; the patient was placed on maintenance boosters every three weeks and remained stable on this regimen for approximately 12 months. Booster injections were then tapered so that she now receives them every two months. Her disease has remained stable. Although she is atypical in terms of age of onset and severe nature of the illness and her treatment was carried out in an uncontrolled fashion, this patient illustrates two major issues and lines of clinical investigation currently being pursued with the use of cyclophosphamide: (1) the need for retreatment when reprogression occurs, and (2) the issue of maintenance therapy following an induction of remission to maintain a remission. Current plans involve continued tapering and discontinuing maintenance boosters over the coming year.

We believe that an important implication of our work with immunosuppression is that multiple sclerosis is an autoimmune disease that may respond to immunosuppressive therapy. Presumably, cyclophosphamide is acting by destroying immunocompetent lymphocytes in the central nervous system and/or peripheral immune system. Cyclophosphamide has been reported to enter the central nervous system in MS patients.[23] Clearly, a more specific form of immunosuppression or immunotherapy with less potential toxicity is needed, plus a laboratory monitor of immune abnormalities to determine who should be treated and when retreatment should be given. In a pilot study, we did not find that removal of cells from the peripheral circulation via lymphocytapheresis was of benefit.[4] A next step we have embarked on is to treat multiple sclerosis using monoclonal antibodies against T cells. At present, we feel that the use of short courses of high-dose cyclophosphamide offers a treatment modality that is available to the neurologist as a therapeutic option in carefully selected patients with actively progressive multiple sclerosis that have not responded to conventional treatment programs.

ACKNOWLEDGMENT

We would like to thank Ms. Pat Lamy-Gilbreath for her excellent help in the preparation of the manuscript.

REFERENCES

1. Weiner, H. L. & D. M. Dawson. 1980. Plasmapheresis in multiple sclerosis: Preliminary study. Neurology **30:** 1029–1033.

2. HAUSER, S. L., M. FOSBURG, S. KEVY & H. L. WEINER. 1982. Plasmapheresis, lymphocytapheresis, and immunosuppressive drug therapy in multiple sclerosis. *In* Therapeutic Apheresis and Plasma Perfusion. R. S. A. Tindall, Ed.: 239–254. Alan R. Liss. New York.

3. HAUSER, S. L., D. M. DAWSON, J. R. LEHRICH, M. F. BEAL, S. V. KEVY, R. D. PROPPER, J. A. MILLS & H. L. WEINER, 1983. Intensive immunosuppression in progressive multiple sclerosis. A randomized, three-arm study of high-dose intravenous cyclophosphamide, plasma exchange, and ACTH. N. Engl. J. Med. **308:** 173–180.

4. HAUSER, S. L., M. FOSBURG, S. V. KEVY & H. L. WEINER. 1984. Lymphocytapheresis in chronic progressive multiple sclerosis: Immunologic and clinical effects. Neurology **34:** 922–926.

5. GONSETTE, R. E., L. DEMONTY & P. DELMOTTE. 1977. Intensive immunosuppression with cyclophosphamide in multiple sclerosis: Follow-up of 110 patients for 2–6 years. J. Neurol. **214:** 173–181.

6. HOMMES, O. R., K. J. B. LAMERS & P. REEKERS, 1980. Effect of intensive immunosuppression on the course of chronic progressive multiple sclerosis. J. Neurol. **223:** 177–190.

7. ELLISON, G. W. & L. W. MYERS. 1978. A review of systemic nonspecific immunosuppressive treatment of multiple sclerosis. Neurology (Minneapolis) **28**(9:Part 2): 132–139.

8. MULLER, R. 1949. Studies on disseminated sclerosis: with special reference to symptomatology, course, and prognosis. Acta Med. Scand. Suppl. **222:** 1–214.

9. MCALPINE, D. & N. COMPSTON. 1952. Some aspects of the natural history of disseminated sclerosis. Q. J. Med. **21:** 135–167.

10. BAUER, J. J., W. FIRNHABER & W. WINKLER. 1965. Prognostic criteria in multiple sclerosis. Ann. N.Y. Acad. Sci. **122:** 542–551.

11. NOSEWORTHY, J., T. WONNACOTT, D. W. PATY & G. C. EBERS. 1983. Markers and prognosis in multiple sclerosis (Abstract). Ann. Neurol. **14:** 114.

12. WEINER, H. L., P. DAU, G. BIRNBAUM, M. FELDSTEIN, B. KHATRI, J. PETAJAN & M. P. MCQUILLEN. 1983. Plasma exchange in acute multiple sclerosis. Design of a cooperative study. Arch. Neurol. **40:** 691–692.

13. DRACHMAN, D. A., P. Y. PATERSON, R. T. SCHMIDT & R. F. SPEHLMANN. 1975. Cyclophosphamide in exacerbations of multiple sclerosis. Therapeutic trial and a strategy for pilot drug studies. J. Neurol. Neurosurg. Psychiat. **38:** 592–597.

14. WEINER, H. L. & G. W. ELLISON. 1983. A working protocol to be used as a guideline for trials in multiple sclerosis. Arch. Neurol. **40:** 704–710.

15. COOPERATING CLINICS COMMITTEE OF THE AMERICAN RHEUMATISM ASSOCIATION. 1970. A controlled trial of cyclophosphamide in rheumatoid arthritis. N. Engl. J. Med. **283:** 883–889.

16. WOLFF, S. M., A. S. FAUCI, R. G. HORN & D. C. DALE. 1974. Wegener's granulomatosis. Ann. Intern. Med. **81:** 513–525.

17. ARBEITSGEMEINSCHAFT FÜR PADIATRISCHE NEPHROLOGIE. 1982. Effect of cytotoxic drugs in frequently relapsing nephrotic syndrome with and without steroid dependence. N. Engl. J. Med. **306:** 451–454.

18. DONADIO, J. V., JR., K. E. HOLLEY, R. H. FERGUSON & D. M. ILSTRUP. 1978. Treatment of diffuse proliferative lupus nephritis with prednisone and combined prednisone and cyclophosphamide. N. Engl. J. Med. **299:** 1151–1155.

19. PLOTZ, P. H., J. H. KLIPPEL, J. L. DECKER *et al.* 1979. Bladder complications in patients receiving cyclophosphamide for systemic lupus erythematosus or rheumatoid arthritis. Ann. Intern. Med. **91:** 221–223.

20. IARC WORKING GROUP ON THE EVALUATION OF THE CARCINOGENIC RISK OF CHEMICALS TO HUMANS. Some antineoplastic and immunosuppressive agents. IARC Monogr. Eval. Carcinogenic Risk Chem. Hum. **26:** 1–387.

21. CASCIATO, D. A. & J. L. SCOTT. 1981. Acute leukemia following prolonged cytotoxic agent therapy. Medicine (Baltimore) **58:** 32–47.

22. STEINBERG, A. D. 1984. Cyclophosphamide. Should it be used daily, monthly, or never? (Editorial). N. Engl. J. Med. **310:** 458–459.

23. HOMMES, O. R., F. AERTS, U. BAHR & H.-R. SCHULTEN. 1983. Cyclophosphamide levels in serum and spinal fluid of multiple sclerosis patients treated with immunosuppression. J. Neurol. Sci. **85:** 297–303.

Clinical Trial of Natural Alpha Interferon in Multiple Sclerosis[a]

ROBERT L. KNOBLER,[b] HILLEL S. PANITCH,[c]
SHERRY L. BRAHENY,[b] JACK C. SIPE,[b]
GEORGE P. A. RICE,[b] JOHN R. HUDDLESTONE,[b]
GORDON S. FRANCIS,[c] CAROL J. HOOPER,[c]
ROBERTA M. KAMIN-LEWIS,[c] KENNETH P. JOHNSON,[c]
MICHAEL B. A. OLDSTONE,[b] AND
THOMAS C. MERIGAN[d]

[b]*Department of Immunology and Division of Neurology*
Scripps Clinic and Research Foundation
La Jolla, California 92093

[c]*Department of Neurology*
University of California
San Francisco, California 94143

[d]*Division of Infectious Diseases*
Department of Medicine
Stanford University
Stanford, California 94305

INTRODUCTION

The present report describes the first controlled trial of natural human alpha interferon (HuIFN-α) in the treatment of multiple sclerosis (MS). Plans for this randomized double-blinded, placebo-controlled crossover study were initiated in 1979, despite limited availability of HuIFN-α,[1] demands for clinical trials in other diseases, and high costs associated with production and quality control which in turn limited the number of patients that could be treated. Nevertheless, preliminary studies implicating deficient IFN production in MS,[2] coupled with observations of immunological aberrations in MS[3,4] confirmed in several laboratories by a variety of techniques,[5,6] and expanding knowledge of the potent immunomodulatory properties of IFN[7] suggested it

[a]This is publication no. 3266 from the Department of Immunology, Scripps Clinic and Research Foundation, La Jolla, California 92037. This work was supported by National Multiple Sclerosis Society Research grant nos. 1285, 1287 and 1307, United States Public Health Service grant nos. NS–12428 and NS–14069, National Institutes of Health grant no. RR00833 to the General Clinical Research Center at Scripps Clinic and Research Foundation, and grants from the Leiper Trust and the McDonald and Hearst Foundations. Robert L. Knobler was the Ralph I. Straus Fellow of the National Multiple Sclerosis Society during this study and currently is a recipient of Teacher Investigator Development Award no. NS–00803, from the National Institute of Neurological and Communicative Disorders and Stroke. George P. A. Rice is a recipient of the Centennial Fellowship from the Medical Research Council of Canada. Gordon S. Francis was the recipient of a Medical Research Council of Canada Fellowship.

could therapeutically alter the course of MS. This study was thus designed primarily to test the efficacy of this preparation administered systemically in reducing the frequency of exacerbations and affecting the clinical status of patients with the exacerbating-remitting form of multiple sclerosis. A second goal was to determine the need for and approach to subsequent trials of IFN in multiple sclerosis. Finally, the study also provided an opportunity for detailed analysis of selected effects of IFN on specific immune functions, as well as the opportunity to study immune parameters in MS patients with an exacerbating-remitting course in order to investigate the relationship of these to disease activity.

STUDY DESIGN

A placebo-controlled, crossover format was adopted to allow each patient to receive treatment with IFN within the course of the study, as well as to provide an internal control for the placebo response and spontaneous remissions known to be prominent in MS.[8] A total of 24 patients with clinically definite MS,[9,10] selected from two independent clinical centers, was involved. Patients were randomized by an unblinded investigator (TCM) according to age, sex and frequency of exacerbations. The code for medication assignment was sent directly to the study pharmacist at each of the two clinical centers, who prepared a separate syringe containing IFN or placebo for each daily injection. A fresh supply of medication, stored on dry ice, was picked up weekly or monthly throughout the study. Patients were instructed to keep all medication frozen until the day of use, to thaw the medication completely and to self-administer the preparations intramuscularly at multiple injection sites.

Interferon was administered systemically rather than intrathecally or intraventricularly. The rationale for selecting the intramuscular route was based on preliminary studies implicating deficient IFN production by peripheral blood leukocytes of MS patients,[2] evidence for systemic immunological aberrations affecting T suppressor cells in MS,[3–6] and lack of evidence that IFN given intrathecally reaches the CNS parenchyma any better than IFN given systemically. In addition, ease of administration was a factor to consider in a trial of a therapeutic agent which, were it to succeed, might require frequent or perhaps daily injection for an indefinite period of time. Finally, safety was a major consideration. The potential for long-term complications of intrathecal therapy such as adhesive arachnoiditis would be unacceptable in treating a disease which often, but unpredictably, runs a relatively benign course permitting long periods of active productive life. The dosage and frequency of IFN administration in this clinical trial were chosen empirically, based upon the amount of IFN available and previous experience with this particular preparation.

Daily injections of either the Cantell[1] preparation of HuIFN-α (5×10^6 IU daily) or placebo were given for six months. A washout period of six months preceded crossover to the opposite treatment for six months, which was then followed by a second six-month washout period. All patients were hospitalized for the first three to four days when beginning treatment, in order to closely monitor their reaction to institution of treatment, and were given 650 mg of acetominophen four times daily throughout this period to minimize febrile reaction to the medication. Great care was taken to treat all patients identically with regard to injection schedules, number of examinations and procedures performed during all phases of the study. Neurological evaluation included a complete neurological examination, lumbar puncture and evoked potential studies—all performed at standardized intervals. Some physicians followed only the patients' clinical status, whereas others were only involved in the research laboratory tests that might reveal the nature of the code. Exacerbations were defined as acute or subacute objective worsening of neurological status with subsequent stabilization and/or recovery of the affected functions.

Patients were instructed to contact study physicians in the event of any problem, including illness other than MS, and not to take any other medications without their prior knowledge and approval. Women were advised against becoming pregnant because of unknown risk to the unborn child of IFN or taking birth control pills because of potential uncontrolled effects on immune functions. In the event of significant toxicity or unexpected illness requiring treatment which could compromise the nature of the study, a telephone conference among physicians at the University of California, San Francisco, Scripps Clinic and Research Foundation and Stanford University would be arranged to decide the course to follow. Conference calls were also made on a few occasions to decide whether patients with particularly severe exacerbations should be treated with short courses of corticosteroids.

PATIENT SELECTION

Twelve patients were selected for participation in this study at each of the two clinical centers in La Jolla and San Francisco. They had experienced two or more documented exacerbations over the two-year period prior to inclusion in the study, and were thus selected on the basis of clinical evidence of acute exacerbating-remitting disease. Patients were interviewed along with important support persons, such as a spouse or parents, to ensure a broad base of support for continuing involvement considering the lifestyle modifications associated with participation in the study. Consideration was also given to other factors that could influence the response of the patients, including their commitment to participate in the protocol, adjustment to MS, geographical accessibility to the treatment center, restriction on taking holidays because of the need to pick up medication periodically and to keep it frozen, adjustment to the lengthy period of observation with repeated invasive procedures such as venipuncture and lumbar puncture, the potential for side effects of the medication, and the possibility that the treatment being tested would not be effective. Informed consent was obtained from all patients.

PATIENT EVALUATION

Evaluation included the standard neurological examination at each scheduled follow-up visit. The examination findings were quantitated retrospectively by the Kurtzke Disability Status Score (DSS)[11] and by the newly developed Scripps Neurological Rating Scale (NRS) for MS.[12] The latter was devised to reflect findings on the neurological examination that commonly occur in MS, and to express these findings quantitatively with a score of 100 points for a normal neurological examination, and point reductions that would correspond to degree of neurological deficit. Serial laboratory tests included hematologic, hepatic and renal profiles during hospitalization and at each clinic visit. Peripheral blood cells were also analyzed for studies on natural killer (NK) cell function, utilizing ^{51}chromium-labeled K-562 target cells in a four-hour assay,[13] as well as analysis of T cell subsets utilizing the OKT4 and OKT8 or Leu 2a and Leu 3a+3b monoclonal antibodies.[14,15] In addition, serum was stored at −70°C for studies of interferon titer, immunoglobulin subclass, immune complexes, classical and alternative complement pathway components and activation as well as other measurements. Cerebrospinal fluid was obtained prior to the onset of each drug phase, during each hospitalization and at periodic intervals thereafter, and was analyzed for cell count, immunoglobulin indices, and oligoclonal bands and stored for later studies. Clinical neurophysiological testing included visual evoked responses, brainstem auditory evoked responses and somatosensory evoked responses, which were performed at the study onset, at six-month intervals and at other times when clinically indicated.

FINDINGS AND DISCUSSION

Fewer exacerbations occurred during both IFN and placebo phases than had occurred during comparable intervals in the prestudy period. When receiving IFN, patients had even fewer exacerbations than when receiving placebo, but this difference was only of borderline statistical significance. Comparing the results with regard to the sequence of treatment (IFN-placebo vs. placebo-IFN), a greater reduction in number of exacerbations was noted during the IFN phase following the placebo phase. This pattern of clinical response associated with treatment sequence in a crossover design suggests a "learning" response by the patient. Despite careful attempts to mask side effects of IFN therapy, their occurrence may have suggested to patients the nature of their drug therapy. Although patients and physicians made a sufficient number of different errors when queried on treatment assignments to suggest blinding was effectively maintained, the occurrence of even minor side effects could have led patients to believe that they would experience either greater or fewer exacerbations in the second treatment phase based upon their perception of the treatment received in the previous phase. The mechanism of this placebo-like "learning" effect would presumably be similar to the more conventional type of placebo response in MS.[8]

The reduction in frequency of exacerbations during IFN treatment was not associated with long-term clinical improvement for the study group as a whole. During IFN treatment and its washout period there was a drop in the mean NRS score per patient for those receiving IFN before placebo, and minimal change for those receiving placebo first. Kurtzke DSS scores reflected similar changes in functional status. However, certain patients seemed to improve or remained stable while others worsened. When patients were segregated according to clinical course, those with strictly exacerbating-remitting disease had the fewest exacerbations with IFN treatment, independently of treatment sequence, and accounted for the overall reduction in exacerbations for the entire patient group.[16] The remaining patients had exacerbations superimposed upon a chronic progressive course, and did less well while on IFN and throughout the study, experiencing either exacerbations or clinical worsening or both.[16] Exacerbation severity, based on change in the Scripps NRS scores and duration, was less severe in the strictly exacerbating-remitting subgroup than in the exacerbating chronic progressive subgroup.[16]

There were no consistent associations observed for clinical course with such factors as age, sex, HLA phenotype or duration of MS.[16] Visual, auditory and somatosensory evoked responses also showed no distinct trends related to IFN treatment (results to be reported elsewhere). Cellular and humoral immune parameters were evaluated. Studies demonstrated that NK cell function was normal in MS, with activation following IFN but not placebo treatment. Suppressor T lymphocytes, marked with the OKT8 or Leu 2a monoclonal antibodies, fluctuated independently of treatment phase and disease activity.[14,15] Circulating immune complexes were detected in association with development of antibody to a contaminant in the IFN preparation, and remained markedly elevated only during the IFN treatment phase.[14] Studies of classical and alternative complement pathway components and activation are currently in progress. Immunoglobulin levels and oligoclonal bands in the CSF were reduced during administration of IFN in some patients, and fluctuated independently of clinical course or treatment in others.[14,15] Occasionally, new bands, usually at the anodal end of the immunoglobulin region, were seen.[15]

IFN levels were assessed at frequent intervals during all phases of the study, but were detectable only during IFN treatment. The mean levels varied greatly and did not correlate with either body weight or clinical response. Using IFN levels as a measure of compliance showed that all patients continued to self-administer IFN despite the occurrence of sometimes unpleasant symptoms. IFN levels in serum during the washout phases and during administration of placebo were invariably nondetectable. In addition, CSF from several patients did not contain detectable levels of IFN even during the treatment period. Studies of IFN administration on endogenous IFN production and cellular responsiveness to IFN were also carried out and will be reported elsewhere.[e]

Side effects of IFN therapy were adequately tolerated, and rapidly reversible upon discontinuation of treatment. They included febrile reaction, granulocytopenia, elevation of hepatic enzymes, fatiguability, hair loss, localized skin reactions at injection sites, weight loss and depression, all of which were transient, though in some cases severe enough to interfere with normal activity. Other isolated problems related to the administration of IFN included symptoms suggesting an occult neoplasm (malaise and weight loss), diffuse lymphadenopathy, fever of unknown origin (opportunistic infection with *Salmonella dublin*), a possible breast mass (an isolated hypertropic lymph node) and altered mental status which required evaluation, but for which no cause other than IFN treatment could be found. The high degree of motivation among MS patients to participate in clinical therapeutic studies contributed greatly to the successful completion of this trial.

The observations of the present study highlight the importance and difficulties inherent in constructing and evaluating a placebo-controlled, blinded, crossover trial of any therapeutic regimen proposed as a treatment for MS. It is in this light that the recent controversy over the effectiveness of IFN in the treatment of MS[17] originated, based upon an earlier, nonblinded study of intrathecal human beta interferon in MS,[18,19] which reported significant reduction in the frequency of exacerbations. However, continuously scheduled intrathecal delivery in the treatment group, compared to infrequently manipulated untreated controls, precluded blinding and quite probably fostered a major placebo effect, which was not accounted for in the final analysis. In contrast, incorporation of a double-blinded placebo treatment phase in the present study clearly allowed us to distinguish the impact of "involved" placebo participation from that of IFN treatment in reducing the occurrence of exacerbations, as had also been demonstrated in an earlier clinical trial of placebo vs. ACTH in multiple sclerosis.[20] These findings underscore the critical importance of trial design in subsequent interpretations of results.

On the other hand, the crossover format may have contributed an additional complication, the placebo-like response of the "learning" effect discussed earlier. The crossover design was utilized to provide each study participant with IFN treatment as well as placebo. At the time the present study was initiated, both high cost and limited availability of IFN restricted its supply to 24 patients, making the crossover design the only feasible alternative. We decided, therefore, to treat 24 patients with both placebo and IFN rather than treat two 24 patient groups with either IFN alone or placebo

[e] See Kamin-Lewis *et al.* 1984. J. Interferon Res. **4:** 423–428.

alone. Presently, the availability of cloned IFN would allow provision of such therapy to even the placebo control group, if proved effective after a formal evaluation, obviating similar future needs for a crossover design.

The clinical response in our patients, as well as changes in CSF immunoglobulin levels and oligoclonal bands in some patients, indicated that the systemic route was effective, and points the way toward design of future clinical trials. Trials of intrathecal or intraventricular IFN in MS require superior results or specific indications in order to be considered clinically preferable. More recent research using recombinant DNA techniques has shown that there are approximately fifteen distinct molecular forms of alpha IFN, as well as single forms of beta and gamma, most of which are now or soon will be available for therapeutic trials in MS and other diseases. Variables of effectiveness, including dosage, route, and frequency of administration must be carefully evaluated for each of these preparations. Our results indicate that additional trials of systemic IFN therapy for MS patients, utilizing placebo-controlled, double-blinded designs without crossover are warranted.

ACKNOWLEDGMENTS

The authors at Scripps Clinic and Research Foundation would like to acknowledge the nursing assistance of Kaye Smith, Stacy Taylor, Margaret Floyd, Nancy Puariea and Mary Kelly, technical assistance of Kendis Cox, Pamela Elliott and Aparna Ewing of the General Clinical Research Center and John Magee of the pharmacy, and Gay L. Wilkins for assistance in manuscript preparation. The authors at the University of California wish to acknowledge the assistance of Donald O. Kimble and William L. Schalker of the Pharmacy Service; the nursing assistance of Kate O'Hare and the staff of the Special Diagnostic and Treatment Unit of the VA Medical Center, San Francisco; the technical assistance of Paula Fukushima and Elena Bleumers; and the secretarial assistance of Regina Flynn. B.W. Brown, Jr. of the Division of Biostatistics, Department of Family, Community and Preventative Medicine, Stanford University provided biostatistical advice and assistance on the analysis and interpretation of some of the results.

The authors also wish to acknowledge the commitment and continued support of the patients and their families who helped to make this study possible.

REFERENCES

1. CANTELL, K. & S. HIRRONAN. 1978. Large-scale production of human leukocyte interferon. J. Gen. Virol. **39:** 541–543.
2. NEIGHBOUR, P. A. & B. R. BLOOM. 1979. Absence of virus-induced lymphocyte suppression and interferon production in multiple sclerosis. Proc. Natl. Acad. Sci. U.S.A. **76:** 476–480.
3. HUDDLESTONE, J. R. & M. B. A. OLDSTONE. 1979. T suppressor (T_G) lymphocytes fluctuate in parallel with changes in the clinical course of patients with multiple sclerosis. J. Immunol. **123:** 1615–1618.
4. ANTEL, J. P., B. G. ARNASON & M. E. MEDOF. 1979. Suppressor cell function in multiple sclerosis: Correlation with clinical disease activity. Ann. Neurol. **5:** 338–342.
5. REINHERZ, E. L., H. L. WEINER, S. L. HAUSER, J. A. COHEN, J. A. DISTASO & S. F. SCHLOSSMAN. 1980. Loss of suppressor T cells in active MS. Analysis with monoclonal antibody. N. Engl. J. Med. **303:** 125–129.
6. COYLE, P. K., B. R. BROOKS, R. L. HIRSCH, S. R. COHEN, P. O'DONNELL, R. T. JOHNSON & J. S. WOLINSKY. 1980. Cerebrospinal-fluid lymphocyte populations and immune complexes in active multiple sclerosis. Lancet **ii:** 229–231.

7. Stiehm, E. R., L. H. Kronenberg, H.M. Rosenblatt, Y. Bryson & T. C. Merigan. 1982. Interferon: Immunobiology and clinical significance. Ann. Intern. Med. **96:** 80–93.
8. McAlpine, D., C. E. Lumsden & E. D. Acheson. 1972. Multiple sclerosis: A reappraisal. 2d ed. Williams and Wilkins. Baltimore.
9. McDonald, W. I. & A. M. Halliday. 1977. Diagnosis and classification of multiple sclerosis. Br. Med. Bull. **3:** 4–9.
10. Poser, C. M., D. W. Paty. L. C. Scheinberg, W. I. McDonald, F. A. Donnis, G. C. Ebers, K. P. Johnson, W. A. Sibley, D. H. Silberberg & W. W. Tourtellotte. 1983. New diagnostic criteria for multiple sclerosis: Guidelines for research protocols. Ann. Neurol. **13:** 227–231.
11. Kurtzke, J. F. 1965. Further notes on disability evaluation in multiple sclerosis, with scale modifications. Neurology **15:** 654–661.
12. Sipe, J. C., R. L. Knobler, S. L. Braheny, G. P. A. Rice, H. S. Panitch & M. B. A. Oldstone. 1984. A neurological rating scale (NRS) for use in multiple sclerosis. Neurology **34:** 1368–1372.
13. Rice, G. P. A., P. Casali, T. C. Merigan & M. B. A. Oldstone. 1983. Natural killer cell activity in patients with multiple sclerosis given alpha interferon. Ann. Neurol. **14:** 333–338.
14. Rice, G. P. A., P. Talbot, E. M. Woelfel, B. Vandvik, S. L. Braheny, R. L. Knobler, J. C. Sipe & M. B. A. Oldstone. 1984. Immunological observations in patients with multiple sclerosis treated with human alpha interferon. Neurology **34**(Suppl. 1):112.
15. Pantich, H. S., G. S. Francis, C. J. Hooper, P. I. Fukushima, E. B. Bleumens & K. P. Johnson. 1984. Serial immunological studies in multiple sclerosis (MS) patients treated with natural alpha interferon (IFN). Neurology **34**(Suppl. 1):111.
16. Knobler, R. L., H. S. Panitch, S. L. Braheny, J. C. Sipe, G. P. A. Rice, J. R. Huddlestone, G. S. Francis, C. J. Hooper, R. M. Kamin-Lewis, J. P. Johnson, M. B. A. Oldstone & T. C. Merigan. 1984. Systemic alpha interferon in multiple sclerosis: A controlled clinical trial. Neurology **34:** 1273–1279.
17. Abb, J., F. Deinhardt, H. Zander, R. B. Tenser, F. Rapp, J. M. Goust, H. H. Fundenberg, J. Vilcek, M. Ho, T. C. Merigan, M. B. A. Oldstone & G. G. Jackson. 1982. Trials of interferon therapy for multiple sclerosis. J. Infect. Dis. **146:** 109–115.
18. Jacobs, L., J. O'Malley, A. Freeman & R. Ekes. 1981. Intrathecal interferon reduces exacerbations of multiple sclerosis. Science **214:** 1026–1028.
19. Jacobs, L., J. O'Malley, A. Freeman & R. Ekes. 1982. Intrathecal interferon in multiple sclerosis. Arch. Neurol. **39:** 609–615.
20. Rose, A. S., J. W. Kuzma, J. F. Kurtzke, N. S. Namerow, W. A. Sibley & W. W. Tourtellotte. 1970. Cooperative study in the evaluation of therapy in multiple sclerosis: ACTH vs. placebo. Final report. Neurology **20**(5, Part 2):1–59.

Plasmapheresis and Combined Immunosuppressive Drug Therapy in Chronic Progressive Multiple Sclerosis

Choosing the Patient Who Should Respond

BHUPENDRA O. KHATRI,[a] MICHAEL P. McQUILLEN,[a] AND SUSAN KOETHE[b]

[a]*Department of Neurology*
[b]*Department of Pathology*
Medical College of Wisconsin
Milwaukee, Wisconsin 53226

INTRODUCTION

Based on the assumptions that multiple sclerosis (MS) is an autoimmune disorder,[1–9] and that plasmapheresis (PP) is an effective means of removing antibodies and other proteins from the circulation,[10] several pilot studies have been undertaken to ascertain the role of PP in patients with MS.[11–14] Encouraging results from these uncontrolled studies and lack of any effective treatment for MS[15] led to a double-blind, randomized, controlled study of immunosuppressive drug therapy with and without plasmapheresis in chronic progressive MS (CPMS). This study[16] demonstrated statistically significant improvement in the Kurtzke Disability Status Scale (DSS)[17] in patients who received PP and immunosuppressive drug therapy, confirming our pilot study observations.[18] A retrospective analysis of this total experience was undertaken first to identify certain clinical and laboratory characteristics of the responders and nonresponders in both the pilot and double-blind study, and second, to determine the statistical significance of each of the characteristics in order eventually to predict those who should respond to this therapy.

METHODS

Patient Population

Only those patients who had participated in our pilot and double-blind studies were included in this analysis. All patients had clinically definite MS[19] with a chronic and progressive course as evidenced by continuous worsening (by one or more steps on the Kurtzke DSS) over the twelve months preceding the first plasmapheresis. These two criteria were followed rigidly for patient eligibility. Whenever there was a question as to either criterion, that question was settled by agreement between the judgements of two independent observing neurologists. Forty-five patients from the pilot study and twenty-six patients from the double-blind study, all of whom had received extensive PP and immunosuppressive drug therapy were thus included in these analyses. The twenty-nine patients who received sham PP and immunosuppressive drug therapy in the double-blind study served as a comparison group.

Treatment Regimen

Pilot Study. The equivalent of the patient's entire plasma volume, calculated as five percent of body weight, was exchanged during each PP procedure. The replacement fluid consisted of five percent albumin and normal saline in an equal ratio. Physiologic concentrations of calcium ions were added to all replacement fluids. In those patients who had either poor vascular access or blood flow ($\leq$ 30 ml/min), we employed a relatively simple technique[20] involving repeated femoral vein catheterization. Plasmapheresis was carried out weekly for up to ten exchanges and thereafter at gradually longer intervals as dictated by the patient's condition, until no further clinical improvement was noted. Ten grams of human serum globulin with local anesthetic solution were administered deeply intramuscular on each of the two days after each plasmapheresis. Immunosuppressive drug therapy consisting of cyclophosphamide (1–1.5 mg/kg body wt/day) and prednisone (1 mg/kg body wt/alternate day in declining dosages) was begun at the onset of PP and continued for a month after the last PP to prevent a rebound increase in the antibodies presumably removed by PP.[21]

Double-Blind Study

The study was designed as a prospective, randomized, double-blind–controlled comparison of immunosuppressive drug therapy, with and without plasma removal. All patients were randomized to receive either PP or sham PP, once a week for twenty weeks, in conjunction with immunosuppressive drug therapy and human serum globulin given in the regimen as described in the pilot study. Apheresis machines were set up in the same fashion for PP and for sham PP; a curtain was placed at all times between the patient and the machine. The sham PP patients received their own plasma back after its separation in the machine, whereas in true PP, the plasma was exchanged with five percent albumin and normal saline in equal ratios.

Neurological Evaluation and Follow-up

Kurtzke DSS[17] was utilized to measure the clinical changes. Each of the two neurologists "blinded" to the randomization evaluated the same patients once every two weeks. Evaluators did not have access to their findings on previous exams; they did not watch the procedures rendered to the patients; and most importantly, they did not function as "primary" physicians to the study patients to maintain complete "blindness." Follow-up evaluations in the pilot study were obtained at six monthly intervals for three years; in the double-blind study, at one, three, and six months post-PP/sham PP therapy.

Laboratory Studies

Computerized tomography of brain, with and without single-dose contrast using a high-resolution scanner (General Electric 8800) and standard visual, somatosensory and auditory evoked responses[22] were performed at entry and at completion of therapy. Suppressor-cell activity stimulated by concanavalin A (Con A) was determined just prior to and after a series of PP.[23] T cell subsets (T4 and T8) were measured in peripheral blood[6] in the double-blind study patients at entry and after a series of PP/sham PP treatments. HLA typing for antigens of the A, B and C loci was performed using the standard NIH-approved microlymphocytotoxicity assay in all patients.

Comparative Analyses

In order to predict responders to plasmapheresis and immunosuppressive drug therapy, several parameters were utilized in a statistical comparison between responders and nonresponders. Responders were defined as those who improved by one step or more in the Kurtzke DSS during the course of treatment. Clinical parameters included gender, age, severity of disease at beginning of treatment, total duration of disease and duration of disease progression, and predominant signs and symptoms. Although by definition all patients had involvement of the central nervous system at two or more sites, we classified them into three clinical groups, depending upon their predominant signs and symptoms (as summarized in TABLE 1). The laboratory parameters analyzed were standard evoked potentials (visual, auditory and somatosensory), computerized tomography of brain (with and without single-dose contrast), HLA typing, T cell subsets, and suppressor-cell functional activity.

TABLE 1. Clinical Categories Based on Predominant Signs and Symptoms

Cerebral[a]	Cerebellar	Spinal
hemiparesis	severe ataxia	para- or tetraparesis with little or no cranial nerve signs or ataxia
marked cognitive dysfunction	dysarthria	
seizures	nystagmus	

[a]Emotional problems alone were not classified as "cerebral MS." Patients receiving psychotropic drugs were evenly distributed among the two groups (PP and sham).

Statistical Analyses

For the pilot study, the Wilcoxon Signed Rank Test was used to compare the differences between Kurtzke DSS at entry, at termination, and at one- and three-year follow-up. Kurtzke DSS in PP and sham PP patients was compared using Student's t test for independent groups. In order to adjust for the possible effects of the age of the patient and duration of disease, these data were used in an analysis of covariants to compare the two treatments. Stepwise multiple regression analysis was used to identify the clinical factors that may predict an improvement in the Kurtzke DSS. Wilcoxon Rank Sum Test and Wilcoxon Signed Rank Test were used to compare the changes in suppressor-cell functional activity and in T cell subsets between the patients and normal controls, and from time to time in the same patients.

RESULTS

There were 13 men and 32 women in the pilot study, ranging in age from 23 to 59 years (mean 37.2) and in duration of disease from one year to 30 years (mean 8). All but one patient required more than 10 PP treatments (range 9 to 34) to reach maximum improvement. Based on the degree of improvement in Kurtzke DSS, the patients were divided into two groups (TABLE 2). Group I included patients who improved by one or more steps; in Group II the patients either remained the same or

TABLE 2. Clinical Characteristics of Pilot Study Patients

	Years				Kurtzke DSS			
							Follow-up	
	Sex	Age	Duration of MS	Duration of Disease Progression	Before	After	1 yr.	3 yrs.
Group I ($n = 28$)	21 F 7 M	35.6	7	1.4	7.1	4[a]	4.7[a]	5.1[a]
Group II ($n = 17$)	11 F 6 M	40.5	9.9	2.5	6.5	6.5	6.9	8.1

[a]Significance of improvement following therapy is at $p < 0.001$.

worsened. Twenty-eight of the 45 patients improved significantly ($p < 0.001$) on the Kurtzke DSS at conclusion of therapy, with improvement well maintained at three-year follow-up ($p < 0.001$). The clinical characteristics of patients in the pilot study are summarized in TABLE 2.

In the double-blind study, 26 patients received PP and 29 sham PP. The clinical characteristics and outcome in these patients are summarized in TABLE 3. There was no statistical difference in age, sex, total duration of illness, duration of disease progression or in severity of illness between the two groups. Of the 26 patients who received PP, 14 improved by one or more steps on the Kurtzke DSS; in the sham group, only eight of 29 patients improved. The degree of improvement was much larger in the PP group (TABLE 4). These differences were significant ($p < 0.007$) at the conclusion of therapy.

A comparison of responders and nonresponders failed to show any significant difference in age, gender, or in severity or duration of progression of disease. The total duration of disease was a significant predictor: patients whose illness had been less than 12 years in duration improved more than those whose illness was longer ($p < 0.05$). TABLE 5 shows the number of patients in each of the three clinical categories. Nineteen of the 21 patients with cerebral form of MS, who received PP, showed significant ($p < 0.0001$) improvement, with improvement well sustained during the follow-up period (TABLE 6). The range of improvement on Kurtzke DSS was by one to nine steps in the pilot study (mean 3.7) and one to four steps in the double-blind study (mean 2.5). On the other hand, in those patients with the cerebral form of MS who received sham PP and immunosuppressive drug therapy, no significant improvement was noted. Although patients with the predominantly cerebellar form of MS improved (3 out of 6 in the pilot study, and 4 out of 6 in the double-blind study), the degree of improvement

TABLE 3. Clinical Characteristics of Double-Blind Study Patients

	Years				Kurtzke DSS		
	Sex	Age	Duration of MS	Duration of Disease Progression	Before	After	Follow-up (11 Months)
PP ($n = 26$)	15 F 11 M	38.7	10.2	2.2	6.6	5.5[a,b]	5.9[a,b]
Sham ($n = 29$)	23 F 6 M	44.4	10.2	2.6	6.3	6.1	6.4

[a]The difference in overall improvement in the PP group as compared to sham group at conclusion is significant at $p < 0.007$.

[b]Improvement in the PP group (pre- vs. follow-up) is significant at $p < 0.07$.

TABLE 4. Changes in Kurtzke DSS: Double-Blind Study

	PP ($n = 26$)	Sham ($n = 29$)
Improvement (DSS)		
Three or more steps	5	—
Two steps	5	3
One step	4	5
Same	11	18
Worse (DSS)		
One step	1	—
Two or more steps	—	3

was not striking and the number of patients too small to do any statistical analysis (TABLE 7). In the spinal category the patients did not appear to improve; there was no statistical difference between the PP and the sham group (TABLE 8).

Of the laboratory parameters studied, we found no statistical difference between responders and nonresponders in pretreatment evoked potentials, computerized tomography of the brain, HLA typing, or in T cell subsets. The suppressor-cell functional activity of patients prior to PP was a significant predictor: the pretreatment suppressor-cell functional activity of 26 responders was significantly ($p < 0.003$) lower than the activity determined in 86 normal controls. Improvement in suppressor-cell activity in these patients following PP was significant ($p < 0.001$) when compared to their pretreatment values.

DISCUSSION

A significant therapeutic role for plasmapheresis with immunosuppressive drug therapy in chronic progressive multiple sclerosis patients was suggested by our open pilot study[18] and verified in our double-blind randomized controlled study.[16] This combination therapy brings about improvement in the Kurtzke Disability Status Scale (DSS) in over sixty percent of CPMS patients, with improvement well sustained in the majority of patients at three-year follow-up.

This degree of improvement in patients with chronic progressive disease has not been demonstrated—to the best of our knowledge—by any other therapeutic modality. Although PP is an expensive procedure, its potential to change the neurological disability (and, as a result, the lifestyle of a patient) outweighs the costs involved in our judgement.[24] The results of these analyses—which define specifically the characteristics of responders—may permit judicious use of PP in patients with chronic progressive multiple sclerosis. Patients with the cerebral or cerebellar forms of MS—as defined by

TABLE 5. Patients with Predominant Signs and Symptoms

	Clinical Categories		
	Cerebral	Cerebellar	Spinal
Pilot Study ($n = 45$)	14	6	25
Double-Blind Study ($n = 55$)			
PP ($n = 26$)	7	6	13
Sham ($n = 29$)	9	9	11

TABLE 6. Outcome by Clinical Categories: Cerebral

	No. of Cerebral MS	Kurtzke DSS Before	After	Follow-up 1 yr.	3 yrs.
Pilot Study ($n = 45$)	14	7.6	3.9[a]	4.3[a]	4.6[a]
Double-Blind Study ($n = 55$)				11 Months	
PP ($n = 26$)	7	7.1	4.6[a]	4.7[a]	
Sham ($n = 29$)	9	6.7	6.6	6.8	

[a]Significance of improvement at completion and follow-up is at $p < 0.0001$.

us—do not respond significantly to long-term prednisone and low-dose cyclophosphamide therapy alone. However, the combination of PP with immunosuppressive drug therapy in these patients may bring about significant and long-lasting improvement. The reasons why patients with a predominantly spinal form of MS do not seem to respond to this therapy are not clear. This may be due to extensive functional involvement of long spinal tracts, brought about by anatomically small lesions in the spinal cord. Perhaps such patients would respond to more frequent and extensive plasmapheresis.

Although remyelination of MS plaques is now known to occur,[25] we have no evidence in support of that sort of explanation for the fact that some of our patients with long-standing neurological disabilities improved with this therapeutic modality. MS patients with active disease have been shown to have a decrease in the numbers and/or functional activity of suppressor T cells.[3-9] In this study, the patients who improved the most clinically had significantly low suppressor-cell functional activity prior to therapy, with return of the activity to normal range following therapy.

CONCLUSION

We conclude from this study that a course of plasmapheresis and immunosuppressive drug therapy leads to sustained improvement or arrest of the disease in the majority of patients suffering from chronic progressive multiple sclerosis. The improvement we have noted is more common than has been reported to occur in this form of multiple sclerosis. Patients with signs and symptoms predominantly of the cerebral form of MS, as defined by us, are more likely to improve, as are patients with total duration of illness less than twelve years. Patients with low suppressor-cell functional activity are also likely to improve with return of suppressor-cell activity to

TABLE 7. Outcome by Clinical Categories: Cerebellar

	No. of Patients	Disability Status (Kurtzke) Before	After	Follow-up 1 yr.	3 yrs.
Pilot Study ($n = 45$)	6	6.2	4.3	4.8	5
Double-Blind Study ($n = 55$)				11 Months	
PP ($n = 26$)	6	6.5	5.5	6.3	
Sham ($n = 29$)	9	5.7	5.8	6.3	

TABLE 8. Outcome by Clinical Categories: Spinal

	No. of Patients	Disability Status (Kurtzke)			
		Before	After	Follow-up 1 yr.	Follow-up 3 yrs.
Pilot Study ($n = 45$)	25	6.6	5.9	6.3	6.7
Double-Blind Study ($n = 55$)				11 Months	
PP ($n = 26$)	13	6.4	6	6.3	
Sham ($n = 29$)	11	6.5	6.1	6.3	

normal. Age, gender, duration of progression of disease, severity of illness, HLA typing, and abnormalities on evoked potentials, CT scan, and T cell subsets were not found to be significant predictors of response to therapy.

ACKNOWLEDGMENTS

The authors thank Dr. Jitendra Baruah, Department of Neurology, and Dr. Sanford Larson, Department of Neurosurgery, Division of Surgery, for electrophysiological studies, Drs. Marilyn Kay, Walter Gager and the Neurophthalmology Section, Department of Ophthalmology, for eye examinations, and the nurses in the Plasmapheresis Unit, Froedtert Memorial Lutheran Hospital, Milwaukee, for rendering excellent services to the patients. Special thanks go to Ms. Donna Schmoll, M.S.S.W., and to Ms. Donna McKenzie, for without their diligent attention to the social and fiscal dimensions of this work, none of it would have been possible.

REFERENCES

1. TOURTELLOTTE, W. W. & J. A. PARKER. 1967. Multiple sclerosis: Brain immunoglobulin-G and albumin. Nature **214:** 683–686.
2. WALSH, M. J., W. W. TOURTELLOTTE, A. R. POTVIN & J. H. POTVIN. 1983. The cerebrospinal fluid in multiple sclerosis. *In* Multiple Sclerosis. J. F. Hallpike, C. M. Adams & W. W. Tourtellotte, Eds.: 275–358. Williams & Wilkins. Baltimore.
3. BACH, M. A., F. PHAN-DINH-TUY, E. TOURNIER *et al.* 1980. Deficit of suppressor T-cells in active multiple sclerosis. Lancet **8206:** 1221–1223.
4. HUDDLESTONE, J. R. & M. A. OLDSTONE. 1979. T suppressor lymphocytes fluctuate in parallel with changes in the clinical course of patients with multiple sclerosis. J. Immunol. **123:** 1615–1618.
5. HUDDLESTONE, J. R. & M. A. OLDSTONE. 1982. Suppressor T-cells are activated *in vivo* in patients with multiple sclerosis coinciding with remission from acute attacks. J. Immunol. **129:** 915–917.
6. REINHERZ, E. L., H. L. WEINER, S. L. HAUSER *et al.* 1980. Loss of suppressor T-cells in active multiple sclerosis. N. Engl. J. Med. **303:** 125–129.
7. KHATRI, B., S. KOETHE, K. MEZRA & M. MCQUILLEN. 1981. Clinical significance of changes in suppressor T-cell function in chronic progressive MS patients undergoing plasmapheresis and immunosuppressive drug therapy (Abstract). Society for Neuroscience **7:** 568.
8. ANGEL, J. P., B. W. ARNASON & M. E. MEDOF. 1978. Suppressor cell function in multiple sclerosis: Correlation with clinical disease activity. Ann. Neurol. **5:** 338–342.
9. GONZALES, R. L., P. C. DAU & L. E. SPITLER. 1979. Altered regulation of mitogen responsiveness by suppressor cells in multiple sclerosis. Clin. Exp. Immunol. **36:** 78–84.

10. LOCKWOOD, C. M. 1979. Experience with plasmapheresis in glomerulonephritis and other allergic diseases. *In* Plasmapheresis and the Immunobiology of Myasthenia Gravis. P. C. Dau, Ed.: 175–185. Houghton Mifflin. Boston.
11. DAU, P. C., J. H. PETAJAN, K. P. JOHNSON, H. S. PANITCH & M. B. BORNSTEIN. 1980. Plasmapheresis and immunosuppressive drug therapy in multiple sclerosis. Neurology (Minneap.) **30:** 1023–1028.
12. WEINER, H. L. & D. M. DAWSON. 1980. Plasmapheresis in multiple sclerosis: Preliminary study. Neurology (Minneap.) **30:** 1029–1033.
13. KHATRI, B., M. P. MCQUILLEN, S. M. KOETHE, C. HUSSEY & A. COOK. 1980. Plasmapheresis in multiple sclerosis: Correlation of clinical improvement with increased suppressor cell activity in peripheral blood. Trans. Am. Neurol. Assoc. **105:** 318–320.
14. SCHAUF, C. L., D. A. STETOSKI, F. A. DAVIS & B. C. MCLEOD. 1979. The application of plasmapheresis to multiple sclerosis. Plasma Ther. **1:** 33–42.
15. WAKSMAN, B. H. 1983. Rationales of current therapies for multiple sclerosis. Arch. Neurol. (special issue on multiple sclerosis) **40**(11): 671–72.
16. KHATRI, B. O., G. J. HARRINGTON, D. SCHMOLL & M. P. MCQUILLEN. 1983. A double-blind randomized controlled study of immunosuppressive drug therapy (IDT) with plasmapheresis (PP) in chronic progressive multiple sclerosis (CPMS). Abstract. Neurology **33** (Suppl. 2): 178.
17. KURTZKE, J. F. 1965. Disability evaluation in multiple sclerosis. Neurology (Minneap.) **15:** 654–661.
18. KHATRI, B. O., S. M. KOETHE & M. P. MCQUILLEN. 1984. Plasmapheresis with immunosuppressive drug therapy in progressive multiple sclerosis. A pilot study. Arch. Neurol. **41:** 734–738.
19. SCHUMACHER, G. A., G. BEEBE, R. F. KIBLER *et al.* 1965. Problems of experimental trials of therapy in multiple sclerosis: Report by the panel on the evaluation of experimental trials of therapy in multiple sclerosis. Ann. N.Y. Acad. Sci. **122:** 552–568.
20. KHATRI, B. O. 1982. A technique for easy vascular access in patients undergoing plasmapheresis. J. Clin. Apheresis **1:** 55.
21. BUSTRYN, J. C., I. SCHENKEIN & J. W. UHR. 1971. A mode for the regulation of antibody synthesis by serum antibody. *In* Progress in Immunology. B. Amos, Ed.: 627–637. Academic Press. New York.
22. SANCES, A., JR., S. J. LARSON, J. F. CUSICK *et al.* 1978. Early somatosensory evoked potentials. Electroencephalogr. Clin. Neurophysiol. **45:** 505–514.
23. KOETHE, S. M., A. COOK, D. P. MCQUILLEN & M. P. MCQUILLEN. 1981. Clinical and immunologic correlations in myasthenia gravis—measurement of Con A stimulated suppressor cell activity. Ann. N.Y. Acad. Sci. **377:** 447–454.
24. MCQUILLEN, M. P. & D. SCHMOLL. 1983. Alternative funding for clinical trials and the quality of life it purchases. Workshop on role of third party payers in clinical trials of new agents: Multiple sclerosis and rheumatoid arthritis as examples. July 6–7, 1983. Airlie House. Airlie, Virginia.
25. PRINEAS, J. W., E. E. KWON, E-S. CHO & L. R. SHARER. 1984. Continual breakdown and regeneration of myelin in progressive multiple sclerosis plaques. This volume.

Total Lymphoid Irradiation in Chronic Progressive Multiple Sclerosis

A Preliminary Report

M. P. HAFSTEIN,[a] C. DEVEREUX,[a] R. TROIANO,[a]
G. ZITO,[a,b] R. VIDAVER,[a] P. C. DOWLING,[a,b]
M. LAVENHAR,[a] AND S. D. COOK[a,b]

[a]*University of Medicine and Dentistry of New Jersey*
New Jersey Medical School
Newark, New Jersey 07103

[b]*Veterans Administration Medical Center*
East Orange, New Jersey 07019

INTRODUCTION

Total lymphoid irradiation (TLI) produces profound and long-lasting immunosuppression in animals and man.[1–6] Preadministration of TLI to mice prolongs allogenic skin grafts and bone marrow transplants, and induces tolerance to soluble protein antigens.[1–6] Total lymphoid irradiation also causes a sustained remission in the autoimmune disease of NZB/NZW mice,[7] and a similar effect is seen with adjunct-induced arthritis in Lewis rats.[8] Patients with Hodgkin's disease and non-Hodgkin's lymphoma have been treated with TLI for over 20 years.[9] Unlike cytotoxic drugs, TLI alone has not been associated with hematologic neoplasia in over 1000 patients with Hodgkin's disease followed for up to 14 years, and few serious side effects have been reported.[9,10] More recently, TLI was successfully used to treat patients with severe rheumatoid arthritis (RA) refractory to steroids, azathioprine, and other drugs.[1,11] After TLI clinical improvement has been sustained, lasting the duration of the follow-up period (over three years in some RA patients).[12]

In view of the long-term effectiveness and safety of TLI as an immunosuppressive therapy, it seemed reasonable to carry out a study using TLI in patients with multiple sclerosis (MS), a chronic disease considered to have an immune-mediated pathogenesis, but with no effective long-term therapy. A prospective, randomized, double-blind study to determine if TLI could inhibit progression of neurologic deficits in patients with chronic progressive MS was initiated in April 1982. Since that time 32 patients have completed TLI or sham therapy. We now report our clinical findings on the initial 19 patients who have been monitored 6 months or more thereafter.

METHODS AND PROCEDURE

Patients

Twenty patients with clinically definite MS entered the trial between April 1982 and March 1983.[13] Inclusion criteria consisted of the following: patients were between 20 and 60 years of age, had MS for at least three years, had progressive neurologic disability (as documented by a neurologist, or the patient and a family member) for at least one year prior to entry into the study, and had a score between 4 and 8 on the Kurtzke Disability Status Scale (DSS).[14] Most patients had previously received steroids, but none had received immunosuppressive drugs. Patients were excluded from the trial for the following reasons: severe psychiatric or psychoneurotic disease; intellectual impairment sufficient to interfere with understanding and participating in the study; low survivability; unavailability for the duration of the follow-up period (at least two years); chronic bacterial infections, *i.e.*, decubiti or urinary tract infections; serious medical illness; prior neoplasm or tuberculosis; leukopenia (white cell count <4500), anemia (hematocrit $<25\%$) or thrombocytopenia (platelet count $<100{,}000$); prior use of immunosuppressive drugs; pregnancy or a desire to become pregnant subsequently. One patient had a urinary catheter at entry into the study, but we subsequently also made this an exclusion criterion.

During an initial interview the trial protocol, including potential risks and benefits, was explained in detail to the patient and at least one family member. Patients were admitted to University Hospital, Newark, or the Veterans Administration Medical Center, East Orange, where comprehensive medical, neurological, and when necessary, psychiatric evaluations were carried out. In addition to routine laboratory tests, a lumbar puncture, evoked potential studies, a CT scan, and a battery of immunologic tests were performed on most patients. A renal scan and spleen scan were done to locate normal tissues during the simulation of radiation fields. On the final day of hospitalization, just prior to receiving therapy, the patient signed informed consent under the guidelines of the research committee of the University of Medicine and Dentistry of New Jersey. A sealed envelope prepared by our statistician was then drawn to determine whether the patient was randomized to the TLI or sham TLI group. Only the patient coordinator (MH) and radiotherapist (CD) were aware of the patient's therapy, although a sealed copy of the code was available to one of us (SC) for possible emergency use (which was not required).

Total Lymphoid Irradiation

Total lymphoid irradiation or sham TLI was administered on an outpatient basis to the 19 patients at Clara Maass Medical Center, an affiliate of the University of Medicine and Dentistry of New Jersey.

The patients were treated on a SL 75–10 Phillips Linear Accelerator with an 8 MeV photon beam using two pairs of treatment fields. A modified mantle was used that extended from the top of the thyroid cartilage superiorly to the bottom of L-1, including the spleen, inferiorly. The patient was placed with the arms extended fully above the head. This position brings the infraclavicular nodes superiorly and enables one to shield more of the lung and yet include these nodes in the treatment field. Custom-made blocks of cerrobend, equivalent to six half-value layers, were designed to shield the lungs anteriorly and posteriorly. A thyroid block was placed anteriorly over the thyroid cartilage and a midline custom spine block was placed posteriorly from the beginning of treatment to keep the dose to the spine below 1000 rad.

The patients were treated using antero-posterior and postero-anterior fields to a total dose of 1980 rads. This was delivered in 11 fractions of 180 rad each. Both anterior and posterior fields were treated five days a week. Following completion of the mantle an inverted "Y" field was treated. Treatment of the inverted "Y" usually began on the twelfth day, although there was an occasional delay of 2–3 days when simulation could not be scheduled optimally. The inverted "Y" was also treated at 180 rad daily fractions to a total dose of 1980 rad in 11 fractions. A 2 cm spine block was used at the superior portion of the posterior field to assure that no excessive radiation was given at the matchline to the spinal cord.

Follow-up and Clinical Assessment

Patients were evaluated by two blinded neurologists before treatment in order to establish a baseline, and the same neurologists assessed the patients' neurological status at monthly intervals for six months after therapy, and at three-month intervals thereafter. Patients were seen in mid-to-late morning in an attempt to avoid diurnal fluctuations of neurological status. At six months post-therapy, patients were readmitted to the hospital where the lumbar puncture, evoked potential studies, CT scan and immunologic tests were repeated. At each visit, a detailed self-evaluation questionnaire

TABLE 1. Patient Questionnaire

	(Circle Best Answer)			
Since Your Last Visit:	Better	Unchanged	Worse	N/A
1. Vision in your left eye is	1	2	3	9
2. Vision in your right eye is	1	2	3	9
3. Double vision is	1	2	3	9
4. Bladder/bowel dysfunction is	1	2	3	9
5. Strength/coordination in left arm and hand is	1	2	3	9
6. Strength/coordination in right arm and hand is	1	2	3	9
7. Strength/coordination in left leg is	1	2	3	9
8. Strength/coordination in right leg is	1	2	3	9
9. Spasticity (spasms/tightness in muscles) is	1	2	3	9
10. Tremors or shaking in left hand is	1	2	3	9
11. Tremors or shaking in right hand is	1	2	3	9
12. Pain, numbness or tingling in left arm is	1	2	3	9
13. Pain, numbness or tingling in right arm is	1	2	3	9
14. Pain, numbness or tingling in left leg is	1	2	3	9
15. Pain, numbness or tingling in right leg is	1	2	3	9
16. Pain, numbness or tingling in face is	1	2	3	9
17. Speech or swallowing is	1	2	3	9
18. Vertigo is	1	2	3	9

was completed (TABLE 1), a comprehensive neurological examination performed, and the DSS score determined. In addition, a practical functional scale developed by one of us (RT), was graded by the examining neurologist (TABLE 2). Ratings in this scale vary from 0 to 12; the greater the functional impairment, the higher the number. Two other blinded neurologists, neither of whom had seen the patients after entry into the study, scored the patients' disease progression based on the written data only. Criteria for progression included: (1) decrease in DSS or functional scale by 1.0 grade or more; (2) decrease in muscle strength in a proximal or distal limb of at least 2 grades (Medical Research Council scale); (3) deterioration on the six month or one year follow-up neurological examination compared to the pretreatment examination by the same neurologist; (4) worsening in the patient's cumulative self-evaluation score (TABLE 1). Data from all these areas were independently reviewed by the blinded neurologists to give each patient a final assessment of either better, unchanged or worse. In this overall

TABLE 2. Troiano Functional Scale

Gait	ADL	Transfers
0 Normal	0 Normal	0 Minimal or no difficulty
1 Abnormal, independent	1 Independent with minimal dysfunction (may choose to use assistance or device for speed and efficiency)	1 Uses arms to shift weight sitting to standing or sitting to sitting from a straight chair (or wheelchair) Transfers are independent
2 Uses unilateral assistance device	2 Routinely uses partial human assistance for some of: —Dexterity functions (writing, managing utensils, buttons, laces, *etc.*) —Dressing and bathing of lower body	2 Routinely uses assistance for most transfers Actively participates
3 Uses bilateral assistance device May use wheelchair for long distance or prolonged mobility Walking is sufficient to serve a variety of routine daily activities	3 Uses substantial human assistance for most of ADL including bathing and dressing lower and upper body Actively participates	3 Dependent for all transfers Passive with no effective participation
4 Depends mainly on wheelchair for mobility May stand and take some steps with bilateral assistance Steps are not very useful for practical purposes throughout the daily routine and are done largely for short transfers and exercise activity and preferably with supervision	4 Dependent for all ADL, passive with no effective participation	
5 No standing or steps excluding active human support or rigid support such as Kim stander		

assessment greatest weight was given to the DSS, functional scores, and muscle testing. Physical therapy, steroids and other drugs (excluding immunosuppressants) were prescribed to patients at the discretion of the blinded neurologists. On no occasion was it necessary for the code to be broken except after the patient was classified as a treatment failure. Patients were considered as treatment failures if they dropped out of the study after completion of therapy, or progressed to such a severe degree that the blinded neurologist felt the patient should no longer be in the trial.

Absolute Lymphocyte Counts

Blood samples were obtained at the time of each clinic visit. The absolute lymphocyte count was calculated from the total leukocyte count based on percentage of lymphocytes.

Statistics

The characteristics of the patients in the sham and TLI groups were compared (TABLE 3) by applying the Wilcoxon Rank Sum Test (numerical data) and Fisher's Exact Test (binary data, *e.g.,* sex). Pre- and post-treatment differences (paired comparisons) were tested for statistical significance by applying the one-tailed Wilcoxon Signed Rank Test. Differences in the mean lymphocyte count by treatment group and by post-treatment time were analyzed using a repeated measures analysis of variance design (TABLE 7). Differences in group means were tested by Duncan's multiple comparisons procedures.

RESULTS

Patient Characteristics

Nine patients were randomized to the TLI group and 11 to the sham group (TABLE 3). One patient in the TLI group dropped out of the study after 12 days of therapy because of nausea. There was no change in his neurological status and he was not included in our analysis for progression. There was no evidence to suggest that the two patient groups differed with respect to sex, age, duration of MS, and entry DSS rating. However, we have not presented data on individual patients in this preliminary report in order to preserve the "blindedness" of the study in the future. Although there was no significant difference in the mean DSS or mean functional scale ratings between the two groups, a mild but not significant disparity in the distribution of patients by DSS and functional scales in the two groups was noted. The TLI group had more patients with an entry DSS of 8 than the sham group. Similarly, a larger number of patients with functional scale ratings greater than 8 were seen in the TLI group, as compared to the controls, and this was reflected in the higher mean functional scale score in the TLI group (7.5) as compared to the controls (6.5).

Assessment for Progression

Assessment for progression using four different rating scales, as well as a final assessment based on all criteria, is seen in TABLES 3 and 4. Significant progression

TABLE 3. Clinical Profile of MS Patients

	Number of Patients	Mean Age	Sex	Mean Kurtzke DSS			Mean Troiano Functional Scale		
				Entry	6 Mos.	12 Mos.[a]	Entry	6 Mos.	12 Mos.[a]
Sham	11	41.9	5F, 6M	6.5 ($n = 11$)	6.7 ($n = 11$)	7.0 ($n = 8$)	6.5 ($n = 11$)	7.5 ($n = 11$)	8.4[b] ($n = 8$)
TLI	8	38.9	4F, 4M	6.8 ($n = 8$)	6.8 ($n = 8$)	6.8 ($n = 5$)	7.5 ($n = 8$)	7.6 ($n = 8$)	8.0 ($n = 5$)

[a]Two sham patients were treatment failures and not seen at the 12-month follow-up. These patients have not been considered in this analysis.
[b]Significant progression from entry value ($p < 0.01$) when 8 sham patients' entry scores are compared to the same 8 patients at 12-month follow-up.

occurred in the sham group in the functional scale score, self-evaluation score, and final assessment. Although trends favoring the TLI group were seen using the DSS and muscle testing scale, these were not significant. In an effort to make the entry functional scale scores between the two groups closer, data were reanalyzed after dropping the two most severely impaired TLI patients from consideration. Even though the 11 sham patients (mean functional scale 6.5) were then quite similar to the remaining 6 TLI patients (new mean functional scale 6.7), a significant difference in progression in the sham *versus* the TLI group was still noted ($p < 0.05$). From entry to 12-month evaluation, the TLI patients as a group have not changed significantly in the functional scale, whereas the sham group deteriorated to a significant degree in this parameter ($p < 0.01$). No significant difference was noted in the number of patients on steroids in either group, and in fact more sham patients than controls were put on steroids at some time during the study by a blinded neurologist because of an acute exacerbation or rapid rate of progression. Similarly, no significant difference was

TABLE 4. Effect of TLI in Chronic Progressive MS[a]

	TLI	Sham	
1. Overall evaluation			
Unchanged	6	2	$p = 0.02$
Worse	2	9	
2. Troiano Functional Scale (≧ 1 grade deterioration)			
Unchanged	7	3	$p = 0.015$
Worse	1	8	
3. Kurtzke Disability Scale (≧ 1 grade deterioration)			
Unchanged	8	7	$p = 0.085$
Worse	0	4	
4. Patient self-evaluation			
Unchanged	6	2	$p = 0.02$
Worse	2	9	
5. Muscle testing			
Unchanged	6	6	$p = 0.337$
Worse	2	5	

[a]Evaluation at last clinic visit (6 months or 1 year).

found between the groups in the number of patients receiving physical therapy or the number of hours of physical therapy received. Two patients left the study as treatment failures. One patient dropped out of the study at six months because he felt he was worse, and another was dropped from the study after six months because of an unacceptable rate of deterioration. Both patients were in the sham group. However, we have not considered these patients as failures in our present analysis of data, but used the same criteria for progression in them as for the other patients.

An effort was made to ascertain if patients were truly blinded as to whether they received TLI or sham therapy. Immediately after treatment, most patients in each group felt they had received TLI (TABLE 5). On their last follow-up visit, the TLI patients continued to believe that they had received TLI; however, most patients in the sham group no longer felt they had received TLI. There was a good correlation between those sham patients who originally thought they had received TLI, but subsequently changed their mind, and progression of their neurological disease.

TABLE 5. Patient Opinion Regarding TLI or Sham

	Early Post-Therapy		Late Post-Therapy	
	TLI	Sham[a]	TLI	Sham[a]
Received TLI	7	6	7	3
Don't know	0	1	0	0
Received sham	1	3	1	7

[a]Information unavailable from one patient who was a treatment failure and dropped from study.

Side Effects

The short-term side effects of TLI and sham therapy in the MS patients are shown in TABLE 6. These symptoms were generally mild and abated shortly after completion of therapy. The only significant difference in the two groups was in transient hair loss, which was seen only in the TLI group. Thrombocytopenia (platelet count <150,000) was seen during treatment in seven of eight patients in the TLI group as compared to none of the 11 control patients. Thrombocytopenia (or leukopenia) was sufficiently severe to interrupt therapy temporarily in three patients in the TLI group. In one TLI patient, treatment was protracted to 52 days because of thrombocytopenia. In an effort to control for this effect, therapy was temporarily interrupted in two control patients. Thrombocytopenia usually resolved by one month after therapy.

To date no neoplasms have developed in either group (mean follow-up post-therapy: one year). Currently, the incidence of infections is similar in the TLI and control groups.

Lymphocyte Counts

Leukopenia ($< 4{,}000/mm^3$) was noted during therapy in seven of eight TLI patients, and an absolute lymphocytopenia ($< 1{,}000\ mm^3$) was noted in all eight TLI

TABLE 6. Side Effects of TLI

Short Term	TLI (9 Patients)[a]	Sham (11 Patients)
Nausea	2	2
Vomiting	0	1
Fatigue	6	6
Noted hair loss	6	0
Dyspepsia	1	0
Menopause	1	0
Weight loss	0	1
Anorexia	0	1
Dysphagia	1	0
Sore throat	2	0
Long Term	**TLI (8 Patients)**	**Sham (11 Patients)**
Cancer	0	0
Infections		
URI	1	1
UTI	3	4
Deep vein thrombosis	1	1

[a]One patient dropped out of study 12 days after treatment started because of nausea. He is included in side effects but is not considered in the study results.

patients. Neither leukopenia, nor lymphocytopenia, was found in the controls. The absolute lymphocytopenia was significant and persisted in the TLI group for at least one year (TABLE 7), although a slight trend toward increased lymphocytes with time was detected.

DISCUSSION

Multiple sclerosis is a chronic demyelinating disease of the central nervous system (CNS) of probable infectious etiology, which may have an immune component to its pathogenesis.[15] On the premise that the immune response may play a role in causing demyelination, we initiated a prospective, randomized double-blind study of the effects of TLI in chronic progressive MS. Patients with chronic progressive MS were chosen because no accepted therapy is available to these patients and they are likely to continue to deteriorate.[16–19] TLI appeared to be an effective, safe form of immunosuppressive therapy.[1,11] We selected a radiation protocol modified from that of Kotzin *et al.*[1] for RA because their regimen produced more sustained lymphocytopenia and clinical improvement in patients than the regimen of Trentham *et al.*[11] However, we added a posterior spinal block to keep the cord dosage to less than 1000 rad in order to prevent possible untoward damage to a spinal cord already compromised by MS. This

TABLE 7. Mean Absolute Lymphocyte Count in TLI Study

	Pretreatment	Last Week during Treatment	Post-Treatment 1 Month	3 Months	6 Months	12 Months
TLI	2357	557[a]	595[a]	686[a]	767[a]	761[a]
Sham	2188	2368	2223	1959	2060	1870

[a] $p < 0.05$ compared to both pretreatment count and sham controls at the same time interval.

belief was based on the following considerations: (1) CNS irradiation may cause damage to vascular endothelium and blood-brain barrier, making it more permeable to proteins and other molecules;[20–22] (2) CNS irradiation can produce spinal cord damage;[23] (3) irradiation of the CNS of Lewis rats who are then recipients of lymph node cells from animals with EAE is associated with paralysis only in the recipients who received radiation of the spinal cord;[24] (4) cellular infiltrates of EAE are more common in the irradiated region of the neuraxis;[24] and (5) transient damage to the blood-brain barrier occurs in patients with chronic progressive MS who received 1200–1800 rad to the CNS.[22]

Our preliminary results show significantly less progression of disease and a sustained absolute lymphocytopenia in the 8 MS patients in the TLI group as compared to the 11 controls. These clinical differences are found using either the patients' own self-evaluations or the clinician-rated functional scales. Although the two groups are not exactly comparable in terms of entry DDS scores and functional scales, more patients with severe disability being randomized into the TLI group, analysis of results still shows significantly less functional loss over time in the TLI group when the two groups are made closer in entry functional scale rating by dropping the two most severely impaired patients on entry from the TLI group. Thus the difference in rate of progression cannot be attributed solely to maldistribution of patients into the two groups by entry functional impairment.

The fact that the difference in the two groups was noted by the patients themselves, as well as by two pairs of "blinded" neurologists—one pair rating the DSS, functional scales, and NE at each visit, the other pair making a retrospective overall evaluation on the basis of all criteria—makes us more confident that these differences may be real. However, the interpretation of the differences between the groups must be considered with caution. Relatively small numbers of patients have been followed and the follow-up period is short. Randomization of just a few patients with more actively progressive disease into the sham group could produce a greater rate of deterioration in the sham than TLI group, and lead to an artifactual conclusion about the benefit of TLI. In an attempt to circumvent potential randomizational difficulties, we plan to enter more patients into the study, possibly stratifying to ensure that DSS and functional scales are comparable in the two groups, and observe patients over a longer period of time.

Total lymphoid irradiation in MS is well tolerated and associated with only mild, short-term side effects. Although transient hair loss at the nape of the neck, axillary regions and midchest (in hirsute men) occurred only in the TLI group, we conclude that the study was blinded. The areas of hair loss were not inspected by the examining neurologists. Both patients and neurologists were instructed not to discuss side effects with each other. Further, there was no difference immediately post-therapy between the two groups as to whether they felt they had received TLI or sham therapy, the only difference between groups occurring much later and being related to clinical status.

A large number of immunosuppressive therapies, mostly studied in uncontrolled settings, has been used to treat MS patients.[25] Short-term therapy with ACTH or steroids accelerates the rate of recovery following acute exacerbations of MS,[26] but it is unclear whether long-term, high-dose steroids are effective in altering the course of the disease. Recently, in a prospective controlled study, Hauser *et al.* compared 20 chronic progressive MS patients receiving high-dose short-term intravenous (IV) cyclophosphamide plus ACTH with 20 similar MS patients receiving ACTH alone, and 18 patients placed on a regimen of plasmapheresis, low-dose oral cyclophosphamide and ACTH.[16] Beneficial effects were seen primarily in the IV cyclophosphamide-ACTH group and no major complications were reported. The experimental design of their study prevented a double-blind trial from being carried out and since all treated patients developed scalp alopecia, it is possible that an inadvertent investigator or patient bias could have influenced the results.[27] Most of the patients who had improved initially developed signs of progressive disease 15 to 24 months following therapy. In another controlled trial, Khatri *et al.* carried out a double-blind study of low-dose oral cytoxan, steroids, and plasmapheresis in patients with chronic progressive MS.[28] They noted a significant beneficial effect on disease course as compared to a second MS group which received the same drugs but sham plasmapheresis. The full details of this study, including duration of beneficial response and side effects, have not yet been published.

Unfortunately immunosuppressive drugs, particularly alkylating agents, have a close therapeutic-toxic ratio and a wide range of distressing side effects.[29-31] Although long-term prospective studies of the risk of malignancy in patients with non-neoplastic disease treated with immunosuppressive drugs have not been reported, the alkylating agent chlorambucil has been associated with a higher than expected incidence of leukemia (0.75%) in 1612 patients with RA who received this drug,[10,32] and a leukemic incidence of 1.3% has been reported in RA patients treated with azathioprine.[33] Thus the risk of cancer is a major concern in patients receiving immunosuppressive drugs over long periods of time. Another problem with immunosuppressive drugs in nonmalignant disease is that beneficial effects may only be transient. For example, cyclophosphamide may transiently relieve symptoms in patients with rheumatoid arthritis, but symptoms recur soon after the drug is discontinued.[30] In contrast to immunosuppressive drugs, TLI has not been shown to be associated with an increased risk of neoplasia and produces few serious side effects in long-term follow-up.

Recently two open trials of TLI in patients with intractable rheumatoid arthritis were carried out. In the Stanford studies by Kotzin *et al.*[1] and Field *et al.*,[12] 11 patients unresponsive to conventional therapy including steroids in 10, and prior azathioprine in 8, were treated with TLI (2000 rad, two regions, five to six weeks duration) and have been followed up to 3½ years thereafter. Nine of the 11 patients showed marked clinical improvement which reached a peak at six to seven months after therapy, and has persisted throughout the follow-up period. Total remission was not observed but mean daily steroid dosage was reduced by 54%. After therapy all patients exhibited a profound T lymphocytopenia and a reversal of their T suppressor to helper cell ratio. Alterations in T cell numbers persisted throughout the entire follow-up period. However, no change in rheumatoid factor or antinuclear antibody titers was found. Side effects were generally mild and transient. One patient required a splenectomy for Felty's syndrome and a 70-year-old female subsequently died of pneumonia associated with rheumatic lung disease. In view of these encouraging results, the authors have undertaken a double-blind trial to further evaluate the role of TLI in rheumatoid arthritis.

In the Harvard RA study by Trentham *et al.*,[11] a different TLI technique was used (3000 rad, 3 regions, 13 to 15 weeks duration). Trentham *et al.* also noted considerable clinical improvement in 8 of 10 patients, associated with reduced blood lymphocyte counts. As in the Stanford study, no reduction in rheumatoid factor titer, antinuclear antibody, or serum immune complexes was seen and immunoglobulin and complement levels were unchanged. However, unlike the Stanford study, partial recrudescence of arthritis occurred about a year after completion of the irradiation and this was paralleled by a return of blood lymphocyte levels towards normal. The difference in clinical results between the Harvard and Stanford studies could be due to the differences in TLI technique, the Harvard protocol perhaps allowing lymphocytes from the untreated region to circulate and repopulate a previously radiated field.[12] Short-term side effects in the study by Trentham *et al.* were also generally mild and transient although one patient required a blood transfusion. In contrast, deaths at later intervals were seen in 4 of 12 patients: one with myocardial infarct 19 months post-TLI, one with a cardiopulmonary arrest (presumed to be secondary to a pulmonary embolus) 12 months post-TLI, and two with staphylococcal sepsis—one secondary to osteomyelitis postjoint surgery—occurring about 20 months post-TLI.[34] The high mortality rate seen was unexpected based on the extensive prior Hodgkin's experience and was not paralleled in the Stanford RA study.

In considering the reasons for the excessive mortality noted by Trentham *et al.* as compared to other TLI studies, the following should be considered: (1) the mean age of the Harvard RA patients was 61, compared to 51.5 in the Stanford RA study (and 38.9 in our MS study); (2) the Harvard group used a different TLI technique with 3000 rad given over a longer period to three regions; (3) all patients were on steroids, and probably other drugs; (4) rheumatoid arthritis is a systemic disease affecting multiple organs; (5) there may be a predilection for infections to occur in patients with severe rheumatoid arthritis.[35] Thus it is probably unlikely that TLI alone given in the manner used by the Stanford group or ourselves is a cause of high mortality. Nevertheless one should be cautious about giving TLI to elderly patients, or patients on high doses of steroids or other immunosuppressive drugs.

In summary, our study data suggest that the treated MS group showed less disease progression than the untreated group based on some, but not all, of the criteria used to assess efficacy. It should be noted that because of the small numbers of subjects followed in this preliminary report, the statistical tests applied had only limited power to detect small or even moderately large group differences. Larger samples are needed before a definitive conclusion may be reached with respect to the overall efficacy of the TLI treatment.

REFERENCES

1. KOTZIN, B. L., S. STROBER, E. G. ENGLEMAN, A. CALIN, R. T. HOPPE, G. S. KANSAS, C. P. TERRELL & H. S. KAPLAN. 1981. Treatment of intractable rheumatoid arthritis with total lymphoid irradiation. N. Engl. J. Med. **305:** 969–976.
2. STROBER, S., S. SLAVIN & M. GOTTLIEB. 1979. Allograft tolerance after total lymphoid irradiation (TLI). Immunol. Rev. **46:** 87–112.
3. SLAVIN, S., S. STROBER, Z. FUKS & H. S. KAPLAN. 1977. Induction of specific tissue transplantation tolerance using fractionated total lymphoid irradiation in adult mice: Long-term survival of allogeneic bone marrow and skin grafts. J. Exp. Med. **146:** 34–48.
4. KING, D. P., S. STROBER & H. S. KAPLAN. 1981. Suppression of the mixed leukocyte response and of graft-vs-host disease by spleen cells following total lymphoid irradiation (TLI). J. Immunol. **126:** 1140–1145.
5. ZAN-BAR, I., S. SLAVIN & S. STROBER. 1978. Induction and mechanism of tolerance to bovine serum albumin in mice given total lymphoid irradiation (TLI). J. Immunol. **121:** 1400–1404.
6. SLAVIN, S., B. REITZ, C. P. BIEBER, H. S. KAPLAN & S. STROBER. 1978. Transplantation tolerance in adult rats using total lymphoid irradiation: Permanent survival of skin, heart, and marrow allografts. J. Exp. Med. **147:** 700–707.
7. KOTZIN, B. L. & S. STROBER. 1979. Reversal of NZB/NZW disease with total lymphoid irradiation. J. Exp. Med. **150:** 371–378.
8. SCHURMAN, D. J., H. P. HIRSHMAN & S. STROBER. 1981. Total lymphoid and local joint irradiation in the treatment of adjuvant arthritis. Arthritis Rheum. **24:** 38–44.
9. KAPLAN, H. S. 1980. Hodgkin's Disease. 2d ed. Harvard University Press. Cambridge. pp. 366–441.
10. STROBER, S., R. T. HOPPE, H. S. KAPLAN & B. L. KOTZIN. 1982. Letter to the editor. N. Engl. J. Med. **307:** 375–376.
11. TRENTHAM, D. E., J. A. BELLI, R. J. ANDERSON, J. A. BUCKLEY, E. J. GOETZL, J. R. DAVID & K. F. AUSTEN. 1981. Clinical and immunologic effects of fractionated total lymphoid irradiation in refractory rheumatoid arthritis. N. Engl. J. Med. **305:** 976–982.
12. FIELD, E. H., S. STROBER, R. T. HOPPE, A. CALIN, E. G. ENGLEMAN, B. L. KOTZIN, A. S. TANAY, H. J. CALIN, C. P. TERRELL & H. S. KAPLAN. 1983. Sustained improvement of intractable rheumatoid arthritis after total lymphoid irradiation. Arthritis Rheum. **26:** 937–946.
13. POSER, C. M., D. W. PATY, L. SCHEINBERG, W. I. MCDONALD, F. A. DAVIS, G. C. EBERS, K. P. JOHNSON, W. A. SIBLEY, D. H. SILBERBERG & W. W. TOURTELLOTTE. 1983. New diagnostic criteria for multiple sclerosis: Guidelines for research protocols. Ann. Neurol. **13:** 227–231.
14. KURTZKE, J. F. 1961. On the evaluation of disability in multiple sclerosis. Neurology (Minneap.) **11:** 686–694.
15. COOK, S. D. & P. C. DOWLING. 1980. Multiple sclerosis and viruses: An overview. Neurology **30**(7): 80–91.
16. HAUSER, S. L., D. M. DAWSON, J. R. LEHRICH, M. F. BEAL, S. V. KEVY, R. D. PROPPER, J. A. MILLS & H. L. WEINER. 1983. Intensive immunosuppression in progressive multiple sclerosis. A randomized, three-arm study of high-dose intravenous cyclophosphamide, plasma exchange, and ACTH. N. Engl. J. Med. **308:** 173–180.
17. MULLER, R. 1949. Studies on disseminated sclerosis: with special reference to symptomatology, course and prognosis. Acta Med. Scand. Suppl. **222:** 1214.
18. MCALPINE, D. & N. COMPSTON. 1952. Some aspects of the natural history of disseminated sclerosis. Q. J. Med. **21:** 135–167.
19. BAUER, H. J., W. FIRNHABER & W. WINKLER. 1965. Prognostic criteria in multiple sclerosis. Ann. N. Y. Acad. Sci. **122:** 542–551.

20. SCHETTLER, L. & N. C. SHEALY. 1970. Experimental selective alteration of the blood-brain-barrier by x-irradiation. J. Neurosurg. **32:** 89–94.
21. OLDENDORF, W. H. & E. M. CORNFORD. 1977. A comparison of total body and local spinal cord irradiation in experimental allergic encephalomyelitis. J. Neuropathol. Exp. Neurol. **36:** 50–61.
22. TOURTELLOTTE, W. W., A. R. POTVIN, R. W. BAUMHEFNER, J. H. POTVIN, I. M. BOOE, K. SYNDULKO & Z. PETROVICH. 1980. Multiple sclerosis de novo CNS IgG synthesis. Effect of CNS irradiation. Arch. Neurol. **37:** 620–624.
23. MASTAGLIA, F. L., W. I. MCDONALD, J. V. WATSON & K. YOGENDRAN. 1976. Effects of X-radiation on the spinal cord: An experimental study of the morphological changes in central nerve fibers. Brain **99:** 101–122.
24. PATERSON, P. Y., W. P. RICHARDSON & D. G. DROBISH. 1975. Cellular transfer of experimental allergic encephalomyelitis: Altered disease pattern in irradiated recipient Lewis rats. Cell. Immunol. **16:** 48–59.
25. ELLISON, G. W. & L. W. MYERS. 1978. A review of systemic nonspecific immunosuppressive treatment of multiple sclerosis. Neurology (Minneap.) **28:**(9, Part 2)**:** 132–139.
26. ROSE, A. S., J. W. KUZMA, J. F. KURTZKE, N. S. NAMEROW, W. A. SIBLEY & W. W. TOURTELLOTTE. 1970. Cooperative study in the evaluation of therapy in multiple sclerosis: ACTH vs placebo: final report. Neurology (Minneap.) **20**(2): 1–59.
27. FISCHBECK, K. H. 1983. Letter to the editor. N. Engl. J. Med. **309:** 239–240.
28. KHATRI, B. O., G. J. HARRINGTON, D. SCHMOLL & M. P. MCQUILLEN. 1983. A double-blind randomized controlled study of immunosuppressive drug therapy with plasmapheresis in chronic progressive multiple sclerosis. Neurology **33**(Suppl. 2)**:** 178–179.
29. KAPLAN, S. R. & P. CALABRESI. 1983. Drug therapy. Immunosuppressive agents. N. Engl. J. Med. **289:** 952–954.
30. TOWNES, A. S., J. M. SOWA & L. E. SHULMAN. 1976. Controlled trial of cyclophosphamide in rheumatoid arthritis. Arthritis Rheum. **19:** 563–573.
31. DAVIS, J. D., H. B. MUSS & R. A. TURNER. 1978. Cytotoxic agents in the treatment of rheumatoid arthritis. South. Med. J. **71:** 58–64.
32. KAHN, M. F., J. ARLET, H. BLOCH-MICHEL, M. CAROIT, Y. CHAOUAT & J. C. RENIER. 1979. Le risque de leucose aiguë après traitement des rheumatismes inflammatoires chroniques et des connectivités par les cytotoxiques à visée immunosuppressive. Rev. Rheum. Mal. Osteoartic. **46:** 163–167.
33. SEIDENFELD, A. M., H. A. SMYTHE, M. A. ORGYZLO, M. B. UROWITZ & D. A. DOTTON. 1976. Acute leukemia in rheumatoid arthritis treated with cytotoxic agents. J. Rheumatol. **3:** 295–304.
34. TRENTHAM, D. E. 1983. Personal communication.
35. BAUM, J. 1971. Infection in rheumatoid arthritis. Arthritis Rheum. **14:** 135–136.

DISCUSSION OF THE PAPER

A. VANDENBARK (Portland, *ORE*): I was just curious if you had any independent way to assess immune function in these patients?

S. D. COOK (*University of Medicine and Dentistry of New Jersey, Newark, NJ*): We have been looking at oligoclonal bands in the spinal fluid with Dr. Mehta and CSF myelin basic protein with Dr. Whitaker. We've also looked at T cell functions but we're not ready to present that data at this point.

Intrathecal IgG Synthesis and IgG Index after Intensive and Chronic Immunosuppressive Treatment of Multiple Sclerosis

O. R. HOMMES, K. J. B. LAMERS, AND W. VAN GEEL

Institute of Neurology
Radboud University Hospital
Nijmegen, the Netherlands

INTRODUCTION

In a previous study[1,2] it was shown that intensive immunosuppressive treatment with cyclophosphamide and prednisone greatly and immediately reduces the total IgG content of the cerebrospinal fluid (CSF). In patients with improvement in the years after treatment this IgG content remained low three months after the end of the treatment; in those with a progressive course the total IgG of the spinal fluid increased clearly after three months. It was concluded that the total IgG content of the spinal fluid three months after the treatment had prognostic value for the course of the disease in the years following the treatment.

Intrathecal IgG synthesis calculations became available to us in 1976. We now report here the effects of intensive and chronic immunosuppressive treatment on clinical condition, intrathecal IgG synthesis and IgG index of 41 patients with chronic progressive multiple sclerosis (MS).

PATIENTS AND METHODS

The criteria for inclusion of chronic progressive MS patients in this study were the same as described earlier.[1,2] Intensive immunosuppressive treatment (IIS) was given to 24 female and 17 male patients. It consisted of 400 mg cyclophosphamide and 100 mg prednisone per day, with a total dose of 8 g cyclophosphamide.

Kurtzke scores of Standard Neurologic Examination, Functional Systems and Disability Status Scale (DSS) were made immediately before (I), immediately after (II) and three months after (III) the treatment, and finally one to five years after the treatment. At (I), (II) and (III) serum and spinal fluid levels of albumin and IgG were determined and the intrathecal IgG synthesis and the IgG index were calculated.[3]

Only the DSS scores were used for calculations. The patients were divided into three groups (see TABLE 1):

- DSS^+: This group of patients showed decrease of one or more points on the DSS scale one to five years after treatment. These patients were called "improved."
- DSS^o: These patients remained at the same DSS level one to five years after the treatment. This group was called "stationary."
- DSS^-: These patients scored one or more points higher on the DSS scale one to five years after treatment. This group was called "progressive."

Chronic immunosuppressive treatment (CIS) was given to a second group of 27 chronic progressive MS patients. They were treated with 100 mg of cyclophosphamide per day over a prolonged period of at least 6 months. Kurtzke scores were made immediately before (I) and after (II) 6 to 18 months of treatment. At these moments serum and spinal fluid determinations were done as described above. The patients were divided into two groups:

- DSS^{o}: A group of patients that showed the same DSS score at (II) as at (I).
- DSS^{+}: A group of patients showing a reduced DSS score at (II) as compared to (I).

The DSS groups as described above (DSS^{+}, DSS^{o}, DSS^{-}) in the IIS and CIS treatments are essentially groups of patients with improvement, stability, or progression in the course of the disease as assessed several years after the IIS or 6 to 18 months after the start of CIS. Comparing data collected before or in the first period of the treatment among these groups or within each group will give prognostic significance to those parameters that show significant differences. Statistical comparison among the groups was done by the Wilcoxon two-sample test, within each group by the Wilcoxon pairs test. The level of statistical significance is chosen at $p \leqslant 0.05$.

TABLE 1. Number of Patients Treated with a Short Course of Immunosuppression in Two Subsequent Series[a]

	Number of Patients	DSS^{+} (Improved)	%	DSS^{o} (Stationary)	%	DSS^{-} (Progressive)	%
Hommes *et al.*, 1980	39	13	33	14	36	12	31
This report	41	14	34	15	37	12	29

[a]The percentages in the DSS groups scored 1 to 5 years after the treatment are the same in both reports.

RESULTS

After intensive immunosuppressive treatment 14 patients showed a reduced DSS score 1–5 years after treatment, 15 patients remained stationary and 12 patients progressed on the DSS scale. These figures are the same as reported in 1980 over a group of 39 patients[1,2] (see TABLE 1) in which the control period after the treatment was of the same duration. It can be concluded that after a mean control period of three years 70% of the patients were stabilized or improved and 30% showed progression of the disease. In the group with improvement (DSS^{+}), the number of female patients is very high.

The results of statistical comparison among the groups is given in TABLE 2. No significant differences among the groups are found, except in comparing the IgG index between the DSS^{+} and the DSS^{-} group. The IgG index before treatment and immediately after treatment is higher in the DSS^{+} than in the DSS^{-} group. No such difference was demonstrated by comparing the IgG index of DSS^{+} and DSS^{-} three months after the IIS. The mean values for the IgG index in the three groups are given in FIGURE 1. It shows how these values for the DSS^{+} and DSS^{o} decrease steeply whereas those of the DSS^{-} group do not. The mean percentage values for serum IgG and intrathecal IgG are given in FIGURE 2, showing no differences among the DSS groups.

TABLE 2. Comparison of CSF and Serum Parameters between Various DSS Groups after Intensive and Chronic Immunosuppressive Treatment

Parameter	Intensive Immunosuppressive Treatment $DSS^+ \rightarrow DSS^o$	$DSS^+ \rightarrow DSS^-$	$DSS^o \rightarrow DSS^-$	Chronic Immuno-suppressive Treatment $DSS^+ \rightarrow DSS^o$
CSF total protein	ns	ns	ns	ns
CSF total IgG	ns	ns	ns	ns
CSF intrathecal IgG	ns	ns	ns	ns
Serum IgG	ns	ns	ns	ns
IgG index	ns	$p < 0.05$ (I), (II)	ns	$p < 0.05$ (I)
Q alb	ns	ns	ns	ns

(I) = comparison of pretreatment values.
(II) = comparison of values immediately after treatment.
ns = no significant differences in comparing values (I), (II) and (III).

The means and the standard deviation of intrathecal IgG synthesis in the three IIS groups are shown in FIGURE 3. The mean starting value of the DSS^+ group (70 mg/l) is higher than that of the DSS^- group (55 mg/l). This difference is not significant, nor are the other differences among the groups significant. IgG percentage at (III) is lower in the DSS^+ than in the DSS^- group. The difference is not statistically significant. These percentages at (III) of DSS^+ are lower than those of DSS^o and DSS^- combined ($0.5 > p > 0.02$), indicating that a higher percentage of starting value at (III) is related

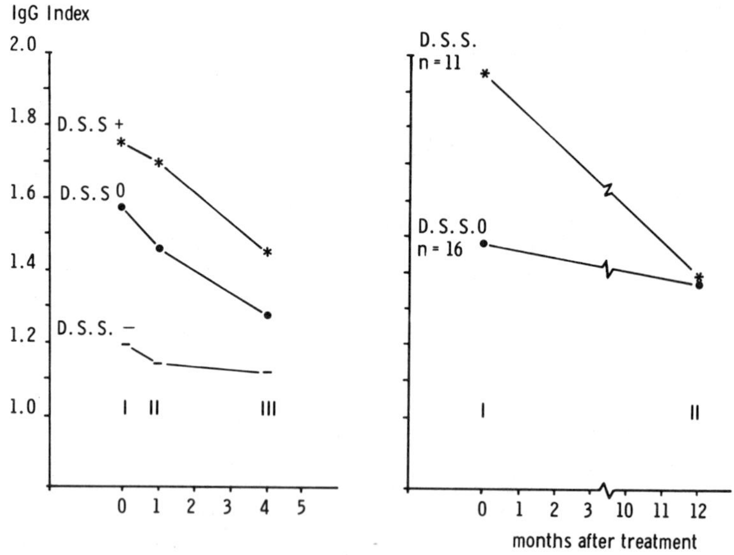

FIGURE 1. The IgG index in various DSS groups after intensive (*left*) and chronic (*right*) immunosuppressive treatment. In the intensive immunosuppressive treatment, DSS^+ at (I) and (II) is significantly different from DSS^- at (I) and (II). In DSS^+ and DSS^o the difference between (I) and (III) is significant. In chronic immunosuppressive treatment significant differences are found between DSS^+ and DSS^o at (I), and between DSS^+ at (I) and (II).

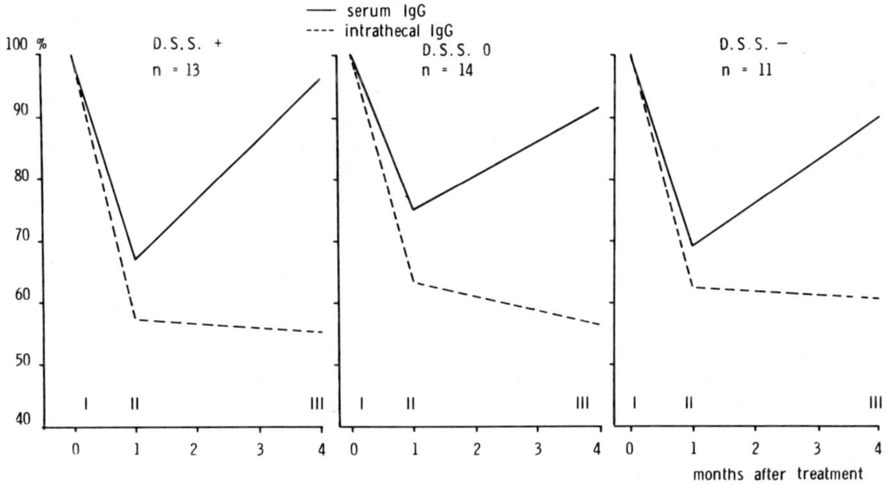

FIGURE 2. Percentages of serum and intrathecal IgG levels at (II) and (III) in various DSS groups after intensive immunosuppressive treatment. Between the groups no differences are found. Within each group there is a significant decrease at (II) for both serum and CSF IgG. Three months after treatment all serum IgG percentages at (III) are higher than the CSF IgG percentages. CSF IgG percentage of DSS^+ at (III) is significantly lower than that of DSS° and DSS^- combined at (III).

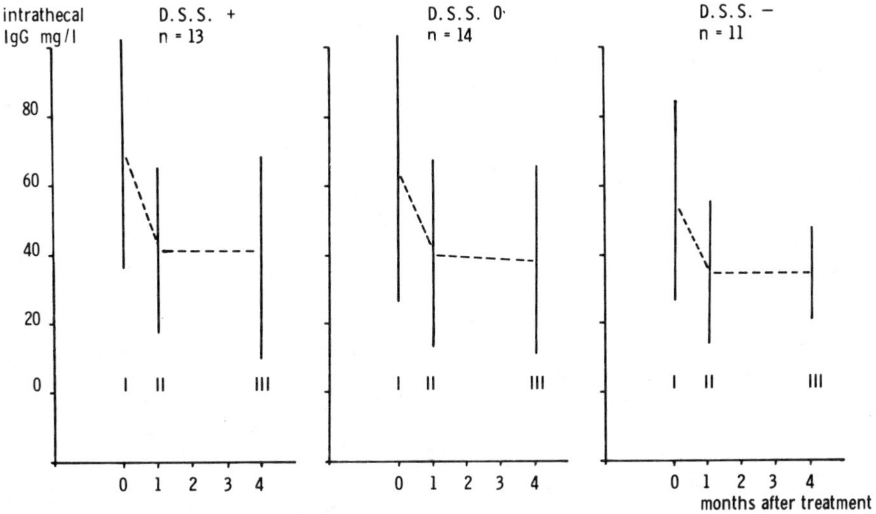

FIGURE 3. Mean intrathecal IgG values with SD of three DSS groups before (I), immediately after (II) and three months after (III) the treatment with intensive immunosuppression. No significant differences are found among the groups.

to more progression. Or, stated in another way, if three months after the IIS intrathecal IgG is low it is a sign of a good prognosis.

Within each of the three DSS groups a significant decrease of CSF and serum parameters is found at (II). At (III) the CSF values are still significantly decreased (TABLE 3, FIG. 3), but serum IgG is not decreased anymore (TABLE 3, FIG. 2). The IgG index shows a significant difference between (I) and (III) only for DSS$^+$ and DSS^o (TABLE 3, FIG. 1), but not for DSS$^-$. Percentages of intrathecal IgG and serum IgG are not different within each group at (I) and (II). However at (III) serum IgG levels are much higher than intrathecal levels. The serum IgG levels have returned close to the starting value, while intrathecal IgG levels remain at post-treatment levels. This trend is of longer duration, as is shown in FIGURE 4, where the intrathecal IgG levels are again determined at 26 months after treatment in nine patients and show the same levels as immediately after treatment.

After low-dose chronic immunosuppression for a period of 6 to 18 months, 16 patients (10 female, 6 male) showed stability and 11 patients (9 female, 2 male) showed improvement of one or more points on the DSS scale. This indicates that a one-year mean duration of chronic immunosuppressive treatment stabilizes or improves the disease.

TABLE 3. Statistical Comparison of Serum and CSF Parameters within DSS Groups of Intensive and Chronic Immunosuppression

	Intensive Immunosuppressive Treatment									Chronic Immunosuppressive Treatment	
	DSS$^+$			DSS^o			DSS$^-$			DSS$^+$	DSS^o
Parameter	I → II	II → III	I → III	I → II	II → III	I → III	I → II	II → III	I → III	I → II	I → II
CSF total protein	–	0	–	–	0	–	–	0	–	0	–
CSF total IgG	–	0	–	–	0	–	–	0	–	0	–
Intrathecal IgG	–	0	–	–	0	–	–	0	–	0	–
Serum IgG	–	+	0	–	+	0	–	+	0	0	0
IgG index	0	0	–	0	0	0	0	0	0	–	0
Q albumin	0	0	–	0	0	0	0	0	0	0	0

– = significant decrease ($p < 0.05$).
\+ = significant increase ($p < 0.05$).
0 = no significant difference.

The results of statistical comparison among the groups is given in TABLE 2. No significant differences in parameters are found, except in comparing the IgG index. As is shown in FIGURE 1 the index is significantly higher in the DSS$^+$ than in the DSS^o group before the treatment. After a low dose of cyclophosphamide for 6 to 18 months this difference is lost and the IgG indexes of the groups are at the same level.

The mean percentage values of intrathecal IgG and serum IgG are given in FIGURE 5. There are no significant differences between the groups. Within each CIS group a significant decrease for CSF parameters is found at (II) for DSS$^+$ and DSS^o. Serum parameters are not different (TABLE 3). In the improved group the number of female patients is again very high. The percentage of serum IgG at (II) in both groups is significantly higher than the percentage of intrathecal IgG at (II), indicating that the tendency for decrease is only present in the intrathecal IgG (FIG. 5, TABLE 3).

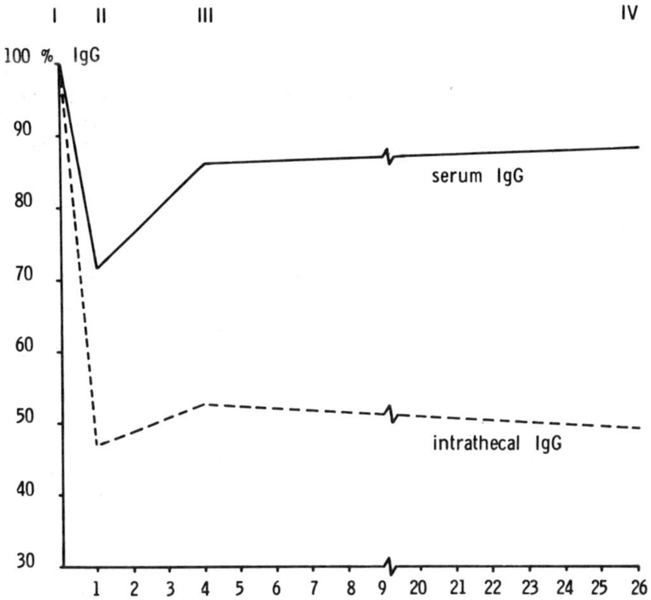

FIGURE 4. Mean percentages of starting values of serum and intrathecal IgG in 9 patients immediately after (II), 3 months after (III) and 26 months after (IV) intensive immunosuppressive treatment. The intrathecal values at (IV) are still significantly lower than before treatment.

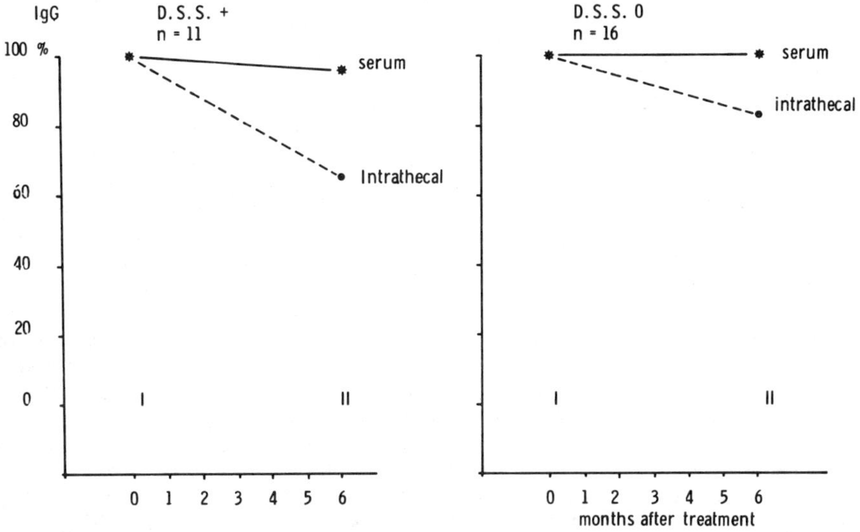

FIGURE 5. Mean percentages of serum and intrathecal IgG in DSS⁺ and DSS° groups of chronic immunosuppressive treatment. The serum values at (II) in both groups are significantly higher than the intrathecal values at (II).

DISCUSSION

The results of this study show that stabilization or improvement over a prolonged period of 1–5 years can be obtained in chronic progressive multiple sclerosis by a short course of intensive immunosuppression. A treatment with low doses of cyclophosphamide over a long period also has such an effect. This study confirms the results of an earlier study.[1,2]

In comparing the various groups formed after a prolonged period of observation with regard to their spinal fluid and serum parameters at an earlier treatment period, only the IgG index showed clear differences. The IgG index of the DSS^+ group before treatment and immediately after treatment was higher than that of the DSS^o group at these moments, and this again was higher than the IgG index of the DSS^- group at (I) and (II). This may also be stated as follows: a high IgG index before and immediately after treatment is connected with a good prognosis after intensive immunosuppression.

The IgG index is an original aspect of MS and as such is not correlated with intrathecal IgG levels[3] as calculated with other formulas; it is said to be a reliable indicator of IgG synthesis in the brain.[4,5] Our results therefore would indicate that as the IgG synthesis in the brain is higher, the effect of intensive immunosuppressive treatment on the course of the disease is better.

The intrathecal IgG levels three months after the treatment also seem to have a connection with prognosis, in the following way: if three months after the treatment the intrathecal IgG remains low, there seems to be improvement of the disease (DSS^+ group). An indication in this direction was found in an earlier study with total IgG content of the spinal fluid.[1] It again relates intracerebral IgG to prognosis in that if the effect of intensive immunosuppression on the intrathecal IgG remains for three months, the disease will probably take a favorable course in the coming years.

Generally the intensive immunosuppressive treatment has a clear effect on CSF parameters and on serum IgG immediately after the treatment at (II). Both serum IgG and intrathecal IgG are reduced to about 50% or 60% of the starting value. After the three-month period without treatment, the serum IgG levels return to normal, but CSF values remain low. If both serum IgG and intrathecal IgG are expressed as percentages of pretreatment values, serum IgG returns to pretreatment levels, but intrathecal IgG does not. This indicates that the intrathecal IgG synthesis is more sensitive to immunosuppressive treatment than the IgG synthesis of the blood. Here again prognosis is of importance as the IgG index remains low for DSS^+ and DSS^o. This aspect was not only demonstrated with intensive, but also with low-dose chronic immunosuppression.

These results may be explained in light of information that has recently been produced with regard to T cell population in brain, CSF and blood of MS patients. The T helper cell probably is the predominant cell in the lesion in the CNS of MS patients.[6,7] The cell population of the CSF consists mainly of T helper cells[8] and is strongly reduced by immunosuppressive treatment.[10,9] As cyclophosphamide[11] and prednisone penetrate the blood-brain barrier, the effects of these drugs may be present directly at the site of the lesion or indirectly via the production of precursor cells in the bone marrow.

This study demonstrates a more intense effect of immunosuppressive treatment on the intrathecally formed IgG than on the serum IgG. This would favor the hypothesis that immunosuppressive treatment acts directly on the intrathecal IgG-producing system. And this in turn may be effected by action on specific oligoclonal precursor cells in the bone marrow, or at the site of the lesion. In our study on immunosuppressive treatment on T cell subpopulation,[8,9] we demonstrated a relatively stronger effect of the treatment on T helper than on T suppressor cells. This effect may also be present intracerebrally and thus produce its therapeutic effect.

REFERENCES

1. HOMMES, O. R., K. J. B. LAMERS & P. REEKERS. 1980a. Effect of intensive immunosuppression on the course of chronic progressive multiple sclerosis. J. Neurol. **223:** 177–190.
2. HOMMES, O. R., K. J. B. LAMERS & P. REEKERS. 1980b. Prognostic factors in intensive immunosuppressive treatment of chronic progressive MS. *In* Progress in Multiple Sclerosis Research. H. J. Bauer, S. Poser & G. Ritter, Eds.: 396–400. Springer. Berlin.
3. LAMERS, K. J. B., W. H. DOESBURG, O. R. HOMMES & W. VAN GEEL. 1984. On the calculation of CSF IgG synthesized in the central nervous system. *In* Immunotherapies in Multiple Sclerosis. O. R. Hommes, J. Mertin & W. W. Tourtellotte, Eds. Clin. Trials J. Suppl. In press.
4. TIBBLING, G., H. LINK & S. OHMAN. 1977. Principles of albumin and IgG analysis in neurological disorders. I. Establishment of reference values. Scan. J. Clin. Lab. Invest. **37:** 385–390.
5. LINK, H. & G. TIBBLING. 1977. Principles of albumin and IgG analysis in neurological disorders. II. Relation of the concentration of proteins in serum and cerebrospinal fluid. Scand. J. Clin. Lab. Invest. **37:** 391–396.
6. BRINKMAN, C. J. J., H. J. TER LAAK, O. R. HOMMES, S. POPPEMA & P. DELMOTTE. 1982. T lymphocyte subpopulations in multiple sclerosis lesions. N. Engl. J. Med. **307:** 1644–1645.
7. NYLAND, H., R. MATRE, S. MØRK, J-R. BJERKE & A. MAESS. 1982. T lymphocyte subpopulations in multiple sclerosis lesions. N. Engl. J. Med. **307:** 1643–1644.
8. BRINKMAN, C. J. J., W. M. NILLESEN & O. R. HOMMES. 1984. The effect of cyclophosphamide on T lymphocyte and T lymphocyte subsets in patients with chronic progressive multiple sclerosis. Acta Neurol. Scand. **69:** 90–96.
9. BRINKMAN, C. J. J., W. M. NILLESEN & O. R. HOMMES. 1984. T cell subpopulations in blood and cerebrospinal fluid of multiple sclerosis patients: Effect of cyclophosphamide. Clin. Immunol. Immunopath. In press.
10. SCHOLTES, F., H. J. TER LAAK & O. R. HOMMES. Effects of intensive immunosuppressive treatment on spinal fluid cells in chronic progressive multiple sclerosis. In preparation.
11. HOMMES, O. R., F. AERTS, U. BAHR & H.-R. SCHULTEN. 1983. Cyclophosphamide levels in serum and spinal fluid of multiple sclerosis patients treated with immunosuppression. J. Neurol. Sci. **85:** 297–303.

Clinical Trials in Multiple Sclerosis

Problems and Opportunities

DONALD H. SILBERBERG

Department of Neurology
University of Pennsylvania School of Medicine
Philadelphia, Pennsylvania 19104

INTRODUCTION

Evidence that suggests immunologic participation in the pathogenesis of multiple sclerosis (MS) and the increasing availability of agents that affect the immune response have contributed to substantial growth in the number of clinical trials of treatment for MS (TABLE 1). This trend will continue.

The fact that potential treatment agents are available, and that therapeutic trials are going on, brings great hope to patients with MS and to their families and friends. Therapeutic trials also hold crucial interest for those conducting research on MS, and for all who pay health insurance premiums and taxes. The considerations involved in designing, conducting and interpreting clinical trials in MS have been reviewed thoroughly in at least four U.S. publications in the last twenty years.[10–13] The landmark communication was delivered at the last New York Academy of Sciences symposium on multiple sclerosis in 1964, by Schumacher and co-workers.[10] Most subsequent statements have added relatively little to that important contribution. I will not review the contents of these comprehensive papers, which are readily available, but rather focus on two issues.

The first relates to the observations that treatment with agents as diverse as immunosuppressants, interferon (an immunomodulator and/or anti-viral agent), plasmapheresis, and copolymer I, all seem to benefit patients with MS. In addition, peer-reviewed reports of the effectiveness of lymphocyte transfer factor[5] and of hyperbaric oxygen[9] in controlled studies add to our dilemma. For the most part, these studies have been carried out with apparent rigor; nevertheless it strains credulity to accept all of these results at face value. Several possible interpretations come to mind, and will be discussed.

The second issue can be expressed as a question: Against the background of what we currently know about the pathogenesis of MS, when is the appropriate time in the development and understanding of a new therapeutic agent to carry out a therapeutic trial? Related to this is our responsibility to prevent widespread application of treatments that are still experimental and sometimes hazardous. These two issues may be shortened to (1) credibility, and (2) propitiousness.

CREDIBILITY

Attempts to understand reports of positive therapeutic effects from diverse treatments lead to questions at several levels: one can (1) question a particular therapeutic trial, or (2) question the validity of the currently available methodologies for conducting and interpreting clinical trials, or (3) further examine the nature of the disease process itself.

Perhaps the most difficult part of any therapeutic trial in MS is the task of assuring both patient and observer objectivity, because the agent used often induces changes that are obvious and dramatic to the patient and physician alike. Examples include fever, weight gain, edema and alopecia. A controlled trial requires assigning the assessment of patients to experienced neurologists who have no way of knowing which patients have received the proposed treatment and which have received the control. This may even necessitate such disguises as the use of wigs, and reliance on the neurologic exam alone, without the patient's description of symptomatic patterns.

The problem caused by the patient's bias is often even more difficult. The patient's awareness of having received the treatment, rather than the control agent, leads the patient to greater effort on the motor exam and minimization of symptoms, the very foundations of our clinical assessment. Since it may not be possible or safe to use control agents that produce side effects similar to the treatment, this problem is sometimes insurmountable. It may be that, at present, any clinical trial of an agent that produces clinically recognizable side effects will appear to show clinical improvement associated with that agent.

TABLE 1. Controlled Clinical Trials in MS

Rationale	Examples	Status		Results
Specific immunologic tolerance	myelin basic protein	completed	P	–
	copolymer I	in progress	FS	
Immunosuppressants	azathioprine	in progress	FS	
		completed[1]	P	±
	cyclophosphamide	completed[2]	P	–
		completed[3]	P	+
Anti-inflammatory	ACTH	completed[4]	FS	+
Biologic response modifiers	transfer factor	completed[5]	FS	+
	levamisole	completed[6,7,8]	p	–
	interferon	in progress	FS	
	plasmapheresis	in progress	P	
Other	hyperbaric oxygen	completed[9]	P	+

P = small scale; pilot study.
FS = larger number of patients; full-scale study

These are crucial stumbling blocks in the conduct of some trials. The overall statistical picture has little meaning if the data itself is in question. This leads to questions regarding the power of our current methods for conducting trials.

Thus, the key problem becomes one of objectivity and the ability to quantify. The several patient examination systems and scales in use attempt to deal with some aspects of this. Unresolved problems that are difficult to solve with these systems are (1) patient cooperation and effort are required, (2) examiners vary in their interpretation, and (3) even patients with fixed, stable deficits have good days and bad days. Surely the answers to these problems will come with the slowly emerging laboratory methods for assessing the extent and severity of tissue damage, and for assessing the impact of lesions on physiologic functioning.

Examples of useful laboratory aids are here already. Proton imaging by nuclear magnetic resonance (NMR) often demonstrates many more areas of demyelination than are expected on the basis of the clinical history and examination. Techniques for computer-generated three-dimensional reconstruction of demyelinated areas visualized by NMR will soon be available. This will permit volume and density measurements of the affected areas throughout the brain and spinal cord of an individual. This one imaging technique alone will completely change our ability to determine whether or not new lesions above a particular size have occurred and whether pre-existing lesions have advanced or receded. The demonstration of leakage of intravascular contrast material into plaques, as seen by high resolution computer-assisted tomographic brain X-ray (CT) scanning, provides an opportunity to study one aspect of the tissue reaction.[14] The blood-brain barrier breakdown apparently occurs only in the early lesion, and disappears with ensuing weeks. Similarly, phosphorous NMR will be used to study energy metabolism within and around plaques, and positron emission tomographic brain scanning will be used to determine blood flow, glucose metabolism, water content, and other biochemical features that may be influenced by a particular treatment.

At present the best available measurement that correlates with concurrently active demyelination is measurement of myelin basic protein (MBP) in the cerebrospinal fluid.[15,16] This is inconvenient and probably underestimates activity in the deeper white matter lesions, but it is safe and reproducible. A blood or urine test for myelin breakdown products would obviously be preferable, and efforts are underway to attempt to make this possible.[17] Serial use of a measurement of current myelin destruction would answer questions of disease activity to supplement the neurologic exam.

Similarly, electrophysiologic assessment of the function of various central nervous system tracts is a relatively recent development. These measurements of the latency of impulse propagation through the visual, auditory-brainstem, and somatosensory systems are sensitive detectors of demyelination. Quantifiable and reproducible results often show clinically unsuspected lesions and can provide a method of assessing function as well as tissue changes.

Thus by combining objective techniques for imaging lesions, measuring disease activity, and measuring physiologic function as supplements to the traditional neurologic history and examination, we may be entering an era in which a smaller number of patients can be studied intensively, and provide more reliable data than is currently available in larger trials.

The third possibility for rationalizing the many recent clinical trial success stories is that these results may be telling us something about the disease process itself. Perhaps lesion pathogenesis depends on many steps, and interference with any one may slow the process. For example, interferon may act effectively as an anti-viral agent, even though it is also a lymphokine which has a number of effects on the immune system, such as enhancing the cytotoxic effects of T cells, macrophages, and natural killer cells, and enhancing the presentation of antigens by macrophages. Some of the so-called immunosuppressants may actually be acting as anti-inflammatory agents; copolymer may be inhibiting proteases, and transfer factor, which has complex activities, may be doing something quite unknown at present. This issue simply points out our need for a more thorough understanding of the cellular and humoral events underlying the MS lesion.

PROPITIOUSNESS

I can do no more than raise this issue for discussion, but I do not want to leave it unsaid. A complex of factors leads the investigator to decide to try a new (or reuse an old) agent as presumptive treatment. Hopefully, the mere existence of an agent with new properties will not alone qualify for trials in MS. For example, we are faced with the availability of many different forms of interferon, each of which could be said to deserve a trial. A clinician-investigator must have a hypothesis to be tested, with a well-developed rationale, or all of the funds for research in MS will soon be devoted to clinical trials. Above all, the investigator must keep in mind the fact that the average patient with MS lives 35 years or more after onset, often productively and relatively free from disability for much of that time. Thus, the preeminence of the risk/benefit ratio. A treatment that requires elegant statistical methods to show a mild beneficial effect may not be worth the specific side effects of that agent.

OPPORTUNITIES

Among the several opportunities that a clinical trial provides is the means to contribute to an understanding of the natural history, and often the pathogenesis, of multiple sclerosis. The group of patients selected for a trial have undergone rigorous scrutiny, have agreed to cooperate, and will be under uniform observation for the duration of the trial. Most will continue to be available after the trial ends. They are ideal subjects in which to investigate the research laboratory correlates of clinical activity, understand psychosocial factors under more controlled conditions, and contribute to improvement in the entire arena of the treatment of individuals with multiple sclerosis.

Clinical trials provide the basis for physician and patient education so as to prevent the widespread application of useless or still-experimental, and sometimes dangerous, approaches. Finally, clinical trials serve to focus attention on the dilemma of patients with MS, which hopefully will lead to better solutions for their vexing problems.

REFERENCES

1. Mertin, J., P. Rudge, M. Kremer, M. J. R. Healey, S. C. Knight, A. Compston, J. R. Batchelor, E. J. Thompson, A. M. Halliday, M. Denman & P. B. Medawar. 1982. Double-blind controlled trial of immunosuppression in the treatment of multiple sclerosis: Final report. Lancet **ii:** 351–354.
2. Millac, P. & H. Miller. 1969. Cyclophosphamide in multiple sclerosis. Lancet **i:** 783.
3. Hauser, S. L., D. M. Dawson & J. R. Lehrich *et al.* 1983. Intensive immunosuppression and progressive multiple sclerosis. N. Eng. J. Med. **308:** 173–180.
4. Rose, A. S., J. W. Kuzma, J. F. Kurtzke *et al.* 1970. Cooperative study in the evaluation of therapy in multiple sclerosis: ACTH vs. placebo. Final report. Neurology **20** (2): 1–159.
5. Basten, A., J. D. Pollard & G. J. Stewart. 1980. Transfer factor in treatment of multiple sclerosis. Lancet **ii:** 931–934.
6. Camenga, D. L. 1977. Safety and efficacy of levamisole in multiple sclerosis (Abstracts). Eleventh World Congress of Neurology. International Congress Series, No. 427. W. A. den Hartog-Jaeger, G. W. Bruyn & A. P. J. Heijstee, Eds.: 331–332. Excerpta Medica. Amsterdam.
7. Ellison, G. W., M. R. Mickey, L. W. Meyers & A. S. Rose. 1980. A pilot study of amantadine treatment of multiple sclerosis. *In* Progress in Multiple Sclerosis. H. J. Bauer & G. Ritter, Eds.: 405–408. Springer. Heidelberg, New York.
8. Gonsette, R. E., L. Demontey, P. Delmotte *et al.* 1982. Modulation of immunity in multiple sclerosis: A double-blind levamisole-placebo controlled study in 85 patients. J. Neurol. **228:** 65.
9. Fischer, B. H., M. Marks & T. Reich. 1983. Hyperbaric-oxygen treatment of multiple sclerosis. A randomized, placebo-controlled, double-blind study. N. Engl. J. Med. **308:** 181–186.
10. Schumacher, G. A., G. Beebe, R. F. Kibler *et al.* 1965. Problems of experimental trials of

therapy in multiple sclerosis: Report by the panel on the evaluation of experimental trials of therapy in multiple sclerosis. Ann. N.Y. Acad. Sci. **122:** 552–568.
11. UNITED STATES DEPARTMENT OF HEALTH, EDUCATION, AND WELFARE. 1974. Report and recommendations of the National Advisory Commission on Multiple Sclerosis. DHEW Publication No. (NIH) 74–534. U.S. Government Printing Office. Washington, D. C. pp. 36–37.
12. BROWN, J. R., G. W. BEEBE, J. F. KURTZKE *et al.* 1979. A design of clinical studies to asses therapeutic efficacy in multiple sclerosis. Neurology **29**(2)**:** 3–23.
13. PROCEEDINGS OF THE INTERNATIONAL CONFERENCE ON THERAPEUTIC TRIALS IN MULTIPLE SCLEROSIS. 1983. Arch. Neurol. **40:** 666–704.
14. LODDER, J., A. W. DE WEERD, J. C. KOETSIER *et al.* 1983. Computed tomography in acute cerebral multiple sclerosis. Arch. Neurol. **40:** 320–322.
15. COHEN, S. R., R. M. HERNDON & G. M. MCKANN. 1976. Radioimmunoassay of myelin basic protein and spinal fluid: An index of active demyelination. N. Engl. J. Med. **295:** 1455–1457.
16. WHITAKER, J. N., R. P. LISAK, R. M. BASHIR *et al.* 1980. Immunoreactive myelin basic protein in the cerebrospinal fluid in neurologic disorders. Ann. Neurol. **7:** 58–64.
17. TROTTER, J. L., C. L. WEGESCHEIDE & W. F. GARVEY. 1983. Immunoreactive myelin proteolipid protein-like activity in cerebrospinal fluid and serum of neurologically impaired patients. Ann. Neurol. **14:** 545–558.

GENERAL DISCUSSION

C. SMITH (*Albert Einstein College of Medicine, Bronx, NY*): I would like to ask questions of those who presented the cyclophosphamide data today. It's not entirely clear from Dr. Weiner's report what the appropriate parameter is that one followed to determine the appropriate dose to give to individuals. Some people in our experience who receive the lower recommended dose, that is 80 mg per kg body weight, do not achieve a leukopenia of the dimensions that he reports in his paper. I want to know if it's the absolute leukopenia that one achieves, or is it the absolute doses that are important in determining what the appropriate amount is for a given individual?

H. L. WEINER (*Harvard Medical School, Boston, MA*): Our studies were based on achieving a certain degree of leukopenia not according to particular dose, so that the doses that people received are generally between 4 grams and 8 or 9 grams and are given in a way that's designed to induce leukopenia of approximately 2,000 or less.

J. FOLEY (*University Hospital, Cleveland, OH*): Is there not a collaborative interferon study going on now, the code of which was supposed to be broken soon?

J. BROWN (*Mayo Medical School, Rochester, MN*): I think the only one, perhaps Dr. Waksman might correct me, was the one that was reported by Dr. Knobler. There's one that's getting started but the one that is to be broken at this time would be the one in California.

B. WAKSMAN (*National Multiple Sclerosis Society, New York, NY*): The trial that you're asking about is the one that Dr. Knobler reported on: the code was broken just a few weeks ago and the analysis is not as yet completed. What you saw were preliminary data from that trial. There are over 20 clinical trials of interferon going on at the present time around the world and almost half of them are well set up trials in the sense of having controls with blinding and so on, and some of them involve intrathecal administration, some of them involve systemic administration, some of them involve natural interferon, some recombinant interferon, some alpha, some beta, some gamma, so the variety is extraordinary. There'll be a lot of new information in another two years.

BROWN: Just a very brief open question, has anybody seen multiple sclerosis in association with AIDS and would anybody comment what might one expect if that were to occur?

J. PRINEAS (*University of Medicine and Dentistry of New Jersey, Newark, NJ*): Amongst the several particles that have been observed in AIDS patients by those people looking for a virus there is a particle that's been reported in *Lancet,* but it's been seen only in AIDS patients and in monkeys with transmissible noninfectious, non-A, non-B hepatitis. And it's an odd particle that might in fact be a virus, it's one of the candidate particles in AIDS; it was observed between lymphocytes and macrophages in one MS patient some years ago. The patient wasn't suspect for AIDS, so there is a sort of an association in that sense that I assume is probably quite irrelevant.

M. P. MCQUILLIN (*Medical College of Wisconsin, Milwaukee, WI*): I would like to ask Dr. Hommes, in the light of the fact that he has such an extensive and long experience with cyclophosphamide, has he among his population of patients observed any of the feared hematologic, oncologic, and other complications from those therapies?

O. R. HOMMES (*Radboud University Hospital, Nijmegen, the Netherlands*): I personally have not found any of these feared consequences. We discussed the problem a year ago at a workshop on immunological treatment in multiple sclerosis and a French group had data on 1500 patients that they followed up for the last seven years, and they did not find that there was an increase of carcinogenesis, compared to a matched control group.

G. W. ELLISON (*UCLA, Los Angeles, CA*): Dr. Hommes, I think that the French group was treated with azathioprine, is that correct?

HOMMES: Yes.

M. B. BORNSTEIN: (*Albert Einstein College of Medicine, Bronx, NY*): Also in response to the last question. I've been using immunosuppression in the form of 6-mercaptopurine, and azathioprine and occasionally alkuran since about 1962. I have known only one patient who developed leukemia and that was after alkuran treatment, and as a matter of fact there's one patient in that group who has been taking 6-mercaptopurine for 18 years, unknown to me, and she has no difficulty whatsover.

R. J. SLATER (*National Multiple Sclerosis Society, New York, NY*): I have a question that bears on the suggestion that we might consider mixed forms of immunosuppression in the future. Is there any evidence that these drugs in combination or in sequence can have a very adverse effect? And if so I think that should be mentioned in these proceedings.

BROWN: Dr. Ellison, I see your head shaking; would you want to comment?

ELLISON: I'm shaking my head because I only have rumors, but the rumor is that it's okay to go from azathioprine to cyclophosphamide but it's not okay to go the other way. If you treat a person with cyclophosphamide and then give azathioprine, the incidence of cancer is supposed to increase but I don't have hard data.

L. SCHEINBERG (*Albert Einstein College of Medicine, Bronx, NY*): I'd like to make one or two closing remarks in a lighter vein. Considering that one is dealing here with very desperate patients, physicians who are often enthusiastic, a usually hopeful national society, an unpredictable disease and crude evaluation methods, it is not unusual that there should be some confusion about therapy in multiple sclerosis.

At an early conference, there was reported in the Annals of the Athenian Academy of Sciences the remark of Euripides to Hippocrates, "Those whom the gods would destroy they first direct to do clinical trials in multiple sclerosis." As if to prove this point a few hundred years later in Jerusalem, there was reported treatment of a patient who had had paralysis for over thirty years. John reports the Kurtzke on that case was 7.5. The patient was treated and his Kurtzke score dropped down to one. The case was lost to follow-up however, after only one day. You know the rest of the story, the therapist was arrested, convicted, and crucified.

Perhaps if the discussion at Calvary had been taped at a later time he might have been heard to say, "Perhaps I should have had controls."

The Current Management of Multiple Sclerosis

RANDALL T. SCHAPIRO,[a] STANLEY VAN DEN NOORT,[b] AND LABE SCHEINBERG[c]

[a]*University of Minnesota Medical School*
Minneapolis, Minnesota 55455
and
Fairview Hospital Multiple Sclerosis Program
Minneapolis, Minnesota 55422

[b]*California College of Medicine*
Irvine, California 92664

[c]*Albert Einstein College of Medicine*
Bronx, New York 10461

Multiple sclerosis (MS) is a demyelinating disease with an unpredictable course. This course is usually characterized as exacerbating and remitting. The clinical spectrum of the disease is, however, much broader. There are several different courses that MS can take.[1,2]

Benign sensory multiple sclerosis often presents as numbness of an area of the body (FIG. 1). This symptom may then clear or remain but the clinical manifestations of the disease do not appear to progress. This form is more common than one would suspect, however is often difficult to diagnose. It may constitute over 10% of diagnosed cases.[3]

Benign relapsing-remitting MS presents with mild neurological symptoms and signs that come and go but fail to produce severe disability (FIG. 2). This type of MS has been estimated at 20–30%.[4]

Chronic progressive MS usually leads to significant disability. The findings slowly and inexorably progress in spite of all measures. This constitutes 10% of MS (FIG. 3).[4]

Sometimes this chronic progression shows fluctuation within the framework of a downhill direction. This may be categorized as *chronic relapsing progressive* multiple sclerosis and accounts for 50–60% of the diagnosed cases (FIG. 4).[4,5]

Very occasionally a rapid, downhill course is seen from the outset. Categorized as *acute rapid progressive* MS, this may lead to severe disability or even death. This may be estimated at less than 10%.

The neurological clinician should be aware that MS can present and progress in a variety of defined manners in order to counsel as well as to treat patients. For similar reasons it is important to understand that certain neurological symptoms herald more problems than others. At times these symptoms may aid in predicting the course of the disease.

Visual symptoms are very common in MS. Decreased vision is a sign of disease in the optic nerve and is seen in 50% of MS patients.[6] The severity of the symptoms may vary from a minor decrease, detectable only by evoked response or color panel testing, to significant blindness. Acute episodes affect one eye at a time. Bilateral acute involvement is exceptional and usually is due to an alternative diagnosis. The symptoms may come on very acutely only to clear just as quickly. They may, however, remain, causing ongoing problems. If decreased vision is the main neurological problem it often improves and may indicate a relatively benign course.[7]

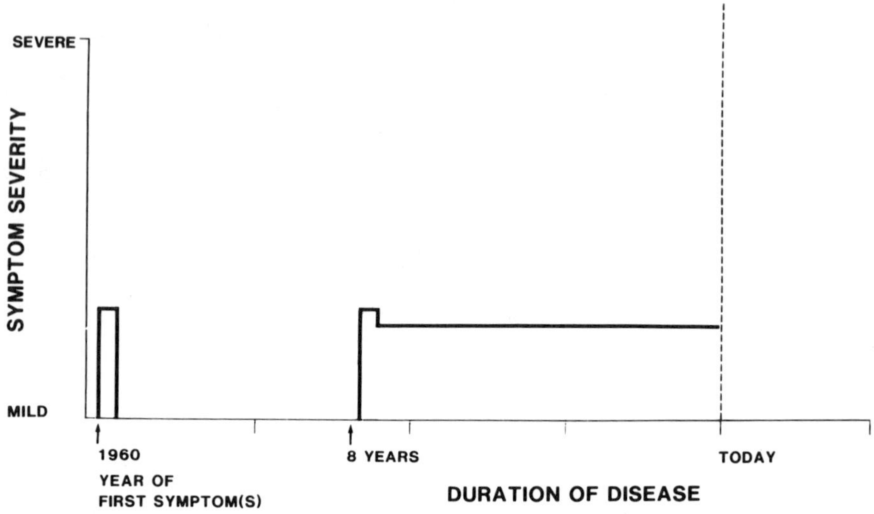

FIGURE 1. The benign course.

Diplopia indicates lesions in the brainstem involving the nerves to the extraocular muscles or their supranuclear and internuclear connections. This indicates brainstem disease. Its frequency has been estimated at 43%.[6] Intention tremor (45%) is also a sign of disease of the brainstem and/or cerebellum. Demyelination in these areas can be the cause of significant disability despite being rather focal and without anatomically large lesions.

Spinal cord demyelination is quite common. It is often seen as the major manifestation of late-onset (age 40–55) multiple sclerosis. The course of this disease presentation is one of progression. The legs are often much more involved than the arms. Patients are

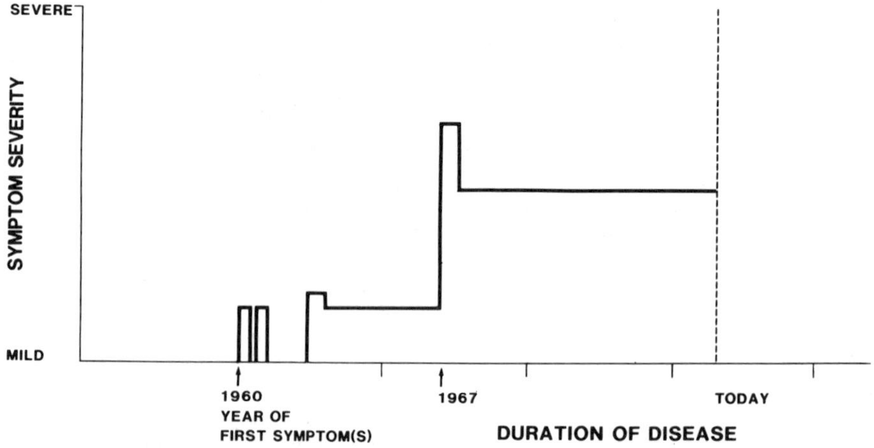

FIGURE 2. The (benign) relapsing/remitting course.

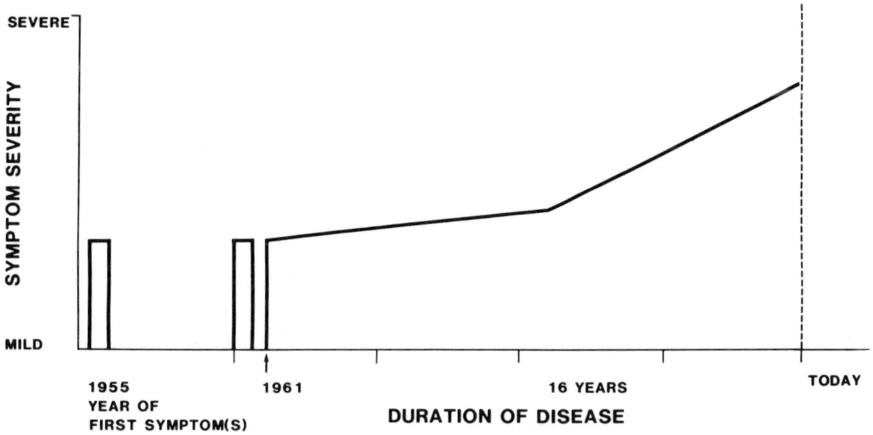

FIGURE 3. The chronic relapsing/progressive course.

often able to function reasonably well because their upper extremities remain strong and coordinated and their thinking is clear.

Cerebral multiple sclerosis as an entity is rare but clearly exists. Manifestations of some cortical involvement may be more common than is generally accorded. Some patients present and progress with cerebral deficits as the primary problem. This leads to significant disability despite lack of long tract signs.

Mixed presentation MS, the most common presentation of multiple sclerosis, is the most unpredictable. As the name implies the demyelination occurs in several areas of the white matter of the cerebrum, brainstem, cerebellum, and spinal cord.

A number of other symptoms are common but do not aid in the predictability of the disease. These include: vertigo, bladder disturbances, handwriting difficulty and Lhermitte's phenomenon.

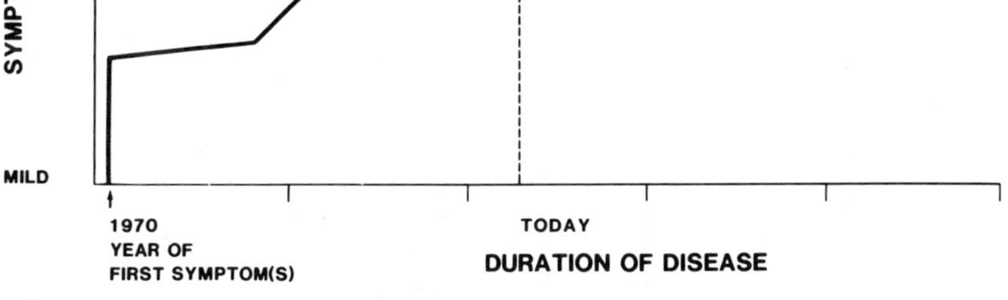

FIGURE 4. The chronic progressive course.

There are other factors that can aid in predicting the course of multiple sclerosis. Often the younger MS patients will lead a more benign course. The older patients develop the spinal cord progressive form and become more disabled in a shorter period of time.[8]

The fewer signs and symptoms occurring in the initial attack of the disease may mean a less severe form. If the symptoms are more sensory than motor there is a better outlook. If recovery from the initial attack is complete a better prognosis is predicted than if significant deficit remains.[9,10]

Cerebellar or brainstem lesions, especially those causing speech problems, are often associated with major difficulties and a poor prognosis for good rehabilitation.

The patient with multiple sclerosis often goes through several medical and psychosocial stages that begin with the first symptoms of the disease. There is often a lag time between the initial symptoms and the time of presentation to the physician for diagnosis (or lack of diagnosis). During this time the patient either denies the symptoms or is waiting for them to disappear spontaneously. The symptoms may be acute or even insidious. They may be disabling or minor.

Eventually because of internal (within the patient) or external (family/friends) pressure the patient seeks medical advice. A diagnosis may or may not be made at that time. However, often the disease goes into remission and the patient sees the problem as not being especially serious.

If the remission fails to come or if another exacerbation follows quickly a diagnosis is usually made and a serious problem is perceived. At that time physician intervention is essential and can make the difference between acceptance and adjustment and lack of acceptance and adjustment. This difference may continue throughout the patient's course. Furthermore, many physicians hide behind the difficulty of diagnosis and delay telling the patient about the working diagnosis until a point at which it is too late to establish a credible relationship with the patient.

In general the management of disease can be divided into four broad categories. These are prophylaxis, curative, restorative, and symptomatic. Despite a growing understanding of the epidemiology of multiple sclerosis there is no knowledge regarding its prophylaxis. Certain facts are known: MS is more common in females (1.8:1 or more); certain HLA types predominate; in temperate geographic areas its incidence is greater; certain races are more at risk.[11] It is conceivable that sometime in the future this knowledge, in combination with future developments, will lead to a breakthrough in the prevention of the disease.

To date no known curative treatment is known for multiple sclerosis. There are, however, some established treatments that appear to hasten remission and some less established treatments that may slow or temporarily slow the course. Corticosteroids or adrenocorticotrophic hormone (ACTH) continue to be the most widely used treatment used to promote remission. Many neurologists use ACTH (either IV or IM). There appears to be little rationale for using ACTH over synthetic corticosteroids and, in fact, there may be reason to choose the synthetic steroids. The bioactivity of ACTH is somewhat unpredictable whereas that of the synthetic steroids is much smoother.[12] Newer methods of production of ACTH have decreased the bioactivity problem somewhat. The value of corticosteroids, however, also lies in the fact that the dosage of cortisone crossing the blood-brain barrier can be much higher than ACTH would consistently produce.

There are a number of dosage regimens, depending upon one's goal. Most clinicians use these medicines as strong anti-edema and anti-inflammatory agents. As such certain rules should be followed. A high-dose, short course regimen is recommended. An example of such a regimen is:

DEXAMETHASONE	16 mg IM, IV, or PO Q.I.D. × 1 day
	8 mg Q.I.D. × 1 day
	4 mg Q.I.D. × 2 days
	2 mg Q.I.D. × 2 days
	1 mg Q.I.D. × 1 day

for a total of seven days. Another example might be less aggressive:

DEXAMETHASONE	4 mg PO Q.I.D. × 3 days
	4 mg PO T.I.D. × 3 days
	4 mg PO B.I.D. × 3 days
	4 mg PO Q.D. × 3 days

Whether appropriate doses of dexamethasone, prednisone, methylprednisolone or others are used matters little. If the anti-edema dose is high enough, anti-inflammatory effect will occur. If the course is short enough (four weeks or less), the complications of steroids are less likely to occur. If a longer course is necessary, a single dose every other day can decrease some of these side effects. One may begin at 100 mg Q.O.D. prednisone and taper over a one-month period of time.

In an attempt to slow the course of the disease immunosuppressant medication is sometimes utilized.[13] This should be reserved for patients with clear chronic progressive or rapid progressive MS that has not responded to high-dose corticosteroid therapy. Occasionally the steroids are used as immunosuppressive drugs. They are then used over longer periods at often lower doses. Steroids are not particularly suited to this use; there are better immunosuppressants. A number of these, including azathioprine, cyclophosphamide, interferon, plasma and lymphocytopheresis are discussed in detail in other papers in this volume. From a practical clinical standpoint azathioprine therapy is often recommended for patients with frequent attacks with poor recovery (chronic relapsing progressive or chronic progressive), rapid progression, poor response to corticosteroids or severe steroid side effects. Such treatment should be undertaken by a neurologist thoroughly familiar with immunosuppressive drugs. The patient should be aware of the complications of treatment. Dosage is usually 1–2.5 mg/kg/day in two divided doses. Dosage should be reduced if the white count falls below 3500.

In patients with chronic progressive MS that has not been amenable to steroids or azathioprine, cyclophosphamide may be tried. A recent pilot study suggests remission for a year or more following a two-week course at 100 mg/kg.[14] There are relatively greater risks with this drug. Alkylating drugs (cyclophosphamide) are also more likely to produce neoplasia than other similar drugs. The complications of damage to the marrow, liver and kidney resemble azathioprine but include alopecia. Another major complication is that of a sterile hemorrhagic cystitis.

Combinations of the above agents are occasionally used to induce remission and slow exacerbations (FIG. 5). Treatments with hyperbaric oxygen, dietary manipulation, protease inhibitors, transfer factor and levamisole lack enough convincing data to recommend their use at this time.

Although restoring the demyelinated nervous system appeals to the imagination, there is no practical means to do so at this time.

The best available therapy today for the MS patient is symptomatic treatment. Disabling symptoms or signs of MS can be categorized as primary (direct), secondary (complicating), or tertiary (psychosocial). Primary signs result directly from a strategically located plaque and include weakness, spasticity, incoordination, visual loss, cognitive abnormalities, sensory disturbances and some urinary abnormalities. Secondary findings include contractures, decubitus ulcers, urinary tract infections, and other intercurrent infections. Tertiary findings include emotional, vocational, social, and marital problems.

Gait problems are frequent primary symptoms of MS. These may be due to spasticity, weakness, ataxia, or any combination. Ataxia carries the gravest prognosis for disability. Only spasticity can be directly affected by treatment. Baclofen is the drug of choice for spasticity. Other drugs (dantrolene sodium, diazapam) are less effective and have unacceptable side effects. Many patients need their spasticity to stand and alleviation results in apparent weakness. The dosage of baclofen should be adjusted by the patient and the physician to the level desired. Fifteen to 200 mg/day in divided doses are often required.

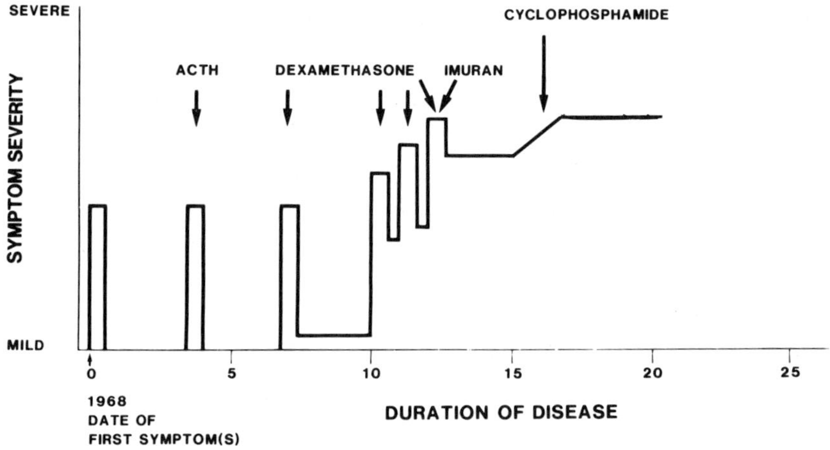

FIGURE 5. Treatment regimen in multiple sclerosis.

Often medical (pharmacologic) intervention is not enough to ameliorate the problem. Combinations of medical, physical, surgical, and psychosocial therapies are often necessary. The later stages of spasticity are often characterized by severe adductor spasm of the hips with flexor spasms of the hips and knees. If unrelieved this may lead to fibrous contractures of these joints with resultant decubiti over the sacrum and hips due to inability to properly position the patient. Contractures may be prevented at this stage by slow, passive stretching exercises done at frequent regular intervals during the day. Neurectomies, motor-point blocks, tenotomy, and intraspinal injection of phenol are occasionally necessary for disabling spasticity. These treatments leave the patient weak and destroy bladder function. Thus these must be used with extreme caution.

The spasms in the arms and legs may occur in a paroxysmal manner. They are often associated with pain and a very insecure subjective feeling. These "paroxysmal spasms" are dystonic and may easily be confused with seizures. They appear to originate at the rostral brainstem and are not epileptic. Treatment with carbamazepine (600–800 mg/d) will usually abolish the spasms immediately. Less often phenytoin sodium (300 mg/d) or baclofen (40–80 mg/d) will be effective. Therapeutic levels of the medications are usually necessary for complete control. After control of the spasms is achieved and the patient is stable these medications may be tapered. The spasms will often remit and not recur.

Physical therapy should accompany any type of spasticity management. This includes slow passive range of motion exercises to all extremities several times daily. This may be preceded by ice packs applied to the spastic extremities for 30 min twice daily. Family members and others should be instructed to administer the therapy.

Gait training may require aids such as a walker, cane, braces, crutches, and parallel bars. A qualified physical therapist is valuable in working with the patients.

Weakness is not directly affected by interventions of any type. Similarly ataxia is not influenced by any interventions. Nonetheless aids for ambulation should be employed for these also. If the gait remains inefficient, even with aids, a wheelchair may be necessary. Certain drugs (propranolol, INH) and surgery (stereotactic thalamotomy and dorsal column stimulation) have proved to be of doubtful therapeutic benefit and carry unacceptable risks.

General conditioning exercises must be employed judiciously. Vigorous exercise may raise the body temperature and aggravates symptoms. In addition, it may so exhaust the patient as to make activities of daily living difficult. Swimming is often of value. It should be done in a tepid pool. The stretching and conditioning accompanying this are often beneficial.

Fatigue and lassitude are common problems for patients with MS and make it difficult for them to be gainfully employed or to carry out activities of daily living. The patient must have regular rest periods with graduated work and exercise activities. These symptoms may or may not be associated with depression. A trial of antidepressant drugs may be attempted. Often low doses are effective in contrast to the dosage regimens of primary psychiatric disease.

Urinary findings in MS may be related to lesions in the spinal cord or to urinary tract infections. It is difficult to differentiate these on the basis of history. A urine culture is necessary. A postvoid residual urine should be determined by catheterization. In the absence of infection the dysfunction can be classified as (1) failure to store (hypertonic, hyperreflexic, small capacity), (2) failure to empty (hypotonic, hyporeflexic, large capacity), or (3) mixed with detrussor-sphincter dyssynergia (increased simultaneous sphincter and detrussor contractions). The determinations may require cystometry. Cystoscopy is rarely necessary. Disease of the upper urinary tract is, surprisingly, rarely present but when suspected intravenous urography and/or computed tomography will assist in assessing calculi, reflux, or dilation.

After evaluation, any significant infection should be specifically treated. The "failure-to-store" bladder usually responds to anticholinergic medications. The tricyclic antidepressant imipramine may also be of benefit (up to 300 mg/day in one bedtime dose). The "failure-to-empty" bladder may respond to intermittent self-catheterization. This is a clean but not sterile technique that can easily be mastered if there is little extremity ataxia. Occasionally lower extremity spasm hampers the technique. The frequency of catheterization and the duration of this type of management will depend on checking residuals regularly. As an accompaniment to this one should administer vitamin C (ascorbic acid, 0.5–1 g four times per day). This acidifies the urine, making bacterial growth less likely. Urinary antisepsis with a number of different antibiotics/antiseptic agents is often necessary (methenamine hippurate, sulfa-trimethoprim, furadantoin.)

Other drugs that might modify the urinary bladder through stimulation (cholinergics) have not proved to be of much clinical use. Urinary diversions (cystostomy, conduits, *etc.*) are seldom necessary unless the bladder cannot be kept from severe infections. Condom catheter drainage system is often useful in male patients.

Once the bladder findings have been managed, the bowel problems are treated by use of adequate fluid intake, diet and occasional suppository or enema. A bowel program that allows for a bowel movement at least every three to four days is satisfactory. Stool softeners given once or twice daily are helpful. If no results occur in three days a glycerine suppository is given after breakfast on the third day. If no results occur, on the fourth day a Dulcolax (stimulatory) suppository is given after breakfast. If still no results occur an enema is utilized. If frequency and urgency of stool is the main problem, bulk formers are administered regularly and sitting at the stool at a prescribed time, after a meal, each day is advised. If no results occur at that sitting, a glycerine suppository is administered with the goal of cleaning out the rectum on a schedule of convenience.

Sexual problems are extremely common and in the male partial or total impotence is quite disturbing. It is possibly slightly less of a problem in the female but may be a major concern.

The various penile prostheses result in a partial solution but these problems not only involve the person with MS but also their "significant other." A differentiation must be realized between the "sexual act" itself and a person's "sexuality." Sexuality refers to the overall scope of sexual function, including psychological as well as physiologial components.

It is important to answer the following questions as part of the sexual history of the MS patient: (1) What are the psychological effects on the MS person? (2) What are the physical effects? (3) What are the psychological effects on the spouse (partner)?[15] Nocturnal penile tumescence monitoring may be of value in separating physical from psychological impotency. The Minnesota Multiphasic Personality Inventory also aids in assessing the impotent person. In developing a therapeutic approach one must be understanding, accepting, empathetic, and knowledgeable. One must not be judgmental or impose one's own values. The general therapeutic plan must be an individualized plan and may involve counseling by an experienced sexual counselor.

Sensory disturbances are common during the course of MS but are rarely disabling. Trigeminal neuralgia may be severe but usually responds to carbamazepine. Paresthesias may be painful and annoying; they may respond to antidepressant and tranquilizing medication.

Other sensory disturbances such as blurred vision, diplopia, and vertigo are self-limited (or are compensated) and respond poorly to treatment. These are usually not disabling. Blindness is very rare.

Mental symptoms, both cognitive and emotional, are common in severe MS. Apparent euphoria sometimes masks an underlying dementia of a pseudobulbar variety. Depression, anger and frustation are common at all stages and should be treated with counselling and medications.

Secondary problems such as decubiti are common in severely disabled MS patients. If a deep, infected, draining decubitus develops, plastic surgery should be undertaken to cover the defect with simultaneous release of any contractures to prevent recurrence. At the same time the patient should be well nourished to maintain positive nitrogen balance. It may be necessary to place a feeding gastrostomy or esophagostomy to maintain to nourishment.

The physician responsible for the comprehensive care of the patient will be greatly assisted by involving nonmedical health professionals in the psychosocial and vocational areas, to provide counselling of the patient and the family members.

General guidelines include: (1) The patient and "significant others" should be informed of the diagnosis in specific terms. This adds to the confidence of the patient in the physician and also maintains the ethics of honesty in the medical profession. The diagnosis should be presented in a realistic manner with clear indication that the disease is frequently mild, and in many instances does not impair productivity or life span. (2) The patient should be given a specific return appointment and not told, "There's no treatment, so go home and learn to live with it." Return appointments give the physician the opportunity to educate and counsel the patient, detect complications early, discuss new developments in treatment and research and allow the physician to familiarize himself (herself) with the patient and the course of the illness. (3) The patient should be encouraged to participate in the management of the illness, *e.g.*, the adjustment of dosage of certain drugs, exercise programs, and counselling programs. (4) The patient should be encouraged to continue activities as long as possible and at the same time make realistic vocational and educational plans. (5) Hospitalization should be only for severe medical complications, interventions, and surgical interventions. (6) The patient should be managed by a group of health professionals which may include neurologists, physiatrists, physical therapists, occupational therapists, social workers, nurses, psychologists and others as the need arises. (7) The patient should have a minimal data record kept by the physician which should record regularly the impairment (neurological examination), disability (incapacity to perform activities of daily living) and handicap (vocational, social, and health care needs).[16]

There are numerous factors involved in the delivery of quality care to MS patients. Questions may be raised about the effectiveness of the various delivery systems. These systems include: (1) family practitioner, internist, neurologist, neurosurgeon, physiatrist, practicing as solo practitioners, (2) MS specialty clinics, (3) general rehabilitation facilities, (4) skilled nursing facilities, (5) home care programs, (6) university programs, (7) private programs, (8) Veterans Administration hospital programs.

It is impossible to draw general conclusions as to the exact total worth of these different approaches. What is clear is that there must be a knowledgeable physician who has an intense interest in the general welfare of the patient. That physician must be aware of the various therapeutic modalities (medical, physical, emotional) available for MS today. This involves education not only of the patient but also of the various allied health professionals who must view MS as a unique neurological disease with its own set of treatments. Because of the large variety of problems found in the complicated MS patient it is often most effective to utilize a team of interested health professionals who can analyze together a patient's difficulties and respond to them appropriately. If there is interest, this can be accomplished in small institutions as well as large. However there have to be enough patients to warrant the formation of a specialized team and pique their interest. Thus, in order to insure the delivery of quality care to the MS patient, the practitioner must be aware of his or her own shortcomings and of the variety of treatment facilities in the region.

No dogmatic statements about the effects of stress and pregnancy on the course of MS can be made. Stress does seem to be detrimental to the MS patient as it is in other chronic illnesses. Pregnancy is a stress but its effect is quite variable and thus counselling must be done on an individual basis.

Multiple sclerosis is a complicated disease with many ramifications. It follows that the clinical management must be of broad spectrum. Although the cause and cure of the disease remain a mystery, the treatment of many aspects of the disease is not. Careful management of the MS patients will result in improvement of their lives.

REFERENCES

1. McAlpine, D., C. Lumsden & E. Acheson. 1972. Multiple sclerosis: A reappraisal. Williams and Wilkins. Baltimore.

2. KRAFT, G. H., J. K. CORYELL, J. E. FREAL, C. L. HANAN & N. CHITNIS. 1979. Multiple Sclerosis: A Handbook for Rehabilitation Counselors. University of Washington.
3. EDITORIAL. 1977. Br. Med. J. 2 July 1977.
4. MCALPINE, D. 1961. Benign forms of MS. Brain **84:** 186–203.
5. PERCY, A. K., F. NOBREGA, H. OKAZAKI, E. GLATTRE & L. KURLAND. 1971. Arch. Neurol. **25:** 105–111.
6. MULLER, R. 1949. Acta Med. Scand. **133**(Suppl. 222): 1–124.
7. LAZARTE, J. A. 1950. Multiple sclerosis. Res. Publ. Assoc. Res. Nerv. Ment. Dis. **28:** 512–23.
8. LEIBOWITZ, U., E. KAHANA & M. ALTER. 1969. Survival and death in multiple sclerosis. Brain **92:** 115–30.
9. KURTZKE, J. F., G. W. BEEBE, B. NAWGLER, T. L. AUTH, L. T. KURLAND & M. D. NEFZGER. 1968. Studies on the natural history of multiple sclerosis. Acta Neurol. Scand. **44:** 467–99.
10. KURTZKE, J. F., G. W. BEEBE, B. NAGLER, L. T. KURLAND & T. L. AUTH. 1977. Studies on the natural history of multiple sclerosis. J. Chronic Dis. **30:** 819–30.
11. KURTZKE, J. F. 1983. Epidemiology of multiple sclerosis. *In* Multiple Sclerosis: Pathology, Diagnosis, and Management. J. F. Hallpike, C. W. M. Adams & W. W. Tourtellotte, Eds. Williams and Wilkins. Baltimore.
12. MAIDER, E. & K. SUMMER. 1979. Differing responses to synthetic ACTH. Neurology **220:** 1943.
13. ROSEN, 1979. Immunosuppression in M.S. J. Neurol. Neurosurg. Psych. **42:** 338.
14. HAUSER, S. L., D. M. DAWSON, J. R. LEHRICH, M. F. BEAL, S. V. KEVY, R. D. PROPPER, J. A. MILLS & H. L. WEINER. 1983. Intensive immunosuppression in progressive multiple sclerosis. N. Engl. J. Med. **4:** 173–80.
15. WABREK, A. J. 1983. Talk at American Academy of Neurology. San Diego, California.
16. SCHEINBERG, L. C., B. S. GIESSER & R. J. SLATER. 1983. Management of the chronic M.S. patient. *In* Neurology and Neurosurgery Update, vol 4. Cont. Prof. Educ. Cent.

DISCUSSION OF THE PAPER

UNIDENTIFIED SPEAKER: This is a serious question and I hope I'll get a serious response. What do you do with the patient who feels there are no other alternatives in medicine and wants to go to some of the alternative healers such as the so-called "psychic surgeons" in the Phillipines or the "miracle workers" in Mexico, and so on?

R. T. SCHAPIRO (*University of Minnesota, Minneapolis, MN*): That's a very good question and deserves a serious response. I think the first thing is that if the patient comes in and really wants to do something that is out of the ordinary and has his or her mind set on it, the best we can do is educate rather than castigate. We can't point a finger at them and start swearing and saying that person is an absolute fool and such treatment is of no value, that gets nowhere. So I tell our patients that if it's safe, if it's cheap and it makes you feel better I'm for it, but if going to some place in Mexico is very costly or if it's not safe then I feel very strongly that I have to inform them that that's how I feel about it. I would hope that the bond that I have created with my patients is such that they will then take my advice and not make that wild leap.

But if they come to me and say I want to go on a peculiar diet that is nutritionally sound, I just say to them, "if it's safe, if it's cheap and it makes you feel better, why not?"

Psychosocial Factors in Multiple Sclerosis and the Role of Stress[a]

NICHOLAS G. LAROCCA

Department of Neurology
Albert Einstein College of Medicine
Bronx, New York 10461

Hans Selye[1] was largely responsible for the development of the modern concept of stress. He conceived of stress as any phenomenon leading to what he termed the "general adaptation syndrome" (GAS). The general adaptation syndrome consists of the body's nonspecific response to any of a variety of external stressors. The GAS is the body's way of adapting to a stressor. Three phases occur in the GAS: alarm, resistance, and exhaustion. If the GAS proves ineffective, a "generalized susceptibility" to illness may ensue. This susceptibility operates in concert with other etiological factors such as genetic predispostions, diet, exposure to viral agents, *etc.* Selye's seminal notion of the importance of physical and chemical stressors has been expanded to include the role of psychosocial phenomena as precipitants of the GAS. In fact, the word "stress" in everyday speech has come to mean psychosocial events almost exclusively. The scientific literature on stress and multiple sclerosis (MS) uses the term "stress" in at least two ways.

First, the term "stress" sometimes refers to any set of circumstances that entails change or readjustment in the individual's life pattern.[2] Such occurrences have come to be known as "stressful life events" and include incidents such as death of a loved one or loss of a job. The second type of stress might not be the result of discrete events and might not involve any change or readjustment in a person's routine.[3] This type of stress, "chronic stress," includes such things as commuting every day in heavy traffic or social isolation. Although chronic stress might not entail change or readjustment in the way event stress does, it does elicit Selye's general adaptation syndrome. In addition, life events (*e.g.*, a serious illness) can lead to chronic stress (*e.g.*, difficulty in getting around).

HISTORICAL PERSPECTIVE

Interest in stress as well as the other psychosocial features of multiple sclerosis dates from the nineteenth century when the ailment was first a subject of scientific study. One of the first descriptions of MS in the literature recorded the appearance of symptoms in Augustus d'Este shortly after he had attended the funeral of a father figure.[4] Charcot, who gave MS its name, observed that grief or anger might precipitate the disease. In Charcot's time conversion hysteria was undergoing intense study in Europe. Certain of the symptoms of hysteria (*e.g.*, paresthesias, visual loss, difficulty walking, lassitude) so closely resembled MS that the two disorders were frequently confused.[5]

[a]The preparation of this manuscript was supported by grants from the National Multiple Sclerosis Society (nos. RG 1135–A–4 and RG 1459–A–7) and the National Institute of Handicapped Research (nos. G008006808 and G008200046).

During the first part of the twentieth century, two schools of thought arose concerning the role of psychosocial factors in MS. The one most prominent in the United States held that certain personality types were MS-prone in the face of emotional stress.[6] The contrasting school of thought, more prominent in Europe, held that the psychological abnormalities seen in MS (*e.g.*, dementia, euphoria, and depression) were either direct effects of the disease or else were reactions to the realities of the illness.[7] Using today's terminology, these two schools of thought might be labeled the stress-illness model (stress leads to illness) and the illness-stress model (illness leads to stress). Although these two models are not necessarily in opposition to one another, each leads to a different line of research. This paper will summarize some of the major findings of these two models and show how they are interrelated.

STRESS-ILLNESS MODEL

One of the earliest concepts derived from the stress-illness model was that of the MS-prone personality. The MS-prone personality was regarded as immature and hysterical. In such individuals emotional distress was thought to cause vascular changes in the central nervous system resulting in the plaque formation characteristic of MS.[8] Jelliffe attributed a causal role in MS to long-standing emotional stress arising from oedipal fixations. Langworthy[6,9] also believed that emotional immaturity was an important feature of MS etiology but ascribed importance to the interaction between the underdeveloped personality and stressful situations. Psychotherapy was even recommended as a prophylaxis for susceptible personalities because character reorganization could combat the psychological defects thought to play a causal role in MS.

The idea of an MS-prone personality was consistent with prevailing psychosomatic theory in the first half of the twentieth century. Specific personality patterns were regarded as causal determinants of specific illnesses.[10] Disease was seen as the result of specific organ vulnerability, a predisposing personality pattern, and an emotional precipitant. The precipitating event was thought to mobilize a central conflict specific to the vulnerable organ while breaking down the primary defenses against the conflict. The illnesses that were thought to be so caused were asthma, peptic ulcer, ulcerative colitis, hypertension, rheumatoid arthritis, neurodermatitis, and thyrotoxicosis. This monoetiological theory of disease causation seems to have evolved from germ theory.[11]

Controlled studies using standardized measures of personality failed to identify a cluster of traits common to MS patients.[12] As a result, the notion of the MS-prone personality fell into disfavor and stress came to be regarded as only one of many possible precipitants of the illness.[13] The stress-illness model of MS has thus evolved from the identification of MS with hysteria to the modern concept of stress as a possible precipitant of disease activity in those individuals predisposed, not by personality, but by exposure to a biological agent.

In modern times, stress-illness research in MS has pursued three main hypotheses: (1) stress precipitates the onset of MS; (2) stress triggers exacerbations and/or hastens progression; and (3) stress transiently (for a few hours) worsens symptoms.

Braceland and Giffin[14] evaluated 75 MS patients using a psychiatric interview and reviewed the records of 200 others. A wide variety of events was cited by patients and their families as precipitants of the disease. However, similar events could be discovered in normal subjects and so the role of psychological trauma in MS remained unclear.

Brickner and Simons[15] studied 50 randomly selected case histories for evidence of emotional factors that had precipitated attacks of MS. In eight patients attacks occurred during periods of tension. In an additional six, there was evidence of attacks following tension within a fairly short period of time. The authors concluded that although emotional stress might sometimes provoke attacks, it could not be regarded as causing the disease.

Grinker[16] reported on 26 cases in most of whom symptoms followed a major life change with which an immature personality could not adequately cope.

Baldwin[17] reviewed the life histories of 34 MS patients and 34 patients with other neurological conditions. She found that non-MS patients had just as many traumatic events as MS patients but that those with MS seemed to have had less stability in their lives.

Pratt[18] compared the case histories of 100 MS patients and 100 patients with other neurological problems. In 38 MS patients and 26 controls, emotional stress had preceeded the onset of the disease and was associated with 58 out of 229 exacerbations of MS. However, the relationship between stress and onset or relapses of MS did not prove to be significant. Despite these negative findings, Pratt was impressed by eight cases in which onset or relapses followed stress so closely in time that it was difficult to discount a causal relationship.

In a study of 40 MS patients, Philippopoulos *et al.*[19] found that traumatic experiences preceded the onset of symptoms in 35 cases. For 31 of those cases, stress was long-standing rather than acute.

During an epidemiologic study of MS in Israel, interviews were conducted with 221 MS patients and 442 controls. Interpersonal trauma before disease onset was more common in the MS group.[20]

The onset of MS has also been linked to the "giving up/given up" complex, a constellation consisting of feeling of helplessness, object loss, and a perceived inability to cope on one's own.[21] In 28 out of 32 MS patients studied, onset was chronologically related to the occurrence of a psychologically stressful event. Such situations were generally experienced as difficulty in coping and feelings of helplessness.

In a study of 100 MS patients and 100 controls, the MS patients were (1) more likely to report that they were under unusual stress during the two years prior to onset, and (2) had a larger number of stressful life events than controls.[4]

There have been 10 studies published since 1950 that have addressed the role of stress in MS disease activity. Excluded are anecdotal reports made on very small numbers of patients and studies whose focus was on strictly physical stressors such as the role of childhood infections in development of MS in adulthood.

Out of these 10 studies, 6 used the case-study method, examining a sample of MS patients but no control group. Four used the case-control method, comparing a sample of MS patients with a control group consisting either of patients with other medical conditions or persons with no medical problems. Whereas the case studies have been 2 to 1 favor of a stress-MS link, the case-control studies have been evenly divided.

Thus, considering the existing research as a whole, results have been inconclusive and the role of stress as a precipitant of disease activity in MS remains unclear. These findings parallel the results of stress research in general, where early optimism about discovering a powerful link between stress and illness has frequently been disappointed by negative, weak, or contradictory findings.

Why have efforts so far led to such ambiguous results? The answer lies in six methodological issues that have not yet been adequately addressed in stress-MS research. Once these issues are addressed, we are likely to have clearer answers.

A brief review of these issues will cast light on some of the problems.

The first is the issue of assessing the "stressfulness" of stressful events.[22] What constitutes stress for a person with MS? Is it the amount of change necessitated by a given event as our current life-event scales suggest? Is it the desirability of an event, that is, do negative events such as losses have effects different from positive events? Is the crucial element how upsetting the event is or perhaps whether or not the event is under the control of the person?

In work underway at Albert Einstein, medical anthropologist Dr. Louise Duval has been finding that the most significant sources of stress for people with MS are not the well-studied life events, but rather the everyday problems and uncertainties that are a part of any chronic disabling illness. If we wish to understand the role of stress after the onset of MS symptoms, then we need to develop new methods for assessing stress.

A second major issue concerns the population of events to be measured. Stressful life events can be of three types: (1) subjective events such as sexual difficulties which may be the result of psychopathology; (2) events which may be the result of illness; (3) exogenous events that are presumably independent of physical or mental illness such as the death of a family member. These three types of events need to be examined separately in any chronic illness where physical and psychological effects may be extensive.

The design of studies of life events raises a third critical issue. Retrospective designs have severe limitations including difficulty in recalling symptoms, problems in pinpointing dates, and the tendency for people to attribute illness to some "cause."[23] Because of the low incidence of MS (less than 5 per 100,000),[24] prospective studies of stress and onset of MS are impractical. Such designs could be employed in studies of stress and MS disease activity.

A fourth major issue in stress research concerns the role of mediating variables. In most studies the relationship between stress and illness has been weak, usually on the order of $r = 0.30$ or less.[11] This weak association very likely reflects the relative neglect of mediating variables. This has been particularly true in MS research. Mediating variables do not act on stressful events themselves but instead operate as buffers by modifying the impact which events have on the organism. Buffers appear to operate in three main arenas: (1) physiological, (2) psychological, and, (3) social.[25] Although the buffering hypothesis has run into problems in stress research generally, mediating factors remain a neglected area in MS.

Stress-MS studies have relied almost exclusively on clinical or subjective measures of disease onset and disease activity. Physiological indicators of disease activity need to be explored.

Similarly, the sixth and last issue is that studies of stress in MS have not generally attempted to integrate their hypotheses with prevailing theories of etiology and pathogenesis. For instance, the role of stress in immunoregulatory deficit of cell-mediated immune response remains unexplored territory in MS.

ILLNESS-STRESS MODEL

Research drawn from the stress-MS model has led to inconclusive findings concerning the possible psychosocial precipitants of the disease. For many years, however, a parallel line of research drawn from the illness-stress model has examined, with some success, not the precipitants but the consequences of MS.

The World Health Organization (WHO) has developed a convenient method for classifying the consequences of illness.[26] First come physical changes in the organism. In MS an example is demyelination in the corticospinal tract resulting in lower extremity weakness. Next come difficulties in functioning in everyday activities. An example would be the restriction on mobility created by weakness in the legs. Lastly, adverse changes in the performance of social roles take effect, for instance, the loss of a job because of mobility restriction and architectural barriers.

MS strikes most people during the peak years of career and family development. Consequences range through the three WHO categories. The physical, psychological, social, and economic repercussions can be extensive and profound. The notion that such a disease can be stressful seems self-evident, and yet the process in which these consequences unfold and how they are dealt with by the individual are not completely understood.

Research conceptualizing MS as a source of stress has experienced its own evolution. Early work on the psychosocial consequences of MS tended to focus on the issue of identifying a set of personality traits common to people with MS. The notion of the personality molded by MS echoed the idea of the MS-prone personality and represented specificity theory turned to the question of adjustment to illness rather than cause. Considerable effort was expended in the search for patterns that might characterize the person with MS. Many such studies were conducted in the United States using the MMPI and other standardized instruments. This approach attempted to examine adjustment to physical illness from the perspective of psychopathology, using measures ordinarily employed to assess psychiatric illness. Not surprisingly, the results of these studies were often inconsistent or contradictory, because adjusting to a chronic illness does not necessarily represent psychopathology in the usual sense.

In recent years the assumption that the stress of MS produced an MS personality or some form of psychopathology has been replaced by a new set of assumptions concerning the process of adjusting to MS.

The first is the assumption of normality. The adjustment process with all its emotional upheaval is basically seen as a normal human response to a catastrophic stress which in only a few cases results in psychiatric illness. The second assumption is that of multifactorial influences. Adjustment is assumed to be the result of a host of factors, including characteristics of the disease, the individual, and the social context. How well a person adjusts is thus determined by the interplay of many forces. The third assumption is a developmental one. Adjustment is seen not as a single event but as a process unfolding over many years in a series of stages and in a constant state of flux.

This exciting line of research has as one of its goals to facilitate the process of adjusting to the stress of chronic illness. Some of the major findings of the illness-stress line of research are as follows:

1. There is no "MS personality." People with MS do have many experiences in common as a result of the illness but do not share any particular personality pattern.[27]
2. Psychological distress is very much a part of MS but is generally not what would ordinarily be termed psychopathology.[28]
3. Depression and/or grief is a frequent experience of people with MS. Grief seems to be especially significant as people with MS go through a process of mourning for losses brought on by the disease.[29]
4. Psychological distress increases when exacerbations occur and abates when there is a remission.[28]
5. Self-esteem may be seriously challenged by the illness but seems to be very resilient. People with MS generally have levels of self-esteem that do not differ greatly from those of the general population.[30,31]
6. Knowing more about the illness seems to assist in the adjustment process.[32]
7. Adjustment does seem to unfold over time and seems never to be complete, as new changes call for adjustments.
8. Adjustment is subject to many influences. For instance, one person who is

severely disabled may have adjusted better than another with only minimal disability. Exciting research is under way to try to understand some of these critical forces and to harness them if possible on the patient's behalf.

INTERRELATIONSHIP OF THE MODELS

Having examined two lines of research, what can we conclude about the role of stress in MS? Is stress a precipitant or a consequence of MS? In the present state of our knowledge, we can state with confidence that stress is a consequence of MS. Whether or not it is a precipitant remains unclear. All things considered, the most accurate model may be one that views stress as both an antecedent and a consequence of illness. If such a model were correct, it would imply that MS is a continuing producer of psychosocial stress that may in turn influence disease activity. Such a circular model represents MS as a self-perpetuating illness, at least on the psychosocial level, if the effects of stress are negative.

How could a psychosocial phenomenon such as stress influence MS pathogenesis? Although the etiology of MS remains unclear, the immune response is clearly involved in pathogenesis. Stress is known to have significant effects on the immune system, including powerful immunosuppressant effects. Some of these effects include release of corticosteroids, loss of tissue from the thymus, decrease in circulating T lymphocytes, and suppression of natural killer cells.[33]

Recognition of these stress-related immunological changes leads to a paradox. While social scientists are studying the hypothesized negative effects of a psychological immunosuppressant (stress), clinical neurologists in the same university may be studying the hypothesized positive effects of a chemical immunosuppressant such as azathioprine.

MS disease activity appears to slow during the course of the disease. Will we someday discover that the effects of stress are at least in part positive, helping to suppress the autoimmune response, and thereby slow the progress of the disease? On the other hand, will the common belief that stress triggers attacks of MS be scientifically verified? We do not know at this time.

Three conclusions are evident: (1) multiple sclerosis is a continuing source of stress; (2) stress affects the immune system; and (3) the immune system is clearly involved in MS. Thus, immunologists and psychologists need to develop collaborative studies that examine important psychological and immunological parameters. The statistical power of clinical studies of immunological changes could be enhanced by incorporation of stress measures. Likewise studies of stress could be improved with monitoring of relevant immunological parameters. Such mutual collaborative efforts could enhance our knowledge not only of the life-stress process but of the immunological system as well.

REFERENCES

1. Selye, H. 1976. The Stress of Life. McGraw-Hill. New York.
2. Holmes, T. H. & R. H. Rahe. 1967. The social readjustment rating scale. J. Psychosom. Res. **11:** 213–218.
3. Kanner, A. D., J. C. Coyne, C. Schaefer & R. S. Lazarus. 1981. Comparison of two modes of stress measurement: Daily hassles and uplifts versus major life events. J. Behav. Med. **4:** 1–39.
4. Warren, S., S. Greenhill & K. G. Warren. 1982. Emotional stress and the development of multiple sclerosis: Case-control evidence of a relationship. J. Chron. Dis. **35:** 821–831

5. Caplan, L. & T. Nadelson. 1980. Multiple sclerosis and hysteria: Lessons learned from their association. J. Am. Med. Assoc. **243:** 418.
6. Langworthy, O. R. 1984. Relation of personality problems to onset and progress of multiple sclerosis. Arch. Neurol. Psychiatry **59:** 13–28.
7. Brown, S. & T. K. Davis. 1921. Mental manifestations and the emotional and psychological factors in multiple sclerosis. Proc. Assoc. Res. Nerv. Ment. Dis. **2:** 75–82.
8. Jelliffe, S. E. 1921. Emotional and psychological factors in multiple sclerosis. Proc. Assoc. Res. Nerv. Ment. Dis. **2:** 82–95.
9. Langworthy, O. R. 1950. A survey of the maladjustment problems in multiple sclerosis and the possibilities of psychotherapy. Res. Publ. Assoc. Res. Nerv. Ment. Dis. **28:** 598–611.
10. Alexander, F. 1950. Psychosomatic Medicine: Its Principles and Applications. W. W. Norton. New York.
11. Rabkin, J. & E. Struening. 1976. Social change, stress, and illness: A selective literature review. Psychoanal. Contemp. Sci. **5:** 573–624
12. Dodge C. R. & R. H. Kalstoe. 1971. The M.M.P.I. in differentiating early multiple sclerosis and conversion hysteria. Psychol. Rep. **29:** 155–159.
13. Lemere, F. 1966. Psychiatric disorders in multiple sclerosis. Am. J. Psychiatry **122:** 55–58.
14. Braceland, F. J. & M. E. Giffin. 1950. The mental changes associated with multiple sclerosis (an interim report). Res. Publ. Assoc. Res. Nerv. Ment. Dis. **28:** 450–455
15. Brickner R. H. & D. J. Simons. 1950. Emotional stress in relation to attacks of multiple sclerosis. Res. Publ. Assoc. Res. Nerv. Ment. Dis. **28:** 143–149.
16. Grinker, R. R., G. C. Ham & F. P. Robbins. 1950. Some psycho-dynamic factors in multiple sclerosis. Res. Publ. Assoc. Res. Nerv. Ment. Dis. **28:** 456–460
17. Baldwin, M. V. 1952. A clinico-experimental investigation into the psychologic aspects of multiple sclerosis. J. Nerv. Ment. Dis. **115:** 299–342.
18. Pratt, R. T. 1951. An investigation of the psychiatric aspects of disseminated sclerosis. J. Neurol. Neurosurg. Psychiatry **14:** 326.
19. Philippopoulos, G. S., E. D. Wittkower & A. Cousineau. 1958. The etiologic significance of emotional factors in onset and excerbations of multiple sclerosis. Psychosom. Med. **20:** 458.
20. Antonovsky, A., V. Leibowitz, J. Medalie, H. Smith, L. Halpern & M. Alter. 1968. Reappraisal of possible etiologic factors in multiple sclerosis. Am. J. Publ. Health **58:** 836.
21. Mei-Tal, V., S. Meyerowitz & G. L. Engel. 1970. The role of psychological process in a somatic disorder: Multiple sclerosis. Psychosom. Med. **32:** 67–86.
22. Dohrenwend, B. S. & B. D. Dohrenwend. 1980. What is a stressful life event? *In* Selye's Guide to Stress Research. H. Selye, Ed. Van Nostrand. New York.
23. Hudgens, R. W. 1974. Personal catastrophe and depression: A consideration of the subject with respect to medically ill adolescents, and a requiem for retrospective life-event studies. *In* Stressful Life Events. Their Nature and Effects. B. S. Dohrenwend & B. P. Dohrenwend, Eds. Wiley. New York.
24. Baum H. M. & B. B. Rothschild. 1981. The incidence and prevalence of reported multiple sclerosis. Ann. Neurol. **10:** 420–428.
25. Dohrenwend B. S. & B. P. Dohrenwend. 1974. Overview and prospects for research on stressful life events. *In* Stressful Life Events: Their Nature and Effects. B. S. Dohrenwend & B. P. Dohrenwend, Eds. Wiley. New York.
26. World Health Organization. 1980. International classification of impairments, disabilities, and handicaps. World Health Organization. Geneva.
27. Peyser, J. M., K. R. Edwards & C. M. Poser. 1980. Psychological profiles in multiple sclerosis patients: A preliminary investigation. Arch. Neurol. **37:** 437–440.
28. Dalos, N. P., P. V. Rabins, B. R. Brooks & P. O'Donnell. 1983. Disease activity and emotional state in multiple sclerosis. Ann. Neurol. **13:** 573–577.
29. Schiffer, R. B., E. D. Caine, K. A. Bamford & S. Levy. 1983. Depressive episodes in patients with multiple sclerosis. Am. J. Psychiatry **140:** 1498–1500.
30. Matson, R. R. & N. A. Brooks. 1977. Adjusting to multiple sclerosis: An exploratory study. Social Science and Medicine **11:** 245–250.

31. BROOKS, N. A. & R. R. MATSON. 1982. Social-psychological adjustment to multiple sclerosis: A longitudinal study. Social Science and Medicine **16:** 2129–2135.
32. COUNTE, M. A., L. A. BIELIAUSKAS & M. PAVLOU. 1983. Stress and personal attitudes in chronic illness. Arch. Phys. Med. Rehab. **64:** 272–275.
33. GOLDBERGER, L. & S. BREZNITZ, Eds. 1982. Handbook of Stress: Theoretical and Clinical Aspects. The Free Press. New York.

DISCUSSION OF THE PAPER

O. R. HOMMES (*Radboud University Hospital, Nijmegen, the Netherlands*): I would like to ask you a question on a subject that has been raised recently on the Pavlovian aspects of the immune system. Rats were given cyclophosphamide and sugar water and their leukocyte counts dropped and after a few test trials the leukocyte count dropped with the sugar water only, now could this be one of the ways that the immune system will be influenced by circumstances and stress?

N. LAROCCA (*Albert Einstein College of Medicine, Bronx, NY*): Sounds very plausible to me.

J. R. BROWN (*Mayo Medical School, Rochester, MN*): A few years ago some colleagues and I did a Minnesota Multiphasic Personality Inventory study of patients with multiple sclerosis. One of the findings that emerged was that those patients who tended to have an elevated hysteria score on the MMPI, tended to be more disabled than those who had an elevation of the psychasthenia score. This suggests to me that in addition to the stressfulness that may occur with a lesion, different people will respond to distress, to stress in different ways.

LAROCCA: Yes I would agree with that and I think that one of the very important mediating variables that we would want to look at are parameters of personality, social supports and all of the influences which would modify the impact and the perception of stress and I think that these will probably prove to be extremely important.

L. SCHEINBERG (*Albert Einstein College of Medicine, Bronx, NY*): One last question Dr. Schapiro.

R. T. SCHAPIRO (*University of Minnesota, Minneapolis, MN*): Just a comment coming from Minnesota and the MMPI was just mentioned. There's a bias built into that test. When given to MS people, because the test stresses a number of different somatic symptoms that either hysterical people have or MS people have, MS people in general will show up high in the hysterical scale, that's just the bias of the testing.

Sexual Dysfunctions in Multiple Sclerosis

GEORGE SZASZ, D. PATY, AND W. L. MAURICE

Faculty of Medicine
The University of British Columbia
Vancouver, British Columbia, Canada

The frequency, nature and enjoyment of sexual practices may be disturbed by acute or chronic illness. Sexual problems may be caused by, among other factors, the nonspecific symptoms of illness, the anxieties over disruption of life-style or the specific impairments caused by a disorder. Patients with, for example, multiple sclerosis are thought to experience sexual problems commonly. In one study, Lilius found that in a group of 284 MS patients, 64% of the men and 39% of the women described their sexual life as "unsatisfactory" or "ceased entirely."[1] Lundberg found that 90% of his MS patients confined to wheelchairs "have major problems with sexual function."[2]

Szasz *et al.* used a Sexual Functioning Scale to study 73 consecutive patients at an MS clinic and found that 45% of the patients were "less sexually active" or "inactive" since the onset of MS. Fifty percent of this group indicated that they were "concerned" about this situation.[3] In a follow-up study, 18 "concerned" MS patients listed their sexual concerns as: "cannot satisfy the partner" (11 patients), "don't feel like sex" (9 patients), "cannot satisfy myself" (11 patients), "cannot be like a man" (4 patients), and "partner does not feel like sex" (2 patients). Fifteen of these patients were men; most were over the age of 40, and most were married. The three women were over the age of 50, and only one was married. Most of these patients had MS for over 10 years. Their rating on the Kurtzke Disability Scale ranged from 1 to 7.[4]

The purpose of this paper is to consider the epidemiology, diagnosis and management of one sexual problem area that may be associated with MS, that of sexual dysfunctions.

CLASSIFICATION

Sexual dysfunctions include erectile and ejaculatory disorders in men, disorders of vaginal lubrication, orgasm and vaginismus in women. Some definitions also include sexual disinterest.[5] The nature and the significance of these dysfunctions vary and are dependent on a variety of factors, including the health and the age of the patient and the presence or absence of a partner.

EPIDEMIOLOGY

Sexual Dysfunctions in the General Population

Kinsey *et al.* estimated that impotence affected 18% of the American male population at the age of 60. Premature ejaculation was not considered a disorder and 9% of women were described as nonorgasmic on a lifetime basis.[6]

Frank *et al.* studied 100 white well-educated couples who were nonpatient volunteers. Forty percent of the men reported erectile or ejaculatory problems. Sixty-three percent of the women described orgasmic dysfunctions. However, 80% of the couples reported that their marital and sexual relations were "happy and satisfying."[7]

Sexual Dysfunction in the Selected Patient Groups

Many studies on the prevalence of sexual dysfunctions in specific patient groups have been described. For example, Kolodny quotes Gastant and Colombo who found that 24 out of 36 men with temporal lobe epilepsy were impotent.[8] Bors *et al.* and others reported reflexogenic erection in over 90% of men with complete high spinal cord lesions. They found, however, that these erections are often not satisfactory for the act of intercourse. The ability to ejaculate normally is lost for most spinal cord-injured men. Some men with incomplete lesions may require a great deal of genital stimulation for orgasmic and ejaculation experiences.[9,10,11] The situation is not clear with regard to the sexual responsivity of spinal cord-injured women. Reports from many of these women suggest that following their injury, they may lose their orgasmic capability in intercourse.[12]

Sexual Dysfunctions in MS

Vas found 3 out of 37 MS patients with complete impotence and 13 with partial impotence. Loss of ejaculation occurred in three completely and four partly impotent men.[13] Lilius studied the sexual situation of 150 male and 134 female MS patients. Eighty percent of the men reported some degree of erection dysfunction and 77% complained of unspecified ejaculation disorders. Thirty-three percent of women noticed loss of their former orgasmic ability. The majority of these patients was between 30 to 40 years of age; over a half had MS for more than 10 years. One-third were able to walk without aid, but 80% reported incontinence.[1]

Lundberg found that 13 out of 25 women with mild MS noted a decrease in sexual interest, unspecified changes in orgasmic response and lack of vaginal lubrication.[2]

ETIOLOGY OF SEXUAL DYSFUNCTIONS

In general, sexual dysfunctions can be divided into two groups: the "situational" disorders which appear on selected occasions (for example, only during intercourse) and the "absolute" or "global" disorders which are not influenced by circumstances. The etiology of the situational disorders is most probably "psychogenic." The theories explaining the chain of events leading to these sexual dysfunctions are varied. Some are "non-specific." "Some have a common fit, others are unique. Some have face validity; others appear exotic."[14]

Fear of failure acquired after a sexual episode and emerging at the time of the next attempt at sexual activity has been stressed by Masters and Johnson.

They noted: "fear of the inadequacy is the greatest known deterrent to effective sexual functioning, simply because it so completely distracts the fearful individual from his or her responsivity by blocking reception of sex stimuli either created by or reflected from the sexual partner."[15]

Other nonspecific causes may include more remote factors, such as deep-seated emotional conflicts, ignorance and misinformation about sexual functioning and beliefs that may limit a person's perception of the range of norms in sex practices.

The Effect of Illness on Sexual Functioning

The effect of chronic illness and the related depression, stress, and fatigue may affect various aspects of sexual behavior and may contribute to sexual dysfunctions. Specific impairments of the genitalia, or of the neurological, endocrine, cardiac and other systems supporting sexual functioning may cause "absolute" or "global" sexual dysfunctions. Differential diagnosis between situational and absolute dysfunctions and their respective etiologies may be difficult, partly because of the poor understanding of sexual response physiology, and partly because of the varied symptomalogy of sexual dysfunctions which are difficult to quantify.

The Effect of MS on Sexual Functioning

Vas suggested that in MS impotence is caused by lesions in the lateral horns of the dorsal-lumbar area of the spinal cord.[13] Hartings *et al.* felt that stresses arising out of the uncertainty of the patient's present and future health status constituted a major source of the sexual dysfunctions.[16]

Szasz *et al.* conducted linear logistic analyses to find variables in the Minimal Record of Disability in MS[17] which might be best predictors of a decrease in or concerns about sexual activity. The analyses indicated that the risk of being in the "less or not sexually active" category of the Sexual Functioning Scale was four times greater for patients who needed devices or human aid in toilet transfer or who experienced occasional urinary incontinence.

The risk of being in the "concerned" category of the Sexual Functioning Scale was over six times greater for patients who required external financial support and four times greater for patients who needed canes, braces or wheelchair. In the linear logistic analyses, none of the other variables of the Minimal Record of Disability in MS was identified as a significant risk factor at the $p = 0.05$ level.[3]

The Effect of the Onset and Course of MS on Sexual Dysfunctions

Ivers and Goldstein reported that impotence was the presenting complaint in four out of 54 men with MS and another 10 admitted to this problem in their initial history.[18] In Vas's study of 37 men with MS, the average duration of MS was 9 years for the "partially" and 12 years for the "completely" impotent group. In the course of the year subsequent to the original survey, one totally impotent and one partially impotent patient improved, but two previously "potent" men developed partial erection problems.[13] In Szasz's review[4] of 18 sexually concerned patients, the recently diagnosed patients seemed to have just as many concerns as the ones diagnosed over 10 years ago. There are no long-range studies to document the natural history of dysfunctions during remissions or relapses characteristic of MS.

DIAGNOSIS OF SEXUAL DYSFUNCTIONS IN MS

The clinician's first task is to find out if the sexual problem is a dysfunction, and if so, what type of dysfunction it is. Did it exist prior to the onset of MS or did it appear after? The next task is to discover whether the present dysfunction is related to the impairments, disabilities and handicaps characteristic of MS, or whether it is essentially unrelated to the MS condition.

History

The patient's (and the partner's) history is essential in the diagnosis of sexual dysfunctions. Physical examination and investigations are less useful as diagnostic tools.

Sex Functional Inquiry

Once the presence and nature of the sexual dysfunction is established and its relationship to the course of MS, to other existing medical, surgical or psychological problems and to the effects of medications is clarified, a "sex functional inquiry" may help to portray the patient's (and the partner's) sexual capabilities and limitations.

Seven "sex-related" areas may need to be explored.

1. Sexual responsivity: the patient's and the partner's genital, extragenital and mental reactions to appropriate stimulation.
2. Motor ability for sex acts: the patient's ability to transfer to bed, assume desired positions, touch self or partner for purposes of sexual arousal.
3. Bowel and bladder control and genital hygiene: patient's ability to exert control over bowel and bladder functions during sex activities; the ability to manipulate catheters, urinary drainage devices, or, for example, menstrual hygiene appliances and to maintain genital cleanliness.
4. Fertility and birth control: the couple's desire to have children; the patient's options for the use of the safest and most effective methods of contraception or birth control.
5. Sexual interest: the degree of motivation to initiate sex activities.
6. Partnership issues: the patient's ability to present himself/herself as a sexually interested person; the ability to "court" and to explain to a partner the degree of MS-related disabilities and impairments; and the ability to guide the partner in a sexual activity.
7. Sexual perspectives: the patient's and partner's knowledge and beliefs about, for example, the significance of intercouse in the sexual partnership; the role of the man in a sex act; or feelings about, for example, sex activities with a disabled person.

The first four areas may well be directly influenced by the impairments and disabilities characteristic of MS. The last three areas represent disadvantages resulting from the physical problems and from personal and cultural factors that may limit the fulfillment of the patient's accustomed sexual lifestyle.

Inquiry from the Partner

Partners sometime insist that the sexual difficulty is not important to them. On the one hand, this may be true. On the other hand, a partner may try to minimize the problem in an attempt to ease the sick person's already heavy burdens. Sexual problems can be ignored, but usually at the cost of the intimate partnership relationship. A sexual history provided by the partner may help the clinician in further clarifying the situation, and in estimating the couple's motivation to work out the problem. Breaking the silence about sexual fears, sadness or anger may also improve a couple's communication with each other and the clinician.

Physical Examination

The sexually focused physical examination has three parts. First, a musculoskeletal survey to define the patient's competency for touching, holding, caressing, or moving in various types of sexual activities. Second, an inspection of the genital area for hygiene and, if applicable, the nature of the urinary conducting devices. Third, a neurological examination of the sexual response potential. This consists of defining the sensory changes over the body and eliciting some of the genital reflexes. Clear perception of pain, heat or cold on the skin of the genitalia and the ability to control voluntarily the anal sphincter usually indicates that orgasmic experiences could unfold in response to appropriate stimulation. Diminished acuity in the perception of pain, temperature change on the genital skin or diminished or absent voluntary anal sphincter control may signal some disturbance (usually delay) in reaching orgasm in response to stimulation associated with intercourse. In complete transection of the spinal cord, the presence of a strong bulbocavernosus reflex and anal tone and the absence of pain sensation in the genital skin may signal potential for reflex erection to physical touch of the penis. In the absence of the bulbocavernosus reflex, anal tone and pain sensation, the possibility of psychogenic erection may exist. There are no reliable physical signs to indicate the range of potential for vaginal lubrication.

Investigations

Investigations and laboratory examinations are of varying degrees of usefulness in the diagnosis of sexual dysfunctions. Evidence of noctural erections obtained in nocturnal penile tumescence studies may help prove the presence of a situational erection dysfunction. Absence of nocturnal tumescence may indicate "absolute" erection dysfunction, but the effects of depression, side effects of certain medications, and laboratory equipment failure must be excluded before the diagnosis is made. Hormone tests, penile blood flow measurements, and sensory evoked potential studies are still unreliable in the diagnosis of the etiology of sexual dysfunctions.

Therapeutic trials are sometimes of value in the differential diagnosis of sexual dysfunctions. The couple is asked to refrain from the act of sexual intercourse for a limited period of time, but they are encouraged to engage in other acceptable forms of sexual activities in the privacy of their home. Sometimes in such situations, the patient's anxiety about "performance" is lowered and often erection, lubrication or orgasmic responses may become possible, demonstrating the situational nature of the dysfunction. The risk of this approach is that the "therapeutic trial" in itself may become a test of performance with attendant anxieties and sexual dysfunctions.

The following case histories illustrate examples of MS patients with sexual problems that are not dysfunctions, dysfunctions that are related to MS but of varied etiology, and sexual problems that are unrelated to MS.

Case 1: Absence of Sexual Dysfunction

A 32-year-old woman with MS was referred to the Sexual Medicine Unit of a university because of her sexual difficulties. Her main complaint was that she could not achieve orgasm since the onset of MS about 2½ years before. Prior to onset, she was reliably orgasmic with vibrator stimulation. MS was diagnosed after a number of convulsive episodes. At the time of the referral, her condition was stable. She had residual signs of spasticity and incoordination in the limbs, and a slight impairment of visual acuity. She felt insecure about her anal sphincter control. Her history revealed that she was terribly upset when the diagnosis of MS was made. She lost her sexual interest and did not use her vibrator for close to a year. When she resumed vibrator stimulation, she experienced sexual arousal but no orgasm. She became discouraged and felt that the MS had affected her sexual responsivity. She said "I was mad at my body—why doesn't it work?" Was she not receiving sufficient stimulation or did she suffer from orgasmic dysfunction, perhaps secondary to the neurological impairments of MS? She was encouraged to explore systematically the limits of her sexual arousability in the privacy of her home. Within a week, she reported orgasms that were comparable to her pre-MS experiences.

In this case it is difficult to say whether or not the patient suffered a neurological impairment of her sexual response system at the onset of her MS. She was seen during remission of her symptoms. The history established that she still experienced some arousal, and this encouraged her to explore her sexual potential.

Case 2: "Situational" and "Absolute" Dysfunctions Coexisting

A 42-year-old man with MS was referred because of erection and ejaculation problems. His MS was diagnosed five years before. Following initial rapid neurological changes, he was now considered stable. He had at this time bilateral optic atrophy. He had increased deep tendon reflexes with extensor plantar responses. Vibratory sense was mildly decreased in both lower extremities. Voluntary anal sphincter control was poor. His main sexual complaints were that his penile swelling was usually (but not always) insufficient for intercourse and that he was unable to experience climax in the act of intercourse. It took him an inordinately long time, with very active manual stimulation, to experience orgasm. These complaints represented major changes in his sexual experiences. As recently as two years before, he had reliable and strong erections, and if anything, he ejaculated more rapidly than he and his partner desired. The sexual history revealed that he had strong erections upon awakening and on occasions during the day, but not at the time of attempts at intercourse.

In this instance, the delayed orgasmic response was thought to be secondary to neurological impairment. The erection dysfunction was considered to be situational, and likely to be secondary to the concerns over the disturbed intercourse pattern. As the history unfolded, both the patient and the partner recognized the chain of events beginning with the ejaculatory delay, and leading to the situational erection problem. Once they understood that their problem was the result of a combination of physical and psychological factors, they were able to deal with it. His erections became reliable, and they were able to rearrange their sexual practices to accommodate to the ejaculatory dysfunction.

Case 3: Sexual Disinterest Unrelated to MS

A 42-year-old woman with MS was referred because of her complete sexual disinterest for the past 10 years. Her MS was first diagnosed 12 years before, following major sensory and locomotor disturbances. For the past eight years, her condition had been stable, with the exception of recurrent sensory changes over various parts of the body.

The sexual history revealed that the disinterest fluctuated, and that it was most noticeable in the latter half of her menstrual periods. During those times, she also complained of depression, abdominal cramps and bloated feelings. When not depressed, and not completely disinterested, she was able to experience orgasms. The cyclic nature of her disinterest raised the possibility of this being part of a premenstrual syndrome. Progesterone suppositories were recommended. The cyclic depression and sexual disinterest lifted within hours and has not returned since her regular use of this medication over the last year. The couple resumed their sexual practices with a frequency similar to that of her pre-MS days, some 12 years before.

This case illustrates that a cause and effect relationship between a disorder (in this instance MS) and sexual dysfunctions cannot be taken for granted.

Case 4: Sexual Dysfunction, Marital Conflict, and MS

A 48-year-old man with MS was referred because of impotence. He and his wife were married for 28 years. He said, "We married too young. Now it's only a marriage of convenience." His MS was first diagnosed 2½ years ago, following symptoms of shooting pain in the legs, tiredness, and fleeting sensory changes. When the diagnosis was made, he felt that "my whole world as I know it was ending." His wife said: "he became intolerable to have around. He found fault in everything, he was arguing all the time and he blamed me for his sexual problem."

His erection problem started a few months after the diagnosis of MS. Although he did not feel sexually interested, he wanted to see "if I am still a man." When he did not have an erection sufficient for intercourse, he blamed his wife for not being more attractive sexually. When their physician first recommended an evaluation of his impotence, she refused to go along. She said: "I will stand by him while he is sick, but there will be nothing sexual; he can try it with someone else." Nocturnal tumescence studies indicated erection capability.

In instances like this, when a couple presents with relationship conflicts, sexual dysfunction, and multiple sclerosis, it is exceedingly difficult to establish cause and effect. Marital friction is not unusual in couples referred for the treatment of sexual dysfunction; one may be a cause of the other, or the two may have coexisted for some years.[19] The relationship may be so discordant that one partner might not be willing even to participate in the history-taking process. Partners, however, often suffer in silence or feel embarrassed or fear judgment in admitting to sexual needs. The onus is on the clinician to know not only which questions to ask, but also how to ask these questions without causing embarrassment either to the patient or to the partner.

MANAGEMENT

Treatment approaches can be visualized as psychological (education, talk and guidance-oriented methods, including sex therapy), physical (using external devices, appliances), medical (involving medications), and surgical (using, for example, penile prosthetic devices). Guidance-oriented methods may require the involvement of a partner. The educational approach might be applied in a group setting.

Whichever method or combination of methods might be implemented eventually, treatment begins when the clinician first reacts to the MS patient's expressions to the clinician of sexual concern. An organized approach to the patient's problem shows acceptance of both the patient and the problem. The historical inquiry itself may be therapeutic because it defines for the patient the activities and emotions with "sexual" connotations. The patient then may begin to put together a realistic inventory of, for example, sexual responsivity capabilities, motor function abilities, partnership skills, and so on. Relevant educational material may be presented while clarifying, for example, the erection, ejaculation, or orgasmic abilities. Statistical or cultural norms can be portrayed while inquiring about the types of frequencies or preferred sex activities.

As the clinician begins to understand the patient's MS-related impairments, disabilities and handicaps, and as the patient begins to appreciate the available sexual abilities and choices, realistic goals can be formulated for a reasonable sexual adjustment.

The selection of the treatment method will depend on a variety of factors, including the nature of the dysfunction, the presumed etiology of the condition, the age of the patient, and the presence, or absence, of a partner. For example, if the dysfunction has preexisted, the onset of MS is clearly situational in nature, and the couple is highly motivated to resolve the problem, "sex therapy" may be considered. An example of this situation might be primary anorgasmia in a woman or premature ejaculation in a man with MS. When the etiology of a sexual dysfunction suggests a medical cause, independent of MS, attention would be focused on *medical management*. For example, an MS patient who also suffers hypertension, and is taking antihypertensive medication, may require a review of the effect of this medication on sexual responsivity. When erection dysfunction is neurologically based, consideration may be given to the *surgical approach*. The insertion of a penile prosthetic device can be of help to selected individuals and couples. The effect of this surgical procedure on the course of MS is not clear yet.

The goal of the *physical approach* is to give technical assistance to patients and partners in the physical aspect of sex activities. On a general level, promotion of independent movement, dressing and undressing, cleanliness, and secure bowel and bladder management are part of this approach. On a more specific level, the patient may need technical advice, for example, about positions in bed, or the use of a vibrator to provide added genital stimulation.

PROGNOSIS

Sexual dysfunction treatment results vary and are dependent on a variety of factors, including the nature of the dysfunction, the etiology of the condition, the age of the patient, past sexual experiences and the presence of a partner. There is some question also about the relative efficiency of various treatment methods. In one controlled study, for example, 65 nondisabled patients with erectile impotence of varying etiology were treated either with chemotherapy or the Masters and Johnson format of sex therapy. A control group was not given any specific treatment. Study subjects whose impotence was related to a psychological or physical trauma experienced a spontaneous remission rate "not far off" the rate of neurosis. Patients with erection problems which had an insidious decline, and had no discernable etiological factors, showed no complete recovery, and those who showed improvement relapsed very soon. Neither chemotherapy nor sex therapy were in any way superior to no treatment. The author concluded that "it is of considerable practical importance to recognize those subjects in whom the prognosis is likely to be poor in order to enable the couple to adjust to the situation, by explanation and support, rather than by lengthy treatments."[20]

In spinal injured patients, the severity of the impairment or disability is not the important determinant of the outcome of sexual rehabilitation. Two factors seem to help the patient to refocus toward realistic sex-related goals. These are active, varied and satisfying sex relationships before the injury, and a present, available, interested and adventurous partner.[21]

Some of these findings may be applicable to MS patients. However, treatment results may be further influenced because of the relapsing-remitting nature of the disorder.

SUMMARY

The nature, incidence, prevalence, etiology and management of sexual problems in MS has not been well defined yet. Sexual dysfunctions in MS seem to be related to a combination of the neurological consequences of MS and the personal, partner and social reactions to this condition. A sexual history is valuable in defining the specific areas of concern, and bringing into focus the patient's and the couple's sexual resources. Physical examination and investigations may assist in clarifying the extent of the sexual impairment and disability, and its relationship to MS. Treatment strategies include: relevant information, education, physical rehabilitation and supportive therapy in combination with medical intervention, and when indicated, surgical treatment or sex therapy. Long-range prognosis with or without treatment is not clear yet.

REFERENCES

1. Lilius, H. G., E. J. Valtonen & J. Wikstrom. 1976. Sexual problems in patients suffering from multiple sclerosis. J. Chron. Dis. **29:** 643–647.
2. Lundberg, P. O. 1978. Sexual dysfunction in patients with multiple sclerosis. Sexuality and Disability **1:** 218–222.
3. Szasz, G., D. Paty, S. Lawton-Speert & K. Eisen. 1983. A sexual functioning scale in multiple sclerosis. Acta Neurol. Scand. Submitted for publication.
4. Szasz, G. 1983. Unpublished material.
5. American Psychiatric Association. 1980. Diagnostic and Statistical Manual of Mental Disorders. 3d ed. Washington, D. C.
6. Kinsey, A. C., W. B. Pomeroy & C. E. Martin. 1948. Sexual Behavior in the Human Male. W. B. Saunders Company. Philadelphia.
7. Frank, E., C. Anderson & D. Rubinstein. 1978. Frequency of sexual dysfunction in "normal" couples. N. Engl. J. Med. **299:** 111–115.
8. Kolodny, R. C., W. H. Masters & V. E. Johnson. 1979. Textbook of Sexual Medicine. Little, Brown and Company. Boston.
9. Bors, E. & A. E. Comarr. 1960. Neurological disturbances of sexual function with special reference to 529 patients with spinal cord injury. Urol. Surv. **10:** 191–222.
10. Comarr, A. E. 1970. Sexual function among patients with spinal cord injury. Urol. Int. **25:** 134–168.
11. Talbot, H. S. 1949. A report on sexual function in paraplegics. J. Urol. **61:** 265–270.
12. Griffith, E. R. & R. B. Trieschmann. 1975. Sexual functioning in women with spinal cord injury. Arch. Phys. Med. Rehab. **56:** 18–21.
13. Vas, C. J. 1969. Sexual impotence and some autonomic disturbances in men with multiple sclerosis. Acta Neurol. Scand. **45:** 166–182.
14. Wagner, G. & R. Green. 1981. Impotence. Plenum. New York.
15. Masters, W. H. & V. E. Johnson. 1970. Human Sexual Inadequacy. Little, Brown and Company. Boston.
16. Hartings, M. F., M. M. Pavlov & F. A. Davis. 1976. Group counselling of MS patients in a program of comprehensive care. J. Chron. Dis. **29:** 63–73.
17. International Federation of Multiple Sclerosis Societies. 1983. Minimal record of disability in multiple sclerosis. Rehabilitation Research and Training Center. Albert Einstein College of Medicine. Bronx, New York.
18. Ivers, R. R. & N. P. Goldstein. 1963. Multiple sclerosis: A current appraisal of symptoms and signs. Mayo Clinic Proc. **38:** 457–466.

19. MAURICE, W. L., F. STUART & G. SZASZ. 1976. Sex therapy: Considerations in the selection of patients. Can. Med. Assoc. J. **115:** 317–320.
20. ANSARI, J. M. A. 1976. Impotence: Prognosis (a controlled study). Brit. J. Psychiat. **128:** 194–198.
21. SZASZ, G. 1983. Sexual health care *In* Management of spinal cord injury. C. M. Zejdlick, Ed.: 125–151. Wadsworth. Belmont, Calif.

DISCUSSION OF THE PAPER

UNIDENTIFIED SPEAKER: Could you elaborate on how men find the penile prostheses satisfactory?

G. SZASZ (*University of British Columbia, Vancouver, BC*): I have very little experience with MS patients and prosthetic devices, but I have plenty of other patients with the same. The device fits inside the corpora cavernosa. There are two types actually, the rigid or semirigid on the one hand, and the inflatable, which is a very elegant method, on the other. Once the devices are activated and inside the penis they provide for a rigidity of the penis which permits sexual intercourse. In the act of intercourse the sensation, if it is okay before the operation, will be exactly the same as before. Orgasm will be experienced in exactly the same way; if ejaculation was possible, ejaculation will also occur. Self-stimulation is possible in exactly the same way and with the same results as just before. If somebody had sensory problems, ejaculation or orgasmic problems or retrograde ejaculation or whatever, that will also continue with this instrument.

The problems with the instruments are that they are instruments and as a consequence they have mechanical breakdowns of various sorts and there's something like a 20–30% reoperation rate for some of these devices; it's a bit better for some other devices.

Actually we are finding a very interesting thing, which is that there are people who desperately want the device but once they have it they don't use it and when we ask them what is going on they tell us, "well I now feel like anybody else, I have all my options. At the moment my option is not to use it." There's a very interesting philosophical thought behind this.

Development and Testing of a Minimal Record of Disability in Multiple Sclerosis[a]

ROBERT J. SLATER,[b,c] NICHOLAS G. LAROCCA,[d] AND LABE C. SCHEINBERG[d]

[b]*National Multiple Sclerosis Society*
New York, New York 10017

[c]*Department of Pediatrics*
Cornell Medical College
New York, New York 10021

[d]*Research and Training Center for Multiple Sclerosis*
Albert Einstein College of Medicine
Bronx, New York 10461

In 1979 the International Federation of Multiple Sclerosis Societies (IFMSS) convened a panel drawn from its twenty-two members to examine ways to improve communication of experiences in the management of individuals afflicted with multiple sclerosis (MS). Comparison of the planning and allocation of resources both locally and nationally was difficult within and among countries. Determination of outcomes in specific functional change and cost-effectiveness in the provision of medical and social services was difficult also because of the varying cultural patterns and social systems prevailing in each country. Furthermore each professional discipline and indeed those in each medical center had their own unique system for coding and recording information. With the advent of computer capability to enhance data retrieval and analysis, the generation of a simple common language to record functional disability in MS was deemed worthwhile.

This project was an extension of a similar endeavor organized by Broman's group[1] in 1972. Commencing with an IFMSS symposium held in Stockholm in 1980,[2] twelve countries have collaborated in nine languages to develop experience: Australia, Belgium, Canada (English and French), Denmark, West Germany, Great Britain, Holland, Italy, Japan, New Zealand, Switzerland and the United States. Subsequent workshops have led to agreement on a simple, widely applicable system of rating to provide indices of functional disability.

The IFMSS Minimal Record of Disability (MRD) is based on the following criteria:

1. It should include the most limited information required for practical assessment of the individual's functional capability and needs for activities of daily living.
2. The descriptors used for various functions should be compatible with the terminology used by the different professionals (in neurology, rehabilitative medicine, nursing, social work, *etc.*), each of whom participate in various aspects of medical and social care.

[a]The preparation of this manuscript was supported in part by a grant from the National Institute of Handicapped Research (no. G008200046).

3. It ought to comprise questions that are adequately inclusive and clearly descriptive of functional disabilities so as to be meaningful when translated into different languages, and ensure a basis for cross-country comparisons.
4. Existing record systems for multiple sclerosis in different centers should be compatible with it, so that the individual MRD components can be readily correlated with methods of assessment already in use.
5. Sufficient items of performance should be included despite possible redundancy to assure their usefulness to community health professionals for planning services.
6. It should be administered by health professionals or volunteers trained and supervised by professionals.

The decision was made to limit the system to multiple sclerosis because it was professionally and politically impractical to attempt to use one record of disability for the variety of physical handicaps resultant to different pathogeneses and administered by different cadres of professionals. However, it was clearly recognized that the system should be linked to the World Health Organization (WHO) conceptual framework of impairment/disability/handicap described by Wood[3] so that later linkage and correlation to comparable data systems used in other forms of handicap could be achieved. Thus, at present, this new system stands on its own to define profiles of dysfunction for the MS population. Over time correlation with other record systems will permit aggregation of data on classes of problems such as employment, transportation, home care management, *etc.,* for which adaptations at the community and national level in matters such as health and social insurance and resource systems are necessary.

DEVELOPMENT OF THE MINIMAL RECORD OF DISABILITY

The current version of the MRD as modified at the 1983 IFMSS symposium[4] is set forth in the Appendix. This three-tier system, which originated at the 1980 symposium, conforms to the WHO hierarchical concept and has the following characteristics.

Impairment. This part of the record quantifies the biological dysfunction and is administered by a physician, usually a neurologist. By international consensus, the rating system recommended by Kurtzke[5] has been accepted and consists of two components. The quantitation by neurological examination of the organic impairment of the neuronal tracts is defined on a scale of 0–5 or 0–6 (normal to nonfunctional) by the Functional Systems (FS). The degree of overall functional disability is estimated on a scale of 0–10, the Disability Status Scale (DSS). Recently a more sensitive indicator of functional disability, the Expanded Disability Status Scale (EDSS) has been described by Kurtzke[5] to improve quantitation of functional changes anticipated in clinical trials of new therapies.

Disability. This part of the record quantifies the individual's physical and mental dysfunction, closely reflecting the activities of daily living. The items are derived from descriptors most commonly used in the field of rehabilitation and have been captioned the Incapacity Status Scale (ISS) by the IFMSS.

Handicap. This third part of the record is likewise derived from systems used in rehabilitative and psychosocial analyses to depict the effect of impairment and disability on the individual's interaction with the social environment. The IFMSS has captioned this part the Environmental Status Scale (ESS). The ESS was derived from a scheme described by Mellerup *et al.*[6] Both ISS and ESS are readily administered under the direction of allied health professionals.

The Incapacity Status Scale was first described by Kurtzke[7,8] in 1980; it was based on the work of Carl Granger and designed to be a summative or linear composite scale for functional assessment of MS patients. In contrast to assessment of the organic neuronal function, the ISS is descriptive of individual abilities or limitations in performance of social roles.

During the initial construction of the Incapacity Status Scale, Granger[9] tested it for correlation with his Long Range Evaluation System (LRES). The LRES was a composite of widely tested functional assessment scales—Barthel, PULSES and ESCROW. For the 39 MS patients tested the correlation of ISS items with Granger's LRES had a coefficient of 0.87.[7] For the Barthel/PULSES index the coefficient of correlation was 0.94.[8]

Field Testing the MRD

Apart from work proceeding in the collaborating IFMSS countries, eight centers[e] in the United States and Canada tested the MRD on 249 patients during 1983 to provide the following measures: (1) qualitative evaluation that included administration and scoring criteria, and (2) quantitative evaluation that included item analysis, reliability and validity.

The 1982 modification[10] of the MRD was used and differed from the 1981[8] version by inclusion in Incapacity Status of a new item, sexual function. (The final 1983 version of the MRD listed in the appendix has essentially the same content.) Furthermore, an interview protocol was developed by LaRocca[11] that was implemented by each of the collaborating centers (and translated by the IFMSS collaboraters) to enhance the reliability of information.

RESULTS

TABLES 1 and 2 summarize the characteristics of the sample evaluated. Close to two-thirds (60.2%) were females. The average age was 41.6 years, with 75% falling between the ages of 20 and 50. Thus the sample consisted mainly of individuals in the middle adult years, the most productive years for family and career development. The average age of onset of symptoms was 29.6, making for an average duration of symptoms of 11.8 years. Onset occurred between the ages of 20 and 40 in 73% of cases.

[e]The eight centers contributing data (investigators listed in parentheses) as of 1 September 1983 were: Albert Einstein College of Medicine, New York, NY (L. Scheinberg, B. Geisser, C. Smith, and W. Traugott); Fairview Deaconess Hospital, Minneapolis, MN (R. Schapiro); University of British Columbia MS Clinic, Vancouver, BC, Canada (D. Paty, S. Hashimoto, V. Hooge, and L. Kastrukoff); Rocky Mountain MS Center, University of Colorado, Denver, CO (G. Franklin and W. Cobble); University of Utah MS Clinic, Salt Lake City, UT (J. Petajan); University of Washington MS Clinic, Seattle, WA (G. Kraft, D. Frankel, and M. Catanzaro); Veterans Administration Clinic/Boston University, Boston, MA (C. Poser); Wadsworth VA Clinic/University of California at Los Angeles, Los Angeles, CA (W. Tourtellotte and W. Baumhefner).

TABLE 1. Characteristics of Study Sample Expressed in Years

	Mean	Median	SD
Age	41.6	39.8	10.7
Age of onset	29.6	28.3	9.5
Duration of MS[a]	11.8	10.5	8.1
Education	13.9	13.3	2.1

[a]Duration of MS indicates time elapsed since diagnosis.

The majority of persons sampled were white (93.2%). Nearly three out of four of those interviewed (70.3%) were married and living with their spouses. Almost everyone sampled had worked at some time in their lives (97.6%), although only 38.5% were employed at the time of evaluation. The occupations of those working were mainly white collar (91.9%) with significant representation among the ranks of executives, professionals and managers (43%). The average educational attainment was 13.9 years, with 33.2% having completed college and 91.5% having completed high school.

Qualitative Evaluation

Administration

Except for the Functional Systems, which require neurological examination, the scales were rated on the basis of questioning by use of the structured interview rather than by direct testing.

Information was sometimes obtained additionally from family members. Some practice was necessary in order to develop proficiency; it was not possible simply to pick up the manual and start interviewing. The assessments were made by physicians, mainly neurologists, as well as by other health professionals. Some physicians conducted all three parts of the MRD, while others rated only the neurological section FS/DSS.

The structured interview proved very important in standardizing administrative procedures. The consensus from the eight study centers was that the rating system was easy to use after some practice. Administrative time was approximately one hour (including the neurological examination) for those beginning to use the MRD. Experience led to reduction of this time to as little as twenty minutes. There was agreement that the MRD provided a worthwhile focus to clinical examination, adding at most ten to twenty minutes to the usual time spent with patients. Patients accepted the use of the MRD and found the questions meaningful.

TABLE 2. Distribution of Patients by Sex[a]

	Frequency	Percent
Male	98	39.4
Female	151	60.6
	249	100.0

[a]The study accepted individuals in sequence but an effort was made to develop a male:female ratio of 2:3 in order to avoid skewing of distribution which might inadvertently occur.

TABLE 3. Item Analysis for Incapacity Status

Item[a]	Corrected Item-Total Correlation[b]
Transfers	0.86
Bathing	0.85
Dressing	0.84
Ambulation	0.83
Stair climbing	0.82
Grooming	0.73
Societal role	0.72
Feeding	0.68
Bladder function	0.62
Fatigability	0.56
Sexual function	0.53
Bowel function	0.52
Vision	0.47
Speech and hearing	0.43
Psychic function	0.41
Physical problems	0.25

[a]Items are those listed in the 1982 version of MRD.
[b]Range of correlations reflects heterogeneity of the item content.

Scoring

Most of the comments offered by raters concerned problems in using the scoring criteria based on correlation of the interview questions to the quantitation of each item. Improvement in the clarity of the interview questions is being developed. In a separate study LaRocca[12] noted that the interrater agreement on examination of 20 patients by two physicians revealed a correlation coefficient of 0.94 for the Incapacity Status Scale and 0.97 for the Environmental Status Scale.

Quantitative Evaluaton

Item Analysis

TABLES 3 and 4 depict the item-total correlations, the correlations of each item with the summed score of the ISS and ESS of which it is a part. TABLE 5 shows that

TABLE 4. Item Analysis for Environmental Status

Item[a]	Corrected Item-Total Correlation
Transportation	0.73
Personal assistance	0.71
Financial/economic status	0.62
Actual work status	0.59
Personal residence/home	0.59
Community health services	0.52

[a]Items are those listed in the 1982 version of MRD.

TABLE 5. Variance Shared with Total Scores

50% or More	25 to 50%	Less than 25%
Transfers	Feeding	Vision
Bathing	Bladder function	Speech and hearing
Dressing	Fatigability	Psychic function
Ambulation	Sexual function	Physical problems
Stair climbing	Bowel function	
Grooming		
Societal role		

three groups of items in the Incapacity Status could be identified. Seven items had the highest correlations with the total scores 0.72 to 0.86, that is had 50% or more of their variance in common. The second group of five items had moderate correlations, 0.52 to 0.68, sharing 25–50% of their variance with total scores. The third group of four items with correlations 0.25 to 0.47 showed less than 25% of their variance in common with total scores.

Most of the items with moderate correlations (25–50% variance in TABLE 5), were mentioned by raters as presenting problems with their scoring criteria. Thus the need for refinement of the scoring criteria is suggested by both qualitative and quantitative analyses. Items with low correlations are likewise candidates for later revision or exclusion because they appear to be measuring something different from the content reflected by total scores. In contrast, TABLE 4 reveals that all items on Environmental Status fell into a narrow band of common variance between 27–53%. Whereas some items need refinement, none appear to be candidates for exclusion.

Reliability

Summary statistics for the MRD scales are presented in TABLE 6. Following the Likert model for linear composite scales, Cronbach's alpha was chosen as a measure of reliability for Incapacity Status and Environmental Status. Alpha is a lower-bounds estimate of reliability and indicates the minimum proportion of true variance in scores. True reliability may actually be higher but cannot be lower. Alphas were 0.93 for Incapacity Status and 0.83 for Environmental Status. These high alphas indicate that at least one fairly homogenous dimension underlies the additive scores of the scales, supporting their use as composite scales. Indeed, the high correlation of many of the

TABLE 6. Summary Statistics for MRD Scales

	Impairment		Disability	Handicap
	DSS	EDSS	Incapacity Status	Environmental Status
Minimum[a]	0	0	0	0
Maximum[a]	9	9.5	57	30
Median	4.0	4.6	15.7	8.0
Mean	4.3	4.6	17.9	8.5
Standard deviation	2.4	2.4	12.5	7.5
Cronbach's alpha[b]	N/A	N/A	0.93	0.83

[a]Minimum and maximum figures represent range of scores from 249 patients studied.
[b]High Chronbach's alpha reflects a high degree of internal consistency.

items suggests that certain pairs of items may be largely redundant (*e.g.*, stair climbing and ambulation, $r = 0.86$, and bathing and dressing, $r = 0.87$) at least when used in aggregated data.

Validity

TABLE 7 shows the intercorrelation of the three MRD rating scales plus the Kurtzke[5] Expanded Status Scale (EDSS). All are high, indicating in excess of 50% common variance. However the pattern of correlations is as interesting as their magnitude. This pattern is consistent with the conceptual scheme upon which the MRD is based, the WHO classification of impairment (DSS), disability (Incapacity Status) and handicap (Environmental Status).

The WHO scheme represents a conceptual hierarchy, suggesting that impairment/disability and disability/handicap should correlate more highly than impairment/handicap. This is exactly the pattern observed in the data of TABLE 7, although the differences are small. Correlation of the two new IFMSS scales (Incapacity/Environmental Status) with the established measure of disease severity (DSS) represents a crude indication of validity. Further studies of validity are planned after scoring criteria and administrative procedures have been refined.

TABLE 7. Intercorrelation of MRD Scales[a]

	EDSS	Incapacity Status	Environmental Status
DSS	0.99	0.81	0.76
EDSS		0.81	0.76
Incapacity status			0.85

[a]The high intercorrelation of the ISS and ESS with the DSS suggests that functional disability does reflect organic involvement.

COMMENTARY

Redundancy and Functional Groupings of Scale Items

In considering the need for a multidimensional rating system to reflect the overall effect of MS, Kurtzke[8] noted that his Functional Systems and Disability Status Score by no means provide a rating of functional disability for universal therapeutic or psychosocial interventions. He emphasized that as an encoded neurological examination, it is an appropriate part of the categorization of the MS patient but is not a sufficient scheme to summarize the MS disabilities. Thus while the neurological professional deals with a coding system to explain the anatomic cause of dysfunction (FS) and its general effects (DSS), the physiatric and other health professionals are most concerned with the type and severity of end-organ impairment and the consequences on a variety of physiological funtions required for activities of daily living. Therefore, inclusion in one composite record system of items designed to satisfy these various anatomic and physiologic functions are clearly going to have some overlap and redundancy.

This redundancy is most apparent, as Kurtzke[13] notes elsewhere in this volume, in the items reflecting motor function. The first nine items of the Incapacity Status Scale reflect involvement of the motor and coordinative functions. Similarly, items reflecting social behavior and interrelation with the environment listed in the ESS will reflect aberrations that are the result of one or more neurological functional deficits that can be located and quantified by the neurological functional system (FS) record.

In another context, Kurtzke[13] points out that major changes in neurological function will be reflected by similar changes in ISS item grades but the converse is not necessarily true; changes in ISS item severity grades can occur without measurable changes in neurologic function. The obvious redundancy among many items in the DSS and the ISS (ambulation, bowel and bladder, visual and cerebral functions) reflects the functional focus and terminology of two different sets of professionals. The high coefficients of correlation delineated in TABLE 7 have the practical implication that assessment of function defined by the ISS and conducted by allied health professionals precludes the need for frequent intervention by a physician to define an FS/DSS for this particular aspect of monitoring patient care needs.

The ISS item analysis correlations and variances in TABLES 3 and 4 revealed three groupings of function. Similar findings were reported by Fog *et al.*[14] Those with correlations of 0.68 and above were all related to the integrity of motor and coordinative function. Items with lower correlations measured other less well-defined functions: excretory, sexual, fatigue, and cerebral. Nevertheless for service interventions these are critical factors and cannot be excluded. The redundancy among motor/coordinative-dependent abilities could be rectified by deletion of several high-correlation items. This might be practical for statistical efficiency but such a change would lose the value to health care personnel of certain critical descriptors of activities of living that enhance the practical assessment of need for service interventions.

In planning to simplify the interpretation of the aggregated item data by summing the scores for an overall number (ISS: 0–64; ESS: 0–42) experience must be gained in order to introduce appropriate weighing for items showing low correlations to item-total scores. Kurtzke[8] noted that while the DSS was originally planned as an ordinal (ranked) scale, experience has shown that it can be treated as a true numerical (equal interval, additive) scale.

Minderhoud *et al.*,[15] examined the data from 184 patients to determine if the ISS and ESS could be sum scored and thus simplify assessment of overall functional disability or main classes of problems. By means of factor analyses, they identified three clusters in the ISS. The first and major cluster was based on motor performance; the second and third smaller clusters were identified with bladder, bowel and sexual function and with communication. Fatigue represented a fourth cluster that did not correlate with any other variable but was a significant problem in 71% of their patients. Minderhoud states that sum scoring which includes less-related variables will conceal important differences. He concludes that if sum scoring of ISS and ESS is to be attempted, the ISS must be reduced to the three variables noted above and then added to the six ESS (1982 version) scores. These findings require comparison with experience in other centers.

Sibley[16] reported a study of 135 MS patients to relate the Disability Status Score with the Incapacity Status Score (1980 version) and the status of employment or dependency. He noted that the DSS and ISS may show considerable variability because different parameters of function may be recorded despite a high correlation on mobility. Thus he noted that a relatively high DSS of 6 can be compatible with a relatively low ISS score of 16 (out of 64). By summing and comparing ISS mean scores, Sibley reported fully employed persons scored approximately 10, half-time employed scored 20 and those receiving Social Security disability benefits scored 30. If the neurological FS/DSS scores low in contrast to a relatively high ISS score, the possibility of a significant psychogenic basis for the disability should be considered.

Potential Uses of the MRD in Clinical Practice and Research

The Minimal Record of Disability shows promise in clinical use as an aid to needs assessment for planning and evaluating specific therapy or services. It provides members of the health professions involved in care of MS individuals with a comprehensive picture of a person's neurological status, activities of daily living, and psychosocial needs. As such the MRD helps to organize the acquisition and recording of this information which in many instances may otherwise be gathered in an erratic and impressionistic manner. In some centers the MRD is being used as a standard patient progress note. Instead of the usual (and at times illegible) paragraph notation, clinical records contain a one page checklist format and retain the familiar commentary by clinical staff while adding the standardized quantitative MRD assessment. The information can be entered into the computer file as core data, compatible with other more extensive information which may be aggregated. The system thus facilitates the clinician's evaluation of changes in the patient's status over time.

Madonna[17] subjected the MRD to field trials in 15 MS chapter/community settings involving review of 160 MS persons in Canada and the United States. They noted that, despite the lack of prior training of personnel, there was acceptance that the MRD would provide useful basis data for planning services and that the ISS/ESS could be administered by a trained and supervised nonprofessional volunteer.

The recommendation has been made by Slater[18] that the MRD be used as a core data set in controlled clinical trials of new therapy. Though individual investigators usually have detailed methods of detecting functional change unique to their own interests, the MRD is the only data system, including the Kurtzke FS/DSS scales, that has been subjected to extensive multinational, multilanguage testing. Because of the protracted nature of the disease and the extended periods required for clinical trials in which coordinated observations are made by a team of professionals, the ISS and ESS provide valuable indices of function and psychosocial adaptation that may not necessarily be recorded by changes in the Kurtzke FS/DSS or other modalities of neurological assessment.

Finally, the MRD is finding use in research where measures of disability are needed. Such projects include studying vocational problems and psychosocial adjustment to chronic illness, planning and evaluating resource allocation, and defining the costs of various forms of intervention basic to determining appropriate medical and social insurance programs. Although it is too early to judge the usefulness of the MRD in all these contexts, the availabilty of a comprehensive and standard instrument applicable to multicenter studies and to the bridging of geopolitical boundaries and languages will help realize maximal comparability of findings.

REFERENCES

1. ANDERSON, O., L. BERGMANN & T. BROMAN, Eds. 1974. The International Symposium on Multiple Sclerosis. Acta Neurol. Scand. **50** (Suppl. 58).
2. SLATER, R. J., T. FOG & L. BERGMANN, Eds. 1981. Functional disability ratings: Medical, social and economic implications. Symposium on Multiple Sclerosis Services. Acta Neurol. Scand. **64** (Suppl. 87).
3. WOOD, P. H. N. 1980. Appreciating the consequences of disease: The international classification of impairments, disabilities and handicaps. WHO Chronicle **34:** 376–380.

4. SLATER, R. J. & N. RAUN, Eds. 1984. A minimal record of disability for multiple sclerosis. Acta Neurol. Scand. **70** (Suppl. 101).
5. KURTZKE, J. F. 1983. Rating neurologic impairment in multiple sclerosis: An expanded disability status scale (EDSS). Neurology **33:** 1444–1452.
6. MELLERUP, E., T. FOG, N. RAUN, P. COLVILLE, B. DE RHAM, B. HANNAH & J. KURTZKE. 1981. The socio-economic scale. Acta. Neurol. Scand. **64** (Suppl. 87): 130–138.
7. KURTZKE, J. F. 1981. Initial proposal for a uniform minimal record of disability. Acta Neurol. Scand. **64** (Suppl. 87): 48–51.
8. KURTZKE, J. F. 1981. A proposal for a uniform minimal record of disability in multiple sclerosis. Acta Neurol. Scand. **64** (Suppl. 87): 110–129.
9. GRANGER, C. V. 1981. Assessment of functional status: A model for multiple sclerosis. Acta Neurol. Scand. **64** (Suppl. 87): 40–47.
10. SLATER, R. J., N. G. LAROCCA & L. SCHEINBERG. 1982. Minimal record of disability: Unpublished test model. MS Clinical Center. Albert Einstein College of Medicine. New York.
11. LAROCCA, N. G. & F. FOLEY. 1984. Development of a structured interview for the IFMSS minimal record of disability. Acta Neurol. Scand. **70** (Suppl. 101): 165–168.
12. LAROCCA, N. G., L. C. SCHEINBERG & R. J. SLATER. 1984. Field testing of a minimal record of disability in multiple sclerosis: The United States and Canada. Acta Neurol. Scand. **70** (Suppl. 101): 126–138.
13. KURTZKE, J. F. 1984. Disability rating scales in multiple sclerosis. This volume.
14. FOG, T., A. HELTBERG, K. KYHN, E. MELLERUP, N. E. RAUN & I. ZEEBERG. 1984. Evaluation of disability, incapacity, and environmental status scales in multiple sclerosis. Acta Neurol. Scand. **70** (Suppl. 101): 77–86.
15. MINDERHOUD, J. M., H. DASSEL & A. J. A. PRANGE. 1984. Proposal for summing the incapacity status or environmental status scores. Acta Neurol. Scand. **70** (Suppl. 101): 87–91.
16. SIBLEY, W. A. & K. CLARK. 1982. The IFMSS incapacity status score and work status in a clinic of 135 patients. IFMSS Rating System Workshop. Unpublished report.
17. MADONNA, M. G., B. HANNAH & N. G. LAROCCA. 1984. Experience in the use of the IFMSS minimal record of disability in multiple sclerosis chapters and community settings. Acta Neurol. Scand. **70** (Suppl. 101): 139–142.
18. SLATER, R. J. 1983. Scoring techniques and problems in the evaluation of change in patients. Arch. Neurol. **40:** 675–677.

APPENDIX

IFMSS Minimal Record of Disability

The following lists outline the IFMSS Minimal Record of Disability as modified for international use at the IFMSS annual meeting at Vancouver, Canada, in September 1983. The complete instructions and structured interview system will be published as a supplement to *Acta Neurologica Scandinavica* in 1984.

Much of the data noted in this report reflects work conducted on earlier versions of the MRD (1981; 1982) in the course of satisfying the integrity of the system and working out international acceptance which has led to this final model. Further adaptations may be recommended by the IFMSS but only after several years of testing in studies on services and of experience in cross-linkage to comparable functional rating systems used in assessment of other types of chronic handicapping disorders.

Kurtzke Functional Systems (FS)
(WHO Impairment)

1. Pyramidal functions
   Grade 0 = normal
   Grade 1 = abnormal signs without disability
   Grade 2 = minimal disability

Grade 3 = mild or moderate paraparesis or hemiparesis; severe monoparesis
Grade 4 = marked paraparesis or hemiparesis; moderate quadriparesis; or monoplegia
Grade 5 = paraplegia, hemiplegia, or marked quadriparesis
Grade 6 = quadriplegia
Grade 9 = unknown

2. Cerebellar functions
   Grade 0 = normal
   Grade 1 = abnormal signs without disability
   Grade 2 = mild ataxia
   Grade 3 = moderate truncal or limb ataxia
   Grade 4 = severe ataxia of all limbs
   Grade 5 = unable to perform coordinated movements due to ataxia
   Grade 9 = unknown
   Grade 7 = use "7" throughout after each number when weakness (grade 3 or more on pyramidal) interferes with testing
3. Brainstem functions
   Grade 0 = normal
   Grade 1 = signs only
   Grade 2 = moderate nystagmus or other mild disability
   Grade 3 = severe nystagmus, marked extraocular weakness, or moderate disability of other cranial nerves
   Grade 4 = marked dysarthria or other marked disability
   Grade 5 = inability to swallow or speak
   Grade 9 = unknown
4. Sensory functions
   Grade 0 = normal
   Grade 1 = vibration or figure-writing decrease only in 1 or 2 limbs
   Grade 2 = mild decrease in touch or pain or position sense, and/or moderate decrease in vibration in 1 or 2 limbs; or vibratory (c/s figure writing) decrease alone in 3 or 4 limbs
   Grade 3 = moderate decrease in touch or pain or position sense, and/or essentially lost vibration in 1 or 2 limbs; or mild decrease in touch or pain and/or moderate decrease in all proprioceptive tests in 3 or 4 limbs
   Grade 4 = marked decrease in touch or pain or proprioception, alone or combined, in 1 or 2 limbs; or moderate decrease in touch or pain and/or severe proprioceptive loss in more than 2 limbs
   Grade 5 = loss (essentially) of sensation in 1 or 2 limbs; or moderate decrease in touch or pain and/or loss of proprioception for most of the body below the head
   Grade 6 = sensation essentially lost below the head
   Grade 9 = unknown
5. Bowel and bladder functions
   Grade 0 = normal
   Grade 1 = mild urinary hesitancy, urgency or retention
   Grade 2 = moderate hesitancy, urgency, retention of bowel or bladder or rare urinary incontinence
   Grade 4 = in need of almost constant catheterization
   Grade 5 = loss of bladder function
   Grade 6 = loss of bowel and bladder function
   Grade 9 = unknown
6. Visual (or optic) functions
   Grade 0 = normal
   Grade 2 = scotoma with visual acuity (corrected) better than 20/30
   Grade 2 = worse eye with scotoma with maximal visual acuity (corrected) of 20/30 to 20/59
   Grade 3 = worse eye with large scotoma, or moderate decrease in fields, but with maximal visual acuity (corrected) of 20/60 to 20/99
   Grade 4 = worse eye with marked decrease of fields and maximal visual acuity (corrected) of 20/100 to 20/200; grade 3 plus maximal acuity of better eye of 20/60 or less
   Grade 5 = worse eye with maximal visual acuity (corrected) less than 20/200; grade 4 plus maximal acuity of better eye of 20/60 or less

Grade 6 = grade 5 plus maximal visual acuity of better eye of 20/60 or less
Grade 9 = unknown
Grade 7 = add after first digit for presence of temporal pallor

7. Cerebral (or mental) functions
   Grade 0 = normal
   Grade 1 = mood alteration only[a]
   Grade 2 = mild decrease in mentation
   Grade 3 = moderate decrease in mentation
   Grade 4 = marked decrease in mentation (chronic brain syndrome, moderate)
   Grade 5 = dementia or chronic brain syndrome—severe or incompetent
   Grade 9 = unknown
8. Other functions
   Grade 0 = none
   Grade 1 = any other neurological findings attributed to MS (specify)
   Grade 9 = unknown

[a]Does not affect DSS score.

Kurtzke Disability Status Scale (DSS) (WHO Impairment)

(In parentheses are listed usual equivalents for defects in the Functional Systems.)

Grade 0 = normal neurological examination (all grade 0 in functional systems)

Grade 1 = no disability and minimal signs such as Babinski sign or vibratory decrease (grade 1 in functional systems)

Grade 2 = minimal disability, for example, slight weakness or mild gait, sensory, visuomotor disturbance (one or two functional systems, grade 2)

Grade 3 = moderate disability though fully ambulatory, for example, monoparesis, moderate ataxia, or combinations of lesser dysfunctions (one or two functional systems, grade 3, or several, grade 2)

Grade 4 = relatively severe disability though fully ambulatory and able to be self-sufficient and up and about for some twelve hours a day (one functional system, grade 4, or several, grade 3 or less)

Grade 5 = disability severe enough to preclude ability to work a full day without special provisions; maximal motor function: walking unaided no more than several blocks (one functional system, grade 5 alone, or combination of lesser grades)

Grade 6 = assistance (canes, crutches, or braces) required for walking (combinations with more than one system, grade 3 or worse)

Grade 7 = restricted to wheelchair but able to wheel self and enter and leave chair alone (combinations with more than one system, grade 4 or worse; very rarely pyramidal system, grade 5 alone)

Grade 8 = restricted to bed but with effective use of arms (combinations usually grade 4 or above in functional systems)

Grade 9 = totally helpless bed patients (combinations usually grade 4 or above in most functional systems)

Grade 10 = death due to multiple sclerosis

Incapacity Status Scale (ISS) (WHO Disability)

1. Stair climbing (ability to ascend and descent a flight of stairs of about 12 steps)
   Grade 0 = normal
   Grade 1 = some difficulty but performed without aid
   Grade 2 = need for canes, brances, prostheses, or dependent upon banister to perform
   Grade 3 = need human assistance to perform
   Grade 4 = unable to perform; includes mechanical lifts

2. Ambulation (ability to walk on level ground or indoors some 50 meters without rest)
   Grade 0 = normal
   Grade 1 = some difficulty but performed without aid
   Grade 2 = need for canes, braces, prostheses to perform
   Grade 3 = need for human assistance or use of manual wheelchair which patient enters, leaves, and maneuvers without aid
   Grade 4 = unable to perform; includes perambulation in a wheelchair and motorized wheelchair
3. Toilet/chair/bed transfer (ability to enter and leave regular toilet and/or chair and/or bed; includes wheelchair transfer as indicated; the worst transfer function determines the grade)
   Grade 0 = normal
   Grade 1 = some difficulty but performed without aid
   Grade 2 = need for adaptive or assistive devices such as trapeze, sling, bars, lift, sliding board to perform
   Grade 3 = requires human aid to perform
   Grade 4 = must be lifted or moved about completely by another person
4. Bowel function
   Grade 0 = normal
   Grade 1 = bowel retention not requiring more than high fiber diets, laxatives, occasional enemas or suppositories, self-administered
   Grade 2 = bowel retention requiring regular laxatives, enemas or suppositories, self-administered in order to induce evacuation; cleanses and disimpacts self
   Grade 3 = bowel retention requiring enemas or suppositories administered by another; disimpacted by another; needs assistance in cleansing; occasional incontinence; presence of colostomy tended by self
   Grade 4 = frequent soiling due either to incontinence or a poorly maintained ostomy device or an ostomy device which patient cannot maintain without assistance
5. Bladder function
   Grade 0 = normal (even if maintained by drugs)
   Grade 1 = occasional hesitancy or urgency; occasional need for drugs
   Grade 2 = frequent hesitancy, urgency, or retention; use of indwelling or external catheter applied and maintained by self; intermittent self-catheterization, manual compression to evacuate bladder, regular use of drugs
   Grade 3 = occasional incontinence; use of indwelling or external catheter applied and maintained by others; ileostomy or suprapubic cystostomy maintained by self; intermittent catheterization by others
   Grade 4 = frequent incontinence; ostomy device which patient cannot maintain without assistance
6. Bathing
   Grade 0 = normal
   Grade 1 = somc difficulty with washing and drying self though performed without aid whether in tub or shower or by sponge bathing, whichever is usual for thc patient
   Grade 2 = need for assistive devices (trapeze, sling, lift, shower or tub bar) in order to bathe self; need to bathe self outside of tub or shower if that is the usual method
   Grade 3 = need for human assistance in bathing parts of the body or in entry/exit/positioning in tub or shower
   Grade 4 = bathing performed by others (aside from face and hands)
7. Dressing
   Grade 0 = normal
   Grade 1 = some difficulty clothing self completely in standard garments, but accomplished by self
   Grade 2 = specially adapted clothing (special closures, elastic-laced shoes, front-closing garments) or devices (long shoe horns, zipper extenders) required to dress self
   Grade 3 = need for human aid to accomplish; performs considerable portion him/herself
   Grade 4 = need for almost complete assistance; unable to dress self
8. Grooming (care of teeth or dentures and hair, shaving, or application of cosmetics)
   Grade 0 = normal

Grade 1 = some difficulty but all tasks performed without aid
Grade 2 = need adaptive devices (electric razors or toothbrushes, special combs or brushes, arm rests or slings) but performed without aid
Grade 3 = need for human aid to perform some of the tasks
Grade 4 = almost all tasks performed by another person

9. Feeding (ingestion, mastication, swallowing of solids and liquids, and manipulation of the appropriate utensils)
Grade 0 = normal
Grade 1 = some difficulty but performed without aid
Grade 2 = need for adaptive devices (special feeding utensils, straws) or special preparation (portions precut or minced, bread buttered) to feed self
Grade 3 = need for human aid in the delivery of food; dysphagia preventing solid diet; esophagostomy or gastrostomy maintained and utilized by self; tube-feeding performed by self
Grade 4 = unable to feed self or to manage ostomies

10. Vision (rate on the basis of the worse of either visual acuity or double vision)
Grade 0 = normal vision (can read standard newsprint with corrective lenses)
Grade 1 = cannot read print finer than standard newsprint with corrective lenses or complains of double vision
Grade 2 = magnifying lenses or large print necessary for reading or double vision interferes with function
Grade 3 = can only read very large print such as major newspaper headlines, constant double vision or movement of objects
Grade 4 = legal blindness

11. Speech and hearing (verbal output and input for interpersonal communication)
Grade 0 = normal; no subjective hearing loss; articulation and language appropriate to the culture
Grade 1 = impaired hearing or articulation not interfering with communication
Grade 2 = deafness sufficient to require hearing aid and/or dysarthria interfering with communication; needs communication aids such as special keyboards, *etc.*
Grade 3 = severe deafness compensated for by sign language or lip reading facility and/or severe dysarthria compensated for by sign language or self-written communication
Grade 4 = severe deafness and/or dysarthria without effective compensation

12. Medical problems (presence of general medical and/or neurological and/or orthopedic disorders; this includes MS and related problems such as decubiti, contractures, and urinary tract infections)
Grade 0 = no significant disorder present
Grade 1 = disorder(s) not requiring active care; may be on maintenance medication; monitoring not required more often than every three months
Grade 2 = disorder(s) requiring occasional monitoring by physician or nurse, more often than every three months but less often than weekly
Grade 3 = disorder(s) requiring regular attention (at least weekly) by physician or nurse
Grade 4 = disorder(s) requiring essentially daily attention by physician or nurse, usually in hospital

13. Mood and thought disturbances (includes anxiety, depression, mood swings, euphoria, delusions, hallucinations, and thought disorder; the rating should reflect current behavior even if the patient is maintained on medication)
Grade 0 = no observable problem
Grade 1 = disturbance is present at times, but does not interfere with day-to-day functioning
Grade 2 = disturbance does interfere with day-to-day functioning, but the person can manage without professional assistance except for occasional visits to maintain medication
Grade 3 = disturbance interferes with day-to-day functioning and consistently requires professional intervention beyond that required to maintain medication, *e.g.*, requires psychotherapy or hospitalization
Grade 4 = despite medication and/or other intervention, disturbance is severe enough to preclude day-to-day functioning

14. Mentation (disturbances in memory, reasoning, calculation, judgment or orientation)
    Grade 0 = no observable problem
    Grade 1 = disturbance is present but does not interfere with performance of everyday activities
    Grade 2 = disturbance interferes with performance of everyday activities; the person may need to use lists or other prompting devices, but manages without the help of other people; the person is likely to be a poor historian
    Grade 3 = disturbance is severe enough to require prompting or assistance from others for performance of everyday activities
    Grade 4 = disturbance precludes the performance of most everyday activities; may include severe confusion, disorientation, or memory loss
15. Fatigability (a sense of overwhelming weakness or lassitude which dramatically alters baseline motor and coordination functions, and occasionally visual or sensory functions; it may be transient or persistent for hours or even days, and occurs at varying frequency; a very common complaint in MS)
    Grade 0 = no fatigability
    Grade 1 = fatigability present but does ot notably interfere with baseline physical function
    Grade 2 = fatigability causing intermittent and generally transient impairment of baseline physical function
    Grade 3 = fatigability causing intermittent transient loss or frequent moderate impairment of baseline physical function
    Grade 4 = fatigability which generally prevents prolonged or sustained physical function
16. Sexual function
    Grade 0 = sexually active as before and/or not experiencing some sexual problems; no changes in patient's usual pattern of sexual activity, for example, no changes in frequency and type of sex activities, and no changes in previous genital sensations, erections, and ejaculation in men, and vaginal lubrication and orgasm in women; this includes persons without previous sexual experience
    Grade 1 = sexually less active than before, and/or now experiencing some sexual problem(s) but *not* concerned; less frequent or less varied sexual activity, and/or some changes in previous genital sensations, erection, and ejaculation in men, and vaginal lubrication and orgasm in women but does not consider this an issue; may be using a prosthesis or sexual aids
    Grade 2 = sexually less active than before, and now experiencing some sexual problems *and* concerned; would like to regain former sexual activity pattern and/or would like to regain previous genital sensations, erection, ejaculations, and/or orgasmic experiences
    Grade 3 = sexually inactive but still concerned; sexual activity has ceased for several months, or years, but wishes to regain previous pattern and functional ability
    Grade 4 = sexually inactive and not concerned; sexual activity has ceased for several weeks, months, or years, but does not consider this an issue

Environmental Status Scale (ESS)
(WHO Handicap)

1. Actual work status (this question applies also to students and homemakers; it describes the overall situation and is not limited to MS-related problems)
    Grade 0 = normal or retired for age, *e.g.*, full-time worker, homemaker, or student
    Grade 1 = works essentially full-time but in less demanding position
    Grade 2 = works more than half-time at job, housework or school
    Grade 3 = works between one-quarter and one-half time at job, housework, or school
    Grade 4 = works less than one quarter time at job, housework, or school
    Grade 5 = unemployed, not able to do any housework or to attend school at all
2. Financial/economic status (MS related)
    Grade 0 = no MS-related financial problems
    Grade 1 = family maintains usual financial standard without external support despite some financial disadvantages resulting from MS

Grade 2 = family maintains usual financial standard with aid of some external financial support
Grade 3 = family maintains usual financial standard by receiving basic disability pension as defined in location of residence
Grade 4 = family maintains usual financial standard only because receiving all available financial assistance
Grade 5 = family is unable to maintain usual financial standard despite receipt of all available financial assistance

3. Personal residence/home (MS related)
Grade 0 = no change necessary
Grade 1 = minor modification necessary
Grade 2 = moderate modification necessary
Grade 3 = major structural alteration or addition necessary
Grade 4 = must move to satisfactory personal home
Grade 5 = must live in facility for dependent care because unable to continue in any personal home (institutionalized)

4. Personal assistance required (MS related)
Grade 0 = none
Grade 1 = minor help; relatives involved but personal independence is maintained
Grade 2 = requires assistance for activities of daily living up to one hour per day from relatives or others in the home
Grade 3 = requires assistance with activities of daily living up to three hours per day from relatives or others in the home
Grade 4 = requires more than three hours of personal assistance per day but is able to live at home and does not need a constant attendant
Grade 5 = requires a constant attendant or care in an institution, *i.e.*, cannot be left alone for more than short periods such as two to three hours

5. Transportation (refers to transportation problems which are attributable to MS and includes difficulties in both the availability and accessibility of transport; if the person with MS does not know how to drive, the questions on driving should be ignored)
Grade 0 = drives or uses public transportation with no problems
Grade 1 = uses all forms of transport available despite minor difficulties or drives with minor difficulty, *e.g.*, needs handicapped parking
Grade 2 = uses some public transport despite difficulties or needs hand controls to drive
Grade 3 = cannot use public transport but can use private transport, cannot drive but may be driven by others
Grade 4 = requires community (public or private agency) transport in a wheelchair
Grade 5 = requires ambulance

6. Community services (MS related; community services may include medical, social, household, personal assistance, or similar services whether administered at home or in an institution)
Grade 0 = none required
Grade 1 = requires service once per month or less frequently
Grade 2 = requires not more than one hour per week
Grade 3 = requires not more than average of one hour per day
Grade 4 = requires one to four hours per day
Grade 5 = requires more than four hours per day or institutionalized

7. Social activity
Grade 0 = socially active as before with no changes in the usual pattern of social activity, and no difficulty in maintaining this pattern
Grade 1 = maintains usual pattern of social activity despite some difficulties
Grade 2 = some restrictions on social activity such as change in type or frequency of some activities or increased dependence on others
Grade 3 = significant restriction of social activity; largely dependent on actions of others but still able to initiate some activity
Grade 4 = socially inactive except for the initiative of others
Grade 5 = no social activity; does not see friends or family; social contact is limited to that provided by community service providers, *e.g.*, visiting nurse

The National Multiple Sclerosis Survey

Background and Economic Impact

FREDERIC D. WEINFELD AND HERBERT M. BAUM

Biometry and Field Studies Branch, IRP
National Institute of Neurological and Communicative Disorders and Stroke
Bethesda, Maryland 20205

Several years ago the National Institute of Neurological and Communicative Disorders and Stroke launched a program of national probability surveys to meet its need for accurate health statistics. The chief goal of the program was to obtain precise national estimates of the incidence, prevalence and economic costs of neurologic disorders. At the outset four disorders were selected: head and spinal cord injuries, stroke, intracranial neoplasms, and multiple sclerosis.

Prior to the current study no precise *national* figures were available on the incidence and prevalence of multiple sclerosis, or on the toll that the disease inflicts on patients and their families. This study was undertaken to reveal the magnitude of the problem and to establish baseline data for the United States.

Many in this audience are familiar with our findings on incidence and prevalence. They were published two years ago in the *Annals of Neurology*. In addition, findings with respect to mobility restriction will be published in the December issue of the *Archives of Physical Medicine and Rehabilitation.* Today we would like to focus attention on the economic impact of the disease. We will describe the data on cost and how they are gathered.

At the outset methodologies were developed to overcome two major problems: (1) how to identify cases efficiently, and (2) how to identify persons diagnosed but unaware of or unwilling to admit their diagnosis. To achieve this a two-stage sampling approach was adopted. In the first stage, a probability sample of physicians and hospitals was drawn and their MS patients were identified. Because of privacy considerations only the first name and last initial of the patient were reported, together with other nonspecific identifying information. No patient was contacted during this stage. All practicing neurologists, neurosurgeons, and hospitals with approved neurological residency programs were included. In addition, a probability sample of other physicians and hospitals was drawn.

The physicians and hospitals were asked to provide us with selected information on each of their MS patients seen between 1 January 1970 and 31 December 1975. Because there was high probability that patients had seen more than one medical provider during the period, duplicate cases were eliminated using the information provided by the physician or hospital.

In the second stage, a probability sample of patients was drawn from the list of all unduplicated patients. Physicians and hospitals were asked to provide the full names and addresses for these individuals. The patients later signed a release form giving permission for the use of their interview data. These patients became the study population. The data provided by the patient has given us additional information on the progression of the disease, and the medical, social and psychological environment.

The survey effort was initiated in early 1976 and data collection efforts were concluded by May 1979. Approximately 8,000 physicians and 790 hospitals were surveyed; over 43,000 unduplicated patients were identified, and 1,200 patients were interviewed.

Patients were given two interviews, approximately 90 days apart. The first, a face-to-face encounter, lasted over an hour and provided baseline disease and economic data. The second interview was conducted by telephone and provided information on changes during the three-month period. During the interval between the interviews, cost diaries were used to gather data on current expenses. It was assumed that gathering these data prospectively would minimize any recall problems. The 1,055 patients alive at the initial interview were requested to complete 90 daily cost diaries. Each patient was provided with 6 books of 15 daily diaries. They were instructed to fill out one diary per day and then to mail in the completed book. The purpose of the diaries was to gather information on the services or products received, from whom they were received, the people or agencies that paid the bills, the total cost, and the household's share of the total.

It was not easy to obtain patient cooperation for this task. Overall response rates were about 70%, whether the patient was reported by a physician or hospital, or whether the patient "knew" he or she had MS. What did surprise us was that a patient who agreed to participate usually did so for the full 90-day period. An average of 5.3 books of diaries (out of a set of 6) were completed by those who agreed to cooperate. This high completion rate was in part due to the continual telephone contacts which were conducted.

The "economic impact" of MS obviously includes physician costs, lost wages, hospital expenses, *etc.* Ideally we would have liked to include estimates of lost professional opportunity, loss of social contact, *etc.* It is, however, impossible to attach a dollar value to these latter items. Of particular importance for the study of economic impact are the data on employment history, medical insurance, patient income, income of spouse, sources of income and progression of disease.

The magnitude of the gross economic costs (direct and indirect) was impressive: $6,527 per patient per year in 1976. Let us put this estimate into perspective by comparing MS to stroke, a disease about 14 times more prevalent than MS. The cost of stroke per patient was only $4,322. Therefore, on a per patient per year basis, the cost of MS was 50% greater than that for stroke. Yet this is only a small measure of the impact of MS because the disease affects people early in their lives and persists for a great many years, whereas stroke mostly occurs among the aging population.

Assuming the average patient contracts MS at age 30, then the expected lifetime cost, in 1981 dollars, is $584,000 for men and $256,000 for women. A 30-year-old male with four years of college, working full-time year round, could expect to earn in his lifetime $1,228,000, according to the data published by the United States Bureau of the Census. A female under the same constraints would earn $694,000. So, MS costs a person nearly 40% of his or her lifetime earnings.

These results raise some important health policy issues. Economic impact is a major dimension in the health policy decision-making process; however the process requires similar data for the other disorders.

GENERAL DISCUSSION

R. J. SLATER (*National Multiple Sclerosis Society, New York, NY*): I have one comment to make. It's interesting if one looks at the 1964 conference held by the Academy on multiple sclerosis in relationship to the 1983 conference. At that time most of the work was given over to research and advances in research because there was so little basic knowledge that there was hardly any way to approach therapy.

Interestingly, at this time 20 years later, a great deal of effort has been allocated to therapeutic modalities. Difficult though they are to interpret we're moving in that direction. I believe the other main point is that because we haven't come up with the pathogenesis or a clear way to treat, we're increasingly having to face the problem of long-term chronic illness mangement, and it's to that point that I simply wanted to address the comment to the last speakers.

In the MS Society we have become increasingly interested in working with our chapters from the base of information that they were able to aggregate through the NINCDS study. You have provided a marvelous understanding of about how much it costs and the breakdown in those costs and we feel now that with the work that Dr. Kurtzke and the International Federation and Dr. Granger and others have done to put together the rating system, we'll be able to develop profiles of how people spend their lives and what their problems are and build on what you've been able to put together as a baseline in order to be able to provide guidance to health care policy makers, the politicians and the like, as to how to implement more effectively health and social programs. So we anticipate moving in the direction of working with the health care planners, the health care economists and so on in the years ahead while we still battle ahead on the whole matter of fundamental pathogenesis that will lead us to some type of maintenance or a cure.

The Future of Funding for MS Research

THOR HANSON

President and Chief Executive Officer
National Multiple Sclerosis Society
New York, New York 10017

I am pleased to be a part of this first conference in 20 years solely about MS. I am also pleased that our society is one of the sponsors.

I want to thank the New York Academy of Sciences for hosting this very fine session. It has brought together concerned people from all over the world.

I have just completed my first year at the Society. It has been an exhilarating one for me, a year of learning—a year of instigating some change in the Society. I would like to talk to you about both of those points.

As to learning—certainly as to research—I have learned that we don't talk about breakthroughs; we don't talk about being that close to finding a cause and cure. As Dr. Cedric Raine put it at lunch today, there aren't any headlines coming out of this conference.

On the other hand, it seems evident that we—and I mean by "we" those of us who have come here for this conference and the members of the Society—know much more than was known 36 years ago at that first medical advisory board meeting that Sylvia Lawry talked about. We now know a lot more about the disease. We understand it better, which of course is obviously terribly important if we're ever going to figure out how to cure it. We certainly know more about how to help improve the lifestyles of the people who have MS, although it's been very evident at this conference that we have much more to learn. The Society has to put a lot more emphasis on that as we look into the future. I'm sure we also know much more about how to conduct a clinical trial.

Certainly the targets have been narrowed in the research field over the past 10 years. The kind of thing that excites me, as a layman, after my first year of meetings with our research advisory committees and after coming to a conference such as this, is the possibility of the convergence of two or three different techniques. For example, if we could combine true early diagnosis—NMR, CAT and PET scans—with a genetic typing that indicated the chronic progressive form of MS and then be able to treat with a nontoxic immunosuppressive drug and arrest the disease before it really begins, that, to me, would be really exciting. We certainly aren't there yet but the possibilities seem achievable if not imminent.

So we have come a long way. I emphasize again that I have been using "we" to refer to the sorts of people who have been here. But in the first year, as I have traveled around the country and visited 26 of our chapters, I have learned another thing. The "we" of the general public has learned very little about MS. There is a very fuzzy image of multiple sclerosis among most people and certainly among many doctors—a great deal of confusion. Basically it is a lack of awareness. And, if you have a lack of awareness, you have a problem in raising money and in funding research and community services.

That really brings me to what I want to talk about in the few minutes left to me. I was billed to talk about the future of MS research, but in this group of scientists I feel more comfortable addressing the future of funding for MS research. I want to relate it to the lack of awareness I mentioned earlier.

First, in considering federal funding for all medical research, it is true that this has doubled since 1970. On the other hand, in constant dollars it's the same in 1984 as it was in 1974! It hasn't increased a whit in 10 years if you adjust for inflation. Inflation has really been hurting medical research these past years.

Another interesting trend in Washington: in the past three years, Administration requests for medical research funding—with inflation factored out—have actually decreased. The key to funding increases is now the Congress. It is the Congress that ensured that the 1983 budget for medical research increased by $355 million during 1982. Similarly, Congress has forced another $450 million increase in 1984. Leverage now is with the Congress, and that is where we must and will put our emphasis.

Now to address the subject of the National Multiple Sclerosis Society. In this next year research funding is going to be fairly austere; let me explain why. Sylvia Lawry mentioned in her talk that the Society over the years has been generous in research funding; it has totalled $73.6 million as a matter of fact, as of this summer. In 1983 we funded $5.6 million of grants and fellowships. On the other hand, in the past 10 years, the rate of increase of funding for research has gone up 1½ times as fast as the rate of increase in income. The Society has been living beyond its means. A result is that in the last five years Society reserves fell from $6 million to $3.5 million. When you consider our annual funding of $5.5–6 million for research, you realize the problem. The Board of Directors and I thus decided to hold our reserves at a minimum of $3.5 million. We don't intend to preside over the demise of the Society.

There are two ways to do that: one is to cut costs, the other to raise income. In the short term we are cutting costs and putting together the organization and ideas needed to increase income. We are budgeting only $5.3 million for research in 1984—a $300,000 cut in funding from 1983 levels. I have also cut $450,000 from our 1983 operating budget. In 1984, we will run the Society with 15% less staff and three fewer regional offices. I'm not implying a cut in effectiveness, but rather the reverse: I've always believed that fewer people—good ones—can do more in less time. I want a lean and efficient organization and we are on that track.

That is the short term; it is austere for the next year. I am, however, optimistic for the longer term and have set a goal to double our income by 1990. We are going to be at the $60–70 million income level without inflation factored in. Hopefully, we will thus be able to fund every approved research grant application. That is the goal.

Is it realistic? Am I aiming for something we can't achieve? I think it is practical because we are doing things to make it happen. I've set up a national development department—a full-time professional team with nothing to do but research development funding—with annual drives in four cities. The San Diego and Houston campaigns are well under way for 1984; we'll have four new cities each year and expect to raise $12 million extra in income for research only over the next five years.

We're also concentrating on raising awareness, that is so key. For instance, to do good direct mail fund raising, there must be awareness. In England direct mail works beautifully. But the Multiple Sclerosis Society there is the third best known health agency in the country—right after heart and cancer. We've got to get up into that bracket, so we can do direct mail nationally, not just locally. We have tended to specialize in special-event fund raising and we have to broaden our approach.

As one new effort, we had a training program in October for 80 of our chapters to introduce a new, imaginative way of using television—not a telethon, but the use of many 30-, 60- and 90-second spots in a one-week period. We call this "Moments for MS." We have put together all the material for this campaign and are hoping to have it in place and on the air in early 1984. It is a program for awareness and for fund raising and it will be the beginning of good direct mail lists.

This is only one of several new initiatives to raise awareness. If the American people really understand this disease, Society fund raising will increase, as will pressure on the Congress for more government funding for medical research in general, for MS in particular. I am optimistic for the future—for the rest of this decade. I'm excited about it, and I want you to know that although the short term is austere, I'm working in every way I know to raise monies to fund all grant applications that can pass the muster and to improve and standardize services in our chapters to help those with multiple sclerosis.

Multiple Sclerosis and Epstein-Barr Virus

Guilt by Association?

HELEN B. WARNER

New York State Institute for Basic Research in Developmental Disabilities Staten Island, New York 10314

Multiple sclerosis (MS) is characterized by remissions and exacerbations; latency and reactivation are typical of the herpes viruses. Epstein-Barr virus (EBV) is a herpes virus. Immune suppression, allogenic stimulation, stress, UV light, *etc.*, which produce exacerbations in MS also reactivate latent herpes. Multiple sclerosis is a late onset disease in affluent societies, as is infectious mononucleosis, a disease caused by EBV. Multiple sclerosis and infectious mononucleosis both affect principally populations of northern European origin. In underdeveloped countries, 99.9% of the population develops a natural immunity to EBV before the age of three years. If EBV were responsible for MS, early immunity to this agent could protect persons who migrated from a low to a high MS risk area before the age of 15.

Central nervous system plaques in MS are heavily populated with plasma cells (activated B lymphocytes). B lymphocytes are almost exclusively the only cells known to harbor a latent EBV infection.

In vivo, B lymphocytes carrying the EBV genome are normally detected and destroyed by cytotoxic T lymphocytes, keeping EBV latency within limits. Cytotoxic T cell activity is depressed during active MS. Regression assays show specifically reduced suppression of EBV-induced transformation in MS. Failure of cytotoxic T cells to destroy EB virus-infected cells during active MS could directly expose oligodendrocytes to an expanded population of EBV-infected cells.

REFERENCES

1. EPSTEIN, M. A. & A. J. MORGAN. 1983. Clinical consequences of Epstein-Barr virus infection and possible control by an anti-viral vaccine. Clin. Exp. Immunol. **53:** 257–271.
2. CRAIG, J. C., M. HAIRE *et al.* 1983. Immunological control of Epstein-Barr virus-transformed lymphocytes in multiple sclerosis. Clin. Immunol. Immunopathol. **29:** 86–93.

Fcγ Receptors in Multiple Sclerosis Brains

HARALD NYLAND,[a,b] SVERRE MØRK,[c]
AND ROALD MATRE[a]

[a]*Broegelmann Research Laboratory for Microbiology*
[b]*Department of Neurology*
[c]*Department of Pathology*
University of Bergen
Bergen, Norway

Receptors for the Fc part of immunoglobulin G (FcγR) are present on a variety of cell types belonging to the lymphoreticular system, *e.g.*, macrophages and monocytes, granulocytes, B lymphocytes, and a subpopulation of T lymphocytes (Tγ cells). In addition, the receptors have been demonstrated on other cell types, *e.g.*, trophoblasts and endothelial cells of fetal stem vessels of the placenta, and on cells infected *in vitro* with different types of viruses. In the normal human central nervous system FcγR are detected on cells in the leptomeninges, the arachnoid granulations, on pericytes and adventitial cells in the perivascular spaces, and on stromal cells and epithelial cells in the choroid plexus. Cultured microglial cells and endothelial cells from cerebral vessels also express FcγR.

We have studied FcγR *in situ* in multiple sclerosis (MS) brains using cryostat sections. Tissue from eight MS brains containing both active demyelinating lesions and chronic burned-out lesions as well as samples of five normal brains were snap frozen in liquid nitrogen and sectioned on a cryostat. The FcγR were demonstrated by three different techniques: hemadsorption of indicator cells prepared by sensitizing sheep erythrocytes with rabbit IgG antibodies (EA), binding of soluble immune complexes of horseradish peroxidase (HRP) and rabbit IgG anti-HRP, and by monoclonal antibody to human placental FcγR using an indirect immunofluorescence technique.

In line with previous data, FcγR were demonstrated on cells in perivascular spaces in sections of normal brain, whereas the white or gray matter did not express FcγR. Similar FcγR activity was demonstrated in the perivascular spaces in sections from chronic MS lesions. No FcγR were found in the neural parenchyma of the burned-out lesions. In contrast, strong FcγR activity was found throughout the active demyelinating lesions. We used soluble immune complexes of HRP and rabbit IgG anti-HRP and the monoclonal antibody to human placental Fcγ to localize FcγR to cells with a morphology of lipid macrophages (FIG. 1). In addition, a small number of the cells in the perivascular cell infiltrates and some lymphocyte-like cells in the parenchyma also expressed FcγR (FIG. 2), while the oligodendrocytes apparently did not stain. Compared with sections of normal brain, an increased FcγR activity was observed in the perivascular spaces outside the active MS lesions. The monoclonal antibody also stained the endothelium in both normal and MS brains (FIG. 3).

The FcγR may be involved in the immunopathogenesis of active MS lesions in several ways: by immunophagocytosis of myelin, in antibody-dependent cytotoxicity and by binding immune complexes. The FcγR on endothelial cells indicate that these cells may participate in the local inflammatory responses.

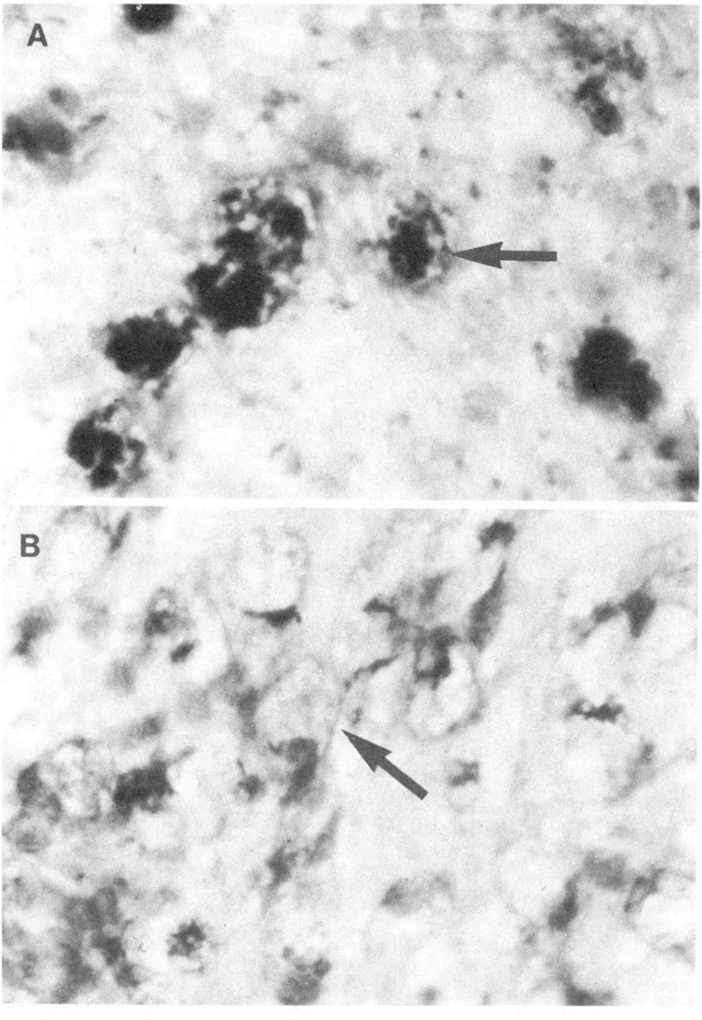

FIGURE 1. Section of an active MS lesion. (**A**) Macrophages stained with nonspecific esterase. (**B**) FcγR (*arrows*) identified by HRP rabbit IgG anti-HRP immune complexes.

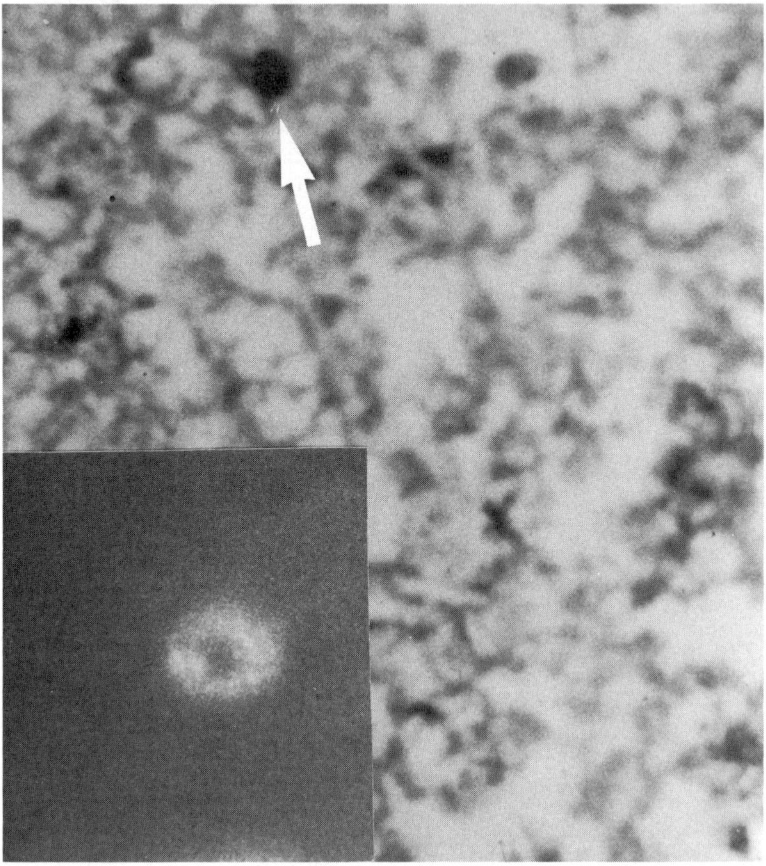

FIGURE 2. T lymphocyte within the neural parenchyma demonstrated by $F(ab')_2$ preparation of rabbit anti-T lymphocyte serum using immunoperoxidase technique (*arrow*). *Insert:* Indirect immunofluorescence test with a mouse monoclonal antibody to human FcγR staining a lymphocyte-like cell within the tissue.

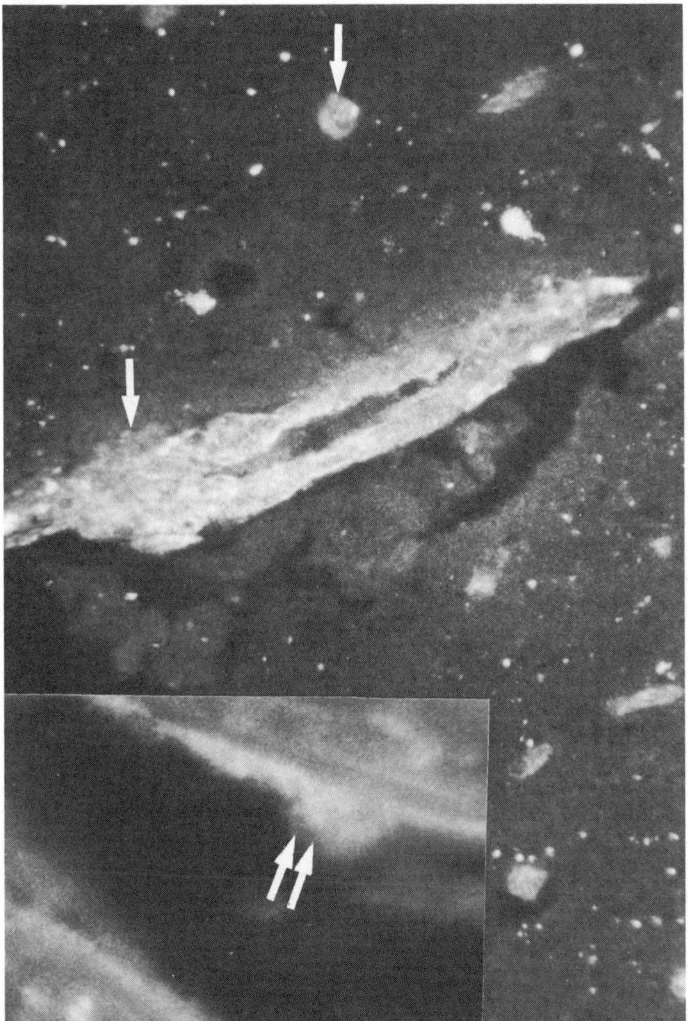

FIGURE 3. Staining of perivascular spaces in unaffected areas of MS brain by a monoclonal antibody to human FcγR (*single arrow*). *Insert:* Staining of the endothelium of a cerebral venule in an MS brain (*double arrow*).

Long-Term Culture of Bulk Isolated Adult Human Oligodendrocytes[a]

SEUNG U. KIM, GIUSEPPE MORETTO, DOO H. SHIN, AND DONALD W. PATY

Division of Neurology
Health Sciences Centre Hospital
University of British Columbia
Vancouver, British Columbia, Canada V6T 1W5

Oligodendrocytes, the cells responsible for the formation and maintenance of the myelin in the central nervous system, are the possible primary target in human demyelinating diseases, including multiple sclerosis. In order to understand the pathogenesis of these diseases, investigation of human oligodendrocytes in isolation is desirable.

We have devised a method by which viable oligodendrocytes were isolated from human brains obtained 3–15 hours postmortem and cultured for a period of up to six months.[1] Oligodendrocytes were prepared from corpus callosum by trypsinization, screening and Percoll density gradient centrifugation. Cells harvested were grown on polylysine- or collagen-coated coverslips. Cell yield was $0.3–1 \times 10^6$ cells/g tissue.

Twenty-four hours after the plating, a large number of small round cells (6–8 μm in diameter) were found to attach to coverslips. Many others formed small aggregates of 10–100 cells, and were released into the medium. These aggregates were collected and seeded again on new coverslips. This procedure, differential adhesion process, was repeated again 24 hours later. After two cycles of differential adhesion process, one could obtain an almost pure population of oligodendrocytes.

By immunofluorescence microscopy, 95–98% of cells were identified as oligodendrocytes by positive reactions to rabbit anti-galactocerebroside antibody 4–7 days after the isolation. These oligodendrocytes also expressed surface or cytoplasmic antigens of myelin basic protein (FIG. 1), 2′,3′-cyclic nucleotide 3′-phosphodiesterase and GM4 ganglioside. These antigens are considered as myelin- and oligodendrocyte-specific markers.[2–4]

Electron microscopic examination revealed that these cultured oligodendrocytes possessed fine structural features of mature oligodendrocytes found *in vivo*. All of the organelles were well preserved; the nucleus contained dense chromatin granules which were at the nuclear envelope, and the electron-dense cytoplasm had large numbers of mitochondria and microtubules.

Recently we have developed serum-free chemically defined media (DM2 and DM3) for the long-term maintenance of human oligodendrocytes in culture. The media are composed of F12 synthetic medium supplemented by hormones, growth factors and trace metals. The oligodendrocytes grown in these media expressed cell-type specific markers, galactocerebroside and myelin basic protein.[5]

We have also studied the possible presence of shared antigen determinants between human oligodendrocytes and lymphocytes. Our results showed that cultured oligoden-

[a]This work was supported by grant no. MA–7700 from the Medical Research Council of Canada.

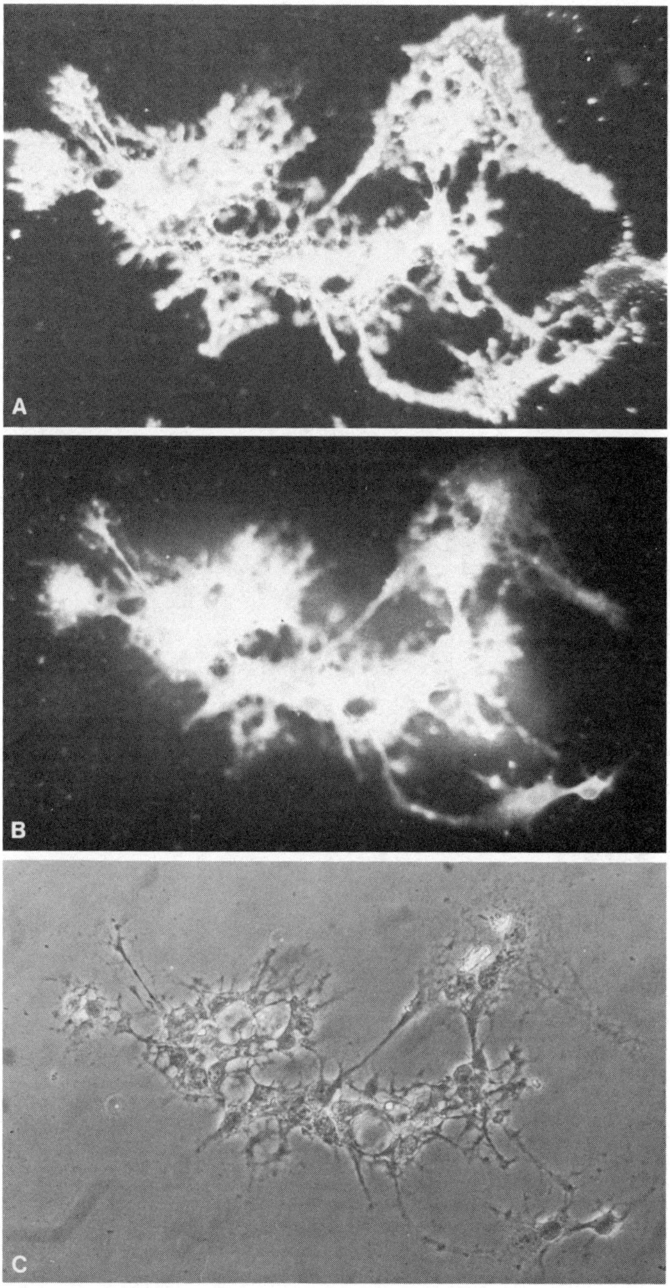

FIGURE 1. Double labeling of cultured human oligodendrocytes by rabbit anti-galactocerebroside serum and anti-myelin basic protein monoclonal antibody. Oligodendrocytes were isolated from 39-year-old female six hours postmortem and were cultured for 65 days. Magnification: ×350; original ×500. (**A**) Galactocerebroside-rhodamine immunofluorescence. (**B**) Myelin basic protein-FITC immunofluorescence. (**C**) Phase contrast microscopy.

drocytes reacted to monoclonal antibodies that recognize human natural killer T cells (Leu 7) and Ia antigen (HLA-DR). No other monoclonal antibodies directed toward subclasses of human lymphocytes stained human oligodendrocytes grown in culture. These included OKT3 and Leu 1 (pan T cell), OKT4 and Leu 3 (helper T cell), OKT6 (thymocyte), OKT8 and Leu 2 (suppressor T cell), and OKM2 (monocyte). The sharing of selected antigens by oligodendrocytes and peripheral lymphocytes suggests that common factors might influence the number and function of these cell types.

REFERENCES

1. KIM, S. U., Y. SATO, D. SILBERBERG, D. PLEASURE & L. RORKE. 1983. Long-term culture of human oligodendrocytes: Isolation, growth and identification. J. Neurol. Sci. **62:** 295–301.
2. RAFF, M., K. FIELDS, S. HAKOMORI, R. MIRSKY, R. PRUSS & J. WINTER. 1979. Cell-type specific markers for distinguishing and studying neurons and major classes of glial cells in culture. Brain Res. **174:** 283–308.
3. SIMS, N. & P. CARNEGIE. 1978. 2′,3′-cyclic nucleotide 3′-phosphodiesterase. *In* Advances in Neurochemistry. B. Agranoff & M. Aprison, Eds.: 1–41. Plenum. New York.
4. YU, R. & K. IQBAL. 1979. Sialosylgalactosyl ceramide as a specific marker for human myelin and oligodendroglial perikarya. J. Neurochem. **32:** 293–300.
5. KIM, S. U., D. H. SHIN & D. PATY. 1984. Long term culture of human oligodendrocytes in serum-free defined medium. *In* Experimental Allergic Encephalitis: A Useful Model for Multiple Sclerosis. E. Alvord, M. Kies & A. Suckling, Eds.: 207–214. Alan R. Liss. New York.

Early Experience in Nuclear Magnetic Resonance Imaging of Multiple Sclerosis

D. LI, J. MAYO, S. FACHE, W. D. ROBERTSON,
D. PATY,[a] AND M. GENTON

Department of Radiology
[a]Department of Medicine
UBC Imaging Research Centre
Faculty of Medicine
University of British Columbia
Vancouver, British Columbia, Canada V6T 2B5

INTRODUCTION

Preliminary studies[1-3] suggest that magnetic resonance imaging (MRI) demonstrates abnormalities in patients with multiple sclerosis in a noninvasive manner on a scale not previously seen except at autopsy. At the UBC Imaging Research Centre, MRI is being used to investigate the appearance, evolution, magnitude and character of the lesions of multiple sclerosis in the central nervous system.

METHODS

Twenty-nine patients with "clinically definite" or "probable" multiple sclerosis have had a total of 37 MRI studies of the brain, using a Picker International Cryogenic 2000 MR Scanner based on a 0.15 Tesla superconducting magnetic. Fifteen studies were complete examinations from the posterior fossa to the supraventricular area with contiguous 10 mm sections. The other 22 studies consisted of noncontiguous sample slices through the cerebellum, pons and midbrain, ventricular and supraventricular levels. Images were obtained with both inversion recovery and spin-echo sequences. Coronal and sagittal images were also obtained in selected cases. In seven patients, CT examinations were performed within the same week, consisting of both noncontrast and double-dose delayed examinations with either a Siemens Somatom DR2 or G.E. CT8800 whole-body scanner.

RESULTS

CT versus *MRI*. The superior sensitivity of MRI compared to CT was confirmed in this small series. In 3 of 7 studies, CT scans were negative whereas MRI studies were positive. In those with positive CT scans, many more lesions were noted on the corresponding MRI examination. (FIG. 1)

Optimizing Pulse Sequences. Although the inversion recovery sequences (IR) gave better anatomical display and gray-white matter differentiation, the spin-echo (SE) sequences showed many more lesions, especially those situated more peripherally at

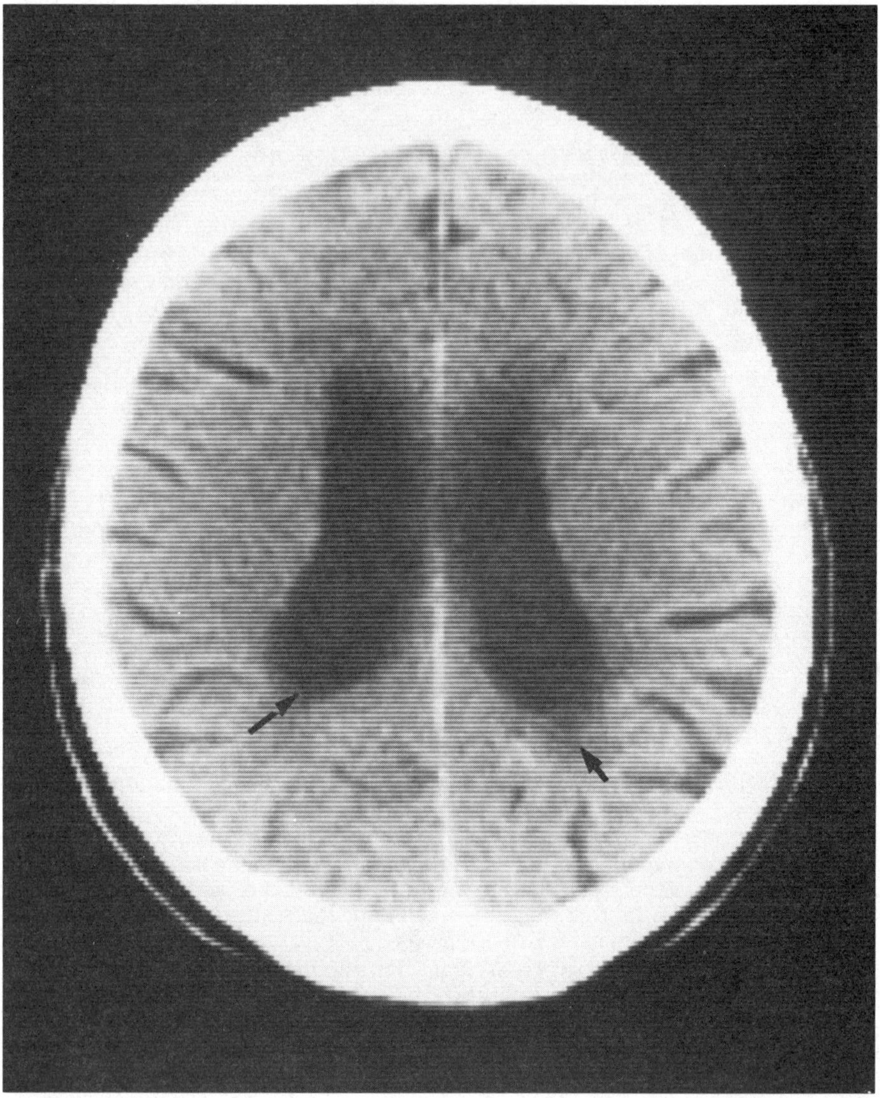

FIGURE 1A. Low-density changes are seen posterior to the ventricles on the double-dose delay CT scan.

the gray-white matter junction. Only on two occasions were abnormalities noted on the IR sequence and not seen on the SE examination.

Serial Studies. Three patients have had follow-up studies. In one patient, monthly follow-up scans revealed an increase in size and number of lesions during the time when the patient was asymptomatic. In two other patients, follow-up studies, after an acute relapse, showed a decrease in size of the lesions.

FUTURE PLANS

A computer program is under development that will allow precise quantitation of the volume of MS lesions detected. A patient-positioning device to allow for accurate repositioning of patients on serial studies is being developed. Clinical pathological correlation of brain specimens of patients who have died from MS is also underway. Basic questions that are being asked include: (1) Can MRI be helpful in the diagnosis of MS? (2) What is the nature of the MRI-detected lesion in MS? (3) Does the accumulation of MRI lesions indicate progression of MS as measured clinically? (4) Can MRI be used as a quantitative measure of the pathological process in the assessment of clinical trials, including therapy?

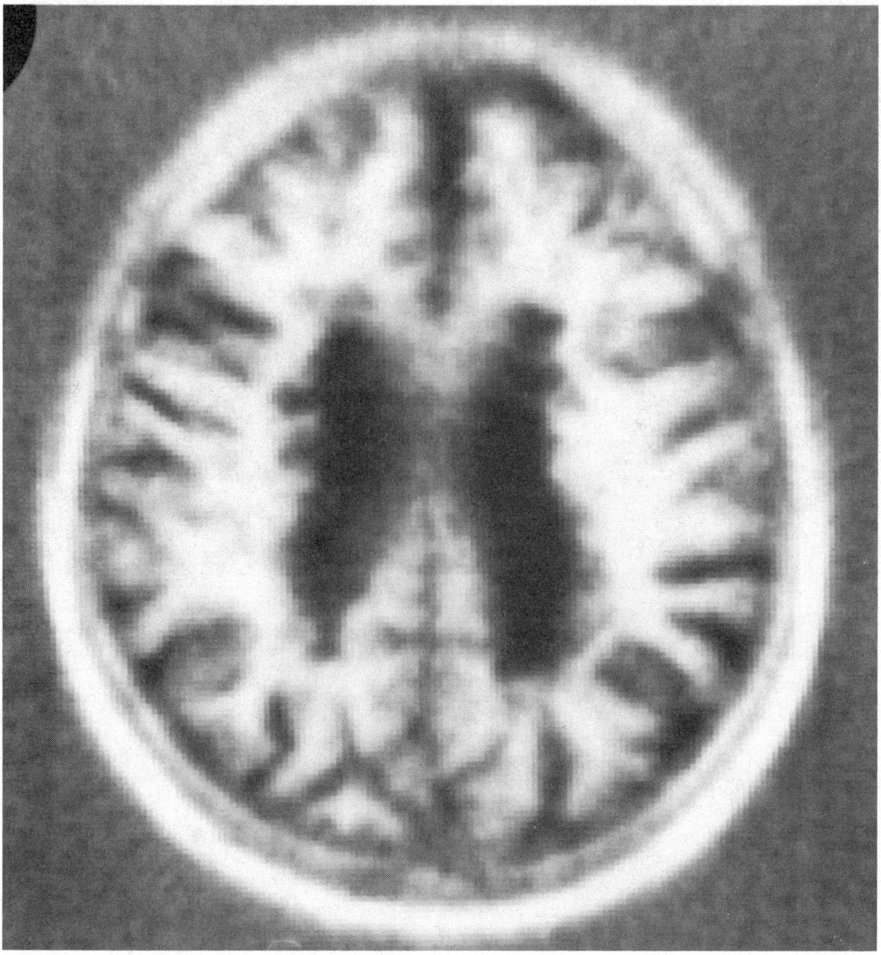

FIGURE 1B. Many more lesions (compare FIGURE 1A) along the entire margin of the ventricles on the IR 1400/400 MRI scan.

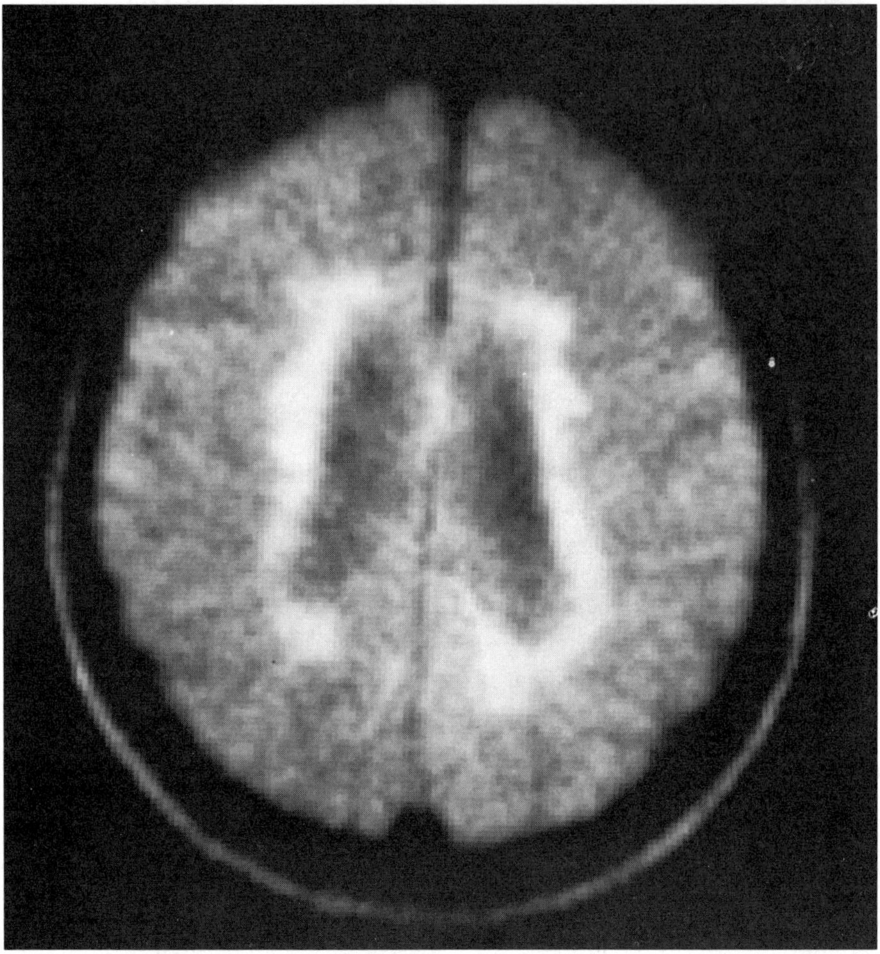

FIGURE 1C. SE 1080/80 MRI scan. Same results as in FIGURE 1B.

REFERENCES

1. YOUNG, I. R., A. S. HALL, E. A. PALLIS, M. J. LEGG, G. M. BYDDER & R. E. STEINER. 1981. Nuclear magnetic resonance imaging of the brain in multiple sclerosis. Lancet **ii:** 1063–1066.
2. BRANT-ZAWADSKI, M., P. L. DAVIS, P. E. CROOKS, C. M. MILLS, D. NORMAN, T. H. NEWTON, P. SHELDON & L. KAUFMAN. 1983. NMR demonstration of cerebral abnormalities. Comparison with CT. A.J.R. **140:** 847–854.
3. YOUNG, I. R., C. P. RANDALL, P. W. KAPLAN, A. JAMES, G. M. BYDDER & R. E. STEINER. 1983. NMR imaging in white matter disease of the brain using spin-echo sequences. J.C.A.T. **7:** 290–294.

Electrophysiological Confirmation of Orientation-specific Contrast Losses in Multiple Sclerosis[a]

MARK J. KUPERSMITH,[b] JEREMIAH I. NELSON, WILLIAM H. SEIPLE, AND RONALD E. CARR

Department of Ophthalmology
[b]Department of Neurology
New York University Medical Center
New York, New York 10016

INTRODUCTION

Visual evoked potentials are often abnormal in patients with multiple sclerosis. Prolongation of the latency of the first major positive wave of the transient visual evoked potential (VEP) reflects the typical conduction defects in the retinocortical pathway in patients without obvious clinical complaints. However, the transient VEP may be delayed less frequently in those patients without retrobulbar neuritis or normal visual system, found with careful neuro-ophthalmic exam. In addition, there is only fair correlation of VEP defects with the typical visual complaints in patients with 20/20 Snellen acuity even when performed with a low-contrast visual pattern.[1]

In contrast to VEP testing, subjective tests of color or contrast are often abnormal in MS patients. These defects in visual performance usually reflect the subjective complaints, so frequently described by patients, of color desaturation or feeling as if the world always appears cloudy.[2] In a clinical setting psychophysical testing of contrast thresholds can be variable and is dependent on the subject's comprehension and cooperation in giving reliable responses. The clinician needs an objective measure of visual performance. The VEP is capable of objectively evaluating the visual system but the typical computer-averaged VEP studies are too slow, they fatigue patients, and are too marred by adaptation[3] to obtain accurate contrast thresholds in a clinical setting. Additionally, the test stimuli (such as checkerboard) used to elicit the pattern VEP are too complex[4] to reflect the functioning of select groups of cortical neurons that may respond to pattern stimuli of a specific spatial frequency or orientation. Bodis-Wollner[5] has advocated the use of reversing sinusoidal bar gratings as a simple stimulus for VEP studies similar to those used to determine contrast sensitivity psychophysically. Camisa[6] has further applied these gratings to demonstrate prolongation in latency which is selective for specific orientations of the bar stimulus. However, a delay in latency of the VEP cannot be related to a visual performance deficit.

Real time retrieval of visual responses to continuously changing, or "swept" stimuli (*e.g.*, contrast levels increasing with time) can give visual performance data. Such methods have been pioneered in the study of evoked potential responses to spatial frequency[7,8] and color[9] and extended by us to swept contrast.[10] We have recently

[a]This work was supported by NEI grant no. 1 P50 EY 02179, a contract from the Naval Air Systems Command, and an unrestricted departmental award from Research to Prevent Blindness, Inc.

reported finding an oblique effect in contrast and acuity threshold using these methods.[11] In this study, we have applied the technique to the study of contrast sensitivity to study objectively whether orientation-selective losses previously reported only with psychophysical methods[12] indeed occur in patients with MS.

RESULTS

Twenty-six patients with probable or definite MS (according to McAlpine's criteria) had evoked potential contrast sensitivity determinations for three spatial frequencies (1, 4, 8 cycles/deg) and four orientations (0, 45, 90, and 135 deg) of sine wave gratings. Contrast threshold deficits (above the 99% confidence interval calculated for controls) were observed for at least one combination of spatial frequency and orientation in all cases. Both eyes were affected in 25 cases. The losses were spotty with respect to stimulus orientation, spatial frequency and viewing eye (FIG. 1). The deficits were the same among 10 patients with or 16 without retrobulbar neuritis except in 4 cases with acuity worse than 20/70 where contrast thresholds were elevated beyond the

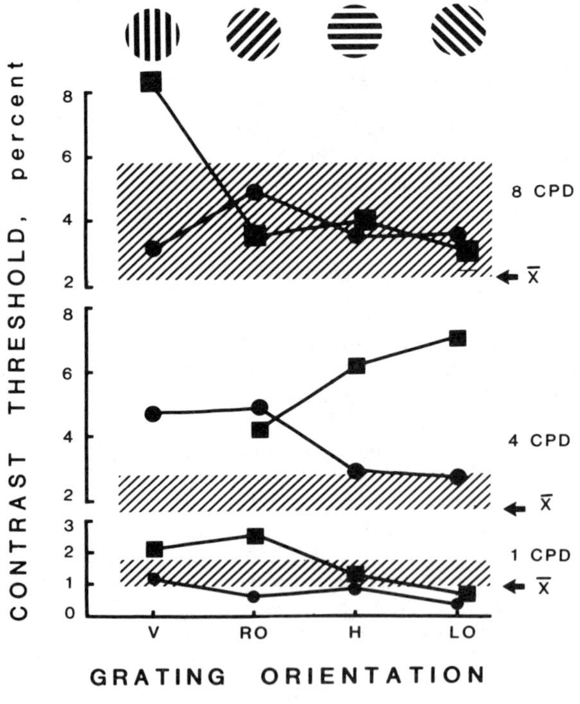

FIGURE 1. Actual contrast thresholds for orientations (*V* = vertical, *RO* = right oblique, *H* = horizontal, *LO* = left oblique) and three spatial frequencies (1, 4 and 8 cycles/deg) for right eye (*circles*) and left eye (*squares*). Cross-hatched region extends from the mean contrast to the 99% confidence limit for controls. Losses are variable with regard to both eye and orientation or spatial frequency changes.

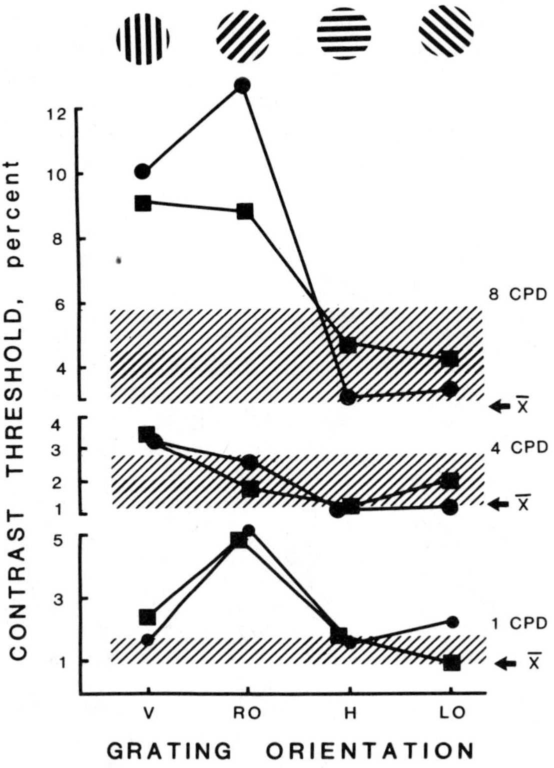

FIGURE 2. Contrast thresholds for a second case, key same as in FIGURE 1. Losses are similar in the two eyes and are selective for orientation but not spatial frequency.

20% contrast tested. Multiple orientations were affected in 24 cases. Orientation-specific losses which were the same in both eyes were found in 18 cases (FIG. 2). Discrete spatial frequency losses were present in only 5 cases and were not selective for orientation in only one case. Contrast abnormalities at 1 cycle/deg occurred twice as frequently as those at 4 or 8 cycles/deg.

In comparison the averaged pattern-evoked potentials (using a reversing checkerboard stimulus[1]) were abnormally prolonged in 14/26 cases. Only 6/16 patients without retrobulbar neuritis had delayed VEP. On clinical exam 16 had 20/20 acuity, 9 dyschromatopsia, 14 abnormal funduscopy of the optic disc or nerve fiber layer, 10 different pupillary defects, and 16 abnormal psychophysical Arden contrast thresholds.

DISCUSSION

Contrast threshold elevations selective for a combination of orientation and spatial frequency were demonstrated by VEP in all patients with multiple sclerosis. These occurred even in those subjects without a history of retrobulbar neuritis or clinical evidence of optic nerve dysfunction. The averaged VEP was less sensitive in identifying visual pathway defects, particularly in those cases without clinical optic neuropathy. The importance of measuring contrast sensitivity by psychophysical methods in this group of MS patients has been previously reported,[1] but now this can be objectively performed.

Orientation-specific losses of contrast sensitivity were as often uniocular as binocular. Discrete spatial frequency losses were rare. These results are similar to and extend those which we described in a previous preliminary report.[13] These findings provide an objective electrophysiological confirmation of psychophysically determined orientation-specific contrast threshold elevations reported by Regan.[12]

In comparison, patients with macula retina lesions or optic neuropathy not secondary to demyelinating disease have contrast threshold elevations which are not orientation-specific. Additionally, three other patients, referred with a wrong diagnosis of MS, had no contrast sensitivity abnormalities. Further evaluation uncovered a glioma of the spinal cord found at surgery, an intrinsic brainstem tumor diagnosed by computed tomography using intrathecal metrizamide and nuclear magnetic resonance scanning, and a hereditary familial spastic spinal paraparesis in each of the three, respectively. VER contrast losses which are not orientation-specific can help distinguish patients with other neurological diseases wrongly suspected of MS.

Orientation-selective contrast deficits in MS strongly suggest cortical involvement in these patients. True orientation tuning in the retino-cortical pathway is first found at the level of the visual cortex, beyond the neurons in layer IV.[14] Columnar organization of orientation-selective neurons in the cortex has been neurophysiologically[15] and anatomically[16,17] demonstrated by Hubel and Wiesel. Additionally, intralaminar cortical fibers, which are myelinated, have recently been revealed to extend up to 4 mm, giving rise to periodic clustered axonal arborizations thought to be related to the columnar architecture. The neurons from which these axons arise also have orientation specificity.[18] Previous electron microscopic study has demonstrated myelination of many axons throughout the neuropil in the cortex.[19]

Though cortical abnormalities are commonly thought to result from plaques at the border between white and gray matter, true lesions of the myelinated fibers in the gray matter alone have been described.[20] Demyelinating plaques which disrupt the myelinated intralaminar cortical axons could disrupt the functional architecture of the visual cortex. Thus, orientation-selective dysfunction could be found in otherwise random, nonselective patchy lesions in the visual cortex.

REFERENCES

1. KUPERSMITH, M. J., J. I. NELSON, W. H. SEIPLE, R. E. CARR & P. WEISS. 1983. The 20/20 eye in multiple sclerosis. Neurology **33:** 1015–1020.
2. REGAN, D., R. SILVER & T. MURRAY. 1977. Visual acuity and contrast sensitivity in multiple sclerosis: Hidden visual loss. Brain **100:** 563–579.
3. CAMPBELL, F. W. & J. J. KULIKOWSKI. 1971. An electrophysiological measure of the psychophysical contrast threshold. J. Physiol. **217:** 54P.
4. DEVALOIS, K. K., R. L. DEVALOIS & E. W. FUND. 1979. Responses of striate cortex cells to gratings and checkerboard patterns. J. Physiol. **291:** 483–505.
5. BODIS-WOLLNER, I., C. HENDLEY, L. H. MYLIN & J. THORNTON. 1978. Visual evoked potentials and the visuogram in multiple sclerosis. Ann. Neurol. **5:** 40–47.
6. CAMISA, J., L. H. MYLIN & I. BODIS-WOLLNER. 1981. The effect of stimulus orientation on the visual evoked potential in multiple sclerosis. Ann. Neurol. **10:** 532–539.

7. REGAN, D. 1973. Rapid objective refraction using evoked brain potentials. Invest. Ophthal. Vis. Sci. **12:** 669–679.
8. TYLER, C., P. APKARIAN, D. LEVI & K. NAKAYAMA. 1979. Rapid assessment of visual function: An electronic sweep technique for the pattern visual evoked potential. Invest. Ophthal. Vis. Sci. **18:** 703–713.
9. REGAN, D. 1975. Colour coding of pattern responses in man investigated by potential feedback and direct plot technique. Vis. Res. **15:** 175–183.
10. NELSON, J. I., W. H. SEIPLE, M. J. KUPERSMITH & R. E. CARR. 1984. Lock-in signal retrieval techniques for swept-parameter visual stimulation. J. Clin. Neurophys. In press.
11. NELSON, J. I., M. J. KUPERSMITH, W. H. SEIPLE, P. A. WEISS & R. E. CARR. 1984. Spatio temporal conditions which elicit or abolish the oblique effect in man: Direct measurement with swept evoked potential. Vision Res. **24:** 579–586.
12. REGAN, D., J. A. WHITLOCK, T. J. MURRAY & K. I. BEVERLEY. 1980. Orientation-specific losses of contrast sensitivity in multiple sclerosis. Invest. Ophthal. Vis. Sci. **19:** 324–328.
13. KUPERSMITH, M. J., W. H. SEIPLE, J. I. NELSON & R. E. CARR. 1984. Contrast spatial loss in multiple sclerosis: Selectivity by eye, orientation and spatial frequency measured with the evoked potential. Invest. Ophthal. Vis. Sci. **25:** 632–639.
14. HUBEL, D. H. & T. N. WIESEL. 1968. Receptive fields and functional architecture of monkey striate cortex. J. Physiol. **195:** 215–243.
15. HUBEL, D. H. & T. N. WIESEL. 1974. Sequence regularity and geometry of orientation columns in the monkey striate cortex. J. Comp. Neurol. **158:** 267–293.
16. HUBEL, D. H., T. N. WIESEL & M. P. STRYKER. 1977. Orientation columns in macaque monkey visual cortex demonstrated by the 2-deoxyglucose autoradiographic technique. Nature **269:** 328–330.
17. HUBEL, D. H., T. N. WIESEL & M. P. STRYKER. 1978. Anatomical demonstration of orientation columns in macaque monkey. J. Comp. Neurol. **177:** 361–380.
18. GILBERT, C. & T. N. WIESEL. 1983. Clustered intrinsic connections in cat visual cortex. J. Neuroscience **3:** 1116–1133.
19. PETERS, A., S. L. PALAY & H. DE F. WEBSTER. 1976. The Fine Structure of the Nervous System. The Neurons and Supporting Cells. Saunders. Philadelphia. pp. 308–315.
20. PETERS, G. 1958. Multiple sklerose. *In* Handbuch der Pathologische Anatomie und Histologie. Zweiter Teil. W. Schotz, Ed.: 525–602. Springer-Verlag. Berlin.

A Monoclonal Antibody for Astrocytes[a]

S. K. MALHOTRA,[b] F. WONG,[b] N. SINHA,[b]
V. MANICKEVAL,[c] T. K. SHNITKA,[c] AND K. G. WARREN[d]

[b]*Biological Sciences Electon Microscopy Laboratory*
and Department of Zoology
[c]*Department of Pathology*
[d]*Department of Medicine*
University of Alberta
Edmonton, Alberta, Canada T6G 2E9

We are involved in the production of monoclonal antibodies that could be utilized in the characterization of multiple sclerosis (MS) tissue. A crude membrane homogenate from the brain or spinal cord obtained at autopsy was used for the immunization of Balb C female mice. Serum obtained by tail-bleeding was tested for antibody production by using ELISA on the nervous tissue homogenate used for immunization. The spleen cells from the immunized mouse were fused with the myeloma NS1-SP2 cells by using 50% polyethylene glycol.[2] The hybridoma clones were selected by growing on HAT medium and tested for antibody secretion by using ELISA and immunofluorescence microscopy. Clones determined to be positive for antibody secretion were subcloned by growing in limiting dilutions. Ascites fluid produced by injecting these clones into pristane-treated mice was used for isotyping antibodies by radioimmune assay using rabbit anti-mouse subclass specific antibodies. One subclone, designated G.3.5, secretes IgM type antibodies that recognize astrocytes in the human brain and rat vermis. This clone was thought to bind to a certain type of nerve fibers, particularly parallel fibers in the rat vermis.[3] However, we have now employed two-fluoro-chrome immunofluorescence on the same cryostat sections of the human brain and rat vermis and compared the distribution of astrocytes (FIG. 1A) with the staining pattern revealed by G.3.5 (FIG. 1B) in these sections. In both cases (human brain and rat vermis), G.3.5 binds to the structures shown to be astrocytes as revealed by polyclonal antiserum for glial fibrillary acidic protein (GFAP). Glial fibrillary acidic protein is characteristic of astrocytes[1] and binds to the intracellular glial filaments in the astrocytes.[4] The specific nature of the astrocytic material that binds the G.3.5 antibody is being investigated. However, cryostat sections were incubated in G.3.5 ascites fluid (1:100 dilution) and goat anti-mouse IgM-FITC (1:100 dilution) before incubation in rabbit anti-human GFAP (1:1000 dilution) and goat anti-rabbit IgG-Rhodamine. As is apparent from FIGURES 1A and 1B, G.3.5 and GFAP reveal the same basic morphological structures. But it is unlikely that the GFAP antibody and G.3.5 clone recognize the same antigenic determinant(s), as prior incubation in anti-GFAP serum did not abolish subsequent immunofluorescence staining due to G.3.5.

[a]This work has been supported by grants awarded to SKM by the MS1 Foundation and NSERC. We are most grateful to Ms. H. Good who assisted in this work in the early stages. Dr. B. Singh has kindly performed radioimmune assay for isotyping monoclonal antibodies.

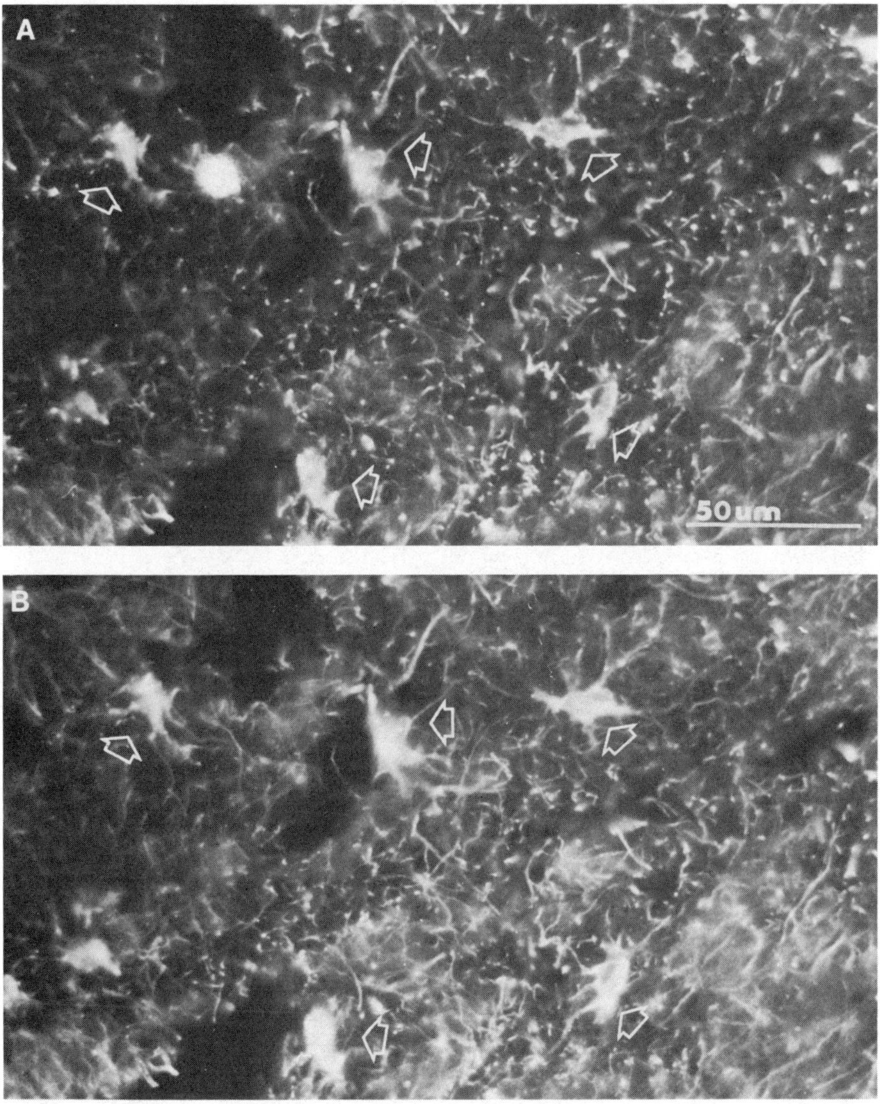

FIGURE 1. Cryostat section of MS brain incubated in the order goat serum (30%), G.3.5 ascites fluid (1:100 dilution), washed in PBS (phosphate buffered saline), goat anti-mouse IgM-FITC (1:100), washed in PBS, goat serum (30%), rabbit anti-human GFAP (1:1000 dilution), washed in PBS, goat anti-rabbit IgG-Rhodamine (1:50 dilution), washed in PBS and mounted in glycerol (with *p*-phenylenediamine). (**A**) Photographed with Rhodamine filter to bring out anti-GFAP fluorescence. (**B**) Photographed with FITC filter to bring out anti-G.3.5 fluorescence.

REFERENCES

1. BIGNAMI, A., L. F. ENG, D. DAHL & C. T. UYEDA. 1972. Localization of the glial fibrillary acidic protein in astrocytes by immunofluorescence. Brain Res. **43:** 429–435.
2. GALFRÉ, G. & C. MILSTEIN. 1981. Preparation of monoclonal antibodies: Strategies and procedures. Methods Enzymol. **73:** 3–75.
3. MALHOTRA, S. K., F. WONG, H. GOOD, N. SINHA, V. MANICKAVEL, T. K. SHNITKA & K. G. WARREN. 1983. Monoclonal antibody for certain nerve fibres in the spinal cord and brain. Microbios. Lett. **24:** 7–16.
4. RAFF, M. C., K. L. FIELDS, S.-I. HAKOMORI, R. MIRSKY, R. M. PRUSS & J. WINTER. 1979. Cell-type specific markers for distinguishing and studying neurons and the major classes of glial cells in culture. Brain Res. **174:** 283–308.

Neuropsychological Studies in Chronic Progressive Multiple Sclerosis

STEPHEN M. RAO, THOMAS A. HAMMEKE, SANDER GLATT, MICHAEL P. McQUILLEN, B. O. KHATRI, ANNE MARIE RHODES, AND SUSAN POLLARD

Department of Neurology
Medical College of Wisconsin
Milwaukee, Wisconsin 53226

In a series of prospective studies, we have assessed cognitive functions in patients with chronic progressive multiple sclerosis (CPMS) and related these findings to neuroanatomic disease-related changes (by CT scan). All CPMS patients met the criteria for clinically definite MS and had a mean Kurtzke Disability Status Score of 6.6 (range: 4 to 9).

In Study 1,[1] 44 patients with CPMS were compared to age- and education-matched patient (chronic pain; $n = 19$) and normal ($n = 15$) control groups on a battery of clinical (Wechsler Memory Scale, WMS) and experimental (Free Verbal Recall Test, FVRT, 7/24 Spatial Recall Test) memory tests. On the WMS, the CPMS patients had significantly lower Memory Quotients than patient controls [mean 100.5 vs. 115.1; $t(61) = 2.67$, $p < 0.01$]. TABLE 1 reports means, standard deviations, and group comparisons for each index derived from the FVRT and 7/24 tests. Significant group differences were observed, with CPMS patients performing inferiorly on most measures of learning, immediate and delayed memory, and proactive/retroactive interference. More striking deficits were observed in the recall of spatial, as opposed to verbal, stimuli. These memory findings were unrelated to degree of visual disturbance, medication effects or personality disturbance.

In Study 2,[2] 38 patients with CPMS were compared to an age- and education-matched patient control group (chronic pain; $n = 19$) on a measure of hypothesis testing and conceptual reasoning (Levine task). CPMS patients were less likely to employ strategies leading to correct solution [58.7% accuracy for CPMS patients vs. 83.6% for controls; $t(50) = 3.16$, $p < 0.01$] and were more likely to perseverate with one strategy despite negative verbal feedback (*i.e.,* CPMS patients made significantly greater lose-shift errors). Significant differences were also observed on focusing scores, with CPMS patients demonstrating lowered efficiency in eliminating irrelevant hypotheses.

In Study 3,[3] 47 patients with CPMS underwent CT scanning and evaluations of verbal intelligence and memory. On the basis of blind subjective ratings of cerebral atrophy, 19 patients were found to have mildly dilated ventricles and another 9 had moderate to severe ventricular enlargement. Learning efficiency on the FVRT and 7/24 tests was found to be related to degree of ventricular enlargement (see FIGURE 1). Three linear measurements of ventricular size (Bifrontal, Bicaudate and Third Ventricle) were also recorded. Using this method, width of the third ventricle proved to be the best indicator of cognitive dysfunction. These findings were unrelated to the effects of age.

In all three studies, neuropsychological test performance did not correlate with length of illness or overall disability as rated by the Kurtzke DSS.

TABLE 1. Results of Experimental Memory Measures

	Multiple Sclerosis (n = 35)	Patient Control (n = 23)	Normal Control (n = 15)	MS vs. PC	MS vs. NC
Free Verbal Recall Test					
List A					
Trial 1	4.0[a] (2.1)[b]	5.2(1.3)	5.8(1.7)	*	*
2	6.5(2.2)	7.1(1.6)	7.6(1.8)		
3	7.4(2.0)	7.7(2.3)	9.0(2.0)		*
4	8.1(2.4)	9.1(2.0)	9.9(1.6)		*
5	8.7(2.1)	9.7(1.8)	10.0(1.4)		
Total recall	34.8(9.5)	38.9(7.4)	42.3(6.8)		*
List B	3.9(1.8)	4.9(1.2)	6.0(1.7)	*	*
List A recall	6.3(3.0)	8.0(2.4)	8.3(1.4)	*	*
List A delayed	5.5(3.2)	7.0(2.8)	7.6(2.6)		*
7/24 Spatial Recall Test					
Design A					
Trial 1	3.8(1.9)	5.0(1.6)	5.4(1.4)	*	*
2	4.7(2.1)	5.9(1.5)	6.1(1.9)	*	*
3	5.4(1.7)	6.4(1.1)	6.8(0.6)	*	*
4	5.9(1.7)	6.7(1.0)	7.0(0.0)	*	*
5	6.0(1.5)	6.9(0.4)	7.0(0.0)	*	*
Total recall	25.8(7.2)	30.4(4.6)	32.5(2.5)	*	*
Design B	3.7(1.8)	4.6(1.6)	4.7(1.8)		
Design A recall	4.5(2.1)	5.7(1.9)	6.5(0.9)	*	*
Design A delayed	4.8(1.9)	5.7(2.0)	6.1(1.5)		*

[a] Mean.
[b] Standard deviation.
*$p < 0.05$, based on Tukey *a posteriori* contrast test.

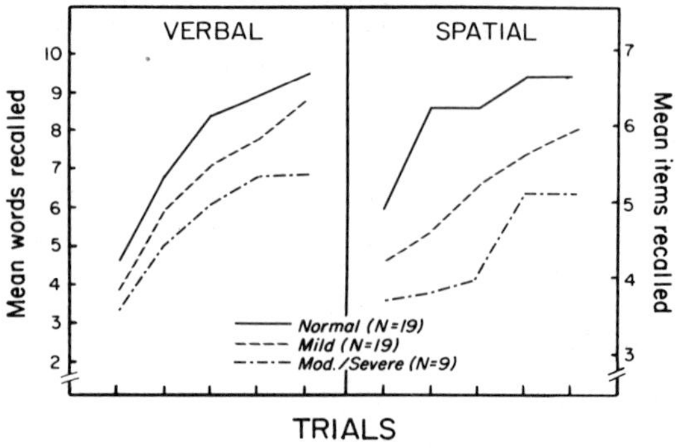

FIGURE 1. Learning curves for the Free Verbal Recall and 7/24 Spatial Recall tests for three CPMS subgroups having normal ventricular size, mild dilatation, and moderate to severe ventricular enlargement.

REFERENCES

1. RAO, S. M., T. A. HAMMEKE, M. P. MCQUILLEN, B. O. KHATRI & D. LLOYD. 1984. Memory disturbance in chronic progressive multiple sclerosis. Arch. Neurol. **41:** 625–631.
2. RAO, S. M. & T. A. HAMMEKE. 1984. Hypothesis testing in chronic progressive multiple sclerosis. Brain Cognition **3:** 94–104.
3. RAO, S. M., S. A. GLATT, T. A. HAMMEKE, M. P. MCQUILLEN, B. O. KHATRI, A. M. RHODES & S. POLLARD. 1985. Chronic progressive multiple sclerosis: Relationship between cerebral ventricular size and neuropsychological impairment. Arch. Neurol. In press.

Copolymer I: Effect on Normal Human Lymphocytes[a]

C. F. BROSNAN, M. LITWAK, P. A. NEIGHBOUR, AND M. B. BORNSTEIN

Albert Einstein College of Medicine
Bronx, New York, 10461

Copolymer I (COP I), a random basic polymer of L-alanine, L-glutamic acid, L-lysine and L-tyrosine, has been shown to function as a nonencephalitogenic peptide that can suppress experimental allergic encephalomyelitis.[1] These results have led to preliminary trials to determine the effectiveness of COP I in the treatment of multiple sclerosis.[2] As part of a double-blind, matched placebo-control pilot study on the effectiveness of treatment with COP I in patients with multiple sclerosis, possible antigenic responses of peripheral blood mononuclear cells (PMBC) to COP I were monitored by standard lymphocyte transformation tests using a six-day stimulation period. It rapidly became apparent, however, that unblinded PBMCs from healthy donors that had been included in the assay procedure as normal controls were proliferating in response to COP I. Stimulation indices in the range of two- to twelvefold (>20,000 cpm above background) were observed in the total PBMC population and occurred in 9 out of 10 individuals.[3] Studies have been undertaken to explore further this response of normal PBMC to COP I. The reactivity of PBMC to a wider dose range of COP I was assessed in both the total and nylon nonadherent (NNA) cell populations. Doubling dilutions, commencing at 50 μg/well were prepared and stimulation periods of three and six days were used. The results from six donors showed that both the total and NNA cells responded to COP I with maximum responses in the NNA with 12 μg/well (60 μg/ml) in a six-day assay. Minimal responses were observed at three days.

Further studies of this response have shown that (1) in contrast to the concanavalin A response that peaks at 3 days, maximal responses to COP I were found at 5 or 6 days; (2) positive transformation assays were found in medium (RPMI 1640) supplemented with either 10% fetal calf serum or human AB serum, with slightly higher responses in human AB serum; (3) no preparation of COP I has failed to induce blastogenesis, but different preparations of COP I have been found to result in different stimulation indices when tested against the same donor PBMC; (4) COP I in the D-form was toxic and this toxicity could not be lost by dialysis against normal saline; and (5) bovine myelin basic protein (MBP) did not stimulate a similar proliferative response when tested at the same concentrations, although a twofold stimulation was observed to MBP in two out of five donors tested. At the end of a six-day culture period the cells were analyzed with monoclonal antibodies against the T cell subsets OKT4 and OKT8, and the natural killer cell marker Leu7. The results showed that following incubation with COP I there was essentially no difference in the T cell subset distribution when the results were compared with cells incubated in medium alone. Analysis of the supernatant fluid from the cells stimulated by COP I detected the presence of interferon that was labile at pH 2.0, suggesting that gamma interferon is induced in

[a]This work was supported by USPHS grant no. NS 11920.

these cultures. We conclude that the PBMC of most normal healthy donors give a proliferative response to COP I *in vitro*. The fact that stimulation indices were generally highest in the NNA cell population suggests that T lymphocytes are responding, but no specificity for a particular T cell subset could be determined.

REFERENCES

1. TEITELBAUM, D., C. WEBB, A. MESHORER, R. ARNON & M. SELA. 1973. Eur. J. Immunol. **3:** 273–79.
2. BORNSTEIN, M. B., A. I. MILLER, V. SPADA, D. TEITELBAUM, R. ARNON & M. SELA. 1982. Ann. Neurol. **11:** 317–19.
3. BROSNAN, C. F., M. LITWAK, P. A. NEIGHBOUR & M. B. BORNSTEIN. 1983. J. Neuropathol. Exp. Neurol. **42:** 356.

Metabolic Pathology of Brain Inflammation

RICHARD J. DiROCCO

Monell Chemical Senses Center
Philadelphia, Pennsylvania 19104

In order to examine the effect of brain inflammation on glycolysis, ^{14}C-deoxyglucose autoradiography was applied to Lewis rats 4, 8 and 12 days after footpad inoculation with myelin basic protein (MBP) and Freund's complete adjuvant.[1] At 12 days when clinical signs of experimental allergic encephalomyelitis (EAE) were evident, discrete foci of intense glycolytic activity were observed (FIG. 1). Metabolic labeling corresponded to the periventricular distribution of inflammatory EAE foci as indicated by the presence of mononuclear cells in H and E stains of the material. One interpretation of this result is that it represents anaerobic glycolysis, precipitated by inflammatory events beginning with increased capillary permeability followed by exudation, edema, hemoconcentration, hemostasis and ischemic hypoxia in the lesion sites. Another contributing factor may be the high metabolic rate of infiltrating mononuclear cells. Unlike EAE lesions, however, gold thioglucose (GTG)-induced lesions of circumventricular organs (CVOs) are not accompanied by the infiltration of significant numbers of monocytes.[2] Moreover, few microglia are evident in CVOs until several days after GTG administration.[3] Therefore, an increase in glycolysis that occurs before this time could not easily be attributed to the accumulation of these cells.

CBA/ki and Balb/c mice were injected with GTG (IP) at doses of 0.4 and 0.8 mg/g respectively. ^{14}C-deoxyglucose (100 μ Ci/kg) was injected (IP) 1, 3, 5 and 7 hrs as well as 2, 8 and 12 days later. Autoradiograms obtained as early as 3 and 5 hrs after GTG revealed intense activation of glycolysis in the ventromedial hypothalamus (VMH). At these early times, no cellular infiltration was evident in H and E-stained lesion material (FIG. 2). At 8 days post-GTG, intense gliosis was observed in the VMH. A contribution of these cells to the cerebral metabolic rate of glucose (CMR_{gl}) in the lesion site can be seen in the 8-day ^{14}C-deoxyglucose autoradiogram. Thus, accumulated macrophages can contribute to the CMR_{gl} in inflammatory brain lesions. However, an increase in the CMR_{gl} in affected regions can occur in the absence of cellular infiltration. In light of Caffyn's[3] clear demonstration that GTG produces an infarctive lesion of the VHM, the increase in CMR_{gl} seen at 3 and 5 hours post-GTG probably represents anaerobic glycolysis precipitated by ischemic hypoxia.

These considerations call attention to the importance of local ischemia and lactate accumulation as determinants of histopathological and clinical mainfestations not only in EAE, but also in other instances of brain inflammation where significant hemostasis occurs. An important consequence of ischemic hypoxia, in addition to anaerobic glycolysis and lactate accumulation, is an increase in cytosolic Ca^{++} levels.[4] This causes an increase in the activity of phospholipase, thereby leading to an increase in free fatty acid levels including arachidonate. When collateral blood flow develops, and reperfusion of ischemic brain matter occurs, the oxidation of arachidonate leads to the production of prostaglandins and leukotrienes.[4] These further stimulate inflammatory sequelae leading to ischemia. This problem may be particularly acute for lesions in cerebral white matter which is less well vascularized than gray matter.[5] Indeed, in this

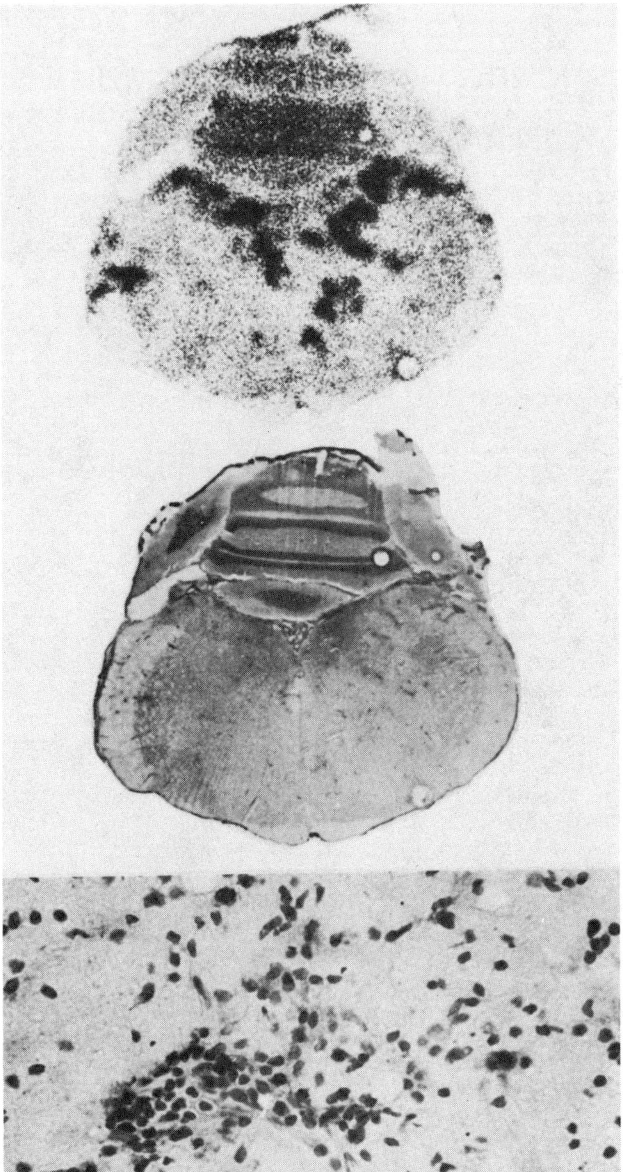

FIGURE 1. *Top:* ^{14}C-deoxyglucose autoradiogram obtained from a rat with EAE. *Middle:* Hematoxylin and (H and E) stain of same section that produced the autoradiogram shown above. Petechial pattern of darkly stained regions indicate perivascular cuffing and parenchymal infiltration of monocytes. Note that regions of intense glycolysis shown above appear to involve areas of tissue beyond the regions containing significant accumulations of monocytes. *Bottom:* H and E stain at higher magnification showing mononuclear aggregate in an inflammatory lesion site.

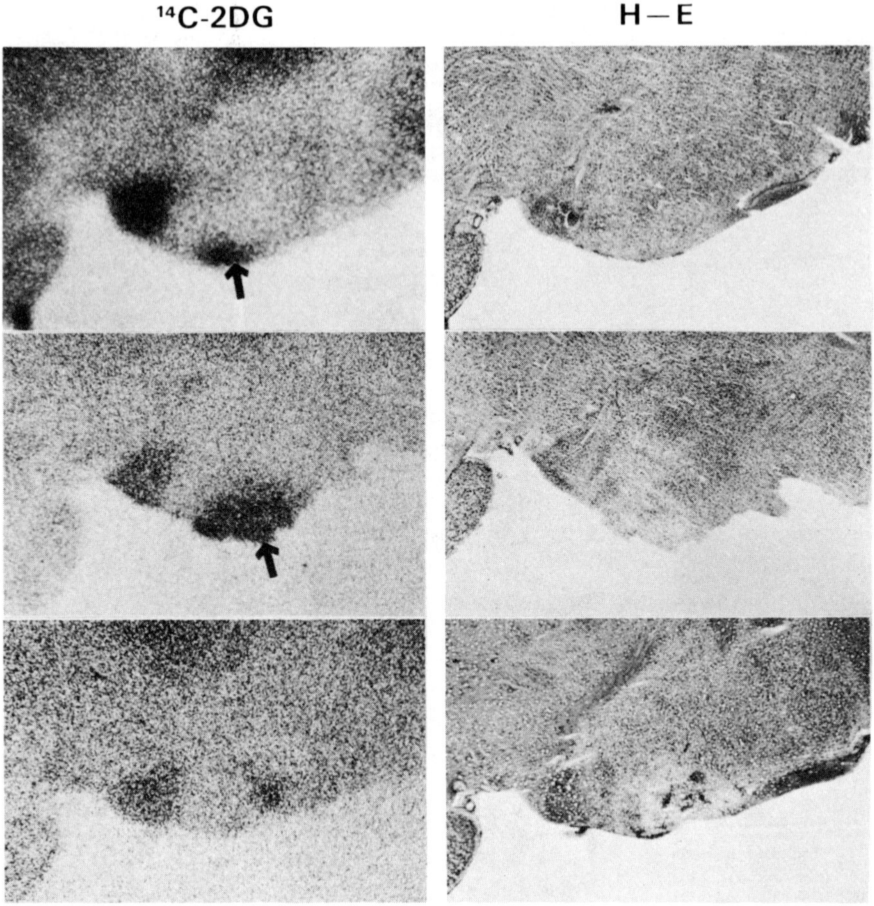

FIGURE 2. ^{14}C-deoxyglucose autoradiograms and hematoxylin and eosin stains of sagittal mouse brain sections obtained at 3 hrs (*top*), 5 hrs (*middle*) and 8 days (*bottom*) after GTG administration. Caudad is leftward in the figure. The region of high metabolic activity at the caudal aspect of the hypothalamus corresponds to the mamillary bodies. This region, which contains the axon terminals of the fornix is typically very active. An increase in glycolysis seen in the VMH (*arrows*) as early as 3–5 hours after GTG, when no cellular infiltration is evident in the stained material, indicates that ischemia alone can trigger an increase in glycolysis. Magnification ×14; original ×19.

respect, the metabolic pathology of postischemic leukoencephalopathy may have some features in common with active white matter lesions of multiple sclerosis.

REFERENCES

1. DiRocco, R. J. & G. A. Hashim. 1983. Increased glucose utilization associated with inflammatory brain lesions of experimental allergic encephalomyelitis. Neurosci. Lett. **37:** 105.

2. FUKUYAMA, U. & R. WATANABE. 1958. On histological changes of the hypothalamus in mice caused by administration of goldthioglucose. Folia Anat. Jap. **31:** 11.
3. CAFFYN, Z. E. X. 1972. Early vascular changes in the brain of the mouse after injections of goldthioglucose and bipiperidyl mustard. J. Path. **106:** 49.
4. SIESJO, B. K. 1981. Cell damage in the brain: A speculative synthesis. J. Cereb. Blood Flow Metab. **1:** 155.
5. PULSINELLI, W. A. & T. E. DUFFY. 1979. Local cerebral glucose metabolism during controlled hypoxemia in rats. Science **204:** 626.

A Murine Model of Herpes Simplex Virus Type 1 of the Nervous System

LORNE F. KASTRUKOFF, ALLEN S. LAU, AND DONALD W. PATY

Division of Neurology
Department of Medicine
Health Sciences Centre Hospital
University of British Columbia
Vancouver, British Columbia, Canada V6T 1W5

Herpes simplex virus type 1 (HSV1) can produce an acute as well as a persistent infection of the human nervous system. This type of infection could have relevance to chronic neurologic diseases such as multiple sclerosis for which an infectious etiology has been postulated. A murine model of HSV1 infection following lip inoculation has been developed.[1] The purpose of this study is to examine the genetics of natural resistance to HSV1 and the influence of genetic differences on the development of latent ganglionic infection in the peripheral nervous system (PNS), in both short- and long-term studies.

Male mice, 10–12 weeks of age, from 12 inbred strains, 6 congenic strains, and 4 Fl hybrids were lip inoculated with serial dilutions of HSV1 as previously described.[1] Animals were observed for 30 days (short term) and 68 weeks (long term) in parallel studies and mortality recorded. Animals were then sacrificed and the presence of latent infection in the trigeminal ganglia identified as previously described.

TABLE 1. Susceptibility of Inbred Strains of Mice to Latent HSV1 Infection in the PNS (Long Term)

	% of Animals with Latent Infection (Short Term)	% of Animals with Latent Infection (Long Term)
Inbred Strains[a]		
Resistant		
C57BL/10	70%	0%
Balb/c	70%	50%
C57BL/6	50%	12%
Moderately susceptible		
SWR/J	87%	50%
Susceptible		
CBA/J	100%	86%
Inbred Strains[b]		
A/J	86%	0%
DBA/1	90%	0%
PL/J	100%	0%
LP/J	100%	14%
DBA/2	100%	37%

[a]Patterns remain short- and long-term.
[b]Patterns dissimilar short- and long-term.

TABLE 2. Long-Term Resistance of Inbred Strains of Mice to HSV1

Inbred Strains	Numbers of Deaths (4–68 Weeks Postinfection)
Resistant	
C57BL/10	0/15
C57BL/6	0/15
DBA/1	0/14
Moderately resistant	
CBA/J	1/13
Balb/c	1/10
DBA/2	1/9
Susceptible	
A/J	2/6
SWR/J	3/9
PL/J	2/5
LP/J	5/12
Very susceptible	
AKR/J	8/9

The results of the short-term studies indicate that 11 inbred strains can be separated into three categories on the basis of resistance: resistant (C57BL/10, C57BL/6, DBA/1, LP/J, CBA/J), neutral (Balb/c, DBA/2, SWR/J, AKR/J), and susceptible (A/J, PL/J). Studies with Fl hybrids and congenic strains indicate that resistance is dominant and unrelated to the major histocompatibility complex (MHC). Resistance to the development of a latent infection in the PNS is dominant, not associated with the MHC, and unlike the pattern observed with resistance to mortality. Classification of inbred strains on the basis of resistance to mortality and susceptibility to latency identifies a number of strains that differ in their resistance to each aspect of infection. This would argue in favor of different mechanisms mediating resistance to mortality and the development of a latent infection.

The results of preliminary long-term studies indicate that generally fewer animals show the presence of latent infection in the PNS than short term. Both inter- and intrastrain variations were observed, along with major changes in latency rates in some strains (TABLE 1). The pattern observed with long-term mortality is similar to that of short-term mortality (TABLE 2). Although these results have yet to be confirmed, they would suggest that long-term mortality might be the result of persistent HSV1 infection.

REFERENCE

1. KASTRUKOFF, L., T. HAMADA, U. SCHUMACHER, C. LONG, P. C. DOHERTY & H. KOPROWSKI. 1982. Central nervous system infection and immune response in mice inoculated into the lip with herpes simplex virus type 1. J. Neuroimmunol. **2:** 295–305.

Reduced OKT8+ and OKT3+ Cells in Blood of Progressive MS Patients

J. OGER,[a] S. JACKEVICIUS, J. P. ANTEL,
AND B. G. ARNASON

Department of Neurology
University of Chicago
Chicago, Illinois 60637

INTRODUCTION

In active multiple sclerosis Con A-induced suppressor-cell function is decreased,[1–2] as well as NK cell function.[3–4] On the other hand, IgG secretion *in vitro* is increased even in stable patients,[5–6] as is intrathecal IgG secretion.[7] Early reports suggested reduction[8–9] or even disappearance[8] of a T cell subset (OKT5+, OKT8+) known to be involved in suppression of immune response *in vitro*. This prompted us to enumerate subsets of mononuclear cells between February 1981 and August 1983. Cells were enumerated using fluorescence microscopy.

TECHNIQUE

Subjects. Sixty-seven healthy controls, 13 noninflammatory neurological diseases and 76 MS patients were studied. MS patients were all clinically definite. They were subdivided into "stable" (no change in neurological signs or symptoms over a six-month period), "progressive" (increased disability for over a six-month period), and "attack" (increased symptoms in the preceding three weeks).

Protocol. Blood was collected on ACD and mononuclear cells separated by Ficoll Hypaque flotation. After three washes, 1×10^6 mononuclear cells were pelleted and resuspended in 50 μl of monoclonal antibody. Monoclonal antibodies were diluted in Hanks to which 0.1% BSA, 0.01% sodium azide and 10% goat serum (diluting solution) had been added so as to obtain final dilutions of 1:40 for OKT3 and OKT8 and 1:20 for OKT4 and OKM1. After 30′ incubation in ice, cells were washed three times, pelleted and resuspended in goat 50 μl anti-mouse FITC-labeled (cappel Fc specific) diluted 1:100 in diluting solution (vide supra). This antibody had previously been absorbed on human IgG and ultracentrifuged (100,000 g × 1 hr). After 30′ incubation on ice, cells were washed three times, pelleted, fixed with 0.3% paraformaldehyde and mounted on slides.

Counting. Counting was done at 1,000× magnification using a Leitz UV microscope. Each of 200 cells was identified under bright light and UV fluorescence then studied. Cells were considered positive if they showed distinct speckles of membrane-bound fluorescence.

[a]Present address: Health Sciences Centre Hospital, University of British Columbia, 2211 Wesbrook Mall, Vancouver, BC, Canada.

RESULTS

Results are presented in TABLE 1. Stable MS patients are not different from healthy individuals. Progressive MS patients have reduced OKT8+ cells but also reduced OKT3+ cells; OKT4+ are slightly lower but not significantly. During attacks OKT8+ are slightly reduced. Proportion of OKM1+ cells tends to be increased.

CONCLUSION

Our results would confirm that a reduced proportion of OKT8+ cells is present in progressive phase of MS, together with a decrease of total T cells. During attacks OKT8+ cells seem to vary. The variations reported need to be studied longitudinally as in ref. 10, but could suggest that modulation by antibody more than cell destruction may be at work in multiple sclerosis. Further work is needed to shed light on the relationship between (1) suppressor cell number and antigen density,[11] and (2) suppressor cell number and suppressor-cell function in multiple sclerosis.[12]

TABLE 1. Percentage Positivity

	T3	T4	T8	M1
Healthy controls	60.5 ± 1.3 (65)	35.5 ± 1.7 (27)	22.8 ± 0.9 (67)	23.9 ± 2.0 (29)
Noninflammatory neurological	52.9 ± 4.8 (13)	34.9 ± 5.1 (11)	22.9 ± 2.6 (11)	27.8 ± 2.6 (10)
MS stable	54.8 ± 2.3 (31)	38.2 ± 1.8 (13)	21.3 ± 1.4 (31)	25.9 ± 4.2 (12)
MS progressive	46.7 ± 2.4 (29)[a]	33.2 ± 2.5 (19)	15.6 ± 1.3 (32)[a]	34.6 ± 7.1 (16)
MS attack	55.6 ± 4.3 (16)	28.2 ± 3.3 (9)	18.6 ± 1.8 (16)[b]	32.5 ± 5.5 (11)

[a] $p < 0.001$ vs. healthy controls.
[b] $p < 0.05$.

REFERENCES

1. ANTEL, J. P., M. WEINRICH & B. G. W. ARNASON. 1978. Neurology **28:** 999–1003.
2. NEIGHBOUR, P. A. & B. R. BLOOM. 1979. Proceed. Natl. Acad. Sci. U.S.A. **76:** 476–480.
3. BENCZUR, M., G. G. PETRANYI *et al.* 1980. Clin. Exp. Immunol. **39:** 657–662.
4. MERRILL, J. E., M. JONDAL *et al.* 1983. Exp. Immunol. **47:** 419–430.
5. OGER J., J. ANTEL & B. G. W. ARNASON. 1982. Ann. Neurol. **11:** 177–181.
6. GOUST, J. M., E. L. HOGAN & P. ARNAUD. 1982. Neurology **32:** 228–234.
7. COHEN, S. & R. BANNISTER. 1967. Lancet **1:** 366.
8. REINHERZ, E. L., H. L. WEINER *et al.* 1980. N. Engl. J. Med. **303:** 125–129.
9. BACH, M. A., F. PHAN-DINH-TUY *et al.* 1980. Lancet **ii:** 1221–1223.
10. KASTRUKOFF, L. F. & D. W. PATY. 1984. Ann. Neurol **15:** 250–256.
11. REDER, T., J. ANTEL, J. OGER *et al.* 1984. Ann. Neurol **16:** 242–249.
12. ROSENKOETTER, P., A. T. REDER, J. OGER *et al.* 1984. J. Immunol. **132:** 1779–1783.

CSF Antibrain Antibodies in Neurologic Diseases

A. A. VANDENBARK,[a] F. VAN ROMPAEY,[b] D. NIJST,[b] H. OFFNER,[a] H. HEYLIGEN,[b] AND J. RAUS[b]

[a]*VA Medical Center Portland, Oregon 97207*

[b]*Dr. L. Willems Institute Diepenbeek, Belgium*

Although the cerebrospinal fluid (CSF) of most multiple sclerosis (MS) patients contains increased IgG levels of restricted clonal origin, the specificity of these antibodies remains largely unknown. This study seeks to evaluate reactivity of CSF IgG to crude membrane extracts of brain using the ELISA procedure.

The results of this study indicate that neat CSF IgG from 80% of 64 MS patients and 30% of 171 patients with other neurological diseases (OND) reacts significantly with crude extracts of brain (TABLE 1). Within the OND group, patients with

TABLE 1. Antibrain IgG Reactivity in Patients with Multiple Sclerosis and Other Neurological Diseases

Patient Group	Antibrain Antibody Activity in CSF Number (+)[a]/Number Tested
MS (confirmed/probable)	51/64 (80%)
OND	
Symptomatic	26/110 (24%)
Possible MS(?)	7/27
Pyramidal syndrome	2/11
Paresis/ataxia	5/12
Motor disturbance	4/13
Headache/dizziness	1/17
Epilepsy	2/7
Other	5/23
Inflammatory/Vascular	22/49 (45%)
Encephalitis	3/6
Meningitis	8/20
Lupus (CNS involvement)	1/1
Optic neuritis	0/3
Guillian-Barré	3/3
Polyneuritis	2/3
Polyradiculoneuritis	1/2
Cerebrovascular accident/trauma	4/11
Degenerative Diseases	3/12 (25%)
Amyotrophic lateral sclerosis	2/2
Parkinson's	0/3
Huntington's chorea	1/1
Atrophy/dementia	0/6

[a](+) by ELISA reactivity (OD 450 $\geq$ 0.01 = 0 + 2 mean standard deviations).

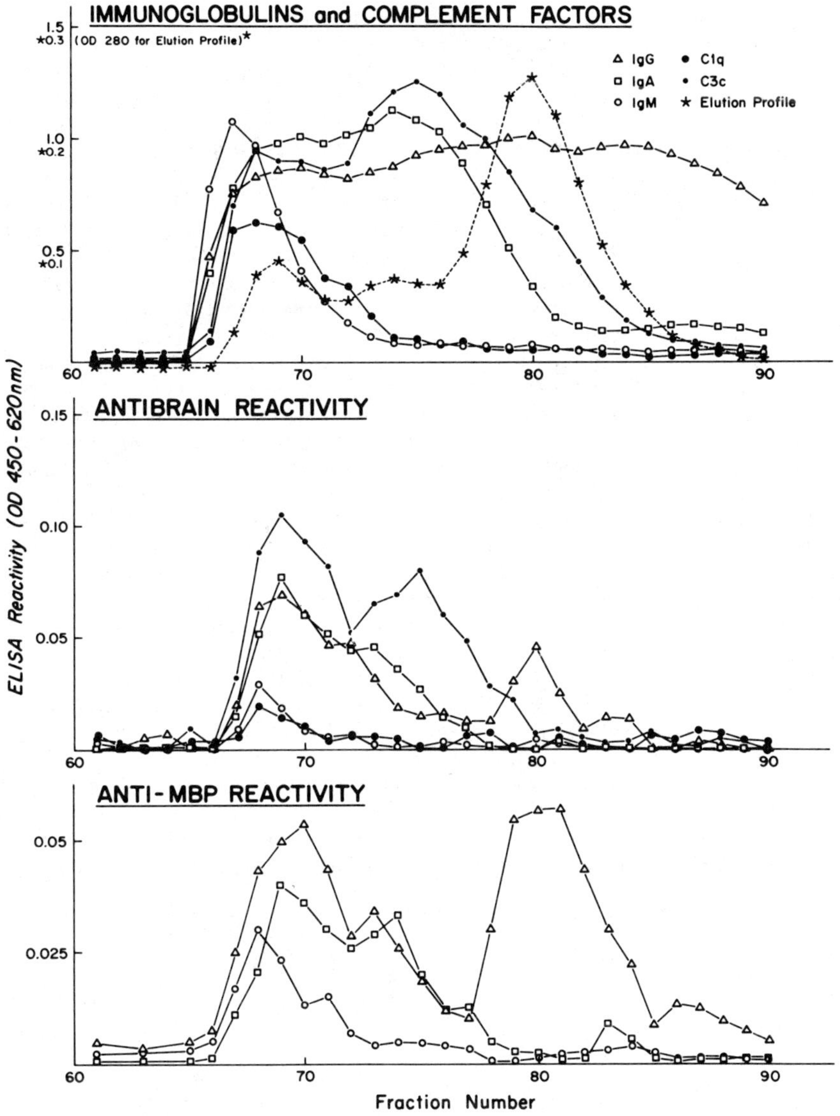

FIGURE 1. G-150 separation of reactive CSF pool.

inflammatory or vascular diseases of the CNS were more likely to have CSF antibrain antibodies (43% positive) than were patients with noninflammatory degenerative disease (25%) or undiagnosed patients with early neurologic symptoms (24%). The antibrain reactivity was significantly greater in patients with increased CSF IgG levels and/or oligoclonal CSF bands. Quantitatively the ELISA reaction was dependent on the brain extract coating concentration as well as the CSF IgG levels.

Reactivity to crude extracts of brain was significantly greater than to extracts of lung, suggesting that the majority of antibody reactivity was directed at brain-associated antigens. Extracts of membrane-associated molecules (3M KCl and butanol) bound more CSF antibody reactivity than extracts of cytosol components (NaCl and perchloric acid). However 3M KCl extracts of different brains (MS, Huntington's or normal) or of various regions of the same brain (of varying degrees of myelination) bound similar levels of CSF IgG. Extracts of plaque regions or of normal-appearing periplaque regions from MS brains also bound similar levels of CSF IgG. Purified myelin bound CSF IgG more efficiently than crude brain extracts, and within myelin subfractions, the ETOH-ether soluble fraction (enriched for lipids) bound CSF IgG more efficiently than the insoluble fractions. Purified myelin basic protein also bound significant CSF IgG. These data suggest that the antibody "targets" include a variety of myelin membrane-associated antigens.

Pooled CSF from antibrain "reactive" patients (where neat CSF gives significant ELISA reactivity—most MS patients and some OND patients) demonstrated approximately twice as much antibrain reactivity per μg IgG as "nonreactive" patients (most OND patients and 20% of MS patients). Separation of the CSF IgG by absorption on a staphylococcal protein A-Sepharose column indicated that this increase in specific activity was in the IgG3-enriched fraction (column pass). The eluted IgG1, IgG2, and IgG4-enriched fraction from both "reactive" and "nonreactive" CSF pools also had significant antibrain activity which was 30–60 times less per μg IgG than the IgG3-enriched fractions. Further evaluation of the CSF Ig using class- and subclass-specific reagents indicated that the antibrain reactive Ig included IgG1, IgG3, IgA, and to a lesser extent, IgM. The reactivity of these immunoglobulins was confirmed by testing fractions of CSF eluted from a Sephadex G150 column. This analysis revealed that both monomeric and complexed forms of IgG and IgA were bound by the brain extract or by myelin basic protein (FIG. 1). Furthermore, the complexed Ig was associated with the complement component C3c but not C1q, suggesting involvement of the alternative complement pathway. These data suggest that antibrain reactivity may involve both specific immunoglobulins and activated immune complexes which are directed at a variety of membrane-associated lipid and protein "targets." These humoral factors are found most frequently in patients with established inflammatory diseases of the CNS and may result from or contribute to progressive disability.

Characterization Of Antigen-specific T Cells in Multiple Sclerosis Twins with Elevated Responses to Measles Virus

J. I. GREENSTEIN, S. JACOBSON, J. R. RICHERT,
AND H. F. McFARLAND

Neuroimmunology Branch
NINCDS
National Institutes of Health
Bethesda, Maryland 20205

The cellular immune response to measles virus as measured by lymphocyte proliferation in normal sero-positive late convalescent individuals is considerably lower than the proliferative responses to either mumps or vaccinia viruses.[1] Significant proliferative responses to measles virus occur after natural infection,[2] but these decline within a few weeks, probably as the result of a failure to maintain a clonally expanded population of antigen-reactive lymphocytes in the circulation.[2] The responses of stable multiple sclerosis (MS) patients to measles virus do not differ significantly from the norm.[3] However, previous studies in twins with MS demonstrated that 20% of affected twins had significantly elevated responses (HR) to measles virus.[4] The differences between HR and unaffected low responders (LR) were unrelated to differences in T cell subsets, the kinetics of the response or differential susceptibility to the effects of *in vitro* infection by measles virus. The specificity of the response was found to reside in an E^+ subpopulation, and the addition of low-responder E^+ cells failed to identify an active LR-suppressor population. These findings suggested the presence of clonally expanded measles-specific T cell populations in the HR. Further characterization of the cellular basis for the elevated responses has utilized rigorous purification of plastic adherent cells (Adh) and separation of T cell subpopulations by affinity plating. The findings demonstrate that both HR and unaffected LR Adh support high responses to measles virus in HR T cells but do not elevate LR T cell responses, indicating that HR T cells are the cells responsible for HR proliferation, and that LR Adh are able to present antigen. The proliferating HR cell to measles virus resides in the $OKT4^+$ subpopulation, and is not suppressed by the addition of autologous $OKT8^+$ cells to primary *in vitro* cultures. The LR in unaffected twins is the result of a quantitatively lower response of $OKT4^+$ cells, rather than a qualitative difference in response. Again, suppression by autologous $OKT8^+$ cells was not demonstrated in LR. Equivalent amounts of interferon (essentially all alpha interferon) are produced by HR and LR, but only HR produce interleukin 2 (I12) in response to measles virus, whereas both HR and LR produce I12 to mumps virus. The HR subset responsible for I12 production resides within the $OKT4^+$ subpopulation (TABLE 1). Thus the cells responsible for producing the elevated measles responses in HR reside in a T cell subset with helper-inducer phenotype and function. These cells are presumably responsible for the clonal expansion of measles-specific T cell populations in the MS HR. The mechanisms involved may have potential relevance to the understanding of immunoregulatory abnormalities in MS.

TABLE 1. Antigen-stimulated Production of Interleukin 2 by Measles High- and Low-Responder Twins

Experiment	Supernatant Source[a]	Cells[b]	Dilutions of Supernatant Added to CT6 Cultures[d] 1:2	1:4	1:8
			(ΔC.P.M. $\times 10^{-3}$)[e]		
1. HR	Measles	E^+	12,759	7,158	4,126
		E^-	0	0	0
	Mumps	E^+	3,281	661	1,537
		E^-	0	0	0
LR	Measles	E^+	0	0	0
		E^-	0	0	0
	Mumps	E^+	5,117	1,870	1,350
		E^-	0	0	0
	Il2 standard		36,378	26,089	18,765
2. HR	Measles	4^+ + MØ[c]	47,259	36,125	22,158
		8^+ + MØ	0	0	0
	Mumps	4^+ + MØ	41,705	24,132	14,860
		8^+ + MØ	0	0	0
	Il2 standard		37,604	32,610	30,006

[a]Supernatants obtained at 48 hrs after stimulation with viral-infected monolayers. No counts obtained above medium control with uninfected Vero cell monolayers.

[b]SRBC rosetted cells. $E^+/E^- = 2 \times 10^5$ cells/well.

[c]T cell subsets 2×10^5 cells + 1×10^4 MØ/well.

[d]CT6 assay for Il2.

[e]+ΔC.P.M. = C.P.M. stimulated − C.P.M. medium control.

REFERENCES

1. McFarland, H. F., C. A. Pedone, E. S. Mingioli & D. E. McFarlin. 1980. The response of human lymphocyte subpopulations to measles, mumps and vaccinia viral antigens. J. Immunol. **125:** 221.
2. Greenstein, J. I. & H. F. McFarland. 1983. Response of human lymphocytes to measles virus after natural infection. Infect. Immun. **40:** 198.
3. McFarland, H. F. & D. E. McFarlin. 1979. Cellular immune response to measles, mumps, and vaccinia viruses in multiple sclerosis. Ann. Neurol. **6:** 101.
4. Greenstein, J. I., H. F. McFarland, E. S. Mingioli & D. E. McFarlin. 1984. The lymphoproliferative response to measles virus in twins with multiple sclerosis. Ann. Neurol. **15:** 79.

The National Neurological Research Bank

A Collection of Cryopreserved Human Neurological Specimens for Neuroscientists[a]

W. W. TOURTELLOTTE, H. H. ITABASHI,[b] I. ROSARIO, AND K. BERMAN

Neurology and Research Services
VAMC West Los Angeles, Wadsworth Division
Los Angeles, California 90073
and
Department of Neurology
Reed Neurological Research Center
University of California at Los Angeles School of Medicine
Los Angeles, California 90024

[b]*Department of Pathology*
Harbor-UCLA Medical Center
Torrance, California 90502

The National Neurological Research Bank (NNRB) is a publicly and privately supported service organization that provides human brain, spinal fluid, serum and other tissues to qualified scientists whose research is directed towards the understanding and eradication of neurological and psychiatric diseases. The Bank, founded in 1961 by Dr. Wallace Tourtellotte and based at the Veterans Administration Wadsworth Medical Center in Los Angeles, acquires human donor tissues through its Gift of Hope Donation Program. These tissues are specially frozen, stored at low temperature and distributed to investigators conducting studies that require nonfixed ice artifact-free tissues.[1-3]

Brain tissue (cerebrum, brain stem and cerebellum) is the mainstay of the Bank's service program. In addition to normal control tissues, brain tissue is acquired and stored from individuals with the diagnoses listed in TABLE 1.

Spinal cord materials (including cauda equina) are available from multiple sclerosis and amyotrophic lateral sclerosis donors. Materials from donors with other neurological and nonneurological diseases are obtainable for comparison.

We have an inventory of other cryopreserved organs, such as lymph nodes, spleen, lung, heart, liver, muscle, kidney, adrenals, pancreas, pituitary and dura.

Cerebrospinal fluid (CSF) and matched serum are available principally for multiple sclerosis research. Samples from 100 MS patients have been collected during the course of the disease; each sample is correlated with clinical type, disease activity and neurological disability. For comparison, a large number of normal, neurological and nonneurological samples are available. Fluids can be pooled to provide enough material to do preparative isolations of components that are present in low concentrations, such as immunoglobulins, so that they may undergo detailed functional analysis.

[a]This work is supported by the National Multiple Sclerosis Society, Hereditary Disease Foundation, California Comprehensive Epilepsy Program, NINCDS/NIMH Intra-Agency Agreement, and the Veterans Administration.

In addition, we have prepared dried-on glass slides and stored frozen CSF and matched blood leukocytes for immunocytohistochemical and virological analyses. A modest number of postmortem samples of CSF and matched serum are also available. In order to eliminate thawing and refreezing of collected samples, CSF and serum is aliquoted into 1 ml portions for storage in airtight screwtop plastic tubes prior to cryopreservation.

Brain and other tissues are generally received in the fresh, nonfixed state. In order to make these tissues suitable for the application of various immunocytochemical and *in situ* hybridization techniques now gaining favor, the entire cerebrum with brain stem removed is secured upon a special table, so that full coronal sections 4–6 mm thick can be cut with an electric knife. These slices are then quick frozen between liquid nitrogen-cooled aluminum (400 g) plates. Midline structures, such as nucleus basalis of Meynert, are remarkably preserved and readily available for precise dissection.[4–8]

TABLE 1. Brain Tissue Samples Available from the National Neurological Research Bank

Multiple sclerosis
Subacute sclerosing panencephalitis
Herpes encephalitis
Huntington's disease
Schizophrenia
Major depression
Bipolar depression
Suicide
Epilepsy
Alzheimer's disease
Dementia (not Alzheimer's disease)
Mental retardation
Down's syndrome
Parkinson's disease
Progressive supranuclear palsy
Tourette syndrome
Tardive dyskinesia
Dystonia musculorum deformans
Hereditary ataxia
Amyotrophic lateral sclerosis
Neurofibromatosis
Tuberous sclerosis
Alcoholism
Drug abuse

In addition, tissues quick frozen by the above method demonstrate minimal ice crystal artifact formation, thus facilitating the correlation of special immunological and virological binding techniques with histopathological classification. In fact, quick frozen sections can be thawed in room temperature formalin between glass plates for further routine histopathological techniques and/or techniques that are enhanced or not affected by formalin fixative.[9] Accordingly, our technique of preparing brain tissue for cryopreservation permits complete anatomical structures of the brain to be examined, offering distinct advantages over tissue preservation methods that involve pulverization or powdering of anatomical structures of the brain.

When the Bank receives intact brain from patients and well-classified clinical cases in the frozen state, these tissues are warmed to −15°C before cutting on an electric meat slicer and are then processed as above for the fresh tissue. Ice artifact in these en bloc frozen tissues makes it nearly impossible to do histochemical correlation studies, but gross lesions and anatomical regions can be dissected for tests of binding sites, enzymes liquid hybridization, *etc.*

Before the freezing process, or after a frozen brain has been cut, photomacrographs are produced to record the gross appearance of each brain section for later reference of the investigator and bank dissectors as they prepare to excise particular structures which have been requested. Investigators may review color prints made from these photomacrographs.

Brain tissue sections are heat sealed in plastic bags and stored in ultra-cold freezers at −70°C. These airtight bags minimize water dessication that would otherwise occur as a result of exposure to air in an ultra-cold freezer environment. This permits expression of result on the basis of gram per fresh brain. Spinal cord, optic nerve, pituitary and other solid tissues are similarly packaged and stored.

All tissue specimens stored in the bank are inspected for gross lesions, and samples of these are submitted for microscopic histopathological classification. Routine sampling for microscopic analysis is undertaken to document any pathology of the cerebral cortex, basal ganglia, substantia nigra, brain stem and spinal cord. Based on these examinations a neuropathological diagnosis is made.

In order to further establish validity of diagnoses, clinical records are obtained and are available to users of bank specimens. Details are recorded concerning the circumstances at the time of death, medications, alcohol and other substance abuse. Efforts are made to determine the cause of death, including drug analysis of tissues. The time from death to the moment the tissue is frozen is also recorded. For psychiatric cases and controls, a detailed structured interview with family and/or "significant others" is carried out by a trained interviewer.

Our collection of quick frozen and cryopreserved brain biopsies continues to enlarge and to become more diversified. Temporal lobe tissue excised to eradicate medically uncontrollable epileptogenic focus and brain tumors are the main entries in this collection.

Requests for special handling or processing of tissue are considered and approved on an individual basis, based upon practical considerations.

Investigators with a research need for central nervous system, cauda equina, CSF and matched serum, CSF and blood leukocytes or other human specimens may write to Dr. Tourtellotte to request (1) the disease entity or entities of interest, (2) the number of cases of each disease state or normal control desired, (3) the specific anatomical area(s) of interest and the quantity needed, and (4) a description of the objective(s) and methodology of the study as concerns the use of the requested tissue; this description may be brief and may be contained in a reprint.

Tissues are provided and shipped worldwide free of charge. All specimens are shipped with a sufficient quantity of dry ice to assure that they will be received in a deep-frozen state.

REFERENCES

1. TOURTELLOTTE, W. W. 1982. Tissue available for neurologic research. Arch. Neurol. **36:** 14.
2. TOURTELLOTTE, W. W. 1982. Tissue available for neurological research. Ann. Neurol. **12:** A40.
3. TOURTELLOTTE, W. W., H. H. ITABASHI, I. ROSARIO, K. BERMAN *et al.* 1983. National

neurological research bank: A collection of cryopreserved human neurological specimens for neuroscientists. Neurology **33** (Suppl. 2): 249.

4. TOURTELLOTTE, W. W. 1970. Avant-propos: A human specimen bank and a brain biopsier. Riv. Patol. Nerv. Ment. **91:** 2155–262.
5. TOURTELLOTTE, W. W., R. C. COHENOUR *et al.* 1978. The NINCDS/NIMH human neurospecimen bank. *In* Neuropsychopharmacology, vol. 2. P. Deniker, C. Radouco-Thomas & A. Villeneuve, Eds: 1593–1595. Pergamon Press. Quebec.
6. COLE, B. 1982. National brain tissue banks: A service for neurological research. News and Features from NIH. U.S. Department of Health and Human Services. March. pp. 10–13.
7. TOURTELLOTTE, W. W. 1982. National brain tissue banks. A service for neurological research. NINCDS Research Currents. February.
8. U.S. DEPARTMENT OF HEALTH AND HUMAN SERVICES. 1983. *In* Human Brain Dissection. Public Health Service. National Institutes of Health. National Institute of Neurological and Communicative Disorders and Stroke. National Institute of Mental Health. U.S. Government Printing Office. 1983–381–132: 3096. 243 pp.
9. ITABASHI, H. H., W. W. TOURTELLOTTE *et al.* 1976. A freezing method for the preservation of nervous tissue for concomitant molecular biological research and histopathological evaluation. J. Neuropathol. Exp. Neurol. **35:** 117.

Index of Contributors

(Italicized page numbers refer to comments made in discussion.)